Mirror of Beryl

The Library of Tibetan Classics is a special series being developed by the Institute of Tibetan Classics aimed at making key classical Tibetan texts part of the global literary and intellectual heritage. Eventually comprising thirty-two large volumes, the collection will contain over two hundred distinct texts by more than a hundred of the best-known Tibetan authors. These texts have been selected in consultation with the preeminent lineage holders of all the schools and other senior Tibetan scholars to represent the Tibetan literary tradition as a whole. The works included in the series span more than a millennium and cover the vast expanse of classical Tibetan knowledge—from the core teachings of the specific schools to such diverse fields as ethics, philosophy, psychology, Buddhist teachings and meditative practices, civic and social responsibilities, linguistics, medicine, astronomy and astrology, folklore, and historiography.

Mirror of Beryl: A Historical Introduction to Tibetan Medicine

Desi Sangyé Gyatso (1653–1705)

Mirror of Beryl is a detailed account of the origins and history of medicine in Tibet through the end of the seventeenth century. Its author, Desi Sangyé Gyatso (1653–1705), was the heart disciple and political successor of the Great Fifth Dalai Lama and the author of several highly regarded works on Tibetan medicine, including *Blue Beryl*, a commentary on the foundational text on Tibetan medical practice, *Four Tantras*. In the present historical introduction, Sangyé Gyatso traces the sources of influence on Tibetan medicine to classical India, China, Central Asia, and beyond and shows how it developed in Tibet through royal patronage and the establishment of practice lineages. He provides an extensive bibliography of works on medicine, many of which are no longer extant; he provides life details on many central figures, such as Yuthok Yönten Gyatso, and critiques the contribution of another influential figure, Surkhar Lodrö Gyalpo.

In addition to his historical survey, Sangyé Gyatso devotes significant portions of his text to other topics as well. He investigates, for instance, the question of whether *Four Tantras* is the word of the Buddha or of a later figure, such as Yuthok. He gives a commentary on the three levels of Buddhist vows—pratimokṣa, bodhisattva, and tantric, giving special attention to the last. Finally, he details the qualities necessary in a master and student of Tibetan medicine.

Written at the very end of his life, Desi Sangyé Gyatso's *Mirror of Beryl* remains today an essential resource for students of medical science in Tibet.

THE LIBRARY OF TIBETAN CLASSICS • VOLUME 28
Thupten Jinpa, General Editor

Mirror of Beryl

A Historical Introduction to Tibetan Medicine

Desi Sangyé Gyatso
Translated by Gavin Kilty

Wisdom Publications • Boston
in association with the Institute of Tibetan Classics

Wisdom Publications
199 Elm Street
Somerville MA 02144 USA
www.wisdompubs.org

Library of Congress Cataloging-in-Publication Data

Saṅs-rgyas-rgya-mtsho, Sde-srid, 1653–1705.
[Bai dūr sṅon po. English]
Mirror of beryl : a historical introduction to Tibetan medicine / Desi Sangyé Gyatso ; translated by Gavin Kilty. — 1st ed.
p. cm. — (The library of Tibetan classics ; v. 28)
Includes translation from Tibetan.
Includes bibliographical references and index.
ISBN 0-86171-467-9 (hardcover : alk. paper)
1. Medicine, Tibetan—History. I. Kilty, Gavin. II. Title.
R127.5.S263513 2009
610—dc22

2009027243

15 14 13 12 11 10
6 5 4 3 2 1

Cover and interior design by Gopa&Ted2. Set in Adobe Garamond Premier Pro 10.5/13.5.

Wisdom Publications' books are printed on acid-free paper and meet the guidelines for permanence and durability of the Production Guidelines for Book Longevity of the Council on Library Resources.

Printed in the United States of America.

This book was produced with environmental mindfulness. We have elected to print this title on 30% PCW recycled paper. As a result, we have saved the following resources: 29 trees, 9 million BTUs of energy, 2,767 lbs. of greenhouse gases, 13,328 gallons of water, and 809 lbs. of solid waste. For more information, please visit our website, www.wisdompubs.org. This paper is also FSC certified. For more information, please visit www.fscus.org.

Message from the Dalai Lama

THE LAST TWO millennia witnessed a tremendous proliferation of cultural and literary development in Tibet, the "Land of Snows." Moreover, due to the inestimable contributions made by Tibet's early spiritual kings, numerous Tibetan translators, and many great Indian *paṇḍitas* over a period of so many centuries, the teachings of the Buddha and the scholastic tradition of ancient India's Nālandā monastic university became firmly rooted in Tibet. As evidenced from the historical writings, this flowering of Buddhist tradition in the country brought about the fulfillment of the deep spiritual aspirations of countless sentient beings. In particular, it contributed to the inner peace and tranquility of the peoples of Tibet, Outer Mongolia—a country historically suffused with Tibetan Buddhism and its culture—the Tuva and Kalmuk regions in present-day Russia, the outer regions of mainland China, and the entire trans-Himalayan areas on the southern side, including Bhutan, Sikkim, Ladakh, Kinnaur, and Spiti. Today this tradition of Buddhism has the potential to make significant contributions to the welfare of the entire human family. I have no doubt that, when combined with the methods and insights of modern science, the Tibetan Buddhist cultural heritage and knowledge will help foster a more enlightened and compassionate human society, a humanity that is at peace with itself, with fellow sentient beings, and with the natural world at large.

It is for this reason I am delighted that the Institute of Tibetan Classics in Montreal, Canada, is compiling a thirty-two volume series containing the works of many great Tibetan teachers, philosophers, scholars, and practitioners representing all major Tibetan schools and traditions. These important writings will be critically edited and annotated and will then be published in modern book format in a reference collection called *The Library of Tibetan Classics,* with their translations into other major languages to be followed later. While expressing my heartfelt commendation for this noble project, I pray and hope that *The Library of Tibetan Classics* will not only make these important Tibetan treatises accessible to scholars of Tibetan studies, but will create a new opportunity for younger Tibetans to study and take interest in their own rich and profound culture. Through translations into other languages, it is my sincere hope that millions of fellow citizens of the wider human family will also be able to share in the joy of engaging with Tibet's classical literary heritage, textual riches that have been such a great source of joy and inspiration to me personally for so long.

The Dalai Lama
The Buddhist monk Tenzin Gyatso

Special Acknowledgments

THE INSTITUTE OF TIBETAN CLASSICS expresses its deep gratitude to Curt Jones and Alice Jones for funding this translation.

We also gratefully acknowledge the Hershey Family Foundation for its generous support of the Institute of Tibetan Classics' project of compiling, editing, translating, and disseminating key classical Tibetan texts through *The Library of Tibetan Classics*. The Institute likewise thanks the Ing Foundation and Nita Ing for their generous help toward the publication of this volume.

Publisher's Acknowledgments

THE PUBLISHER wishes to extend a heartfelt thanks to the following people who, by subscribing to *The Library of Tibetan Classics*, have become benefactors of this entire translation series.

Tenzin Dorjee
Steven D. Hearst
Heidi Kaiter
Arnold Possick
The Randall-Gonzales Family Foundation
Jonathan and Diana Rose
Claudia Wellnitz
Robert White
Eva and Jeff Wild

Table of Contents

General Editor's Preface

It is a joy and a source of deep satisfaction to see the publication in English today of *Mirror of Beryl*, an important classic of Tibetan literature composed by the prolific seventeenth-century author Desi Sangyé Gyatso. A historical work outlining the various strands in the development of Tibet's rich system of medical science, profiling the major figures and texts, the book also contains a detailed commentary on the three sets of Buddhist vows and a discussion of the ideal relationship between master physician and disciple. This book is one of three key works composed by Desi on the Tibetan medical system, the other two being the two-volume exposition of the four medical tantras entitled *Blue Beryl*, and *A Sword to Cut the Noose of Untimely Death*, an important work on diagnosis and treatment methods. From a literary-historical point of view, one of the greatest values of *Mirror of Beryl* is its meticulous recording and citing of numerous important works on medicine, many of which are no longer extant.

Among Tibet's great classical authors, Desi's position is unique. Though not a monk, he was groomed by the Great Fifth Dalai Lama from an early age, and he acquired in this way an impressive intellectual and cultural education—eclectic in its breadth and steeped in the love of poetry and literature that was a hallmark of the Great Fifth. Taking over rule of Tibet as regent following the Great Fifth's death, Desi saw through the construction of the monumental reliquary of his predecessor inside the Potala Palace, penned the conclusion of the Great Fifth's acclaimed autobiography, *Silken Robe*, and more importantly, took charge of discovering and bringing up of the Sixth Dalai Lama, Tsangyang Gyatso. The fates of these two figures—the loyal regent and the young incarnation of his mentor—would become intertwined in a profound tragedy involving the unfortunate death of both. Often the full extent of Desi's contribution to Tibet's rich intellectual heritage is not appreciated. So to see Desi's *Mirror of Beryl* featured in *The Library of Tibetan Classics* is, for me at least, a source of special satisfaction.

Two primary objectives have driven the creation and development of *The Library of Tibetan Classics*. The first aim is to help revitalize the appreciation and the study of the Tibetan classical heritage within Tibetan-speaking communities worldwide. The younger generation in particular struggle with the tension between traditional Tibetan culture and the realities of modern consumerism. To this end, efforts have been made to develop a comprehensive yet manageable body of texts, one that features the works of Tibet's best-known authors and covers the gamut of classical Tibetan knowledge. The second objective of *The Library of Tibetan Classics* is to help make these texts part of global literary and intellectual heritage. In this regard, we have tried to make the English translation reader-friendly and, as much as possible, keep the body of the text free of scholarly apparatus, which can intimidate general readers. For specialists who wish to compare the translation with the Tibetan original, page references of the critical edition of the Tibetan text are provided in brackets.

The texts in this thirty-two-volume series span more than a millennium—from the development of the Tibetan script in the seventh century to the first part of the twentieth century, when Tibetan society and culture first encountered industrial modernity. The volumes are thematically organized and cover many of the categories of classical Tibetan knowledge—from the teachings specific to each Tibetan school to the classical works on philosophy, psychology, and phenomenology. The first category includes teachings of the Kadam, Nyingma, Sakya, Kagyü, Geluk, and Jonang schools, of miscellaneous Buddhist lineages, and of the Bön school. The texts in these volumes have been selected largely by senior lineage holders of the individual schools. Texts in the other categories have been selected primarily in recognition of the historical reality of the individual disciplines. For example, in the field of epistemology, works from the Sakya and Geluk schools have been selected, while the volume on buddha nature features the writings of Butön Rinchen Drup and various Kagyü masters. Where fields are of more common interest, such as the three codes of conduct or the bodhisattva ideal, efforts have been made to present the perspectives of all four major schools. *The Library of Tibetan Classics* can function as a comprehensive library of the Tibetan literary heritage for libraries, educational and cultural institutions, and interested individuals.

I offer my deep gratitude first and foremost to His Holiness the Dalai Lama for always being such a shining exemplar and an advocate of Tibet's great classical heritage. I thank the translator of this volume, Gavin Kilty, for doing such a magnificent job in making this important work accessible to the modern reader. In Gavin I have found a real comrade, someone who is always ready to take on the most arduous of the translation projects from *The Library of Tibetan Classics* and then proceeds with remarkable efficiency and success. I owe heartfelt thanks to David Kittelstrom of Wisdom Publications for being, as usual, a most incisive editor; to the Central Institute of Higher Tibetan Studies, Sarnath, for providing full access to its library to my Tibetan colleagues who created the critical edition of the Tibetan text; and to my wife, Sophie Boyer-Langri, for taking on the numerous administrative chores that are part of such a collaborative project. Finally, I express my heartfelt thanks to Curt and Alice Jones, who most generously provided the funding for this translation project, the Ing Foundation for its grant for publishing this volume, and to the Hershey Family Foundation for its longstanding support of the Institute of Tibetan Classics, without which *The Library of Tibetan Classics* series simply would not have become a reality.

It is my sincere hope that the publication of this volume will benefit many and that it will provide a valuable resource to help people better understand and appreciate the richness of Tibet's classical intellectual and spiritual heritage. May the efforts of all those who have been part of this endeavor help alleviate the sufferings of all beings; may they especially help us humans become wiser so that we may make this world a more caring and a more peaceful place for all.

Thupten Jinpa
Montreal, 2009

Translator's Introduction

THE MEDICAL SYSTEM referred to as "Tibetan medicine" has found its way from its longtime home in Tibet to many parts of the modern world, where it has settled successfully alongside other alternative systems of medical practice. Physicians trained in this medical system and offering traditional Tibetan treatments can now be found in many countries worldwide. Moreover not all practitioners of this medical system are Tibetan nationals; its theory and methodology have attracted students from other countries. Many books have appeared on Tibetan medicine, most offering an overview of its theory and practices, a few giving brief accounts of its history, and even one or two presenting translations of medical texts.[1]

Mirror of Beryl is a detailed traditional account of the origins, theoretical bases, and practices of this ancient and wide-ranging medical system. It was composed by Desi Sangyé Gyatso (1653–1705), a student of the Fifth Dalai Lama and, beginning in 1679, his political successor as well. Much of the historical narrative in the introduction below is summarized from Sangyé Gyatso's text, a work that, from the time it was written at the beginning of the eighteenth century, has been regarded as the leading authority on the development of medicine in Tibet.[2]

Origins of the Tibetan Medical System

Tibetan medicine as it is practiced today is closely connected with Tibetan Buddhism, but its roots may predate the arrival of the Buddhadharma in Tibet in the seventh and eighth centuries. Some commentators mention the existence of a system of medicine—crediting it with varying degrees of sophistication—within the indigenous Bön or pre-Buddhist culture that flourished in Tibet. Kachuwa Chölothar, for example, in his hitherto untranslated analysis on the origins of Tibetan medicine, puts forward evidence for the existence of a Bön medical system.[3] Some Bön documents say that their founder,

Tönpa Shenrap, who was contemporaneous with the Buddha, preached thirteen volumes of medical teachings. One work on Bön history claims his son Chebu Trishé memorized 21,000 medical works.

In Darmo Menrampa's (1638–1710) *Brilliant Jewel Treasury,* in answer to a question from an Indian doctor on the kinds of medical practice in Tibet, the eighth-century medical scholar Yuthok mentions medical texts on purgatives, fomentation, balneology, and ointments found in the Shangshung Bön and Yungdrung Bön traditions. Also, *Four Tantras,*[4] the principal medical reference and subject of study in Tibetan medical training up to the present day, contains a few names of medicines, medicinal compounds, and illnesses that are said to be from the ancient Shangshung language. The concluding chapter of *Four Tantras* lists mantras that come from Bön religious practice. Some commentators have even suggested that *Four Tantras* itself is of Bön origin, and that the translator Vairocana, rather than translating it from Indian sources as others have suggested, took it from Bön medical literature. Kachuwa Chölothar says that these days many scholars recognize several principles taught in *Four Tantras* as being developments of the basic medical practices that existed during the Bön phase of Tibetan history.

From the seventh century onward, evidence suggests that Tibetan medicine developed from three distinct non-indigenous sources. A passage from a work called *Weapons of Fearlessness,* cited in *Mirror of Beryl,*[5] talks of three great medical systems, and that ignorance of any of them would exclude one from being counted among the great physicians. The passage continues by naming the purveyors of these systems in Tibet as Bharadhaja, Galenos, and Hsüan Yüan Huang. These three physicians, says Desi Sangyé Gyatso, came respectively from India, "Trom," and China. India, as is clear from the extensive accounts of Āyurvedic medical literature and practices, is easily identifiable as the Indian subcontinent. China during the seventh century, when these physicians were in Tibet, was under the Tang dynasty with its capital at Chang-an (Xian). The third locale is harder to identify.

Much has been written on the identification of Trom *(khrom* or *phrom).* Geographically, it seems to refer to the Central Asian lands west of Tibet whose inroads into Tibet were via the Silk Route. Culturally, it seems to refer to the Greek or Persian culture that had permeated so far east by the eighth century. It can be no coincidence that the Galenos from Trom named above bore the same name as the celebrated Greek physician who graced the Roman courts in the second century B.C.E. Because of this, Beckwith identifies Trom with Rome.[6] Desi Sangé Gyatso and others equate Trom with Taksik *(stag gzigs, ta zig),* which is tempting to identify with Tajikistan. However, the *Five Chronicles,* cited by Jampa Trinlé,[7] disputes the identity of Trom with Taksik, stating that Taksik is in the west and Trom in the north. Trinlé goes on to say that some commentators place Taksik to the west of Xinjiang and north of Afghanistan, and that the Bön tradition speaks of regions called Taksik Trom and Taksik Olmo Lungring. Pawo Tsuklak Trengwa talks of the "Hor (Mongolians) similar to the barbarian Taksik or Turks."[8] It may be that there is an overlap between Trom and the ancient land of Shangshung, from whence came the Bön practices. One of the medicines listed in *Four Tantras* mentioned above is *daryakan,* a name said to be from the Shangshung language. This is an ambrosia-like panacea with twenty-five types. However, according to Beckwith:

> The word *daryakan* is patently non-Tibetan in origin, and it is in fact said by Jampal Dorjé to be a Shangshung term. His etymology is rendered most probable in the light of the form *taryak,* the name of a "Persian" remedy for snake-bite in Swat, land of ancient Shangshung and Tibetan cultural contacts. Since there can be no doubt but that taryak is identical to *teryak* or *deryak*, i.e., Arabic *tiryaq(un)* or *diryaq(un)*, Islamic forms of the word theriac, then (regardless of the actual pathways followed by the drug's name on its way to Tibet) it is undoubtedly also true that *daryakan* was originally the compound drug theriac, a very ancient Greek medicinal concoction (*theriakon harmakon,* or *theriake*), prepared with snake's flesh, honey, and numerous other ingredients. Theriac proper was ordinarily a cure-all, but was supposed to be especially good against snake-bite.[9]

These three sources, or "great rivers," brought their own strains of medical knowledge to Tibet. It seems that Trom in the west, personified by the physician Galenos, brought much anatomical knowledge to Tibet during those early times, in the form of medical works on dissection. Galenos himself stayed on in Tibet and composed several medical works. Through his sons his medical lineage grew and flourished. This medical influence from the west seems to have been predominant around the time of Songtsen Gampo, as evidenced by the fact that Galenos and another physician, Tsenpashilaha, also from Trom, were rewarded with titles and commendations from the king. Tsenpashilaha was also known as Biji, and the lineage of Galenos was known as the Biji lineage, and according to Beckwith, this term is a transcription of a Sogdian word meaning "doctor."[10] In the succeeding centuries, the Trom influence seems to have waned.

The influence of China in medical matters also appears to have been dominant in the seventh and eighth centuries in Tibet and may have lasted longer than the Trom influence. The Chinese bride of Songtsen Gampo brought an extensive medical text with her from China as a gift for the king. This was translated into Tibetan by Hvashang Mahādeva and Dharmakośa. Later, in the eighth century, the Chinese queen of Jangtsa Lhabön brought many medical and astrological works to Tibet. The Chinese translators Hvashang Mahāyāna, Hvashang Mahākyinda, Hsüan Yüan Huang, and Hvashang Penatseta compiled and translated many medical texts in to Tibetan. These include the renowned *Somarāja,* whose influence was still evident in the seventeenth century, when Desi Sangyé Gyatso included its teachings on diagnoses from urine and cauterization points in his famous collections of medical paintings. Trinlé states (p. 31) that the great physician, the later Yuthok Yönten Gönpo, in the eleventh century incorporated some of the principles of *Somarāja* into the edition of *Four Tantras* that he was supplementing. Dr. Tsering Thakchoe Drungtso, in his recent *Tibetan Medicine: The Healing Science of Tibet,* also describes urine diagnostic techniques taken from the *Somarāja.*[11]

Somarāja, translated from Chinese and sometimes attributed to Nāgārjuna, includes chapters on many of the principal treatments found in Tibetan medicine to this day, including purgatives, emetics, channel cleansing, pulse and urine analysis, enemas, suppositories, and bloodletting. However, it also has a chapter on *daryakan,* which, as asserted above, is of Shangshung derivation. Therefore, it cannot be established that this work or other Chinese compositions are the sources of these diagnostic techniques or therapies. Nevertheless, a passage from *Four Tantras* cited in *Mirror of Beryl* states that cauterization and channel cleansing come primarily from China.[12] Also, several works translated from the Chinese deal with pulse and urine analysis. Dr. Tsering Thakchoe Drungtso stresses the differences between traditional Chinese and Tibetan medicine, while admitting similarities in medical theory and practices as well as in diagnostic techniques. Urine divination techniques using a turtle grid described by Dr. Drungtso are distinctly Chinese.

The influence of the Indian or Āyurveda medical system in Tibet was more extensive. From the eighth century onward, inspired by the aspirations of King Trisong Detsen, Tibetan translators and scholars visited India regularly in pursuit of Buddhist literature and teachings. In doing so they brought back compositions on medicine by great practitioners of Āyurveda. The translator Vairocana in the eighth century traveled to India and translated many works on medicine, astronomy, and the Great Perfection, among other topics. According to those who hold it to be of Indian origin, he was the translator of *Four Tantras*. The *Lotus Chronicles*, cited in *Mirror of Beryl*, said of him:

> Never has there been a translator like Vairocana,
> and there never will be again.
> In the future those who speak the languages of India
> may be called translators,
> but they will come nowhere near Vairocana.
> He was called a translator,
> in reality he was a pandit.
> Generations hence will look on his work
> with immense gratitude.[13]

Translator Rinchen Sangpo in the tenth century also traveled to India. He translated *Essence of Eight Branches* by Śūra, or Vāgbhaṭa, and its extensive commentary *Moonlight* by the Kashmiri Candranandana. These are found in the Tengyur, the canon of works by Indian masters translated into Tibetan, and became widespread and influential in the medical systems of Tibet. The physician Shangtön Siji Bar in the eleventh century also journeyed to India and returned with many teachings on medicine. Indian physicians also visited Tibet where they introduced various traditions. The last physician to visit Tibet from India was reputed to be Pandit Vanaratna in the fifteenth century.

The Tengyur includes about twenty-two translations of Indian medical works. These include compositions on comprehensive theory and practice of the eight branches of Āyurveda, works on herbal preparations, elixirs, and the alchemical preparation of mercury, and even a veterinary work on the treatment of horses.

Of these Indian compositions, the *Essence of Eight Branches* or *Treatise of Eight Branches (Aṣṭāṅgahṛdayasaṃhitanāma)* is regarded within Indian Āyurveda as one of the great works on medicine. The eight branches of Āyurveda are: physical or internal disorders *(kāya)*, children's disorders *(bāla)*, women's disorders *(mātṛ roga)*, demonic disorders *(bhūta vidyā)*, surgery for injuries from weapons or wounds *(śalyatantra),* antidotes to poisons *(agada),* remedies for aging *(jarā),* and aphrodisiacs and cures for impotence *(vājikaraṇa).* The same or very similar eight branches are mentioned in *Four Tantras* as subjects to be studied.

A passage in *Four Tantras* describing the origins of the branches of Tibetan medicine says that India was mainly responsible for the preparation or compounding of medicinal plants and minerals. Medicinal substances used as ingredients in compounds are chosen for the powers and tastes effective in combating disorders. These disorders in turn are classified according to their basic cause, which is a disturbance, excess, or depletion of the three humors *(doṣa),* which are wind *(vāyu, vāta),* bile *(pitta),* and phlegm *(kapha).* Therefore, renowned Indian medical works, such as *Eight Branches,* the *Caraka Saṃhita,* and the *Suśruta Saṃhita,* describe in detail the three-humor pathology, the powers and tastes of single-ingredient medicines, and the compounding of these ingredients. Such detail is mirrored in *Four Tantras* and other indigenous Tibetan medical compositions. The five therapies *(pañcakarma)* renowned in Āyurveda have also found their way into the Tibetan medical system and are described in *Four Tantras.*

Therefore, the principal origins of the medical system in Tibet were those of the indigenous Bön culture, the Greco-Arab cultures to the west, China, and India. Other sources of influence can also be detected. Tibetan sources talk of the "nine royal physicians from surrounding countries." Alongside Trom, China, and India, these surrounding countries include Kashmir, Drugu,[14] Dolpo,[15] and Nepal. Other sources talk of ten medical traditions, listing Khotan, Minyak, Hor or Mongolia, and Oḍḍiyāna in addition to the above.

Four Tantras

The full name of *Four Tantras* is *Essence of Ambrosia Secret-Instruction Tantra on Eight Branches.* This work is the bible of the Tibetan medical science and is met with great praise from all established Tibetan medical traditions. As a single text it contains four main sections or tantras. The first or Root Tantra is an enumeration and overview of the chapters of the other three tantras and an introduction to the three-humor theory. The second or Explanatory Tantra covers embryology, physiology of the human body, causes and classification of disease, diet, medicines, diagnosis, criteria for becoming a doctor, and so on. The third or Instruction Tantra is primarily a comprehensive medical manual for the treatment of specific disorders. The fourth or Final Tantra covers pulse and urine diagnosis; various medicine forms such as pills, pastes, decoctions, powders, mineral medicines; the five cleansing therapies, such as purgatives and emetics; and the five external therapies, such as bloodletting and cauterization.

The format of these tantras is that of a dialogue. Rishi Manasija, a manifestation of the Buddha's speech, requests the individual chapters from Rishi Vidyājñāna, the manifestation of Buddha's mind. A rishi *(ṛṣi)* is a sage, and *Four Tantras* is a tantra not in the commonly understood sense as an esoteric Vajrayana manual, but in its other meaning of "treatise," especially as one on the ancient sciences of India, such as medicine, grammar, and the arts. Throughout the tantra, Medicine Buddha, although present, is silent. The discourse takes place in the beautiful medicine city of Sudarśana, surrounded by the four medicine mountains of Gandhamārdana, Himavat, Vindhya, and Malaya or Malabar. The audience consists of Buddhist and non-Buddhist gods usually associated with India, such as Avalokiteśvara, Brahmā, etc., as well as human and celestial physicians and rishis.

At first glance this great medical work appears to be a standard Indian composition or teaching of the Buddha that was eventually translated into Tibetan. The surroundings and the audience are distinctly Indian in name and description. All four mountains are identifiable as ranges in the east, north, middle, and the western ghats of India. All the rishis present in the audience are found in ancient Indian literature. However, a sizeable number of Tibetan medical scholars doubt its Indian origins. They point out that although the text follows generally the principles of the eight branches of Āyurveda, much of the content of the medical work is deliberately geared toward the climate and environment of Tibet. Some chapters, such as those on pulse and urine diagnosis, are decidedly non-Indian. They claim that certain substances mentioned in the text such as white china bowls and tea were not in existence during the time of the Buddha. Substances such as yak meat and roasted barley porridge are distinctly Tibetan foods. Even the clothing described is Tibetan in style. The references to the mother-son and friend-enemy cycles in the chapter on pulse analysis follow the thinking of the *Somarāja,* which was translated from the Chinese. Moreover, there is no reference to this work in the great canon of translations from India—the Kangyur and Tengyur—and there is no trace of there ever having been a Sanskrit version of the text.

These doubts have given rise to much debate and discussion over the centuries as to the author or authors of *Four Tantras.* Some commentators consider it to be primarily the word of the Buddha with additions and supplementary material by the later Yuthok. The identification of Sudarśana, its place of teaching, has been identified with Bodhgāya in northern India or Oḍḍiyāna in the west of India. Others maintain it is solely a Tibetan composition, the author being variously the eighth-century translator Vairocana, the elder and younger Yuthok, or the eleventh-century treasure revealer Drapa Ngönshé. Desi Sangyé Gyatso, the author of this work, asserts that *Four Tantras* was originally taught in Oḍḍiyāna (often identified with the Swat Valley in Pakistan) by the Buddha manifest as the blue Medicine Buddha. It was preserved, some say as a treasure later revealed by Nāgārjuna and Śūra, and eventually translated and brought to Tibet by Vairocana. From there it was either concealed in a pillar at Samyé Monastery by King Trisong Desten or his son to be revealed later by Drapa Ngönshé, or passed on through Padmasambhava as a part of the Transmission tradition. Eventually it came into the hands of the later Yuthok, who revised the work and supplemented it with other medical traditions existing in Tibet at that time, thereby attuning it to the demands of the Tibetan environment.

Most modern Tibetan scholars maintain the tantra to be primarily the work of Yuthok the elder and younger. Troru Tsenam, for example, says that Yuthok the elder took the medical translations made by Vairocana as a basis, added much from his own experience and from the teachings he received from the Kashmiri Candranandana, together with already established indigenous Tibetan medical science, and produced an early version of *Four Tantras.* This was concealed as a treasure to be later revealed by Drapa Ngönshé and finally reaching Yuthok the younger. Taking this composition as a basis, he supplemented it with teachings from the Āyurvedic *Essence of Eight Branches* and its commentary and added medical practices and oral-tradition techniques that had developed in Tibet since the time of his ancestor. This work was undertaken accompanied by a pure vision of Medicine Buddha and takes the form of a question-and-answer dialogue between Rishi Manasija and Rishi Vidyājñāna in the manifested medical city of Sudarśana. Because of these exalted credentials, Troru Tsenam says, this work is inseparable from the teachings of the Buddha himself.[16]

Other scholars diverge in various ways from this account, but all Tibetan medical practitioners agree that this composition is the foundation on which later medical science in Tibet was built. The work's creation may well be the major turning point in the history of Tibetan medicine, when it went from being a purely derivative tradition to being an innovator of medical science in its own right.

Buddhist Influence

As we have seen, the origins of the medical system in Tibet were by no means exclusively Buddhist. Medical practices from the old Bön culture and from the Greco-Arab traditions, for instance, were clearly not Buddhist. Although many of the medical texts translated from India begin with homage to Medicine Buddha, Āyurveda itself is said to predate the Buddha, and to have begun at the instigation of the god Brahmā, and developed by the god Indra, the rishis, and brahman-caste physicians. Nevertheless, medicine arrived in a Tibet that was embracing the Buddhist doctrine, and the science and the religion have become linked. Such a relationship between medicine and religion was inevitable in the world before the advent of modern scientific thinking, and Tibet was no exception.

Buddhism teaches that the root of all suffering lies in ignorance, aversion, and desire. These three states of mind are known as the *three poisons,* depicted in paintings of the wheel of life as a pig, snake, and chicken, respectively. Illness is an obvious form of suffering. Therefore, although Tibetan medical texts place the three humors at the root of all disease, the deeper root is that of the three poisons. The deep root of phlegm disorder is the pig-like poison of ignorance. The root of bile disorder is the snake-like poison of aversion or anger. The root of wind disorder is the chicken-like poison of desire.

With Buddhism as its spiritual philosophy, Tibetan medicine says that the true path to perfect and permanent health is Buddhist practice aimed at eliminating the three poisons, whereas following medical treatments can alleviate the suffering of illness only temporarily as long as the three poisons reside in the mind. The Buddha is the culmination and final accomplishment of Buddhist practice and is therefore permanently free of any humor imbalance or illness. The accounts in scripture of the Buddha becoming sick toward the end of his life are thus interpreted as mere displays of illness for a pedagogical purpose.

According to the Mahayana Buddhism of Tibet, a buddha is the product of the wisdom of omniscience, total compassion, and unobstructed power. Therefore, a buddha would not only know every disease, the cause of every disease, and the perfect remedy for every disease, but would work effortlessly and compassionately to free living beings of disease. For having such wisdom and compassion, the Buddha is said to be the perfect physician. Desi Sangyé Gyatso himself states:

> The physician who eliminates desire, aversion, and confusion, the ignorance that causes these three poisons, together with the wind, bile, and phlegm disorders that result from the three poisons is the blessed Buddha. He is the physician surpassed by no one.

Because of the unobstructed power of this perfect physician, the Buddha is appealed to in his form as Medicine Buddha. Many ritual-based meditative practices and initiations have appeared, focusing on Medicine Buddha, that aim to enhance the physician's power, overcome disease, lengthen lifespan, and so on. One of the most famous of these is Yuthok Yönten Gönpo's *Heartdrop.* This work describes the initiation or empowerment processes in great detail, including, for example, the medical instruments initiation and the ambrosia longevity initiation, followed by the associated generation and completion-stage practices. With these features, it is a practice on a par with those of highest yoga tantra.

In the practice of Mahayana Buddhism, knowledge is pursued to better equip ourselves to help others. On this bodhisattva path, knowledge of the science of medicine is considered a necessary supplement. Because of this, even those who are not medical practitioners will request and receive the Medicine Buddha initiation, with the aim of planting the seeds for future skill in healing. Others will request and receive the initiation when ill in order to supplement medical treatment. It is not an uncommon practice for those suffering from illness to recite with deep faith the Medicine Buddha mantra or to visualize Medicine Buddha at the site of the illness. There are many recorded testimonials to these rituals' efficacy.

The doctrine of karma is a central pillar of Buddhist philosophy. Essentially, this doctrine preaches that all thoughts and deeds leave imprints on the stream of consciousness that intended them, and those imprints ripen in this and future lives in diverse ways. Our body type, with its strengths and weaknesses and its general constitution, the fortunes and misfortunes we meet through life, and even the environments we find ourselves in, all have their root causes in thoughts and deeds carried out in previous lives. The immediate circumstances that may precipitate pain and pleasure are regarded as mere conditions or triggers that cause the karmic effects to ripen.

Sickness is often brought on by immediate circumstances and conditions

—such as poor diet, unhealthy lifestyle, or contagions in the environment—but its deeper, direct cause is said to be karma. This view is not mere fatalism. Illness may have its deeper cause in the past actions of the patient, but it was triggered by particular circumstances. Similarly, the deeper cause of the cure may be the patient's karma, but the immediate condition for bringing the cure about is the doctor and the medicine. Because of this relationship between illness, remedy, and karma, a patient will often attempt to find a doctor, medicine, or even medical system with which they have a karmic relationship. Medicine will work for some and not for others. Doctors successfully treat some patients and have little success with others. A simple ailment is cured for some but becomes chronic with others. Some recover quickly; some do not. And some do not recover at all. In the world of medicine informed by Buddhism, the seemingly unexplainable course of an illness is attributed to the deeper roots of karma.

Taking into consideration the part that karma plays in the treatment of illness, a physician will sometimes consult the patient's horoscopes to determine the karmic influence on the illness. If it is thereby determined that no amount of conventional treatment will be effective, the patient often resorts to rituals indicated by an astrological calculation or by the divination of an appropriate lama. Physicians will resort to astrology for other reasons also. Desi Sangyé Gyatso states:

> Using [astrology] one calculates the times, directions, and dates when the collecting, preparation, and taking of medicines becomes effective and auspicious. There is a great difference between these benefits and the disastrous consequences that come from not knowing this astrology.[17]

Because of this, medicine and astrology in Tibet enjoy a close relationship.

Yuthok Yönten Gönpo the Elder and Younger

After the introduction of medical systems from abroad and the development of indigenous medicine that occurred in the second half of the first millennium, Tibet saw the appearance of learned physicians of their own. This had its beginnings with the call from King Trisong Detsen in the eighth century for bright young men to engage in the study of medicine, resulting in the arrival of the "nine wise Tibetan physicians." Among them was Drangti

Gyalsang, whose lineage ultimately merged into the Sakya medical lineage; Nyawa Chösang, whose lineage continued well into the time of Desi Sangyé Gyatso in the seventeenth century; and Yuthok Yönten Gönpo the elder.

Yuthok was an almost mythical figure who had made a striking impression as a young man during a conference of foreign doctors held at Samyé Monastery under the auspices of the king. In later years he traveled to India and to other lands to seek out medical teachings, which he brought back to Tibet. Once he brought back from his travels a statue of Medicine Buddha specially made for him by the supernatural serpent-like creatures called *nāgas* in gratitude for curing their queen. This statue was still in the Potala palace in Lhasa in the seventeenth century during the time of the Fifth Dalai Lama, who prayed before it when suffering with an eye condition and met a successful outcome. Yuthok was the composer of many a work on medicine and founded the first medical college in Kongpo. He is said to have lived 125 years.

Yuthok Yönten Gönpo the younger was a descendent of the elder Yuthok and was born in the eleventh century. Although preceded by several great physicians, such as Drapa Ngönshé, Shangtön Siji Bar, and his own mentor, Roktön Könchok Kyap, his contribution to establishing medicine as a truly Tibetan science was immense. His prolific output of teaching and composition established what were among the first son and disciple medical lineages in Tibet. He reputedly traveled to India six times. He is spoken of in glowing terms as a true incarnation of Medicine Buddha. The Fifth Dalai Lama said of him:

> Fusion of all buddha families of the three enlightened bodies,
> the lord of medicine, Vajradhara,
> in the dance performed according to the minds of disciples,
> appears the one renowned as Yuthok Yönten Gönpo,
> in reality the naturally arising lord of myriad mandalas.[18]

He was especially influential in the propagation of *Four Tantras* (or, according to many commentators, its composition).

Consolidation of Medical Science after Yuthok

The later Yuthok Yönten Gönpo left a disciple lineage that begins with the great twelfth-century physician Sumtön Yeshé Sung, as well as a lineage beginning with his son that includes Palden Tsojé of the famous Drangti lineage; the celebrated royal physician Minyima Thongwa Dönden, of the Jang lineage; and Tashi Palsang, in whom the Treasure and Transmission lineages of *Four Tantras* combined.

As well as producing one lineage of *Four Tantras,* the revealed Treasure tradition produced a wealth of oral-instruction treatments for a variety of disorders. The most famous of these are the medical treasures revealed by Guru Chökyi Wangchuk and Dorbum Chökyi Drakpa.

The fifteenth century saw the dawn of two of the greatest medical lineages in Tibet—the Jang and the Sur. The Jang tradition began with Jangpa Namgyal Draksang, whose aristocratic father had been honored by the Mongolian emperor Kublai Khan. In later years he himself was awarded the title of Tai Situ by the emperor. He wrote many authoritative works and was especially knowledgeable on the Kālacakra tantra. He had both tantric disciples, including the famous Palden Chökyong, and medical disciples, including Minyima Thongwa Dönden.

The Sur lineage began with Surkhar Nyamnyi Dorjé. It is said that he received a vision of Yuthok, who gave him oral-tradition teachings and pointed out where later commentators had erred in their understanding of *Four Tantras* and Yuthok's *Heartdrop.* His compositions included many definitive reference works on the tastes, powers, post-digestive tastes, natures, etymologies, and functions of various medicines, as well as the famous *Relic of Millions,* a vast collection of oral-tradition treatments. He was also a dedicated practitioner of tantra and often meditated naked from the waist up using meditation straps to hold his posture. His lineage has produced many worthy physicians. These include Surkhar Lodrö Gyalpo, who produced the first major redaction of *Four Tantras* and some other works that, while not highly regarded by Desi Sangyé Gyatso, were nonetheless quite influential.

Desi Sangyé Gyatso

Both these lineages were eventually merged by Desi Sangyé Gyatso, the author of the present work, in the seventeenth century during the time of the Fifth Dalai Lama. Ngawang Losang Gyatso, the Fifth Dalai Lama, was not a physician, nor did he concentrate on the study of medicine, but he made a significant contribution to the growth and establishment of this science through patronizing medical schools, encouraging the publication of medical works, arranging the translation of Indian texts, inviting Tibetan physicians from far away to pass on their oral traditions, and generally seeing that all conducive conditions for the above were in place. This he was able to do because of the great political power he now possessed, having nullified the challenge of the Tsang rulers to the west of Lhasa with the help of the Mongolian chieftain Gushri Khan.

Desi Sangyé Gyatso had looked at the redaction of *Four Tantras* made by Surkhar Lodrö Gyalpo, decided that it was not up to standard, and suggested to the Dalai Lama that he attempt a new redaction. He also came to the conclusion, contrary to other opinion at the time, that the Jang and Sur lineages were not incompatible. Therefore, beginning around 1690, he set to work on producing a new and revised edition of *Four Tantras,* using a variety of source and reference works; a comprehensive commentary to *Four Tantras,* known as *Blue Beryl;* and a supplement to the Instruction Tantra, the longest of the four tantras. These works form a substantial basis of the study of Tibetan medicine even today. He was also responsible for commissioning a remarkable collection of seventy-nine annotated medical and anatomical paintings that illustrate the chapters of *Four Tantras.* These are still extant and have been published in book form.[19]

In 1696, inspired by a vision of the site as resembling Sudarśana and motivated by the wishes of the Fifth Dalai Lama, who had by then passed away, he founded the famous medical college on Chakpo Hill in Lhasa. There he would sometimes teach the classes himself, and he established the annual expedition to neighboring areas to identify medical plants. He also had great expertise in astrology and composed *White Beryl,* an authoritative work on all aspects of astronomical and elemental calculation and divination practiced in Tibet at that time. Although he was not a trained physician, he was without doubt an extraordinary scholar, and lived an extraordinary life.

He was born near Lhasa in 1653 as a descendent of Desi Trinlé Gyatso, a former viceroy of the Dalai Lama. He came into contact with the Dalai Lama at a very young age. According to the short account of his life by Dr. Losang Tenzin, when the Dalai Lama visited his family, the four-year-old child clung on to the Dalai Lama's robe and wanted to go away with him.[20] From the age of eight he was part of the retinue of the Fifth Dalai Lama, who conferred upon him the layman's vows. Despite depictions of him as an ordained monk, Desi Sangyé Gyatso remained a layman his entire life, something he makes very clear in the present work. From the age of eight he spent much of his time in the Dalai Lama's presence, benefiting from his vast knowledge.

Although he studied with other teachers, the Fifth Dalai Lama became his root guru and bestowed on him many tantra empowerments.

In 1679 the Dalai Lama retired from political life and handed over the reins of power to Desi Sangyé Gyatso, who was only twenty-six years old. And it was a considerable power to fall on such young shoulders. A legal inscription stating that this young man was to be regarded as of equal political status to the Dalai Lama can still be seen in the Potala palace.

He seems to have been very thorough in his administration of the country's institutions. With the monasteries of Ganden, Sera, Drepung, Tashi Lhünpo, and Mindröling, he overhauled and reviewed their monastic regulations, estates, and sources of income. In the lay community he conducted a census of households and levied taxes where appropriate. In the government he set up many new institutions.

The consolidation of Tibet as a land under a single power residing in the Potala palace at Lhasa was not yet forty years old. Because of this, together with the perceived designs of the Manchu and the instability among the Mongolians, not to mention other internal disputes, the young ruler of Tibet, in keeping with the wishes of the Fifth, decided to conceal from the Tibetan community the death of the Dalai Lama four years later. This secret was maintained for about thirteen years. By the time it was revealed in 1694, the incarnation of the Dalai Lama, Tsangyang Gyatso, was already eleven years old. The subsequent problems involving the Sixth Dalai Lama's unwillingness to pursue a monastic life are well documented elsewhere.[21]

In 1701 the new Mongolian chieftain was Lhasang Khan, who succeeded his father Tenzin Dali Khan, the eldest son of Gushri Khan, who had been poisoned and died. Together with Desi Sangyé Gyatso he ruled Tibet. However, it seems that Lhasang wanted complete rule of the country. To fulfill this aim he stirred up trouble between Desi and the monasteries of Drepung, Sera, and Ganden and launched personal attacks on the character of the teenage Sixth Dalai Lama. This resulted in a delegation from the monasteries persuading Desi to step down from his position in 1702 and to appoint his son Ngawang Rinchen in his place.

However, this did not placate Lhasang Khan, and in 1704 hostilities again broke out. The monasteries, together with the Sixth Dalai Lama and the First Jamyang Shepa, mediated, resulting in Lhasang agreeing to return to Mongolia. However, Lhasang did not keep his word. He divided his army into two divisions—one headed by his wife Tsering Tashi or Tsewang Gyalmo, the other headed by Lhasang himself—and converged on Lhasa. Desi decided to surrender to Tsering Tashi, calculating that to surrender to Lhasang would endanger his life. However, Tsering Tashi seized Desi Sangyé Gyatso and immediately had him beheaded. When he was found, it was said that the body was still warm. This was in the summer of 1705.[22]

Two years earlier he had completed the present text on the history of Tibetan medicine. He had concluded that previous histories of medicine were not comprehensive or were unduly biased toward the tradition of the author. He first conceived the idea of composing his own history of medicine when he was thirty, however, as he had been suddenly thrust into the time-consuming administrative role of ruling Tibet, this undertaking was postponed until 1703, when he was fifty. It was to be his last composition.

Theory and Practice of Tibetan Medicine

From the diverse origins described above, a science of medicine developed in Tibet from the seventh to around the twelfth centuries displaying the characteristics of these influences. The fundamental theory behind its practices is that of the elements. In his work on Tibetan medicine, Khenrab Gyatso[23] quotes a verse from *Four Tantras:*

> The body is formed from the four elements,
> illness to be cured is created by the four elements,
> medicine too has the nature of the four elements,
> body, disease, and medicine are of similar natures.

The elements here are those of earth, water, fire, and air together with the element of space. These are the elemental constituents of the body. The text continues:

> From earth comes flesh and bones;
> from water comes blood, the sense of taste, and liquids;
> from fire comes warmth, complexion, the sense of sight;
> from air comes breath and the sense of touch;
> from space comes the cavities and sense of hearing.

Essentially, nothing in the makeup of the body is outside these five elements, and therefore, all physical disorders are also of these elements. Although these five elements exist in the outer world as well, here the term refers exclusively to the "inner" elements that make up the body. In medical terms the elements of earth and water are together known as *phlegm,* the element of fire is called *bile,* and the element of air is called *wind.* The element of space pervades the other three. These three are literally the three "faults" *(doṣa)* but are often translated as the "three humors." As noted above, disturbance, deficiency, or excess of any or all of these humors results in disease.

The humors, or inner elements, share characteristics with their corresponding outer elements. Bile, being the element of fire, is hot, sharp, and so on. Phlegm, having the nature of earth and water, is heavy and cold. Wind with its nature of air is light and mobile. The factors that act upon these inner elements and thereby alter their balance are primarily medicine, diet, and behavior. The external influences of medicine and diet are not different in nature from the five outer elements and so possess characteristics similar to the inner elements or humors.

Medicine, therefore, is prescribed to counter imbalances among the inner elements. Medicine to be taken internally can be single-ingredient medicine or, more commonly, multi-ingredient compounds. These are in the form of pills, powders, pastes, decoctions, and so on. Medicinal ingredients are mineral, herbal, and animal. Likewise, everyday food and drink possesses similar elemental properties that work upon the corresponding inner elements. Even behavior and personal routines can affect the humor balance. Therefore, treatment in the Tibetan medical system may include a combination of medicinal compounds, changes in diet, and harmonious behavior. The theory behind this is summed up in the line taken from *Four Tantras* and cited above: "Body, disease, and medicine are of similar natures."

Other treatments are in the form of therapeutics. They include the five cleansing therapies *(pañcakarma)* and the five external therapies. The first five are found in Indian Āyurveda. They are purgatives, emetics, nasal purgatives, suppositories, and enemas. The five external therapies are bloodletting or venesection, cauterization or moxabustion, fomentation or compress therapy, balneology or embrocating, and the application of lotions and ointments. Other therapies used are the preliminary internal and external oil therapies and channel cleansing therapy.

Treatment using charms, mantras, blessed substances, rituals, and astrological calculations are also common. *Four Tantras* offer a fourfold classification of the 404 categories of disease, 101 of which are caused by external demonic influence. It is these disorders that are primarily treated with such approaches, but non-demonic imbalances of the humors can also be aided with these treatments. Medicines are blessed or consecrated to increase their potency, and there are elaborate rituals for accomplishing this. Relics that include tiny fragments of the bones, teeth, hair, and robes of great accomplished masters are used as ingredients of special pills or used in fumigation processes. Patients may be required to wear an amulet containing a mantra whose power will aid in curing them of the illness. Often they will invite the monastic community to their home to perform particular rituals, or will request the monks to recite certain scriptures or prayers in the monastery on their behalf. The particular mantra to wear or recite, or the ritual to be performed, is more often than not determined by the patient's lama rather than his or her doctor. These same lamas can be requested to perform a divination ritual in order to determine the best kind of treatment, the most suitable doctor, and even the prognosis.

Diagnosis

Diagnosis in the Tibetan medical system is said to be by visual examination, contact, and questioning. The first refers to the doctor taking note of and examining various physical features of the patient. These include complexion, eyes, tongue, nails, and, in particular, urine. *Contact* primarily refers to reading the pulse. A visit to a Tibetan doctor often involves bringing a sample of that morning's first urination for examination followed by a reading of the pulse on both hands. Dr. Tsering Thakchoe Drungtso quotes the fifteenth-century commentator Taktsang Lotsāwa Sherap Rinchen as asserting that pulse and urine diagnosis are distinctly Tibetan and did not originate in India.[24] However, as discussed above, these diagnostic techniques appear in medical works translated from the Chinese and are also found in Āyurveda. It may be that these techniques are not as developed in these countries as they are in Tibet, where undoubtedly they are sophisticated and highly skilled practices.

Urine is said to resemble a mirror, reflecting the nature of bodily disorder. Important considerations in its examination include the time when the urine is passed, the time it is analyzed, and the food and drink taken by the patient the previous evening. Actual examination involves analyzing the color, vapor, bubbles, smell, sediment, and changes in the urine. Analysis detects the status of the humors, and in connection with various diagrams can also detect the presence of spirits.

As with urine analysis, pulse examination is a sophisticated process that may require various dietary and other restrictions for at least a day before the consultation. The time of pulse analysis is important, the best time being early morning. The location for analysis is usually the radial artery running through the wrist. The artery on both wrists is examined by the doctor using three fingers on each hand to determine the condition of the bodily organs and to determine the balance of the humors. Different fingers read different organs.

The pulse is read by observing its characteristics. These can be, for example, weak, hollow, sunken, trembling, fluctuating, slow, fast, tight, and so forth. The pulse is also described using a variety of similes, such as like the bite of a toothless dog, a river flowing from on high, a boiling hot spring, flames, and a thorn. There are types of pulse according to physical constitution. There also seasonal pulses that relate to the elements of wood, earth, fire, metal, and water. Interpretation of these pulses requires the knowledge of the elemental relationships often referred to as mother-child and friend-enemy relationships.

Like urine analysis the pulse can be used for divination. There are seven types of pulse used for divination, known as the seven wonderful pulses. Unlike in other pulse analysis, the subject is healthy when these are read. The *family pulse* is read on a senior member of the family to foretell important occurrences that may befall the household. The *guest pulse* provides information on a guest about to visit the family. The *enemy pulse* predicts the outcome of attacking an enemy. The *friend pulse* provides information about the wealth of the family. The *evil-spirit pulse* discloses the malevolent presence of a spirit affecting the household. The *substitution pulse* is read on a healthy member of the family to provide diagnosis of another member unable to reach the doctor. The son's pulse could be read in order to diagnose the father, for example. The *pregnancy pulse* is used to determine the sex of an unborn child.

Urine and pulse analysis are discussed at length in *Four Tantras* and constitute the main diagnostic techniques in the medical system of Tibet.

Physicians

In Tibet physicians were the products of a one-to-one lineage passed from parent to child, uncle to nephew, or master to disciple, or they were graduates from medical colleges established by celebrated physicians. Family lineages include the Sakya uncle-nephew lineage, the Drangti lineage, and the Tsarong lineage. The celebrated Jang and Sur lineages that began in the fifteenth century contained father-to-son as well as master-to-disciple transmissions.

One of the most famous medical colleges was that of Chakpori in Lhasa set up by Desi Sangyé Gyatso himself.

Four Tantras lists the characteristics expected of a physician. They include possessing an honorable character in line with Buddhist criteria, intelligence, an ethical vow, compassion and skill with patients, and good familiarity with the different aspects of medical science. These technical aspects include urine and pulse diagnosis, a grasp of the medical literature, the experience of having observed one's teacher, and proficiency in prognosis, the use of surgical instruments, different treatments, dietary factors, the five therapies, and the identification of medical substances.

Physicians are strongly urged to avoid becoming tainted with those characteristics that render them "butchers of lives."[25] These include treating patients only after calculating the benefit they can bring; relying on meager learning; prescribing treatments that are unsafe and untried, ineffective, or based on hearsay; and being "little more than a salesman," peddling general tonics as targeted cures.

Development of Tibetan Medicine up to the Present

The present work deals with the history of medical science up to the end of the seventeenth century. However, contemporary sources such as the great scholar and preserver of the Tibetan medical tradition, Jampa Trinlé (b. 1928), director of the Lhasa Astro-Medical Institute, whose work was cited above, and the equally accomplished physician and teacher, Troru Tsenam (b. 1926), have composed biographies of important physicians and short histories of Tibetan medical science up to and including the occupation of Tibet by the Chinese.[26]

Influential physicians after Desi Sangyé Gyatso, whose biographies are described in the above two works, include the eighteenth-century Deumar Tenzin Phüntsok, who composed a renowned and very detailed Tibetan materia medica that is still in use today. Also in the eighteenth century Situ Künkhyen Chökyi Jungné, a prolific traveler, journeyed to India, China, Nepal, and Sri Lanka in search of knowledge of the five sciences,[27] including medical traditions and practices. These he translated into Tibetan, sparing himself no hardship in his efforts to enhance the traditions of Tibet. In his later life he founded an educational institute in Palpung Thupten Chökhor in eastern Tibet, attracting students from Amdo and Kham, including

Karma Ngelek Tenzin, Khamtrül Chökyi Nyima, Degé Gyalpo Tenpa Tsering, many of whom became renowned physicians in their own right. Of these, Tenpa Tsering recognized the value of propagating in Kham the *Four Tantras* redacted by Desi Sangyé Gyatso and his *Blue Beryl* commentary and so took on the task of reprinting and distributing these works in eastern Tibet.

In the nineteenth century Situ Chökyi Gyatso rejuvenated the medical college of the famous Nyingma monastery Kathok Dorjé Den in the Degé district of Kham, while Jamyang Khyentsé Wangpo set up the study of medicine and the other sciences in Degé and at Tashi Lhatsé Monastery in Dzongsar. Kongtrül Yönten Gyatso studied in Kham at the time of the great Rimé movement and became a physician renowned for his magical powers. The renowned Mipham Namgyal Gyatso, or Ju Mipham, also from Degé, includes, in his thirty-five volumes of compositions, commentaries on *Four Tantras;* instructions on compounding medicines; compositions on anatomy; oral-tradition teachings on rabies; treatments for the ears, voice, and eyes; medical teachings from China; and treatments for cattle.

In the latter part of the nineteenth century, Orgyen Tenzin Gyatso, physician to the Thirteenth Dalai Lama, reprinted *Four Tantras* and other medical compositions and helped restore the fortunes of the Chakpori Medical College established by Desi Sangyé Gyatso. Karma Jikmé Chökyi Sengé, born in Kham and a student at the Nyingma monastery of Kathok, became such a renowned medical practitioner that he was invited to Lhasa by Orgyen Tenzin Gyatso, where he taught and raised the profile of many works connected with the Nyingma tradition, the early treasure revealers, and in particular Yuthok's seminal work on combining medicine and tantric ritual, the *Heart-drop.* He also reprinted many medical works. Trekhang Jampa Thupwang and Jabukpa Damchö Palden, physicians to the Thirteenth Dalai Lama, taught bright students chosen from Chakpori Medical College.

Among these students was Khyenrap Norbu (1883–1962), who became the director of Chakpori Medical College and the Lhasa Astro-Medical Institute, founded in 1916 by the Thirteenth Dalai Lama. Khyenrap Norbu was personal physician to the Dalai Lama and is revered in Tibetan medical circles today. He nurtured about a thousand disciples in the two medical colleges of Lhasa, not only with medical science but with the Dharma, poetry, and grammar. He encouraged women, exemplified by the celebrated female doctor Yangchen Lhamo, to undertake the study of medicine and to halt the decline in interest in gynecology and pediatrics. He also composed many works on medicine. His students were numerous and include many of the doctors who fled into exile in India after the 1959 uprising against the Chinese occupation of Tibet, as well as Jampa Trinlé, the author of a history of Tibetan medicine mentioned above.

Concerning the status of indigenous Tibetan medicine after the Cultural Revolution enforced by the Communist Chinese in the 1960s, both Jampa Trinlé writing in 1988 as director of Lhasa Astro-Medical Institute and Troru Tsenam writing in 1996, probably from eastern Tibet, have no criticism of the state of medical science in Tibet after the Chinese occupation. Troru Tsenam says that after the democratic reforms in Tibet, Chakpori Medical College and the Lhasa Astro-Medical Institute merged to become one. But he makes no mention of the fact that Chakpori was shelled by the Chinese during the Cultural Revolution and damaged almost beyond repair. He talks of health centers and Tibetan medical schools being built in Central Tibet, Shigatsé, and in Kham and Amdo, thereby relieving the hardship of there being no local doctors, of large medical conventions and of the opening of the Lhasa school of Tibetan medicine in 1986. He says that these new schools maintain the principles of traditional Tibetan medicine found in Chakpori and the Lhasa Astro-Medical Institute alongside modern medical knowledge.[28]

Outside Tibet, the Fourteenth Dalai Lama established the Tibetan Astro-Medical Institute in Dharamsala in the foothills of the Himalayas in 1961. It was housed in Dharamsala in a rundown wooden building probably built during the days of the British Raj. Dr. Yeshi Dönden and Ven. Lodrö Gyatso were appointed to run the medical and astrological sections. At its inception it had only two students, but it gradually developed as the stock of medicinal ingredients grew and the number of rooms, staff, and students increased. Dr. Khenrab, writing in 2004, says that twelve batches of medical students and six batches of astrological students have graduated over the past forty-three years, resulting in an output of over two hundred doctors and forty astrologers, who now work at the institute, at one of nearly forty branch clinics, or in private practices in India and overseas. Since its beginning, the Tibetan Astro-Medical Institute in exile has had pharmaceutical, research and development, materia medica, and editorial and publication departments. The astrology department produces annual almanacs, calendars, amulets, and horoscopes. Its office in New Delhi exports products all over the world. The staff now numbers 350, and doctors and astrologers from the institute regularly travel worldwide for conferences, consultations, and seminars.

Dr. Dönden opened his own practice in Dharamsala, as did the female doctor Losang Drölma Khangkar, known as Ama Losang. I remember these two doctors fondly and with gratitude. It would not be an exaggeration to say that on more than one occasion Dr. Dönden rescued my wife and me from dreadful illnesses, including hepatitis and pneumonia, during our long stay in Dharamsala in the 1970s. For the home birth of our children in the forests above Dharamsala, Ama Losang gave me detailed instruction on midwifery, and during the birth of our first child she personally trekked up the mountain to prescribe medicine to bring on birth during a long and protracted labor. Our son was born within half an hour of my wife taking her medicine. There are many accounts of these two great doctors delivering health care to the Tibetan refugees, local Indians, and Western travelers and expatriots in and around Dharamsala.

Tibetan medical science has been on a long journey. In the distant past medical systems from other parts of the world converged in Tibet. Together with extant medical practices, they developed into an indigenous medical system that was practiced behind the Himalayas for well over a thousand years. Now that very same medical system, having survived a few threats to its survival, is spreading through the rest of the world as an alternative approach to medical treatment. It brings with it a great variety of treatments and diagnostic techniques, along with a vast stock of compound medicines, all of which testify to those great scholars and practitioners of the past who developed and preserve this unique system. This present work reveals their story.

Structure of the Text

Mirror of Beryl[29] begins with an appraisal of the importance of the five major sciences, especially the science of medicine, and traces the origins of this science in its celestial beginnings. Part 1 then examines the root medical lineages of ancient India. It briefly documents the arising of the Indian Āyurvedic system and recounts the biographies of great medical scholars and practitioners such as Jivaka, a contemporary of the Buddha.

Part 2, on the earlier development of medicine in Tibet, initially focuses on the eighth century, and on such luminaries as King Trisong Detsen, Padmasambhava, and Vairocana. As well as showing the Indian antecedents, the author also examines the considerable influences on Tibetan medicine from China and Central Asia at this time. Part 2 goes on to deal with the propagation of medicine from the eleventh century for the next four hundred years, and recounts the lives of renowned medical practitioners such as Yuthok Yönten Gönpo. Because of the controversy surrounding the authorship of

Four Tantras, and its strong association with Yuthok, much of this section is taken up with an examination of its origins. Consequently many pages are spent on a presentation of the main definitions of *word of the Buddha (buddhavacana)* and subsequent treatises *(śāstra)* by Indian masters.

Beginning from the fifteenth century, part 3 of the book charts the development of the Jang and Sur lineages, the two main indigenous traditions of Tibetan medicine, and consists primarily of the biographies of the main propagators. After these accounts, the author focuses on the condition and development of medical science during his own lifetime. Here he details the Fifth Dalai Lama's contribution to the spread of medical science as well as other contemporary scholars and physicians. As Desi Sangyé Gyatso was himself a great medical scholar, as well as interim ruler of Tibet, he describes his own considerable efforts to propagate medical science, both through composition and administrative establishment.

The final topics of the book are in the Tibetan all grouped under the heading "Study of Medicine." This appears to have been an arbitrary division inserted by a later editor. The section focuses on the fundamental Buddhist practice of devotion to a master, followed by a long and detailed presentation of the three main categories of Buddhist precepts. Although linked to the topic of the study of medicine, this feels like a deliberate departure. This work was Desi Sangyé Gyatso's last composition and was completed in 1703. It was at this time that twenty-year-old Tsangyang Gyatso, the Sixth Dalai Lama, began to show signs of not wanting to enter the monastic life, and I wonder if the two are not connected.

This text concludes with a brief presentation on the ethical behavior of physicians, the correct attitudes of the student, the author's own medical practices, and a bibliography of medical histories.

Acknowledgments

For research and answers to the many queries I had with this project, I spent three months at the Central Institute of Higher Tibetan Studies, Sarnath, India. There I was fortunate to meet with scholars in various fields and to access the excellent facilities there. The obvious dedication of the staff and students has created an almost tangible atmosphere of the love of learning, and in its facilities it is surely the foremost resource for the preservation and continual development of the Tibetan sciences.

Although this is primarily a work on the history of Tibetan medicine, the text nonetheless contains a great number of medical terms, such as the names of diseases, treatments, therapies, medicinal substances, as well as titles of many ancient medical works. Help in identification and translation of these terms has come from Professor Losang Tenzin Rakdho, dean of the faculty of medicine in the Tibetan Medicine Department at the institute. Although a busy doctor involved in teaching consultation and administration, the professor gave freely of his time during my stay in Sarnath. His warmth and kindness extended to frequent invitations to his house for family meals, helping me find accommodation in the institute, and even ministering to me when I came down with a nasty case of food poisoning.

Help in nonmedical areas of the text was provided by Geshé Losang Chödar, also of the Sarnath institute. This included translation queries in areas of Dharma, history, and politics. Geshé-la is the Tibetan editor at the Institute of Tibetan Classics responsible for the critical editions of the Tibetan text. This medical history contains hundreds of citations, and his patient efforts in tracking down the source of these has saved me many months of work. Geshé-la also took it upon himself to make sure I had all requirements for my stay in Sarnath, even down to the essential thermos flask. He was always cheerfully available for queries on identification and location of texts within the vast library complex at Sarnath. His contribution to the completion of this translation has been enormous.

Desi Sangyé Gyatso frequently analyzes the etymology of Indic terms—and in one instance an entire Sanskrit verse—resulting in pages explaining Sanskrit roots, affixes, and case endings. For assistance in this field I turned to the eminent Sanskrit scholar, Venerable Losang Norbu Shastri, director of research and translation at Sarnath and Hindi translator for the Dalai Lama. I am very grateful to him for helping me with these complicated rules, even though he was not well at the time, and for identifying the main Sanskrit grammar work used by Desi in his explanations.

Remaining translation queries were cleared up through Skype discussions with Geshé Thupten Jinpa, president of the Institute of Tibetan Classics in Montreal, Canada. More generally, I am ever grateful to Thupten Jinpa for the privilege of working on the monumental enterprise he has envisioned with the Institute of Tibetan Classics.

I thank my editor at Wisdom Publications, David Kittelstrom, for casting his critical eye over the translation and rendering into clear and comprehensible English those passages where obfuscation had gotten the better of me.

Technical Note

THE THREE TIBETAN TEXTS of *Mirror of Beryl* used for the translation were (1) the critical edition prepared and published by the Institute of Tibetan Classics in New Delhi under the title *Gso ba rig pa'i khog 'bugs vaidūrya'i me long* (2008, ISBN 81-89165-28-3) as volume 28 of the *Bod kyi gtsug lag gces btus* series, (2) the Lhasa Shöl edition reproduced by Tashi Yangpal Tashigang in 1970 from L. P. Lhalungpa's print, and (3) the edition printed by the Tibetan Astro-Medical Institute, Dharamsala, in 1994.

Bracketed numbers embedded in the text refer to page numbers of the critical edition. All Tibetan names in the main body of text are rendered phonetically in accordance with the style sheet developed by the Institute of Tibetan Classics and Wisdom Publications especially for the *Library of Tibetan Classics* series. Transliterated spellings for these names can be found under the relevant entry in the index. Sanskrit diacritics are used throughout, except for naturalized Sanskrit terms such as sutra, mandala, and nirvana.

Where the book form of a Tibetan text is used for referencing, as opposed to standard Tibetan folio text, the reference is chapter, page, line. For example, 2.3.7 means chapter 2, page 3, line 7. When only two numbers are present, it refers to page and line numbers.

For some illnesses, no clear translation was available, and the term has been rendered in phoneticized Tibetan, e.g., *gyuser*. In such cases, the glossary contains descriptions and/or translations, with sources where available.

The glossary also contains the various remedies Desi mentions. Where major variations in identification occur or only one source was traced, the sources are cited. A separate materia medica cross-references these glossary entries to their rendering in Tibetan for easier access by researchers.

Pronunciation of Tibetan phonetics

ph and *th* are aspirated *p* and *t*, as in *pet* and *tip*.

ö is similar to the *eu* in French *seul*.

ü is similar to the *ü* in the German *füllen.*
ai is similar to the *e* in *bet.*
é is similar to the *e* in *prey.*

Pronunciation of Sanskrit
Palatal *ś* and retroflex *ṣ* is similar to the English unvoiced *sh.*
c is an unaspirated *ch* similar to the *ch* in *chill.*
The vowel *ṛ* is similar to the American *r* in *pretty.*
ñ is somewhat similar to a nasalized *ny* in *canyon.*
ṅ is similar to the *ng* in *sing* or *anger.*

Mirror of Beryl

A Well-Explained History of the Glorious Science of Medicine, A Feast to Delight the Rishis

Desi Sangyé Gyatso
1653–1705

Introduction

1. Homage and Verses of Auspiciousness[30]

Of the nature of every buddha,
an exalted gnosis all-pervading,
on the hundred-petal lotus of the navel,
in complete and perfect enlightenment,
omniscient of past, present, and future,
of the lotus family, tathāgata, god of gods,
light from your enlightened features
arises everywhere in all worlds,
immediately opening the gates
to shine on the supreme level,
great king of glory upon glory[31]
for the realms of sentient beings in general,
tormented by the five degenerations,
and specifically for those of the snowy land of Tibet,
you are the creator of all happiness and welfare.
With great compassion you perform the dance
of the red-robes, a vow-holding monk and king,
my root guru, Ngawang Losang Gyatso,
deliberately come again for the doctrine and sentient beings,
Great Sixth born of the celestially descended Nyöpa lineage,
in this life, as promised by your previous incarnation,
care for us and grant us all the happiness of samsara and nirvana.

Amid the stars of fully enlightened and perfect buddhas,
the light of your exalted wisdom of insight and abandonment,
which fill the skies of pure bodhi-mind prayers
reaching all beings fallen into the night of the five dark degenerations,
your full moon of compassion brighter than that of other tathāgatas,
supreme among the eight medicine buddhas,

from the glorious throat of Ṣaṣṭimukti
you taught the medical sutras in eight hundred verses,
medicine for the disease of ignorance,
and in the manifested place of Sudarśana,[32]
a city of qualities beautiful to behold,
you taught the gods, rishis, insiders, and outsiders
the truths of the eight branches of medical science.
Guru of medicine, grant all auspiciousness.

From the pure innate tones
representing the five types of gnosis,
which are born from the nonconceptual realm
found at the five secret places of his body,
the five rishis appear individually,
like separate water reflections of the moon.
Vidyājñāna, **gnosis perceiving** ultimate truth
and in essence the four brothers;
and Manasija, **born from the mind,**
the manifestation of enlightened speech;
by the illusion of manifestation
you are companions carrying out the Conqueror's deeds, [4]
of benefit to others, wearers of the brahman thread,
you five great rishis,[33] drench all realms and all living beings
who seek long life, Dharma, wealth, and happiness
with the rains of the ambrosia of medical science.

Four-faced Caturmukha[34] blessed by the Buddha
to recall the supreme Āyurveda,
Prajāpati, Aśvinīputra, and other gods,
the eight rishis,[35] Ātreya and so forth,
of the scriptural traditions of methods
of maintaining good health, of living long
and of curing disease;
outsiders such as Brahmā, patriarch and creator of all worlds,
the insider entourage of Mañjuśrī, Avalokiteśvara, and others,
who show the path to sentient beings in these degenerate times,
all present as requestors of the teachings;
let the carriage of sentient beings be heavy with the load of happiness.

Born into the Videhan race, named because of their lofty qualities
found at the very pinnacle of the human race,[36]
the son of the householder queen of Bimbisāra, king of Magadha.
His instincts, by the power of training in former lives,
brought him to seek out and study the Āyurveda,
and perfect every branch of medical science.
He was known as Kumāra Bhṛtya,[37]
raised like a son by his elder brother
to become the greatest of physicians.
Grant us happiness and virtue in the three worlds.

Born in the southern region of Veta,
a great and precious source for the understanding
of sutras and tantras, old and new,
his Dharma is peace, free of fabrication,
destroying the torments of samsara and nirvana,
ripening fully as uncontaminated ambrosia essence,
and in his practice of medicine for all living beings,
he is as kind as the supreme buddha of beryl light.
Prophesied by the Buddha, master of the profound path,
Nāgārjuna, grant us the great ambrosia of immortality.

Born in the west, son of the purely practicing brahman doctor Saṃghagupta,
the ripening of previous faith and prayer at a shrine of Īśvara
meant that he first became learned and practiced in outsider doctrine.
Finally, his wrong views of true existence conquered by Āryadeva,
he saw the words of the Buddha, found faith in cause and effect, [5]
and became a follower of the Buddha and a great scholar of India.
Śūra, grant us confidence in Āyurveda.

Great grandson[38] in the pure lineage of the above, son of Kāmānandana,
in the sacred **moon** of his waxing mind of enlightenement,
the gift of the well-written teachings of Śūra sent as far as **Abhirati.**[39]
His **moonlight** perfectly illuminating the jasmine treasury,
the smile at the very **essence** of the **eight** lotus-petal **branch**
of working for the welfare of others.
May we be nourished by these beings,
who spread far and wide the science of medicine.

Your own form that of Amitābha,
born magically within a supreme lotus,
making the lives and health of others as strong as vajras,
not only through the medical science of Āyurveda
but also with the source of the four rivers of enlightened deeds.
Second Buddha, your Manasarovar lake of vast kindness
is of a depth hard to fathom;
watch over us Padmākara.

Master and father of every buddha, hair tied in five places,
deliberately come to and perform the dance of the robed monk
with wisdom, discipline, and goodness
to plant the code of morality within the minds of all beings.
Master of the doctrine of the perfect Buddha,
Losang Drakpa, I bow to you with the crown of my head.

Sun manifested from the gnosis of Vairocana in Akaniṣṭha,
known in the world as a translator
but in reality a pandit master of the five sciences,
I bow to Vairocana, illuminator of the Buddha's doctrine.

Sugata, guide of the world, crown of the conquerors,
Rasmi Samudgata Śrīku Rāja in the form of a king,
deliberately come to protect the people of Tibet,
object of homage, flower of the god Brahmā.[40]

In reality the sugata Vimaladhvaja,
provisionally a bodhisattva on the path,
working for the welfare of beings,
lord of Purgyal, of an exceptional and virtuous mind,
I bow to you, Muné Tsenpo.[41]

Skilled in opening the lotus gates to profound treasures
that remained a long time in the ambrosia of immortality,
their taste dripping into the honey of virtuous Dharma,
you were the incarnation of Vairocana,
discoverer of certainty, Drapa Ngönshé Wangchuk,[42]
friend to the teachings and to living beings.

Great redactor who cleaned the face of the tantra
according to the time and place in Tibet, [6]
king of physicians, Yuthok Yönten Gönpo,
in whom all tathāgata lineages are gathered,
I bow to you with reverence.

Lokeśvara, **revealing three** times a dance
in a pure birth under the control of compassion,
a holy being fully accomplished
in the supreme **meditative retention** of life and **gnosis**,
you too are a venerable object of homage.[43]

Of the lineage of a minister who recited
secret words with Dharma king Aktsom Chen,[44]
and from a family of royal physicians,
Palden Tsojé of the Drangti line,
master of healing, I prostrate before you.

Born into the Tongkhün[45] race from Minyak,
who with his vast knowledge in general
and of medicine in particular was of great kindness
in restoring the welfare and happiness of all beings,
truly a king of physicians,
I bow to you, Jangdak Namgyal Drakpa Sangpo.[46]

Of the lineage of the great Tibetan Dharma kings,
Holding the three great refuges as supreme,
a layman who avoided meat and alcohol like poison,
sun-like friend to the hundred-petal lotus of medical science,
Jangpa physician, Minyima, to you I bow.[47]

Trisong Detsen having taken upon his shoulders
worldly affairs and the Dharma of men and gods,
Chösang was a master physician by royal appointment.
From this physician on down to the one named Dorjé:
how could one not have faith in this lineage
of practice and the discovery of medicines?[48]

Blessed with a vision of Yönten Gönpo,
coming from the region of **Surkar**,
holding self and others as **equal**,
well possessed of the **vajra** of life,[49]
I bow to the lamas of the support transmission
up to Terdak Lingpa, who drank to satisfaction
from the vase of Dharma.

By the power of protector Rājānaka Vajra Mārajit,
who was entrusted with the tantra by Buddha and Padmākara,
may the host of māras be crushed like jewels,
and with feats such as the gift of removing fear,
accomplish the four activities.[50]

You with qualities of a treasure protector
and with the nature of Shingja Chen;
wrathful Apsé, like a butcher slaughtering a sheep,
your function to kill those with broken vows;
Red Jackal Face, the color of your enemy's blood:
these and other protectors, fulfill all wishes without hindrance.[51] [7]

In particular, doctrine protectors of the profound heartdrop,
the supreme and final path of this tradition,
the nine oath-bound guardians, too, protecting like a vajra canopy:
in this and future lives ensure the accomplishment
of a host of virtuous activities.

To find freedom from samsara's constant rain of suffering
and reach the supreme level of omniscience,
you need to study the sciences.
And from among Buddha's teachings, as vast as an ocean,
the science that brings to this hard-to-find human form
of opportunity and leisure—albeit only temporarily—
good health, respite from the suffering of sickness, and long life,
bringing even the vigor of youth to the elderly
and ultimately the achievement of the gnosis
of perfect enlightenment, the state of a buddha,

is a great science more precious and essential than the others,
this science of medicine that cares for all beings.

Drawing from various accounts of its history
the uncorrupted literary traditions of the science of life,
with the excellent credentials of rishi practices,
made even purer with untainted scripture
and the complete process of detailed reasoning,
this **good explanation** that **erects** the **structure**
of the **glorious medical science** tradition,
as it was done by the king of medicine,
a stainless **mirror of beryl**
reflecting the faces of the **delighted** Āyurveda[52] **rishis,**
with their mandalas of manifest virtue;
this great offering of the ambrosia of life,
may it become a glorious spring **feast,** granting long life
to all living beings here and now.[53]

2. Medical Science

The importance of the five sciences

[9] IT IS SAID that even the Tathāgata Trikālajña offered praise in poetic verse before generating the bodhi mind. Also, for any kind of treatise, offering words of auspiciousness to the lamas and deities ensures that their compassionate blessings of wisdom are easily granted. Therefore, for these and other reasons Daṇḍin says:

> Words of auspiciousness and homage
> and a synopsis of the text—
> this is the door.[54]

With the words of auspiciousness to the lamas, medicine buddhas, and the lineages, the urging of the protectors to do their duties and a synopsis of the work, all found in the above thirty *śloka* (stanzas)—a word constructed from the root *ślokṛ,* meaning "to compile"—the door has been opened. In the fifth chapter of the *Uttaratantra,* the noble Maitreya says:

> Relying upon trustworthy scripture and reasoning,
> I teach this solely to purify myself
> and to nourish those with faith
> and with minds possessed of great virtue.[55]

With this verse in mind, I will begin. In the *Sutra of Repaying the Kindness of the Skillful Buddha,* it says in the ninth chapter, on devotion:

> If a bodhisattva does not first train in the five sciences, he can never attain the gnosis of omniscience, the highest and perfect enlightenment. Therefore, in order to attain the highest enlightenment, train in the five sciences. For a bodhisattva, gratitude and

> repaying kindness are expressed by explaining to sentient beings the things to be explained and by teaching them. How should they teach? They should teach by possessing the five sciences in order to attain the highest and perfect enlightenment.[56]

Also *Ornament to Mahayana Sutras* says in the twelfth chapter, "Searching for the Mahayana":

> If efforts are not made in the five sciences,
> even great ārya beings will not attain omniscience.
> Therefore, to refute and to nourish,
> and to attain omniscience, make effort in the sciences.[57]

Ārya Asaṅga states in *Stages of the Yogacaryā,* from his five treatises on the stages, in the second chapter on the words of the Buddha: [10]

> What level of knowledge is born from listening? In brief, it is as follows. Whichever of the five sciences is being studied, the mind is initially applied to the letters and words, and word forms, and one listens, keeps them in the mind, retains, recites, and recalls them. The understanding that arises from this gathering of letters, words, and word forms is the level of knowledge born from listening. What are the five sciences? They are inner science [i.e., Buddhism], medicine, logic, language, and arts and crafts.[58]

In the eighth chapter, "Types of Powers," of Asaṅga's *Stages of the Bodhisattva from Stages of the Yogacaryā,* it says:

> The bodhisattva seeks out a Dharma. What does he seek out? How does he search? Why does he search? In brief, the bodhisattva seeks out the bodhisattva canon, the śrāvaka canon, the treatises of the outsiders, and the arts and crafts of the world. From the twelve branches of scripture[59] that comprise the teachings, the *extensive canon* is the bodhisattva canon. The remaining scriptures should be known as the śrāvaka canon. The treatises of the outsiders are of three types: those on logic, those on language, and those on medicine. The arts and crafts of the world are many and varied. They include, for example, the crafts of goldsmiths,

> blacksmiths, and jewelers. All this knowledge can be classified under the five sciences, which are inner science, logic, language, medicine, and arts and crafts. Whatever the bodhisattva seeks is contained within these five sciences. Therefore, he seeks out all sciences.[60]

Also:

> How does the bodhisattva search? [11] The bodhisattva adopts an attitude of great reverence and goes in search of well-taught, well-explained Dharma. In brief, he maintains his reverence for the teachings in the following ways. The bodhisattva in search of just one good teaching would happily walk over a searing hot surface with a mind of great reverence if not doing so meant that he would not receive that teaching. If that is true, need we mention it is the same for a bodhisattva seeking many teachings?[61]

Also:

> Why does the bodhisattva seek out the study of the teachings? The bodhisattva seeks out the word of the Buddha so that he may truly practice with diligence in accord with the Dharma, and that he may teach others purely and extensively. The bodhisattva seeks out the science of logic in order to understand exactly the faults found in texts and in the spoken word, to defeat others in debate, to induce faith in those who have no faith in this doctrine, and to increase the faith of those who do. The bodhisattva seeks out teachings on language because with his excellent use of language that is definitive in it use of words and syllables, he will be able to compose his utterances well, and those who delight in speech will develop faith in him. Moreover, using various etymological analyses for a single meaning he will be able to make use of terminology. The bodhisattva seeks out the scriptures on medicine in order to cure living beings of their various illnesses and to benefit large communities. The bodhisattva seeks out knowledge of the arts and crafts of this world so that with little difficulty, he can create more pleasures for other beings. Also he will be valued greatly, and knowledge of arts and craft aids the practice of giving.

> Moreover, the bodhisattva seeks out all five sciences in order to complete the great gnosis accumulation for perfect enlightenment, [12] because were he not to train in all of them, he would not attain the unobscured gnosis of omniscience.[62]

In chapter 14, the "Wisdom" chapter, of *Stages of the Bodhisattva from Stages of the Yogacaryā,* it says:

> What is the wisdom of the bodhisattva? It is that which is engaging in all existing knowledge and that which is engaged in all existing knowledge.[63] It is the discernment of phenomena and focuses on and engages in the five sciences of inner science, logic, healing, language, and arts and crafts. This is the nature of the wisdom of the bodhisattva. What are the types of bodhisattva wisdom? They can be condensed into two types: those on the levels of mundane wisdom and transcendent wisdom.[64]

Also:

> What is the wisdom of the bodhisattva that brings happiness here and elsewhere? It should be known as being of nine kinds: the wisdom that is well trained in and abides in the inner science; the wisdom that is well trained in, but does not abide in, the science of healing, the science of logic, the science of language, and the science of worldly arts and crafts, and, in dependence on being well trained in these five sciences, the wisdom of the bodhisattva that brings the true teaching, true concentration, true encouragement, and true joy to, respectively, those disciples who are confused, heedless, discouraged, and engaged in the true path.[65]

Also in the seventeenth chapter, "Enlightenment":

> What does it mean to know the bodhisattva scriptures? From the five sciences, the bodhisattva receives the Dharma from others in the form of a collection of letters, words, and word forms that he retains and recites well. The meanings of the Dharma too he receives from others. Alternatively, he contemplates and analyzes their meanings himself. [13] In this way the bodhisattva knows

> the Dharma and knows their meanings. In order not to forget the Dharma and its meanings and to learn new Dharma and new meanings, he perseveres in his endeavors.[66]

Jamyang Sakya Paṇḍita says:

> All the bright minds in this snow mountain land
> would never outshine the five great sciences;
> even the light of a million stars combined
> would find it hard to outshine the sun.[67]

Sasang Mati Paṇchen says:

> Those who desire enlightenment
> should know the five sciences.[68]

Rinpung Sachö Wangpo says:

> Slaying all wrong views in the arena of knowledge
> with the wrathful sciences of language and logic;
> flawlessly bringing the manifest benefits
> of the caring sciences of medicine and the arts;
> tying the net of Dharma, kings of the orators of inner reality,
> to you masters and practitioners of the five great sciences,
> universal sovereigns who turn your great wheels in the
> three times,
> I offer my joyful praise.[69]

My lama the Great Fifth, definitively an omniscient one, also said:

> In the field of the doctrine of the Buddha,
> his soil made fertile by the doctrine of *pratimokṣa* ethics;
> the shoots, leaves, and flowers of transmission and insight
> grown by language, healing, logic, arts, and the three baskets,
> weighed down by harvest of method and wisdom union,
> on the definitively secret path of Vajrayana,
> this sun of the five sciences correctly applied,
> pulled by the horses of merit gathered in the past....[70]

Therefore, the five great sciences, praised often in the teachings of the Buddha and in reputable treatises, are comprised of language and logic to defeat perverse teachers, medicine and arts to care for and nourish others, and the inner science to understand the ultimate reality of all phenomena. Together with their five secondary sciences[71] to make up the ten sciences, they are indispensable for all who wish to become wise. They should, therefore, be studied. [14]

Features of the science of healing

On the science of healing, the *Sutra of Repaying the Kindness of the Skillful Buddha* says:

> Why do bodhisattvas study scriptures of the science of medicine? They do it to free living beings from the 404 diseases of non-virtue.[72] They do it because they have great love and compassion for all living beings and want to generate faith in the minds of living beings. Freed of illness, the minds of living beings will be filled with joy, and they will constantly remember the Buddha. Then with great compassion, the bodhisattvas will bring living beings to the perfections. This is why they train in the science of medicine.[73]

Also, in *Stages of the Yogacaryā* from the *Stage of Wisdom from Hearing* chapter:

> What is the science of healing? It should be regarded as having four divisions: knowledge of diseases, knowledge of the origin of diseases, knowledge of how to eradicate the disease, knowledge of how to prevent the disease from reoccurring. The wise should learn these divisions exactly as they are taught in the sutras.[74]

In the eighth chapter [of Asaṅga's *Stages of the Bodhisattva*]:

> The medical scriptures have four main aspects: imparting knowledge of disease; knowledge of the origins of disease; knowledge of the eradication of disease; and knowledge of the prevention of disease reoccurring.[75]

In the Root Tantra of the *Four Tantras* it says:

> Those who wish to remain free of illness and to cure disease should study the teachings on the science of healing. Those who wish to live a long life should study the teachings on the science of healing. Those who wish for Dharma, wealth, and happiness should study the teachings on the science of healing. Those who wish to free living beings from the miseries of illness and who wish to be respected by others should study the teachings on the science of healing.[76]

In the Explanatory Tantra of the *Four Medical Tantras* it says: [15]

> For those with human birth,
> chief among the six types of beings,
> to remain free of illness, to be cured of disease,
> for long life, Dharma, wealth, and happiness,
> the science of healing....[77]

In the Final Tantra of the *Four Medical Tantras* it says:

> This [medical science] is a protection cord without mantra,
> a magic charm to destroy the *māras* of the lord of death,
> the warrior who defeats the army of disease,
> the holder of the public purse who balances
> the excesses and deficiency in the constituents,[78]
> a sword that cuts the noose of untimely death,
> a hammer that crushes the pain of illness,
> a hook that pulls us from the swamp of suffering.
> By giving us protection from death,
> it is the generosity that grants freedom from fear.[79]

Pitṛceṭa, crown jewel of millions of scholars, states:

> Those who wish for a long life,
> for Dharma, wealth, and happiness,
> should revere the teachings
> of the Āyurveda.[80]

My master lama, the Great Fifth, crown jewel of samsara and nirvana, said:

> A treasure of ambrosia, the elixir of life
> bringing longevity lasting eons without end,
> opening the door to a gift of fearlessness,
> gained through the currency of merit,
> available to all living beings without exception....[81]

Rinchen Pungpa says:

> The quickening rasping gasps of one's life in one's throat,
> wrought from the pain of being squeezed
> into the lord of death's gaping mouth,
> all to be relieved by the science of life,
> recalled by Brahmā through his memory.[82]

Taktsang Lotsāwa says:

> All beings are tormented by illness.
> To not seek out the science of healing, therefore,
> is to fall to the extreme of samsara;
> and to strive in this second science
> thus accomplishes the great good of caring.[83]

Since time without beginning living beings have been tormented by the five poisonous mental afflictions and have thereby accumulated a great store of black karma. When the fruits of these actions come into contact with a variety of immediate conditions and circumstances, they bring about disturbances in the four constituents,[84] resulting in illness. These illnesses have been classified as fourfold: 101 ailments that disappear by themselves and need no treatment, 101 illnesses caused by spirits that are cured when treated, 101 illnesses that are cured if treated but not if left untreated, and 101 illnesses that even treatment cannot cure. The treatments for these illnesses free living beings from the noose of Yama, the lord of death, thereby bestowing on all beings the powerful gift of fearlessness.

Therefore, it is definitely part of bodhisattva conduct and a field of endeavor for the wise. In Sanskrit this science is known as *āyurveda*. [16] "Lifespan" *(tshe, āyuṣ)* and "life force" *(srog, prāṇā)* are synonyms. "Life" *('tsho ba, jīva)* is the basis for consciousness. In the desire and form realms, it is the basis for warmth and consciousness, whereas in the formless realms it is only the basis for consciousness. Knowledge of this life is the science of life. The Sanskrit term *cikitsitā* means "expertise in healing." It is the expertise in balancing the disordered elements or constituents of the body. It is also referred to as the "science of healing," or *cikitsā vidyā*.

3. Origins of the Science of Healing in the Celestial Realms

[17] A TREATISE STATES:

Sāmaveda, Yajurveda, Atharvaveda, and Ṛgveda:
these are the four Vedic sciences.
Articulation, grammar, metrics,
astronomy, etymology, and rites:
these are the branches,[85]
together with treatises on love and Dharma.[86]

The Vedas, together with the six branches and the two subsidiaries, all emerged from the faces of Brahmā, because of which the text continues:

Therefore, from the central face of Brahmā came Āyurveda;
the Sāmaveda, Ṛgveda, and Yajurveda,
were spoken from the other faces.[87]

Also:

From his mouth came the brahman priestly caste,
from the shoulders the kṣatriya lordly caste,
from the thighs the vaiśya merchant class,
from the feet came the śūdra lower class.[88]

Therefore, the religion of the brahman caste, whose place of birth has the highest status, is the Vedas. It is said that because they were not created by anyone, the Vedas are permanent. Uncorrupted by effort and endeavor they are said to be self-arisen. Because they are able to speak of all things, they are said to be valid. In his *Essence of Eight Branches,* the master scholar Śūra said, "The Āyurveda was recalled by Brahmā."[89] How he recalled it is taught in *Commentary on Praise of the Exalted* by Prajñāvarman:

In this way the gods came to churn the ocean. From the ocean arose many things, including the *kaustubha* jewel and Hayagrīva. After a while some poison also surfaced. Viṣṇu was standing nearby, and the poison turned his skin black. Mahādeva took the poison and swallowed it without fear. The poison stayed in his throat, moving neither up nor down. Because of this his throat glistened with the colors of the peacock. The gods exclaimed, "How beautiful this is! From now on, it is only fitting that his throat remain this way."[90]

Also:

The gods churned the mighty ocean of milk until ambrosia appeared. However, it was stolen by the *asura* Rāhu, who began to use it. Viṣṇu thought, "If he drinks it, even the gods will not be able to defeat him." [18] So with his mighty weapon wheel, he cut off Rāhu's head, and the gods retrieved the nectar. However, some of the nectar had reached Rāhu's throat, and although the body below his throat was dead, he was still alive, and he set off to wreak havoc among gods and men. From that time onward, he has eclipsed the sun and moon that light up the three worlds.[91]

Also, in *Commentary on Praises from the Gods* by the same author:

This I have also heard. Under the orders of Brahmā the gods were gathered in one direction, the demigods in another. Viṣṇu took hold of Mount Mandara from above, the nāga king Vāsuki used himself as the churning rope, and the mountain was supported from below by the back of the great turtle. In this way they churned the ocean of milk.

Suddenly a terrifying personification of the *kālakūṭa* poison appeared. Viṣṇu took it and swallowed it, whereupon he lost consciousness, fell to the ground, and lay speechless. Mahādeva took the poison from Viṣṇu and placed it in his throat, which then turned blue. Then a crescent moon appeared, which Mahādeva took and placed upon his own head. Then Śrī appeared, who proclaimed herself to be the bride of Viṣṇu. After her appeared Hayagrīva and the *pārijāta* wish-fulfilling tree. These were taken by Indra and the other gods. Then a very beautiful woman appeared from the ocean. "Who are you?" they asked. "I am *surā*. If you drink me, you will become intoxicated, lose your senses, and become arrogant." The demigods were afraid to drink and so were known as *asura*. The gods, however, readily partook of the drink and so were known as *sura*.[92]

Then ambrosia arose from the ocean, and the demigods carried it off in eight great containers. The gods became greatly distressed. So Viṣṇu manifested as a very beautiful woman and went to the demigods, while Indra became invisible and waited in the skies. [19] The demigods thought that the woman was one of them and gave her the ambrosia to guard, saying "We are going to bathe. As it says in the Dharma Śāstra:

> Without washing one is not clean,
> so one does not eat before washing."

They went off to bathe. Viṣṇu and Indra took the nectar and carried it to Indra's palace. When the demigods returned after bathing, they could not find the ambrosia and set off in search of it. When they heard that the gods had taken it, they thought, "Now, surely the gods will rise above us." Meanwhile, the gods gathered to partake of the ambrosia. However, Rāhu had taken on the form of a god, and in their company he was able to drink a portion of nectar. Sūrya, the sun god, recognized him and said to Viṣṇu, "That is Rāhu!" Viṣṇu immediately threw his mighty wheel and cut off Rāhu's head. However, the head had tasted the ambrosia and is still alive today. The rest of the body died. From then on Rāhu became the enemy of Sūrya, and from time to time he covers and obscures the disc of the sun. This is the story.[93]

Also, in the same text it says:

This I have also heard. After the theft of the ambrosia, the gods and the demigods became enemies and were spoiling for battle. However, the gods could not attack because they had no weapons. Bṛhaspati said to the gods, "There is a great rishi called Vacasucara.[94] His son Dadhici has dwelled in ascetic conduct for seventy million years, and his bones have become as strong as vajras. With these bones as weapons you will be victorious in the three worlds. Take them and you will defeat the demigods." The gods approached the rishi and requested him accordingly. In response the rishi assisted them by encouraging them to lick his flesh until only his bones remained, which he then donated to the gods. From his ribs Viśvakarman fashioned a vajra and gave it to Indra. From the bones of the lower leg he made a club, which was taken by Viṣṇu.

Sūrya, the sun god, took Reṇukā,[95] the daughter of Viśvakarman, [20] for his wife, but because his form was so dazzling, she was unable to bear the brightness and did not enjoy his company. Kuṣmāṇḍa and other celestial maidens also could not bear the brightness of Sūrya. They all fled, and she returned to her father's house. The father became upset. This distressed Reṇukā, who then assumed the form of a mare and went to Mount Kailash to perform ascetic practices. Sūrya meanwhile had set out to search for his wife, and when he learned of her actions, he went to her in the form of a horse and forced himself upon her. She protested, saying, "I will not become pregnant by another man!" Sūrya laughed and revealed his true form, saying, "It is from me your child will be born." From her nostrils the two sons of Aśvinī were born.

On hearing this Viśvakarman said to Sūrya, "If you can tolerate it, I can make you more attractive. When something has become unbearable, it has to be discarded." Sūrya agreed. Viśvakarman tied him down. A wheel was fashioned into twelve blades and his radiance was sheared off as far as his ankles. The shorn off part was thrown to earth. From then on Sūrya was known as He of Unshorn Feet. The pieces of brightness cast away were gathered and made into a wheel. This wheel was of an intense brightness and so was called *sudarśana*, "beautiful to behold." Indra gave it to Viṣṇu, and this was the wheel Viṣṇu used to cut off the head of Rāhu after he had stolen and drunk the nectar.[96]

In the fourth chapter of *Horse Āyurveda Compiled by Rishi Śālihotra* it says:

During the churning of the ocean,
the horse arose with the ambrosia;

its name was Uccaiḥ Śravas.
Its sound was like that of thunder,
and as it rose powerfully into the skies,
the demigod Bala and the god Akula seized its hind legs.
Gripped by these two powerful forces,
its hind quarters were a little weakened.
Because of this, even now, hind quarters of horses
do not move quickly, and when standing still,
they slowly lift each hind leg.[97]

This is a synopsis. The more extensive account is as follows:

When living beings first arose,
the world they lived in was a peaceful place. [21]
Then in the realms of gods and demigods,
Brahmā caused a pervasive drought.
Again the creatures of the world fled.
The gods, demigods, the *gandharva* spirits,
the *mahoraga* serpents, and the *rākṣa* demons
were also gripped and tormented by terrible thirst,
unable to enjoy their food and sleep.
Reflecting on this, the thought arose,
"By that which abides in the heart of water,
will we quench our thirst."

Therefore, the celebrated Mandara was the churning rod,
and the nāga king Ananta tied on to it as churning rope.
With the gods gathered in one place and the demigods in another,
the rope was pulled and the ocean churned,
provoking a fearsome sound.
Roots and leaves, the medicines of gods and men,
together with milk were cast into the ocean;
medicine bright and radiant, full of taste, full of virtue,
yellow flower, white sister, *aṅgulacarya*[98]
bright *jātisāra,* medicine that denies death and
cures wounds, elixirs manifested by Brahmā,
medicines strong and of unimaginable power,
all were cast into the ocean, and the waters churned.

From the waters first appeared Śrī and others;
the eight *śubha* jewels, which when prayed to in the morning,
banish the fearful prophecies of bad dreams and so forth;
then the horses that pulled the sun's chariot;
surā, drink of the gods; the *kaustubha* jewel; beautiful earrings;
medicine known as ambrosia, and ambrosia itself;
the physician Dhavantari, supreme holder of all scriptures;
and the horse Uccaiḥ Śravas, brave and strong,
with a sound *(śravas)* like thunder, like a drum,
or like a conch, like the great celestial drum,
a high-pitched *(uccaiḥ)* roar giving birth to his name,
so that the gods and demigods christened him Uccaiḥ Śravas.
His body the color of the white clouds,
this swift horse rose from the ambrosia,
from the bright ocean and into the skies,
and Bala, son of Bhānu, seized its legs. [22]
Then all the demigods left Mandara and the nāga king,
and holding on to the precious horse,
left Milk Ocean and came to this world.[99]

In *The Wish-Fulfilling Cow: A Commentary to the Treasury of Immortality* by Subhūticandra it says:

> *Elixir (bcud len, rasa):* When the gods and demigods were churning the ocean, Lakṣmī arose and was carried off by Viṣṇu. A crescent moon arose and was worn by Īśvara on his crown. A vase full of poison arose. Īśvara placed it in his throat and his neck turned blue. A vase of alcohol arose and was taken by the gods. They are therefore known as *sura sura,* which means alcohol, essence of the ocean, or ambrosia.[100]

In *Wish-Fulfilling Tree of the Bodhisattva's Lives,* using the *vibhāvana* poetic device[101] to illustrate an effect seemingly without a cause, it says:

Without the churning of the ambrosia ocean
and the untiring effort of Vāsuki in binding the mountain,
who created this elephant?[102]

In chapter 89 of the Instruction Tantra of *Four Tantras* it says:

> In ancient times the gods and demigods sought out the ambrosia,
> and from their churning of the ocean arose a man of fair hair,
> fire blazing from his eyes and of terrifying form.
> Brahmā chanted *hūṃ,* the illusion vanished,
> and it absorbed into animate and inanimate forms.[103]

And in the *Essence of Eight Branches:*

> In earlier times in their search for ambrosia
> the gods and demigods churned the ocean,
> but before the ambrosia appeared,
> there arose a man of terrifying form,
> with fair hair, fire-spitting eyes,
> and four glistening fangs.
> Seeing him all were filled with fear.
> With Brahmā's *hūṃ* the illusion vanished,
> and the poison took on
> animate and inanimate forms.[104]

Concerning all the above citations, the *Kālacakra Tantra*, in verse 82 of the Gnosis chapter:

> The goddess Śrī, the horse Uccaiḥ Śravas,
> the celestial tree, the lord of elephants,
> the *apsaras* goddess,[105] the *kaustubha* jewel,
> the moon, and the ambrosia—
> if these all arose in the celestial realms
> during the churning of the ocean in the reign of Bala,
> there would have been no moon in the reign of Andhaka
> and therefore no lunar or planetary division of time.[106]

Also in the first chapter of *Treatise of Valid Cognition* by Dharmakīrti:

> They assert the Vedas to be valid,
> they speak in contradictions, [23]
> they claim bathing to be Dharma,

they are arrogant in spouting their knowledge,
they torture themselves to be free of sin:
these are five reasons why they are fools.[107]

Clearly, the Vedas are presented as objects of refutation in the Kālacakra, the literature on valid cognition, and elsewhere. However, if the previous citations that comment on the Vedas' own position and the essential meaning of the traditional explanations found in the guru lineages are brought together, we arrive at the following understanding.

In the eighteenth chapter of the *Mañjuśrī Root Tantra* it says:

During the era of perfection[108]
living beings had their own light,
they flew through the skies,
and old age and death were unknown.
At that time there were no planets,
no sun, moon, or stars,
and no realms of gods and demigods.[109]

Also:

Then the times degenerated,
and their world became unsuitable.
Impelled by previous karma,
they fell to the earth.[110]

Also:

Then came the solar day
and the light from the moon and the planets.[111]

At the end of the age of perfection, living beings began to partake of natural-earth[112] ambrosia and the like, diminishing their miraculous powers and natural luminosity, and the human world was plunged into darkness. At that time, in the midst of the great Milk Ocean, a shining crystal vase sat filled with ambrosia, the elixir of immortality. It was seen by Rāhu as he traveled around the four continents. He addressed the gods and demigods, "Friends! In the still depths of the great ocean I have seen a precious vase filled with ambrosia." The gods and demigods wanted this ambrosia and set out to retrieve it. In an alternative version of this story, they were tormented by a great and increasing thirst, which they realized on investigation could be alleviated by "that which abides in the essence of water." Therefore, they cast medicine and various essences into the ocean, and because they wanted its essence, they needed to churn the ocean. Viṣṇu used Mount Mandara or Mount Meru as a churning stick, the nāga king Vāsuki—or the *nāgarṣi* Nemindhara manifesting in the form of Vāsuki—transformed his body into the churning rope, while Brahmā held down Vāsuki's head. Below, the back of the giant turtle Kūrma acted as a base. Together they churned the great ocean.

First an object made of precious fire-crystal appeared. Accompanied by seven horses, it gave light to the world. Living beings were overjoyed *(nyi)* and exclaimed, "It is the mother *(ma)*." Therefore, it was named "sun" *(nyi ma)*. [24] Again the mighty ocean churned, and from it appeared a disk made of water-crystal and accompanied by five horses. People exclaimed, "It is the companion *(zla bo)* of the sun. Therefore, it became known as the moon *(zla ba)*, and the god Īśvara took it for his crown ornament. Then came the great elephant Airāvata, which the god Indra took for his mount. The wish-fulfilling, or *pārijāta*, tree appeared, which the gods claimed for themselves. The goddess Śrī, or Lakṣmī, appeared and proclaimed herself the wife of Viṣṇu. Then a very beautiful girl appeared. "Who are you?" they asked. "I am Surā," she replied. If you drink me, you will become intoxicated, lose your senses, become crazy with arrogance." The demigods could not drink it but the gods partook of it. In Sanskrit "god" is *sura* and the prefix *a* is a negating particle, and so these two classes of beings are known as *sura* and *asura*.

Next to appear were substances such the eight *śubha* jewels, which eliminate disease, demons, and all misfortune; the *kausthubha* jewel; the beautiful jeweled earrings; and ambrosia and ambrosia-like medicine. These became wealth to be utilized by all.

Then appeared the horse, known by various names such as Uccaiḥ Śravas and Hayagrīva. It was able to move through the skies and was the color of the white clouds. The gods and the demigods all scrambled to gain this horse, and finally the demigod Bala grasped its two hind legs and fled to his abode.

Again the ocean was churned. From it arose a fearsome creature, the personification of the poison *kālakūta*, with nine heads, fair hair, and fire shooting from his eyes. Viṣṇu swallowed his poison but was unable to digest it, and he fell to the ground and lay there speechless. Then Mahādava took the poison from Viṣṇu and placed it in his own mouth, which turned his throat blue. No one could overcome this creature, and so they turned and prayed to the god Brahmā. He in turn recalled a teaching of the past in which Buddha Mahāśākyamuni had conquered a similar creature with the mantra *hūṃ*. Brahmā uttered the syllable *hūṃ* and raised the threatening gesture. The body of the creature broke up and dissolved into the bodies of poisonous creatures, such as snakes, rabid dogs, and *rākṣa* demons, and into inanimate poisons such as aconite and *datura*.

Then the ambrosia appeared, contained in eight great containers. [25] According to Drapa Sherap Rinchen[113] and others, the ambrosia was taken by Brahmā for his personal use, because of which Rāhu threw his wheel at Brahmā and injured his forehead. However, Ācārya Prajñāvarman,[114] in agreement with most other commentators, say that the ambrosia was taken by the demigods. This upset the gods enormously. Viṣṇu transformed himself to a beautiful and alluring woman and went to the abode of the demigods, while Indra remained unseen in the skies above. The demigods thought that this woman was one of theirs and so entrusted her to look after the ambrosia while they went to bathe. Indra and Viṣṇu then stole the vases of ambrosia and took them to Indra's palace, Vaijayanta. When the demigods returned from bathing, they could not find the vases and so set out in search of them. When they heard that the gods had taken them, they thought, "Now surely the gods will rise above us."

When the gods had gathered to enjoy the ambrosia, Rāhu took on the form of a god and joined them. Only after he had received his share of ambrosia was he recognized by Candra, the moon god, who called out to the other gods, "It's Rāhu, king of the demigods!" Rāhu fled. Indra took his vajra, Skanda took his spear, Balabhadra took his plow-like *halāyudha,* and with whatever other weapons were at hand, the gods set out in pursuit.

The vajra that Viṣṇu carried in his hands had been fashioned from the bones of the rishi Dadhici. It was hard, reliable, unstoppable, and unconquerable. In short, it destroyed everything in its path but could not be destroyed in return. Viṣṇu also carried a wheel fashioned by Viśvakarman from the shards of the sun. It carried four guarantees. Whoever it was thrown at, it could not fail to hit. Whoever it hit, it could not fail to injure. Whoever it injured would not fail to die. Whoever died when struck by this wheel would not fail to fall to the lower realms.

As they closed in upon Rāhu, Viṣṇu threw the wheel and cut off his head. As it says in the *Essence of Eight Branches,* "When Rāhu stole the ambrosia, Viṣṇu cut off his head."[115] However, although his body was generally dead, by the power of the ambrosia he had drunk, his head did not die, [26] and he was able to throw the wheel back and wound Brahmā's forehead or cheek. During the fight a drop of ambrosia mixed with the blood of this demigod king fell to the ground, and from this sprang myrobalan[116] and garlic. From that time on, Rāhu became the enemy of the moon, and it is said that his habit of eclipsing and veiling the face of the full moon dates from this time also.

From the pain of his wound and from compassion for the decapitated Rāhu, Brahmā entered the samādhi of peace, and by the force of having listened to a medical tantra from Buddha Mahāśākyamuni in the past, the sound *oṃ ātha*[117] emerged from the wound. This was the start of Āyurveda teachings, and all four Vedas and their branches followed. In *Moonlight: A Commentary on the Essence of Eight Branches,* it says:

> The two syllables *oṃ* and *ātha*
> arose from the cheeks of Brahmā;
> these, therefore, are for auspiciousness.[118]

It is said that in the practice of recitation, the syllable *oṃ* should be recited as if it possessed the measure of the *Ṛg Veda,* the letter *u* as having the measure of the *Sāma Veda,* the letter *e* as the measure of *Atharva Veda,* and the letter *a* as having the measure of the *Yajur Veda.*

The formulation of the syllable *oṃ* according to the *Sarasvatī Grammar Sutra* is as follows. The *Dhātusūtra* says, "*Ava* means to protect, to guard." This is the root. "The *a* at the end of the root is elided." Therefore, the life-letter *a* of *va* is dropped. Then "*uṇ* and so forth always" [The *uṇ* category of affixes, and so on, can always be added to roots, regardless of tense and case]. Therefore, the affix *muku* is added. "The *ya, va, ra* of *yaj,* and so on, added to *ka anubandha* take *samprasāraṇa* into *i, u, ṛt*" [When roots such as *yaj* meet *anubandha* affixes such as *ka,* then the *ya, va,* and *ra* of those roots perform a vowel interchange, or *samprasāraṇa,* with *i, u,* and *ṛ*]. Therefore, by the process of *saṃprasāraṇa, v* becomes *u. Ku* follows the same rule and is elided. *U* is for purposes of pronunciation and is elided. *A* and *u* merge to become *o.* Then an *anusvāra* is added to *m* to form *oṃ.* Therefore, *oṃ* has the meaning of "protect."[119]

In the *Vajraśekhara Tantra* it says:

> The meaning of *oṃ* is this:
> it has the qualities of being supreme,

of being the granter of wealth,
of glory, auspiciousness, and merit;
it is a sacred pledge and it is good fortune,
the essence of *maṇidhārin,* holder of the jewel.[120]

In the *Extensive Commentary on Basic Vinaya* it says:

That with the letter *oṃ*
is three and a half measures
and is spoken pleasingly.[121]

Therefore, *oṃ* is spoken of in terms of esteem, respect, and praise. A passage from the Vedas quoted in *Blaze of Reasoning* states:

The syllable *oṃ* is the mystical song
of Brahmā and Vasudeva.
This syllable of Brahmā pervades all things.
It possesses the clarity of three measures
and is taught to be very subtle.
The first cause is the letter *a,*
comprising speech, *sattva,* fire, and earth [27]
and also body[122] and space.
Mind, *rajas,* and *sattva* possess the letter *u.*
The letter *m,* the creating letter, is the third—
life and *tamas*—which gathers all beings
and causes the great sleep.[123]

Also:

With senses and their objects
withdrawn like a turtle's limbs,
the self will be freed by worship while
recalling and reciting the letter *oṃ.*[124]

The syllable *oṃ,* of the nature of the three letters—*a* Viṣṇu, *u* Īśvara, and *m* Brahmā—is a formulation from the euphonic amalgamation of these three letters. This is its provisional meaning. Definitively it is described in the *Root Kālacakra Tantra:*

Brahmā is the body vajra holder,
the speech vajra is Maheśvara,
the mind vajra of the conqueror
is manifest as Viṣṇu.[125]

These three gods are also discussed in the *Hevajra Tantra*:

Brahmā, Viṣṇu, Śiva, and the others
are spoken of as being the Buddha;
Brahmā *(tshangs pa)* means free of impurity *(tshangs)*
and so refers to the Buddha;
Because he engages *('jug)*
he is spoken of as Viṣṇu *(khyab 'jug)*.[126]

Also in the *Commentary to the Saṃpuṭa Tantra* by Kāyastha it says:

The letter *a* is Nairātmyā,
the letter *u* is Vajrayoginī,
the letter *m* is Akśobhyavajra,
therefore, *oṃ* is the three vajras.
The letter *a* is the speech vajra,
the letter *u* is the body vajra,
the letter *m* is the mind vajra.
The three vajras of one nature is *oṃ*.
Being the first of the syllables,
it is the foremost syllable.[127]

The *Kālacakra Root Tantra* states "Glorious holder of the body vajra!"[128] thereby assigning *a* to the body vajra, *u* to the speech vajra, and *m* to the mind vajra to form the syllable *oṃ* as the representation of the three vajras as the entity of the Buddha. This concept can be further elaborated on using the reasoning that establishes the meaning of the syllables *evaṃ* and is seen in countless phenomena, such as the drops, moon-bodhicitta, fluid, and the bases of correspondence for the outer, inner, and other Kālacakra.

Bright Lamp says: "*Oṃ* is the gathering of merit."[129] In *Treatise on Various Terms* it says "*Oṃ* means great praise; it is the unchanging mantra of Brahmā."[130] Therefore, it is taught that *oṃ* means many things—auspiciousness, praise, respect, the gathering of merit, the entity of the Buddha, and so on.

The *Moon Sutra,* translated by by Tharpa Lotsāwa, talks of how the moon sought refuge in the Tathāgata out of fear of being eclipsed on the fifteenth day as revenge by Rāhu for the moon informing on his theft of the ambrosia.[131] [28]

In the *Sutra of the Great Mantra Protection* from the five great dhāraṇīs[132] it says:

> "By the moon going for refuge to the sugatas,
> who are destroyers of the enemies of the world,
> save the moon, enlightened ones,
> out of compassion for the world!
> Rāhu, release the moon, dispeller of darkness,
> let its light shine in the pure skies again,
> bright and shining, aglow with pure light,
> unfettered in the pure skies,
> set free this light of living beings."
> Accordingly, Rāhu begins to sweat;
> he becomes afraid and, like a sick man,
> suddenly leaves and releases the moon.[133]

The Yungdrung Bön work known as the *Mottled Nāga Collection*[134] says the same. In some scriptures it says that the sun and moon are eclipsed by a wolf. The *Sutra of Remembering the Sacred Dharma* states that it is the hand of the king of the demigods that causes the eclipses. There are many such provisional and conventional explanations of this phenomenon.

Also, concerning the eclipsing of the sun on the day of the empty sky,[135] some accounts describe it being primarily the moon, but brought about by sun and moon being in conjunction. These are merely observations made by the minds of ordinary disciples. The real significance is that Rāhu, in the aspect of the intermediate existence, acts upon the sun and moon in the forms of essences of bodily elements. Moreover, there is no textual evidence that counteracts the description of Rāhu's head and tail casting beryl-colored shadows upon the moon and sun's brightly vivid water-crystal and fire-crystal discs as they make their way through the *gola*[136] firmament. The mother and son *White Beryl* texts extensively explain the way that the central channel as Rāhu and the left and right channels as the sun and moon are used in the correspondences of the inner, outer, and other Kālacakra.[137]

The grandfather Brahmā taught the science to Prajāpati, the second

Brahmā. He in turn taught it to the Aśvinī sons, who are said to be last two of King Pāṇḍu's five sons: Yudhiṣṭhira, Bhīma, Arjuna, Sahadeva, and Nakula. They in turn passed the science of healing to Indra, king of the gods, and from then on it became widespread. [29]

PART 1

THE SCIENCE OF HEALING IN INDIA

4. Early Indian Medical Traditions

WHEN HUMAN BEINGS were first created ages ago in this world of Jampudvīpa, they subsisted for a long time on the joys of meditative concentration, and even the name of coarse and ordinary food did not exist. Because they radiated their own light, there was no sun, moon, stars, or planets, no day and no night. They had the power to fly, and they enjoyed their bodies and pleasures on a par with with the gods of light. After some time, instincts of craving awoke in those of the race known as Manu,[138] who were the first to be born in the human realm, and they began to partake of natural-earth ambrosia, which gave them indigestion. Brahmā heard their cries of pain, and moved by pity for the beings that he is said to have created, he conceived the idea of giving them boiled water as medicine for the indigestion. Alternatively, some say that he remembered a teaching from the *Hundred Thousand Versed Science of Healing Collection* taught by Mahāśākyamuni Buddha at an earlier time, which prescribed boiled water as a cure for indigestion. Whatever the origin, Brahmā taught them the preparation of boiled water, and the indigestion was cured. From this it is well known in the world that the first illness was indigestion, the first patients were the Manu, the first medicine was boiled water, and the first doctor was Brahmā.

When the affix *an* is added to denote a descendent and the vowel *a* of *bra* is lengthened, one arrives at the term Brāhmaṇa, meaning the "children of Brahmā" commonly known as brahmans, who are asserted to be his descendents. Through their high-birth physicians, the brahmans developed and spread the transmission of Āyurveda. This can be seen in the widespread Fortunate Eon Deva tradition and the Vidyādhara Rishi tradition. These will be explained later.

The Buddhist scriptural tradition

The tradition known as the Buddhist scriptural tradition is explained as follows. In this particular eon, the fortunate eon, we cannot say with certainty that teachings given by the buddhas and the commentaries on them by others up to the era of Buddha Kāśyapa have entirely disappeared, [30] but these days we cannot identify them with any certainty. As for Buddha Śākyamuni, concurrent with teaching the four truths during the first turning of the wheel of Dharma at Vārāṇasī, it is believed that he also taught the *Vimalagutra Medical Collection in 72,000 Chapters*[139] and the *Eight Branches in 20,000 Fascicles*. The *Basic Vinaya* on the topic of medicine says, "A sick monk should approach a doctor and follow his advice."[140] Expanding on this somewhat, the third section of this Vinaya work talks a little on medicines, suppositories, and so on, whereas the bulk of the teaching can be illustrated by the following summarizing verse:

> On medicine: that which is permitted,
> medicinal fats, medicine for scabrous skin,
> eye medicines, medicine for the insane, for the monk Pilinda,
> for the monk Revati, and acidic juice.[141]

Therefore, when the Buddha was dwelling in the Anāthapiṇḍada retreat in Jeta Grove and the monks became pale through autumnal illnesses, he allowed them to rely on specific remedies, but he did not allow medicines to be taken beyond specific times. The monks remained pale:

> Ānanda, therefore, the following is permitted. Monks should rely on four types of medicine: taken at the right times, taken at specific times, seven-day medicines, and life-long medicines.[142] Foods to be eaten at the right times include pastes, boiled rice, gruel, meat, and fried or baked breads. Drinks that are to be taken at specific times include the juices from the fruit of the *chocha* tree, plantains, Indian juniper, *aśvattha* figs, *udumbara* figs, *parūṣaka* berries, grapes, and dates. Seven-day medicines include ghee, sesame oil, molasses, honey, and white sugar.
>
> Life-long medicines are of nine kinds: roots, stems, leaves, flowers, fruits, the five resin decoctions, the five powders, the five salts, and the five astringents. Root medicines include nutgrass, sweet flag, turmeric, wild ginger, white aconite, and any other medicinal roots that are not normally used for food. Stem or trunk medicines include sandalwood, clematis, juniper, deodar, heart-leaved moonseed, Indian barberry, [31] and any other stems

> not used for food. Leaf medicines include the leaves of *paṭola, vāśaka,* the neem tree, *kośātaka,* and the seven-leaved *saptaparṇa,* and any other leaves not normally used for food. Flower medicines include *vāśaka* flowers, the neem tree, coriander, *śata,* and lotus filament, and any other flowers not normally used for food. Fruit medicines include chebulic myrobalan, emblic myrobalan, beleric myrobalan, black pepper, long pepper, and any other fruits not normally used for food. The five resin decoctions are asafetida, sal tree resin, lac, beeswax, and black pepper. The five powders are those made from barley, barley husk, corn smut, sesame, and aloe wood. The five salts are rock salt, brown salt, sanchal salt, white salt, and sea salt. The five astringents come from the mango, neem, *jambū, śiriṣa,* and *kośam* trees.[143]

This and further passages teach the use of medicine and the consecration of the medicine.

At the time of the middle turning of the wheel of Dharma, the "phenomena devoid of signs" turning on Vulture's Peak, the Buddha taught the *Hundred Thousand Versed Science of Healing Collection* to the supreme god Brahmā. During the same period, when King Padmaśrī had invited the Buddha for the rainy-season retreat in Matkuṇa Grove in the southern town of Sukhakara, the Buddha taught the *Clearly Seeing Knowledge Tantra* of a hundred thousand verses in 3,500 chapters to Avalokiteśvara, Brahmā, Śāriputra, and others of the Mahayana family. It is also asserted that this work is the same as the *Hundred Thousand Versed Science of Healing Collection.*

In the *Sutra of Golden Light: King of the Supremely Victorious Sutras,* which was also taught on Vulture's Peak but during the period of the third turning, it says in chapter 24 on the elimination of illness in the version translated from the Chinese:

> Goddess of the family, at a time in the past countless eons ago, [32] Buddha Ratnacūḍa, the tathāgata, the destroyer, the perfect buddha, perfectly enlightened, with an enlightenment built on the foundation of the three trainings, the sugata, knower of the world, the greatest of all beings, the charioteer, teacher of gods and men, the bhagavān buddha, came to this world. When his doctrine had become a mere reflection, there lived in the land of King Sureśvaraprabhā the merchant Jalada, who was very learned

in medicine, who had fully comprehended the eight branches of knowledge, and who tended to living beings and protected them from the sufferings of illness caused by an imbalance in the four great elements. This merchant had a son called Jalavāhana, who was fair of face and of handsome build, so that all gazed upon him with great delight. By nature he was of a quick mind. He soon mastered the scriptures, and there was nothing he did not understand in matters of language, the arts, astronomy, and arithmetic.

At that time thousands upon thousands of the citizens of that kingdom were being tormented by sufferings brought on by all manner of diseases, so much so that a joyful mind was not to be found anywhere. Jalavāhana, the son of the merchant, felt great pity for them and thought to himself, "My father, the great doctor, is now very old and is unable to tend to so great a number of sick people. I will ask him if I may study the secret science of healing from him and by so doing cure all these beings of their illnesses and bring them the joys of a long life." With these thoughts he approached his father, prostrated, and made his request in verse:

To protect living beings,
I ask for teachings on medicine;
loving father, with your great compassion,
teach me with your words.

His father heard his request and answered with the following verses:

Relying upon the science of medicine
from the essence of the Rishi tradition,
these things I will gradually teach you;
listen well and protect all beings.

Three months is the time of spring,
three months lasts the summer,
three months is the autumn,
three months the months of winter.

This is the time of a single year
explained in sets of three.

Taking two months as a single set, [33]
the seasons number six.
The first two comprise the season of flowers,
the third and the fourth the hot season,
the fifth and sixth the rains,
the seventh and eighth are autumn,
the ninth and tenth the cold months,
and the last two are the time of snow.

If you know these specifics,
you will administer medicine without fault.
Food and drink taken in accord with the seasons
produces ease of digestion in the stomach,
and many an illness will not occur.
Going against the dictates of the seasons
produces shifts in the four elements
that if not remedied by medicine,
will surely bring the pains of illness.
A doctor knows the four seasons
and must also know the six.

Knowing the seven bodily constituents,
you will administer food and medicine correctly.
When illness enters the essence, the element,
blood, flesh, bones, marrow, and fatty tissue,[144]
you must know if it is curable or not.

Disease is of four types:
wind, bile, phlegm, and their combinations;
you should know the times of their movements.
In spring phlegm is on the move,
in summer wind illnesses arise,
in autumn bile increases,
and in winter all three arise together.

In spring take food that is hot, coarse, and warm;
in summer take that which is oily, warm, salty, and sour;
in autumn take that which is cold, sweet, and oily;
and in winter take that which is coarse, sour, oily, and sweet.
If food, drink, and medicine taken at these four times
accords with the above, few illnesses will arise.

After eating, phlegm disorders have power,
during digestion bile disorders arise,
after digestion the power of wind is strong;
know illness in conjunction with its time.

Knowing the root of the illness,
administer medicine accordingly.
Illnesses may have different forms,
but first know the root.

For a wind illness give oily food,
for bile a purgative is good,
for phlegm give an emetic.
Wind, bile, and phlegm arising together
is known as a combination;
for such give all three treatments.

Though you know the times that illnesses arise,
you should also know their natures.
Therefore examine in this way, and when you know,
administer the medicine appropriate to the time.
Food, drink, and medicine all appropriate—
this is the sign of a wise doctor.

Knowing the eight branches,
you will cover the entire practice of medicine. [34]
Comprehending these well,
you will cure living beings of their illnesses.

Bloodletting, wounds, internal illnesses,
demonic influence, poisons, infant illnesses,
longevity, and potency are the eight.[145]

First examine their complexion and their speech,
then question them on their dreams,
and you will learn about their wind, bile, and phlegm.

Thin, with bad hair,
a mind not firm or stable,
excessive talk, and dreams of flying:
these possess the nature of wind.

Prematurely gray hair,
excessive perspiration, much moisture,
a strong spirit, and dreams of fire:
these are of the nature of bile.

Stable minds, bodies well balanced and erect,
precision in thought, head oily and moist,
water and white in their dreams:
these possess the nature of phlegm.

Among those with a combination,
some will have two, some will have all three;
whichever predominates will be their nature.

Having comprehended their natures,
administer medicine accordingly.
If the signs of death are absent,
that person will recover.

Distorted sensory perceptions,
abuse of one's guru or doctor,
hostility toward friends and relatives:
know these as signs of death.

The eyes become crossed, the whites showing,
the tongue turns black, nostrils flaring,
the ears change their position, the lips hang down:
these are signs of death.

Myrobalan, a single **form** of all six tastes,
eliminating all disease without fault,
the **king** of medicines.[146]

The three fruits and the three spices[147]
are among medicines easy to obtain.
Molasses, honey, milk, and ghee
have the power to cure many an ailment.
Other medicines should be compounded
according to the illness.

From the outset have a compassionate mind,
do not look to wealth or gain.
I have explained to you the precious principles
of the science of healing.[148]

The *Sutra of Golden Light: Mighty King of Sutras* in twenty-nine chapters translated by Yeshé Dé and the *Sutra of Golden Light* in twenty-one chapters give similar accounts.[149] In these two versions the name of Tathāgata Ratnacūḍa is given as Ratnaśikhin, and the father of Jalavāhana is rendered as Jaṭiṃdhara. As for content, these latter two versions say, for example:

Three months are summer, three are autumn, [35]
three are winter, and three are spring.

There are quite big differences in length and translation between these versions. Nevertheless, in all versions our Teacher recalls a time when, born as Jalavāhana, he learned the science of medicine from his father Jaṭiṃdhara.

At this time too the Buddha taught the *Essence of Ambrosia: The Secret Instruction Tantra on Eight Branches,* the very heart of all aspects of the science of healing, in a place called Sudarśana. Concerning the location of Sudarśana, Dza[150] and other early Tibetans place it in the western land of Oḍḍiyāna.[151] Biji[152] and others maintain that it refers to the Sudarśana situated in the center of Trāyastriṃśa heaven on the summit of Mount Meru. Ukpa Dong Nakpa from Tongmi Nyak and others say that it is in the realm of the Buddha Himasaras and is one part of the place known as Foundation and Essence Adorned with Flowers. Dong Nakpa and others say, "Amid the mountain ranges Himavat, Vindhya, etc...."[153] and go on to describe in detail the palace, the four mountains, and the respective dimensions. Dakchenpa and others identify the four mountains[154] with the four mountains taught in the *Treasury of Abhidharma*. Drangti Palden Tsojé says that because Sudarśana is in the middle of the four mountains, Vindhya, and so on, it cannot be seen by ordinary beings. The Dharma lord Jangpa asserts it to be exclusively in Bodhgāya.[155] The master Surkhar Dharmaswāmi says, "The glorious four tantras, supreme among all medical literature..." thereby staking his position by simply leaving the text as it is without entering into discussions on the location of Sudarśana or on whether *Four Tantras* is the word of the Buddha.[156] Tsomé Khenchen and Jarpo Panchen agree with Dza that Sudarśana is located in Oḍḍiyāna. Jarpo talks of one tradition with outer, inner, and secret aspects: the outer celestial city of Sudarśana, the inner Sudarśana of Bodhgāya, as asserted by Jangpa, and the secret Sudarśana identified with one's own mind. Lata Tsewang follows the outer, inner, and secret division as taught by Medicine Buddha to Yuthok Gönpo. Drukpa Pema Karpo says that our Teacher took the physician Jivaka Kumāra[157] to Gandhamārdana Mountain[158] to humble his pride and taught him *Four Tantras* through repetition.[159]

However, some scholars say that this place has no physical materiality, because it was the sphere of perception enjoyed by the nonconceptual gnosis that is the mind of our Teacher as Medicine Buddha appearing in that form. Also, Medicine Buddha, who was the dominant cause for the creation of the speaker of the tantras, was Śākyamuni Buddha appearing in a form suitable for taming disciples.

Sokdok Lodrö Gyaltsen says, "In the lower region the world called Shining Like Beryl with Medicine Buddha, [36] and in this world Yönten Gönpo..." thereby asserting that it is known to be a manifested place and claiming that it was created from virtues accumulated during the pursuit of bodhisattva practices. These claims do not stand up to scripture or reasoning. Some assert it to be in the eastern realm of Beryl Light. There are so many assertions.

Surkhar Lodrö Gyalpo in his *Oral Transmission of Our Ancestors* rejects all these assertions[160] and then quotes a passage—which can be found in Buton's *History of the Dharma* and other works—from the *Great Ocean of Specific Explanation (Mahāvibhāṣa)*, which some people say was written by Vasubandhu but which actually has been extracted from the seven categories of knowledge composed by the seven arhats:

> In the places of turning the wheel of Dharma,
> in Vaiśālī, Paṇḍubhūmi, the celestial realms,

Bālaghna, Kauśāmbī, the wilderness,
in Uśīragiri and the Bamboo Grove,
in Saśabda and Kapilavastu,
the greatest of all beings
spent a single year in each.
In Śrāvastī twenty-three years,
four in the medicine forest, two in Indraśaila,
five in Rajgir, six in ascetic practice,
and twenty-nine years in the palace.
In this way the Conqueror spent his eighty years
and then passed into supreme nirvana.[161]

Thus, he asserts the whereabouts of Sudarśana by relying on this scripture alone. If this establishes the whereabouts of Sudarśana, however, then consider this passage from the introduction to the *Beryl Light Dhāraṇī Developing the Power of the Tathāgata Meditative Concentration.* This text is found in the precious Gyantsé Thempangma Kangyur[162] in the *tha* volume on tantra, and was translated by Shang Yeshé Dé and edited and revised by Jowo Jé and the monk Tsültrim Gyalwa:

> The Bhagavān was staying in the place of medicine together with a great gathering of monks and a great gathering of bodhisattvas. At that time the Bhagavān was dwelling in the meditative concentration known as *invoking buddhafields.* Suddenly every world in the great trichiliocosmic universe shook, and celestial sandalwood dust and countless flowers rained down from above. The seven tathāgatas with their vast entourages appeared in this world and sat upon lion thrones created from their previous merits [37] and surrounded by the bodhisattvas, gods, nāgas, yakṣas, gandharvas, demigods, garudas, kinnaras, mahoragas, kings, ministers, brahmans, and lay people. Then, by the power of the Buddha, Mañjuśrī rose from his seat, put his palms together, and said, "Tathāgatas, hear this request. Purify all beings from their wrong deeds, cure them of their illnesses, fulfill their hopes."[163]

To this request our Teacher pays homage to the eight tathāgatas, the great mother,[164] the sixteen bodhisattvas—Mañjuśrī and so forth—Śāriputra and Maudgalyāyana, Brahmā, Indra, the four great kings,[165] the great nāga upāsakas, and the twelve yakṣa chieftains. Then the seven medicine buddhas and our Teacher teach the dhāraṇī in unison. If you assert that the medical tantras were taught at this time, then apart from the previous citation, such an assertion can be nothing but stubborn insistence, because the actual tantra begins, "The abode of rishis, the city known as Sudarśana."

There are many "abodes of rishis." Soon after he was born, Kumāra Siddhartha—"he who accomplishes all aims"—was named. According to the *Sutra of Great Play* he was named by Rishi Asita from the slopes of the Himalaya, the king of mountain ranges.[166] According to the *Short Vinaya* he was named by Rishi Asita from Kiskindana Mountain.[167] According to the *Basic Vinaya* and the *Sutra of Going Forth* a Rishi Araṇa who lived on Ādhara Mountain came with his retinue to Kapilavastu. He examined the signs on the prince and announced, "Mighty ruler, those who examined are wrong! Universal sovereigns do not appear in the kaliyuga," thereby prophesizing the young prince's enlightenment.[168] Twelve leagues[169] from the city of Kapilavastu was the abode of Rishi Bhṛgu, blessed with the most beautiful fruits and flowers. There the palmyra tree held its golden flowers and its fruits for twelve years uninterrupted. From the day Kumāra Siddhartha went forth into homelessness, this tree became an ordinary tree. During his years of asceticism, he went to stay in a community of rishis who lived very close to Vulture's Peak. [38] There he underwent ascetic practices, such as standing on one leg and enduring the torment of the five fires, to twice the amount required. During the display of miracles, five hundred forest-dwelling rishis who were summoned as companions by the six non-Buddhist teachers developed great insights. Once while five hundred rishis[170] were performing fire offerings in the middle of a dense forest near Śrāvastī, our Teacher manifested his footprint in the hearth and by its power prevented the fire from blazing. In the story of the householder Ghoṣila, five hundred rishis came from the south to the Anāthapiṇḍada retreat in Magadha and became monks under the ordination injunction, "Come here." In the latter part of his life, when he was preparing to entrust the doctrine to Kāśyapa, the Buddha was staying in an *udumbara* forest. In the daytime he went to a pool by the Mandākinī River, and there lived Rishi Kenavaputra with his retinue, who on hearing the teaching attained the level of nonreturner. Rishi Parvata and his retinue of five hundred disciples developed great faith in the Buddha and became ordained.

Therefore, in the accounts of our Teacher's life are mentioned many "abodes of rishis" in India and as many retinues. Moreover, from the vast ocean of

Buddha's teaching, the tiny drop of teachings translated into Tibetan contains sutras such as the *Sutra Requested by the Rishi Vyāsa,* which talk about the deer forest or *udumbara* forest where the rishis fell to earth. However, the argument that in one of these "abodes of rishis" our Teacher Śākyamuni arose in the form of Medicine Buddha, manifested the mountains, city, and the palace for the eyes of the audience gathered there, and then taught the medical tantras is unfounded.

In the twenty-fourth chapter of the *Chronicles of Ministers* from the *Five Chronicles* it says:

> For the curing of those in the clutches of illness,
> the *Essence of Ambrosia Tantra* and *Instruction Tantra*
> came from Medicine Buddha and Jivaka Kumāra
> in the lotus land of India.[171]

This describes the place of the teaching as being in the lotus land of India. However, in his *Stream of Ganges: An Account of Teachings Received,* as well as in his compositions on constitutional documents and cataloging of scripture, my lama, Ngawang Losang Gyatso, in reality an omniscient buddha, asserts it to be in the land of Oḍḍiyāna. According to Surkhar Lodrö Gyalpo, "Asserting Oḍḍiyāna to be the place where this tantra was taught is a mistake [39] that arises from holding that this scripture is a tantra of secret mantra because most tantras were taught in Oḍḍiyāna."[172] This statement is a refutation without considering a proper proof, for what certainty is there on the locale where the tantras were taught? Some tantras, such as the *Vairocana Enlightenment Tantra* were taught on the summit of Mount Meru, and according to the *Kālacakra Tantra,* all tantras were taught in the great stupa of Dhānyakaṭaka. Therefore, we cannot be so conclusive. Also, when this science of medicine tantra is classified in a particular scriptural basket, it belongs to the basket of sutra. The *Medicine Sutras in Eight Hundred Verses* are action tantras, and there is much assertion and refutation around the topic of self-generation when classifying them this way. However, my lama says in his *Monastic Regulations:*

> Without the hardship of trying to categorize the *Profound Heart-drop* and related texts as action tantras, they can be placed into the category of the *Supreme Ambrosia Tantras* from among the eight classifications of generation-stage Mahāyoga practice.[173]

Also, as explained above, he asserts the the tantra was taught exclusively in Oḍḍiyāna.

Concerning the time in Buddha's life when the tantra was taught, the twenty-fourth chapter of the *Sutra of Golden Light* talks of a previous age during the existence of the doctrine of Buddha Ratnaśikhin when the Śākya king Daṇḍapāṇi was born as king Sureśvaraprabhā, and when the Buddha's father Śuddhodana was born as the merchant Jaṭiṃdhara, a physician and healer skilled in the workings of the bodily constituents[174] and possessed of the eight branches of Āyurveda. At that time our Teacher was born as his son Jalavāhana, and during the life of this pure father and pure son there occurred a great epidemic that brought much suffering to the beings of the land. Therefore, the son Jalavāhana decided to learn the science of medicine from his father. The tantra was taught around the time this story of past events was taught on Vulture's Peak to the goddess Bodhisamuccayā.[175] In the introduction to this sutra, the bodhisattva Ruciraketu sees that the Bhagavān Śākyamuni will live to be eighty and thinks this is too short a lifespan. Also the ācārya and soothsayer brahman Kauṇḍinya hears that the Tathāgata will soon pass away and requests a relic the size of a mustard seed.

Based on this we can say that in the latter part of our Teacher's life, a little before the passing of Śāriputra and Maudgalyāyana, in the land of Śrī Oḍḍiyāṇa, in the midst of the medicine forest known as the abode of rishis, on the summit of a four-sided mountain[176] eight leagues long and three leagues high, [40] our Teacher manifested a place as smooth as one's palm, free of all obstructions such as stones and gravel, a wide open area glowing with light and light rays blurring the distinction between day and night, soft and springy to the touch, and pervaded by the sweet smell of incense. In its midst was the city of Sudarśana, boasting a palace built entirely from the precious stones of the human realm—gold, silver, white and red pearls, and beryl—and from the five precious wish-fulfilling jewels. The palace has four sides and four doors, and its ornamented walls are five layers thick. At each door stands one of the great king guardians. The palace's decorations include various medicinal jewels adorning parts of the palace. Five types of celestial jewels adorn the parapets, forming a crisscross pattern of garlands and half garlands. Five types of bodhisattva jewels adorn the tops of the victory standards on the roof and the *ghaṭa*.[177] At all times these jewels glow and radiate light, and they have the power to explain the inner meaning of external signs and the outer meaning of inner signs. The master Ārya Nāgārjuna said:

> Precious jewels and stones of the human realm have a purity of color and possess seven qualities, including eliminating the sufferings of poison, demons, darkness, swellings, and fever. Celestial jewels possess these qualities, too, as well as continuously accom panying the body of the celestial being being perfectly pure, having the ability to talk, and being light in weight. Therefore they possess eleven qualities. Bodhisattva jewels have these eleven qualities and are furthermore able to tell when living beings will pass away and when their births will be at an end, and are able to communicate the Dharma in various languages. Thus they possess these fourteen qualities.[178]

Therefore, these jewels or precious stones possessing these powers and abilities can eliminate the 404 types of illness that arise from the disorders of wind, bile, phlegm, dual combinations, and triple combinations. For hot disorders they become cool and dispel the fever. For cold disorders they develop the power of heat and banish the cold. In this way this precious jeweled palace guards and protects from all harmful forces by pacifying the eighty thousand hindrances that plague the body and mind and so forth, [41] while at the same time granting and fulfilling one's needs and wishes as soon as these appear to the mind.

To the south of the city lies a mountain range "endowed with the power of the sun"[179] on which can be found medicines of hot power that eliminate cold disorders. To the north grow medicinal plants of cold power that eliminate hot disorders. In the east grow the five or seven types of chebulic myrobalan. To the west are found the six excellent plants—calcite, bitumen, and so on—as well as hot springs and medicinal water, all of five varieties. On the tops of the medicinal trees, birds sing sweet songs, while elephants, bears, musk deer, and other creatures whose bodies contain good medicine roam on the floor of the forest surrounding this perfect palace.

Within the palace on a throne made of various precious stones and white, yellow, and blue beryl, supported by lions, elephants, thoroughbred horses, garudas, and peacocks, sat the Teacher of this Dharma on a cushion of priceless celestial cloth. Generally, it is said that the term *medicine buddha (sman bla)* can be applied to Medicine Buddha as lord of the seven sugatas, as described in the passage from the greater and lesser versions of the *Medicine Sutras in Eight Hundred Verses* beginning, "Mañjuśrī, east of this buddha realm, beyond buddha realms as many as grains of sand in the Ganges..." up to "dwelled the teacher of gods and men, the bhagavān, the buddha, the lord of blue beryl light."[180] It can also be applied to the medicine buddhas found among the thousand buddhas of this fortunate eon, to the description of Medicine Buddha as found in the *Illusory Net Tantra,* and to our Teacher, the son of Śuddhodana, as Medicine Buddha.

There are quite a few questions and many scriptural references on whether these forms described above are emanation bodies or enjoyment bodies and, because of having a form the color of beryl—blue—whether the major and minor marks of enlightenment are complete or not. However, because this would take up a lot of space, it has been dealt with elsewhere. The definitive position is found in the seventh fascicle of the *Mine of Jewels Sutra:*

> Mañjuśrī, in these different forms, while I am working in these different buddha realms, at those times sentient beings know me by different names. However, even if they were to quote them for an eon they would never be able to perceive the end of the buddha realms of the east. [42] Similarly, in the buddha realms of the other directions sentient beings know me as tathāgatas of different names. However, if they were to quote them for an inconceivable number of eons, they would not easily perceive the end of all the different buddha realms.[181]

Also, in the fourth chapter of the *Samādhi of Śūraṅgama Sutra* when Mañjuśrī asked the Buddha about "the tathāgata, the arhat, the perfectly enlightened buddha, Vikurvānarāja dwelling beyond this buddha realm, beyond as many buddha realms as there are in sixty times the number of grains of sand in the Ganges, in the upper direction, in the world of Ekadipa," the Buddha replied:

> The buddha realms of the bhagavān buddhas are inconceivable. That buddha is me. Mañjuśrī, in this way the billions of buddha realms are worlds that I engage in. There the śrāvakas and pratyekabuddhas do not enter.[182]

And in the fifth chapter:

> In the east, thirty-two thousand buddha realms beyond this buddha realm, in the world known as Vijaya, dwells Tathāgata Vairocana Prabhāmaya. This buddha too is me.[183]

There are other similar passages, and most Mahayana sutras talk along similar lines.

In *Bright Lamp* by Candrakīrti, a commentary on the father tantra Guhyasamāja, a passage is cited from the *Mahāguhya Yogatantra,*[184] running from, "It is like this: Mañjuśrī was King Śuddhodana..." up to "Mahāvairocana was the perfectly enlightened buddha Śākyamuni."[185] No buddha realm is excluded from the "foundation and essence adorned with flowers" ocean of realms,[186] and the limitless and varied enlightened forms that dwell there emanate from the same enjoyment body. Therefore wondering—from the standpoint of Medicine Buddha being solely a manifestation of our Teacher—whether the seven brothers are also medicine buddhas, and wondering—from the standpoint of *Medicine Buddha* referring to a separate being—whether specific instances of medicine buddhas mentioned in other scriptural references are the same, become unnecessary doubts. [43]

This point can also be understood by the forms of his appearance. In the *Destruction of the Great Thousand Sutra* it says:

> At the time of the perfect enlightenment,
> the guardians of the world held aloft
> four bowls from the four directions
> and offered them to the Sugata,
> by whose power they became a single bowl.
>
> These supreme celestial bowls,
> holding supreme ambrosia-like medicine,
> sit in the hands of the Teacher.
> By the power of these words of truth,
> may all medicine become ambrosia.
>
> Likewise the goddess Harī held aloft
> the celestial and wonderful myrobalan
> and offered it to the Teacher.
>
> The supreme ambrosia-like medicine
> now sits in the hands of the Teacher.
> By the power of these words of truth,
> may the sick be cured of their illness,
> may all faults be driven out,
> may all medicine become ambrosia.[187]

Here the Buddha reveals himself as Medicine Buddha. In the *Illusion-Like Samādhi Sutra* it says, "In order to tame others he shows countless forms."[188] In the *Saṃghāṭa Sutra* it says, "Sarvaśūra, I teach the Dharma in whatever form is necessary for the taming of others."[189] In *Questions of Mañjuśrī* it says:

> With his forms the Tathāgata pervades all worlds. By whatever color, shape, or aspect of behavior living beings will be tamed, the Tathāgata in that color, shape, or aspect of behavior will be seen by living beings.[190]

In the eighth chapter of the *Ornament of Realization,* the Mahayana treatise by the noble Maitreya, it says:

> When the causes come to fruition,
> then to whomever, as whatever,
> and whenever it will be of help,
> to that being, in that form, he appears.[191]

In the fifth chapter of the *Yoga Equal to All Buddhas Later Tantra* it says:

> To tame sentient beings,
> to create every happiness,
> that yoga of the Bhagavān
> is manifest as every buddha.[192]

From the same tantra:

> The one perfect state[193]
> appears as desired.[194]

In the thirty-fifth chapter of the *Abhidhana Later Tantra* it says:

> All knowing and all things,
> holding forms as desired....[195]

In the eleventh chapter of the *Tantra of the Fierce and Wrathful* it says: [44]

> I take on different forms
> to tame living beings.[196]

Therefore, these citations are saying that to appear as a teacher in forms appropriate to those to be tamed is the skillful means of the tathāgata gnosis. Were that not the case, it would be difficult to reconcile the fact of there being one doctrine but not two teachers with the fact of Ānanda, Kumāra Jivaka Bhṛtya, and others who made up the four circles of medical disciples being the disciples of another.

Therefore, our Teacher, the son of Śuddhodana, arose in the form of the Bhagavān, the physician, the buddha of medicine, the lord of beryl light. The vast audience included the circle of gods such as Prajāpati, the circle of rishis such as Ātreya, the circle of outsiders such as Brahmā, and the circle of insiders such as Avalokita. At that time, the five rishi brothers emerged from the five aspects of enlightened body, speech, mind, qualities, and activities as the innate tones of the five kinds of gnosis. One became the manifestation of enlightened speech and was the requestor of the teaching, while the other four manifested as the teacher of the tantra. Each circle of disciples understood the teaching as their own tradition. The gods understood it as the *Science of Healing Collection.* The rishis heard it as the *Caraka Aṣṭavarga.* The outsiders heard it as the *Black Īśvara Tantra.* The insiders heard it as the *Guardian of the Three Lineages Collection.* As it says in the Entrustment chapter from *Four Tantras:*

> For the sake of living beings,
> the emanations of the Sugata
> taught the preparation of medicine in India,
> cauterization and channel cleansing in China,
> mainly bloodletting in the land of Dölpo,[197]
> pulse and urine diagnosis in Tibet,
> the *Science of Healing Collection* to the gods,
> the *Caraka Aṣṭavarga* to the rishis,
> the *Black Īśvara Tantra* to the *tīrthika* outsiders,
> and the *Guardian of the Three Lineages* to the insiders.
>
> All these are included in this medical tantra;
> there is no medical practice not within it.
> The great compassion has no partiality,
> but things appear according to individual disposition.
> Just as a single moon in the sky
> appears as individual moons in every water urn,

> one teaching was delivered,
> but many were understood.[198]

In the understanding of Manasija,[199] the speech-emanation rishi, whose own form is that of Amitāyus, the teaching received was the *Essence of Ambrosia: The Secret Instruction Tantra on Eight Branches.* [45] This teaching was *Four Tantras,* comprising most of the Explanatory Tantra, large parts of the Root Tantra, and parts of the Instruction and Final Tantras, and which was said to cover the eight branches, the eleven topics, the fifteen fields of practice, and the four compilations, with the whole work consisting of 156 chapters and more than 5,900 verses. The original text, written down on sheets of pure gold in beryl ink, is supposedly kept in Oḍḍiyāna ḍākinī land.

Guru Chökyi Wangchuk of the old translation school, in his revealed treasures, says that a hidden enlightened-mind treasure from the mind of the four immeasurables of the Teacher and Sugata was revealed as *Medicine Buddha Lord of Beryl Light.* The medical tantras were mind treasures that became part of the Transmission tradition[200] because the *Caraka Aṣṭavarga* great tantra, *Tantra of Eight Branches,* the eighteen *Ambrosia Drop Tantras,* and others were taught by the Buddha and were then compiled by the great rishi Śaṅkacūḍa and others from the twenty-one rishis, as well as by the youth Avadhūta, Manasija, and so on, and were widely disseminated. Then, to keep them safe and secure, they were put in containers and hidden as treasure in the Bodhgāya forests in India, in the beryl stupa in Oḍḍiyāna, in the secret Asura cave, in Swayambhu in Nepal, and in the Gaudeshan cave in China. Ācārya Padmasambhava, Nāgārjuna Hṛdaya, Tīrthika Munirāj, and others unearthed these treasures and, for the sake of living beings, transmitted them in a one-to-one lineage.

According to Drangti Palden Tsojé's *Illumination of Knowledge,* during the third turning of the wheel, while the Tathāgata was teaching the Dharma to his retinue in the place of the yakṣa Vajrapāṇi, a horde of māras, such as the paranirmita-vaśavartins,[201] arrived and fired a black, nine-headed *yantra,* causing Bakula and Jambala to flee to the Buddha. Bakula died and Jambala was in great pain. Light of the five nectars radiated from the coil of hair between the Buddha's eyebrows, easing Jambala's pain. The Buddha then taught the *Crystal Mirror Medicine Tantra* in fifty chapters to gods such as Brahmā and to human rishis such as Kumāra Jivaka.[202]

In the second chapter of the *Great Nirvana Sutra* taught in the town of Kuśanagar, [46] in the version translated from Chinese,[203] while Upāsaka Cunda, the son of a woodworker from Kuśanagar, together with fifty-one like-minded companions was performing an offering of food, the monks asked:

> "The Bhagavān has said that we should persist through the power of all dharmas being without self and in so doing, we will be freed from pride and pass beyond sorrow. What is the meaning of that?"
>
> The Bhagavān replied, "It is like this. Say there is an unwise king—a man of little knowledge—and an equally unwise and foolish doctor. The king in his ignorance bestows gifts upon this doctor. The foolish doctor, for his part, treats all illnesses with milk, having no idea of the origins of the illness. He does not even use milk as medicine properly, treating with milk all disorders, whether wind, bile, or phlegm in nature. The king, not knowing what makes a good doctor, cannot even distinguish between good and bad milk.
>
> From another land comes another doctor, one possessing the eight sciences, skilled in the art of curing all diseases, and master of all medical practices. The stupid doctor does not question or learn from this wise doctor but instead develops thoughts of superiority and arrogance. The wise doctor, on the other hand, devotes himself to the stupid doctor and regards him as his teacher. So that he may learn any secret medical knowledge he makes a request:
>
> "I beseech you to be my master. Show me and teach me the medical practices."
>
> In reply the other doctor commands, "If you serve me for forty-eight years, I will teach you the practices."
>
> The wise doctor accedes to the demands of the foolish doctor saying, "I will do as you command and do all I can to serve you."
>
> Then the stupid doctor takes the new doctor to the palace to meet the king. There the wise doctor talks about various medical techniques, about many kinds of skills and arts, about how to protect the country, and about remedies for different illnesses, saying, "Great king, you should learn and understand these." [47]

The king listens and realizes that the old doctor is not at all a wise doctor and expels him from the land. From then on he pays great honor and respect to this new doctor.

The doctor thinks to himself, "The time has come to teach the king," and says, "Great king, if you think highly of me, please grant me a request."

The king replies, "From my right arm to every other part of my body, take all that you desire. I willingly offer it all to you."

The doctor replies, "Although your majesty willingly grants every part of his body to me, I cannot accept his offer. I do not seek much. All I ask is that from now on, you issue a decree saying that all the people of this country should cease the practice of taking milk as medicine, as was prescribed by the old doctor. Why? Because that medicine is harmful and will cause the death of many. If you issue a proclamation saying that anyone caught administering this medicine will be beheaded, the practice of using milk as medicine will be halted, there will be no untimely death, and everybody will be happy. Please grant me this request."

The king replies, "This request of yours will be of great benefit. From now on if there is sickness in the land, no one will be allowed to take milk as medicine. If there is anyone who does, they will be beheaded."

After the proclamation the wise doctor prepares medicines of various tastes—hot, bitter, sour, sweet, salty, and so on. When they are administered to the sick, there are none who do not recover. Not long after, the king himself becomes sick and summons the doctor. "I am in great pain," he said, "How can I be helped?"

The doctor examines the king, and it is clear the king needs milk as medicine. He says, "Your majesty, if this illness is to be treated, you should take milk as your medicine. Previously when I said it was not right to take milk as medicine, it was not true. There is no better medicine than milk. [48] Because your illness arises from a hot disorder, you should take milk as medicine."

"Doctor, have you gone mad?" asks the king. "You are saying that when one is suffering from a heat disorder, milk will help? Previously you said milk was poisonous. How can I possibly drink it now! Are you deceiving me?[204] You said that which was praised by a previous doctor was actually poisonous, because of which he was expelled. Now you are saying that milk makes for good medicine. I can see that the old doctor was certainly much wiser than you!"

Then the doctor says to the king, "Your majesty, please don't say such things. Let me explain with an example. A wood-eating insect can leave a trail carved in the wood that resembles a letter. It does not know that it is a letter, and any intelligent person who saw it would not utter in amazement, 'Oh look, this insect knows how to write!' Great king, the former doctor was like this; he did not understand illness. His giving of milk as medicine to everyone is like the insect forming a letter in the wood, because he does not know the difference between good and bad milk, or when it is suitable and when it is unsuitable."

The king asks, "Exactly what did he not understand?"

The doctor replies, "Milk as medicine is both poison and ambrosia. How can it be both harmful and ambrosia? I will explain. If a cow does not eat leftover grain, cut grass, and husks or chaff; if its calf is well behaved; if it lives neither high in the mountains nor low in the forests; if its drinking water comes from a clear-flowing stream and is not too sweet; if, while not living[205] close to the bull, it grazes contentedly and is generally content whether moving or sitting; then the milk of that cow is good for all kinds of illness and is ambrosia. Any other kind of milk is harmful."

The king listens and says, "Excellent, doctor, very well said! Now I know the difference between good and bad milk, and when it is suitable and unsuitable."

The doctor gives him the milk medicine and he recovers. The king issues an order to his people saying that from then on, milk should be given as medicine. When the people hear this they complain, "What is wrong with the king. Has he been possessed by ghosts? [49] Has he gone mad? He is deceiving us by telling us to use milk as medicine."

They became angry and came before the king. "Do not blame me," said the king. "The suitability or unsuitability to take milk as medicine has been decided by this doctor. I have done nothing wrong."

The king and his people were pleased and redoubled their

> reverence and service to the doctor. All who were given milk as medicine were cured.[206]

In the twenty-fifth chapter of the same sutra it says:

> A wise doctor, well versed in the eight branches of knowledge, first investigates the illness for its type. Illness is of three types: wind, bile, and phlegm. For a wind illness he gives ghee, for a bile illness he gives white sugar, and for a phlegm illness he gives a ginger extract. Therefore, treating illness on the basis of understanding the illness is a mark of a good doctor.[207]

And in the forty-first chapter:

> There are three types of illness in the world: bile, wind, and phlegm. These three types of illness are to be treated with three types of medicine. Bile disorder is treated with ghee, wind disorder is helped with oil, phlegm disorder is helped with honey.[208]

Here and elsewhere many passages teach the science of healing through the gathering, arising, and pacifying of illness, and by way of examples. It is also reputed that the Buddha taught the eight branches of medicine in 1002 fascicles.

In the forty-ninth chapter of the mother tantra, the *Vajraḍāka,* it says:

> In the distant past, during the mahāsukha first eon,
> dwelled the great Vajrasattva, great god of gods.
> When seen by the demigods, siddhas, and others,
> as well as by the host of gods, they were afraid.
> The buddhas assembled and beseeched me.
> Great goddess, they had melted into drops,
> to be scattered everywhere by the māras,
> the great stupefier of all, hailed as quicksilver;
> its inferior kind is found in the ocean depths,
> the superior kind on mountains.[209]

Also:

Myrobalan is found in the Vindhya forests
and on the Mahendra mountains.
The best is by the waters of Narmadā,
others are middling or inferior. [50]
Oval, Fearless, Life-giving, Ambrosia, Purity,
Increase, and Victorious are its seven types.[210]
Pointed myrobalan has three sides, Fearless has five;
Life-giving is also known as Golden, Ambrosia as Fleshy;
Purity is known as Fleshless, Increase as Pale Yellow;
Victorious is like the *kuva* fruit.
Āmla is fleshy, with little inner structure,
of strong taste, and found on rocky hills;
well-ripened fruit is the best.
Baleric myrobalan is found on
ordinary hills and elsewhere.[211]

These passages describe general locations of medicines, superior and inferior types, and so on. In the same work it says:

Gold is good for complexion,
silver is good for teeth,
pearl is a purifier,
lapis is good for hair,
diamond turns away thunderbolts,
iron resists water and weapons.[212]

This passage describes the benefits of wearing various substances. Also:

Long pepper and saffron
taken in spring in equal measures,
followed by a drink of warm urine,
will aid appetite and digestion.

Nirguṇḍi juice with urine taken as nose drops
eliminates disorders arising from phlegm;
when mixed with lotus aroma and applied as a lotion,
it cures bull sores.[213]

The root of *markata* mixed
with ground nails and teeth:
to first wash the wound with ghee
and then apply this medicine
is the best cure for a wound.

Brick dust and greater cardamom
mixed into the juice of *girikarṇā*
and rubbed onto the eyes
is best for curing poor vision.[214]

The passages from the above tantra speak of the elixir preparation of mercury, and so on, and in general terms of the gathering, arising, and pacifying of disorders.

In the thirty-eighth chapter of the *Ḍāka Ocean Tantra* it says:

Black zedorary and turmeric combined in whey,
two measures boiled until they become one;
drink this, and in seven days
it will become the complete elixir.[215]

This and other verses describe different types of elixirs.

In the second chapter of the *Saṃvarodaya Tantra* it says:

The initial form is coagulation, [51]
the second is a mass,
the third becomes elongated,
the fourth is solid.[216]

This is the forming of the embryo. In the nineteenth chapter:

One who sneezes while defecating and urinating
will die within a year.[217]

This and other verses talks of the various stages of the signs of death. Also:

With the proper instructions,
death will be bought off.[218]

This talks of the ritual for cheating death.[219] In the twenty-fifth chapter:

> Colored brick dust, mud,
> *nirguṇḍi, avalguja, unmatta* decoction,
> musk with sandalwood, *bālaka,* and angelica,
> when rubbed into the body,
> will eliminate all illness,
> leaving one free of poisons with a healthy glow.
>
> The three fruits, powdered sandal,
> and musk, taken for a year
> with cool medicine, will eliminate illness
> and aging as well.[220]

These verses talk of the curing of various illnesses and rejuvenation therapy.

The Inner chapter of the *Condensed Kālacakra Tantra*[221] says:

> The accumulated constituents of this body
> arise from food and drink endowed with six tastes;
> the six tastes also arise from the elements,
> and the manifest, arising elements
> are within the element of space.[222]

This is describing the formation of the body. Also:

> Firstly, this all-conquering body
> is praised as a source of siddhi
> and should therefore be protected.
> With no body there will be no siddhi,
> and no attainment of supreme bliss in this life.
> Therefore, for the sake of the body
> one should practice channel yoga daily;
> for if this can be accomplished,
> other siddhis of the three worlds
> will be at your service.[223]

This and many other passages talk of protecting the body as a source of worldly and non-worldly siddhi. Also:

Blocking sun and moon channels, with their even and uneven courses,
the flow is brought within the central Kalāgni channel.
If the life-sustaining and downward-expelling winds
dwell there, too, for one day,
the yogi will have cheated untimely death.[224]

This verse talks about cheating untimely death. Also:

With the downward-expelling wind withdrawn,
desires will be met, and in this excellent body
all wind disorders will be pacified.
Prāṇāyāma is for phlegm disorders, [52]
while expelling the winds again
will eliminate all disorders of bile.

Blocking above and below brings bliss,
pacifying complex disorders and infectious fever.
This is because the life-sustaining wind
destroys all illness above the navel;
the downward-expelling wind at the navel
destroys all others.[225]

These two verses describe how the downward-expelling and other winds pacify wind, bile, phlegm, and complex disorders. The next verse talks of curing stomach ailments with wind yoga:

The downward-expelling is withdrawn from its three pathways,
the life-sustaining likewise is withdrawn from above;
for as long as they are joined, the power of the fire pervades the body,
and tumor-like concretions, *muchu,* and hemorrhoids
are cured with a month of this wind yoga.
Respiratory and bronchial illnesses, the three types of poisons,
eye diseases, and others are also cured.[226]

Another verse talks of relieving back pain:

Legs in the vajra position,
grasped by the lotus of the hands,

will relieve all pain in the back.
Feet upward and head downward
will cure all phlegm disorders.
Blocking the winds for a few days
will cure diarrhea and urinary disorders.
At dawn, without water in the mouth,
rubbing the teeth with the ring fingers
will become medicine for the eyes.
Splashing with water will also cure the disorder.[227]

A further verse talks of the elimination of leprosy and other diseases:

The mantra practitioners in union with the consort
cause the bodhicitta to fall but halt it with the winds,
and in half a year, in this excellent body,
they will have destroyed even white leprosy,
to say nothing of other diseases.
Old age of seventy years with its white hair
will also be vanquished after two years.
After a few days[228] of joining mind and path,
the siddhi of the consort will also be attained.[229]

A further verse talks of medicine for the ascetic yogi:

Lukewarm urine[230] cures mouth ailments and toothache;
ingesting urine at dawn cures headaches, as does water;
pouring warm and cold urine into ears and eyes
will cure the ailments of both.
Drinking urine with the three hot foods[231] [53]
relieves the torment of elemental spirits[232] and bites.[233]

Another verse talks of lengthening life, and how the yoga of the five nectars, ingesting a young girl's flowers,[234] and the five lamps will destroy disease and make the old young again:

Excrement, urine, semen, blood, and human flesh
when eaten will give and lengthen life.
Ingesting flowers with meditative absorption

will eliminate aging of the body with its white hair.
The five lamps mixed with bee vomit,
when eaten, will destroy all disease.
Śukra mixed with a young girl's flowers
and eaten for a year will destroy old age.[235]

The next verse speaks of medicine for wind, bile, and phlegm disorders:

Salty and sour foods combat wind,
sweet and astringent foods are the enemy of bile,
all bitter and hot foods combat phlegm;
these medicines can be either solid or liquid.
Goat milk with the three hot foods combats phlegm,
buffalo milk is the enemy of bile,
camel milk, too, will combat wind;
these are the milks combating the three disorders.
Ghee has similar properties.[236]

The next verse talks of boiled medicines for mouth ailments, and so on:

The warmed juice of boiled nutmeg
cures mouth ailments and relieves toothaches.
Sesame oil and goat urine boiled
with the three hot foods and salt
cures ailments of the ears.
Ghee and milk boiled with *nāgakesara* and saffron
cures ailments of the nose.
Karkoṭī, lāṅgalī, indravāruṇī, and donkey urine
applied as a lotion will cure swellings.[237]

The next verse says:

Hands hanging down, lotuses of the feet together,
halting the winds through vase yoga,
again and again while in samādhi—
for as long as one does not fall to the ground,
and for as long as the fever is not released—
this destroys the vajra thorns that bring fear of death.

Meditate also on Viśvamātā pure as the moon
upon a moon disc in the lotus of the heart.[238]

This verse talks of curing "vajra thorns" or smallpox by wind yoga and Viśvamātā meditation and recitation. The next verse says:

Crushed lentils drunk with cold water
destroys the thorns of those pierced with fever. [54]
With the fever subsided, ground skull mixed with urine
and drunk will destroy the fear.
For the mantra, *oṃ* before water, fire, and air,
then *vajra* are the first words.[239]
Meditate with these as protection
in the head, throat, heart, navel, secret place, and so on.[240]

This verse talks of medicine, mantra, and protection for smallpox. The next verse says:

Equal measures of ground *dhātri* fruit and coriander,
likewise powdered petals of the *tintirā* flower,
in water free of impurities, touched by sun and moon,
boiled down to a quarter, mixed with sugar,
drank for three days after the following day,
relieves life-threatening sunstroke
caused by the sun in the hot season
and other ailments caused by heat
that also affect the seven constituents.[241]

This verse talks about alleviating sunburn and other heat-related disorders that arise in the hot season. The following verses describe the making of intermediate-grade elixir:

Gold with copper, lodestone, mica, and iron,
are finely ground with iron pyrites to form the base.[242]
To two measures of the seed is added purified mercury
to form a mass of six measures.[243]
Cow's buttermilk destroyed by a fierce fire until its clear
essence remains

is boiled together with the golden mass in a lodestone vessel
until half remains and is then removed.
Mix this with eight or nine measures of pure sugar
and take at all times for as long as you have given up eating.
In six months you will gain the ambrosia of having the body
of a god,
with no gray hair and all wrinkles vanished.
Therefore, drink this every day,
though it decreases the golden mass.

Take the same amount of the above king of bases
or half as much mixed with mercury.
Work in salts and acids, many medicines, until they become one.
Bile and acids can also be worked into mercury-like substances,
such as sulphur and so forth, *darada,* and realgar.
Rub this into silver leaf and it becomes gold;
matured by fire this is known as semigold.[244]

Iron, mica, yellow orpiment, salt,
potash, sal-tree resin,
are gradually increased and immersed to one taste
in twice the amount of copper, and
the remaining copper is burned away and then
cleaned with salt, softened with buttermilk, and so on. [55]
A third the quantity of silver is added,
and by kneading and stretching,
pure flower petals are produced.[245]

The next and following verses describe the ingredients for incense and aromas as offerings to the Three Jewels:

Cardamom, camphor, the *mālā* flower,[246]
silhaka powder, nutgrass, the *priyaṅgu* flower,
black aloe, *śaileya,* the *kakkola* plant,
siṃhamūtra, costus root, nutmeg and musk,
saffron, the *murā* plant, *putrakeśa,*
nāgakesara, sandalwood, the *uśīra* plant,
tamāla petals, the *māṃsī* plant, *bālaka,*

musk creeper, *bheruṇḍa* bird droppings,
and the *piṇḍitailaka* flower;
make aromas with these five sets of substances,
incense with musk and camphor, and so on,
scents with flowers, purifiers for alcohol.[247]

A later verse describes a yantra for ensuring an easy birth:

Mountains, sun, moon, *manu,*
eyes, desire, jewels, wrathful,
kings, fires, direction, elements,
openings, seasons, dates, and oceans:[248]
place these in the diagram
and the count of four circles is thirty-four.
Draw the circles on the back of a measuring dish and
show it to the mother-to-be as birth draws near.[249]

A further verse describes medicine for a woman in labor:

Costus root, *uśīra, kaśeru, tagara* root,
utpala root, and lotus filament
pulped in cool water, praised by vajra,[250]
and placed upon the pain.
If the womb is rigid,
take eight hairs from a mongoose
and eight strands from a peacock tail,
soak in cool water, and perform as above.[251]

These passages, and others such as those on the movement of the life force, and so on, from the *Kāmaśāstra* collection, *Scripture on Tastes, Protecting the Country,* and other works that follow the Vedas, the scholars of the past have called the Buddhist scriptural tradition.

The Bodhisattva, Deva, and Rishi medical traditions

In the *Heap of Jewels* it says:

On the magically created Five Peaks Mountain in China,
Mañjuśrī taught in the form of a parrot;
in Vajrāsana and on Kukkuṭaka mountain,
Avalokiteśvara taught in the form of a rishi; [56]
in Gauśānti in the land of Oḍḍiyāna,
Vajrapāṇi taught in the form of Māra.[252]

In *Drop from the Heart of Mañjuśrī* it says:

From India, China, and the upper regions
come three traditions of great enlightenment;
the Vidyādhara transmission of all medical knowledge
began with the three protectors.[253]

Therefore, from noble Mañjuśrī, master of the tenth level, come:

- *Alms Bowl of Ambrosia: Treatment of Head Ailments*
- *Jeweled Box*
- *Charms for the Abdomen*
- *Supreme Magic: A Treatment of Womb Disorders*
- *Five Jewel Treasuries*
- *Special Treatment of Head Ailments*
- *Three Sections of the Greater and Lesser Mineral Tantra*
- *Ocean of Ambrosia: A Treatment of Head Ailments*
- *Quintessence: The Magic Fourfold Collection*
- *Clear and Concise Manuscript on Diagnosis*
- *Life Treatment: Opening the Mouths of the Mute*
- *Somarāja Medical Text*
- *Medical Plants Collection*

From Ārya Avalokiteśvara:

- *Supreme Victory Standard: Treatise on Head Ailments*
- *Essential Surgery*
- *Drop of Ambrosia*
- *Supreme Adornment*
- *Greater and Lesser Stream of Ambrosia*
- *Red and Black Treatise on the Abdomen*
- *Greater and Lesser Commentary on Fundamental Topics*

- *Clear Mirror*
- *Clearly Understanding on Seeing*

From the glorious Vajrapāṇi comes:

- *Settling Arguments over Head Ailments*
- *Magic Mirror of Anatomy*
- *Precious Wheel of the Eight Planets*
- *Black Jaṭila*
- *The Upturned Lotus*
- *Charms for Pain*
- *Curing All Miscellaneous Disorders*

From the Noble Tārā comes:

- *Six Methods for Dealing with Pain*
- *Preparing Medicinal Plants*
- *Illustrative Work on Medicinal Plants in 120 Chapters*

These works are reputed to have been composed by these bodhisattvas, and therefore they belong to the Bodhisattva medical tradition.

Fortunate Eon Deva tradition

Brahmā composed the *Guṇaśāstra* in three hundred chapters and the *Guhyagarbha Saṃhita;* Prajāpati composed *Magic Mirror;* the two Aśvinī sons composed *Siddhasāra Saṃhita;* Indra composed *Condensed Siddhasāra* and *Structure of the Abdomen: A Radiant Light of Teachings;* and the medicine goddess Vasudhāra composed *Precious Garland.*

Vidyādhara Rishi tradition

There were seven rishi disciples of Indra who, like the Pāṇḍava sons, had celestial fathers. They are Ātri, Marīci, Pulastya, Aṅgirā, Kaiṭabhajit, Vasiṣṭha, and Kratu.[254] These were known as the seven topknot rishis. [57] Those rishis born in dependence upon a human mother include Ātreya, Agniveśa, Dhanvantari, Dvitapaścaraṇa, Nemindhara, Jagannathauta, and Punarvasu. The words "and so on"[255] include Haladhara. These eight rishis each composed a commentary on the Āyurveda tantra after hearing it from Indra. These commentaries are the *Carved Collection,*[256] *Fundamentals Collection, Great Ambrosia*

Collection, Weapons of Fearlessness Collection, Ambrosia Accomplishment Collection, Box of Life Collection, Preparation of Medicine Collection, and *Five Therapy Collection.* These total 425 chapters and are known collectively as the *Eight Caraka Collections.*

Rishi Śrīmālā wrote a commentary to the first part of the *Eight Caraka Collections* called *Replicating*[257] *Sun and Moon* in eighty fascicles and a commentary to the second part called *Magic Key* in forty fascicles. These one hundred twenty fascicles comprise six hundred chapters. Likewise, there were rishis such as Bheḍa, Jatukarṇa, Parāśara, Kṣārapāṇi, Śrīsaṃpanna, Sūryagarbha, Candragarbha, Candraprabhā, and others. In the *Great Peacock Tantra* it says:

> Ānanda, know them by their names such as rishis, those of ancient conduct, practitioners of mantra, those of blazing renown, mountain and valley dwellers, possessors of the weapon of curses, those of extreme asceticism, possessors of magic, masters of the five kinds of clairvoyance, and travelers through space.[258]

This lists several synonyms of this tradition's name. Therefore, rishis such as Marīci, Jagannathauta, Ātreya, and so on, appeared in the world at a time before our Teacher. The tradition was widely propagated by the many extensive works on Āyurveda composed by Śālihotra, Suśruta, Jajaya, and others. In later times the tradition came down to the physician Ātreya of Takṣaśila, who had crossed the vast ocean of Āyurveda and who was elevated by royal decree by the king Padmaśrī in a document that proclaimed his virtues far and wide.

The later tradition of the tīrthika outsiders arose as follows. On the entreaties of his followers—Viṣṇu, Krenavama,[259] Rāhula, Umā, Yakṣakala, and others—Mahādeva Maheśvara produced from his crown ornament the *Profound and Secret Black and White Tantras.* From his ear ornaments he produced the *Fast-Moving Tantra.* From his neck ornaments emerged the *Red and Blue Life-Channel Tantra.* [58] From his belt came the *Heroic Rescuer Tantra.* From his shoulder ornaments came the *Wheel of Fire Tantra.* From the ornaments on his feet came the *Black and White Frog Tantra.* Many such similar works on Āyurveda were produced.

Vajra Voice, Mountain Stack, Blazing Like Fire, and *Matted Hair* are reputed to have been composed by Deva Sarvajña. Ralpatra wrote three tantras known *Black Volume, Black Tome,* and *Black Moonlight.* These are later traditions. As it has been said, "The emanations of the Sugata taught the *Black Īśvara Tantra* to the tīrthika outsiders."[260] [59]

5. Kumāra Jivaka

IN THE *Vinaya Flower Garland* it says:

> Śrāvastī, Sāketa, Campā,
> Vārāṇasī, Vaiśālī, Rājagṛha:
> these are the six great cities.[261]

These are the six great cities of India. The most important king of these six cities was Bimbisāra, one of the four kings alive during the time of our Teacher, the Lion of the Śākya, and the son of Mahāpadma, king of Rājagṛha in Magadha. He was named Bimbisāra, "he whose essence is the form of the sun," because at his birth all worlds shone like the sun. He took Vaidehī as a wife, and a son, Ajātaśatru, was born. From his liaison with Āmrapālī, a trader in medicine from Vaiśālī who possessed most of the signs of a being a "jewel of a woman,"[262] a son, Kumāra Abhaya, was born.

Mention in some of the shorter sutras of the phrase "requested by Ratnacandra, the son of King Bimbisāra" is not relevant here.

The life of Jivaka is found in the medicine section of the four volumes of Vinaya transmission, and I will relate generally what is written there.

King Bimbisāra was very attracted to the wives of others and would often take his elephant and ride through the streets of the towns casting his eyes about. At that time in Rājagṛha there was a wealthy merchant who had just taken a wife of the same class. After they had enjoyed each other's company, the merchant gathered merchandise and then set off to the other side of the country. His wife was very attached to good food and nice clothes and was consequently often tormented by her desires. King Bimbisāra rode his elephant by her house as she was sitting by the window, and she cast a garland of flowers to the king. "Come here," said the king.

The merchant's wife replied, "Majesty, I am too shy, you please come in." The king entered the house, where they enjoyed each other's company.

Noticing the cessation of her menstrual cycle, she realized she had conceived a child and said to the king, "Majesty, I am pregnant."

The king gave her some fine cloth and a ring seal and said, [60] "If the child is a girl, she is yours. If it is a boy, however, wrap him in this cloth, put the seal ring around his neck, and bring him to me."

After some time the merchant finished his business and set off for home. When he was close to Rājagṛha he sent a letter to his wife telling her he would be home in a few days. She thought to herself, "I have done this shameful deed. When he returns what am I going to do?" At a loss she explained the problem to the king.

He replied, "Do not worry. I will do all I can to delay his arrival." So saying, he sent a message to the merchant, which read, "Merchant, I need this and that jewel. Do not return without them." Accordingly the merchant turned round and set out on a long journey to find the jewels.

After nine months the merchant's wife gave birth to a beautiful and healthy baby boy. She fed him on ghee and honey, and when he had grown a little she tied the seal ring around his neck, wrapped him in the fine cloth, and put him in a box. To a female servant she said, "Go, take this box to the gates of the king's palace, build a fire, and wait to one side until the box is taken away."

The servant did as she was asked. The king with Kumāra Abhaya went to the upper palace and saw the fire burning. He turned to some workers and said, "Men, there is a fire by the palace gates. Go and see what it is."

The workers returned and said, "Majesty, it is a box."

"Bring it," said the king.

Kumāra Abhaya said, "Whatever is in the box, please give it to me."

"Very well," promised the king.

The box was brought to the king who ordered it to be open. Inside was a child. "What is this?" cried the king. "Is he dead or alive?"

"Majesty, the child is alive," replied the workers.

The king then recognized the cloth and the seal ring and gave the child to Kumāra Abhaya. [61] Because he was raised by Kumāra Abhaya, the child was known as Kumāra Bhṛtya—"Raised by Kumāra."

When he had grown, Kumāra Abhaya said to him, "Ajātaśatru has been destined for the throne since birth. You and I must learn the arts and crafts."

Later when Kumāra Bhṛtya saw men dressed in white he asked, "Who are these people?"

His father replied, "They are known as doctors, and they relieve the sufferings of illness."

Through the force of instincts from the past he said, "I too wish to be like them."

His request was granted, and he began to study medicine. However, he had not learned surgery on the human skull. Having discovered that Ātreya,[263] a master physician in Takṣaśila, had mastered this subject, Kumāra Bhṛtya desired to study under him, and armed with a letter from his father addressed to Padmagarbha,[264] the king of Takṣaśila, he set off to meet him. After his arrival the master had only to teach him a few times before he mastered it especially well.

On one occasion when the master went to treat a patient, he took Kumāra Jivaka[265] with him. He gave the patient medicine and they returned home. Jivaka thought to himself, "My master has a made a mistake. If the patient takes that medicine it will adversely affect him and he will die. The medicine my master has given is not good. I must do something."

He returned to the patient and said, "My master says not to take the previous medicine but to take these instead." Therefore in a skillful way he turned the situation around.

Later the master visited the patient and asked how he was. "I am better," he replied.

"You still have to take the medicine," said the doctor.

"The first or the second medicine?" asked the patient.

"I did not give you two medicines," said the master.

"You gave me the first and Jivaka gave me the second," replied the patient.

The master thought to himself, "I made a mistake. Jivaka is very wise." He was pleased with Jivaka and nearly always took him wherever he went.

The other students said to the master, "Master, because he is the son of a king you take delight in Jivaka and give teachings to him and not to us."

The master replied, "Jivaka is highly intelligent. Whatever I teach him he is able to comprehend. You cannot."

"How do you know this master," said the students, "let us see evidence of that."

So the master told them, "All of you, go to the market. Each of you, find out the prices of such and such item on sale and come back here." [62] When they returned the master questioned them on what they had learned. They only knew the prices of items they were asked to inquire of. Jivaka was able to recite the prices of all the items.

On another occasion they were sent to a pine forest on a hill and told to bring back everything that was not medicinal. The other students returned with many substances they thought were non-medicinal. Jivaka, however, realized that no substances there were not medicinal. However, he did pick up the root of arrow-reed grass and a piece of stone. On the road they met a shepherdess carrying a curd pot and whey sediment on her way to see the master. Seeing that she had great pain in her eyes, Jivaka cured her with medicine growing close at hand. In gratitude she offered him the pot of curd. Jivaka took the sediment instead and told her to keep the curd.

Further on the brahman students of Ātreya saw elephant footprints in the middle of the road and stopped to examine them. Jivaka also looked at them and asked, "What animal's footprints are these?"

"They are bull elephant's footprints," they replied.

"They are not," said Jivaka. "They are the footprints of a cow elephant. Furthermore, this cow is blind in the right eye, and today it will give birth to a male calf. It was being ridden by a lady who is also blind in her right eye and who will also give birth today to a son."

With these remarks they returned to the master. The brahman students showed their non-medicinal substances to him. "These are all medicines," said the master, and he proceeded to name the medicines and list the illnesses they treated.

Jivaka said, "All the substances were medicinal and so I have not brought any back. However, I do have these three items with me."

"What do they do?" they asked.

"If one has been stung by a scorpion, fumigating with the smoke of the arrow-reed root and treating the bite with whey sediment will relieve it. And this stone will crack a curd pot in the autumn."

At this the master smiled and the others thought, "The master is not pleased with Jivaka," and so they said, "Master, listen, not only this, but on the road he did not recognize a bull elephant's footprint but instead said the following." They related Jivaka's description.

"Is what you say true?" asked the master.

"It is true," replied Jivaka.

"How can you be so sure?" [63]

"Master," replied Jivaka, "I am from a royal family. Why should I not know these things? The footprint of a bull-elephant is circular, that of a female elephant is elongated. That it was blind in the right eye can be known from the fact that it ate grass from the left side. It is pregnant because the hind leg footprints were deeper than the front leg footprints. It will give birth today because its urine contained natal mucus. The calf will be male because the imprint of the right footprint was deeper than the left. That a lady was riding it can be known from the footprints she made when she dismounted to pass urine. She too is blind in her right eye because she picked flowers on the left side of the road. She is pregnant because the imprints of her heels were particularly impressed. She will give birth today because her urine contained sediment. If you do not believe me please go and make inquiries."

A student was sent to make inquiries and saw that everything was as Jivaka had described it. The master said to the other students, "Listen, this is how intelligent Jivaka is." The master then proceeded to teach Jivaka everything except skull surgery.

Once, someone who was suffering from a brain illness requested the master to treat him. "Today prepare a pit and some dung; I will come tomorrow," said the master.

On hearing this, Jivaka went to the man's house. "Whatever little I have learned," he said, "it is solely for the benefit of others. However, I have not been able to study the skull surgery. Hide me somewhere in your house so I can see how the operation is performed."

The patient agreed. The following day Ātreya arrived at the house. He opened the man's skull and with pincers began to extract an insect whose legs were firmly lodged to the man's brain. Jivaka cried out, "Master, do not do it in such a hurried way. This good man will die this very day."

"Well, how should it taken out?" asked the master.

"Master, heat the pincers, touch the insect on the back and its legs will withdraw. Then you will be able to remove it."

The pincers were heated as Jivaka suggested. The insect's mouth and legs were embedded in the brain but when it came into contact with the hot pincers, it was unable to maintain its hold and was gently removed from the brain, and the patient recovered.

His master was pleased with Jivaka and taught him everything about skull surgery. However, he said, "This is how I make my living. It would be best if you went and practiced somewhere else."

Jivaka prostrated to his master and went before King Padmagarbha before setting off. [64] The king told him, "There is distant land called Pāṇḍu that is in revolt against me. Go and subdue it."

Jivaka agreed and with a four-division army[266] gained surrender and extracted guarantees. The many gifts he received as tribute he gave to his master.

Later he went to the city of Bhadraṃkara, where he spent the rainy season. He studied the treatise, *Understanding the Language of All Creatures.* On his way out of the city he met a man carrying wood who was perspiring heavily and had been reduced to skin and bone. Jivaka asked him the reason for his condition: "I don't know. It happened when I picked up this wood," he replied.

Jivaka examined the bundle of wood and discovered in it a jewel that makes beings transparent. "Sell me this wood," said Jivaka. "How much do you want for it?"

"Five hundred *kārṣāpaṇa,*"[267] said the wood seller.

Jivaka paid him and took the jewel. Like a lamp that illuminates everything in a house, the quality of this jewel was that when it was placed before a sick person, the illness would at once be visible to the physician.

After some time he arrived at the city of Udumbara. There he saw a man striking his head with a measuring bowl. On being asked the reason for his behavior, the man told Jivaka he had an itching sensation in his brain. Jivaka examined the man with the jewel and saw an insect inside his brain. He performed the same operation he had seen his master perform and the man recovered. Jivaka was paid five hundred *kārṣāpaṇa,* which he sent to his teacher.

He traveled on to the country of Rohitaka. There a householder who had been very attached to his beautiful garden had died and been reborn as a ghost in the garden. There he killed many people, and as a result the garden had become deserted. After a while a person suffering from *muchu*[268] whom the doctors had given up on went to the garden to die.

That evening Jivaka stayed in the garden as well. There the ghost went to attack the sick man. However, the demon that caused the sickness appeared and said, "As I have already got him, what harm can you do? You have not been fumigated with the smoke of burnt goat hairs. If you were, you would have to flee for twelve leagues, wouldn't you?"

The ghost replied, "And no one has given you radish seeds mixed with buttermilk. If they had, you would have been broken into pieces, wouldn't you?"

Jivaka heard this discussion and subsequently gave the treatment to the sick person and the fumigation procedure to the son of the former householder. For his successful treatment, he received five hundred *kārṣāpaṇa,* which he immediately sent to his master.

He then traveled to the region of Mathurā. [65] One day he was resting under a tree. A wrestler had been injured in a fight that had severely disturbed his inner organs, and he had died. While his body was being carried out of his house, a vulture was sitting on a tree with her young. "I need food," said the young bird.

"Where will it come from?" said the mother.

"From the corpse of that wrestler."

"But Jivaka will bring him back to life."

"How?"

"By treating him with powders."

Jivaka listened to this discussion. He looked into his jewel, took his medicinal pipe, and administered powders to the man, who recovered as soon as the powder reached his internal organs. For this treatment he received five hundred *kārṣāpaṇa,* which he sent back to his teacher.

In Mathurā a householder died. He had been very attached to his beautiful wife, and so he was reborn as an insect inside her womb. From then on any man she had relations with would die, and therefore no one could touch her. She was brought to Jivaka. She took off her clothes and Jivaka placed a piece of meat by her vagina. The insect, attracted by meat, emerged and was disposed of. The woman recovered and Jivaka received five hundred *kārṣāpaṇa,* which he again sent to his teacher.

He traveled on to the river Yamunā. There he saw a fish tugging on the feet of a corpse, causing its eyes to open and shut. This led him to examine the connections between the sinews of the body. He traveled on to Vaiśālī. There a wrestler had thrust his hand into the face of another and put his eye out of socket. Jivaka pulled on the man's ankle, and the eye was restored to its socket. For this he received five hundred *kārṣāpaṇa,* which he gave to Āmrapālī, mother of his elder stepbrother, Kumāra Abhaya.

In Vaiśālī an insect had lodged itself in a man's ear and had given birth to about seven hundred baby insects, giving the man great cause for concern. Jivaka thought to himself, "Previously, I followed the technique taught by my master, but now I will follow my own idea."

He covered a palm leaf hut with a blue cloth. Inside he placed a drum, made the ground warm, and laid the man down. He sprinkled the ground with water and banged the drum. The insects thought it was the onset of summer, and some emerged from the ear. A piece of meat had been placed by the ear, and they returned into the ear to call the others. As they began to eat the meat they were disposed of. The man recovered and paid Jivaka five hundred *kārṣāpaṇa,* which he sent to Āmrapālī.

Jivaka traveled on to Rājagṛha, where he was to be welcomed by Ajātaśatru, but the two did not meet, and Jivaka entered the city through another gate.

At another time he was surrounded by a large crowd and became distracted. A brahman with an eye problem asked him for medicine. Irritated, Jivaka dismissed him by telling him to use dust. The man put the dust on his eyes and was cured. Later this man met with another. "Where are you going?" he asked. [66]

"I am on my way to see Jivaka for medicine."

"His medicine is dust," replied the former patient. Consequently, the man put dust on his eyes and was blinded.

Around that time, Jivaka's father, the king, developed an abscess on top of his head. He called his doctors and told them to treat it. "Your majesty," they replied, "When the master of medicine, Jivaka, is here, what could we possibly do?"

Jivaka was called and told to treat the abscess. "I will do as you ask if I may be permitted to give you your bath."

The king gave permission. Jivaka anointed the abscess with emblic myrobalan and prepared various ripening substances, which he added to five hundred vases of water. These he poured over the king's body. As the abscess matured, he was able to burst it with just a single strand of hair without the king feeling anything. Then he mixed healing substances with five hundred vases of water and poured them over the king's body. The king was completely healed, and his hair had even grown back on the spot. After the bath, the king said, "Begin the treatment."

"Your majesty, please have some food first," replied Jivaka.

Having eaten, the king again said, "Begin the treatment."

"Your majesty," said Jivaka, "The treatment is complete."

The king did not believe him and felt for the abscess with his hand but could not find it. He looked in the mirror but did not see it. He asked his queen but she could not find it. He was amazed and told his ministers to promote Jivaka to the level of master physician.

The man who had gone blind by applying dust to his eyes approached the king. "Your majesty, did you promote your son out of affection for him or because he is a wise doctor? If you did it because of his great skills, then those skills have made me blind."

"I have not seen you before," said Jivaka.

"That is true," replied the blind man; "But I was told by another who had followed your instructions."

"His constitution is one thing and your constitution is another. Now, follow my instructions," said Jivaka.

The blind man did as Jivaka asked and soon recovered his sight. He said to the king, "Majesty, he is truly a wise doctor; please honor him again."

Jivaka was placed upon an elephant, and with an array of offerings he was honored and hailed as great master physician.

In Rājagṛha lived a person suffering from a tumor for which the ordinary doctors could do nothing. He came to Jivaka to beg for treatment. When Jivaka told him that the particular medicine he needed was difficult to find, he thought, "Even Jivaka has abandoned me," and wandered off to the cemetery. There he ate the flesh of a mongoose and an iguana that had been fighting and fell into a blazing pyre, and drank the water that ran in the cemetery. Then he drank rancid ghee and *kodrava* grain mash found in a cattle enclosure. The tumor burst; he vomited and excreted, and was cured.

One time queen Vaidehī developed an abscess on her genitals. [67] "Treat your stepmother," said the king. Jivaka prepared some soft dough and asked the queen to sit on it. When removed he examined it and placed a porous cloth bag of ripening medicine in the dough and asked the queen to sit on it as before. The abscess burst and was cleaned with astringent water. Healing medicine was prepared, applied as before, and the queen was cured.

"Have you treated her?" asked the king.

"I have, your majesty," replied Jivaka.

"Did you see her unclothed body?"

"I did not," he replied, and explained the procedure.

The king was pleased and honored Jivaka once again.

The person who previously had the tumor came to the king and, like the person blinded by the dust, demurred at Jivaka's honor. "I did not treat this disease," said Jivaka, "because medicine for this illness is difficult to find."

"What are the difficulties?" asked the patient. Jivaka explained how one had to go to the cemetery on the fourteenth day of the waning moon, to the burning corpse of a pale skinned man, and so forth.

"Excellent," he exclaimed. "This is exactly what I did. Majesty, honor Jivaka in stone." Jivaka was duly honored.

Later, Ajātaśatru, urged on by Devadatta, killed his own father. Some time afterward he developed a tumor. He summoned many doctors but they were unable to help him. Therefore, Jivaka came to him and said, "You should eat the flesh of your son Udayibhadra."

"Are you after my kingdom?" he asked.

"There is no other cure," replied Jivaka.

Because Ajātaśatru had no regard for anyone but himself, he agreed. However, Jivaka hid the child, prepared some other human flesh, and gave it to Ajātaśatru. As he was about to eat it, Jivaka snatched it from him, hit him over the head with it, and said contemptuously, "How stupid you are! You kill your father and now you eat your own son."

Ajātaśatru became enraged. The swelling suddenly burst, he vomited and excreted, and he was cured. His son was returned to him and he was overjoyed. And Jivaka was honored for the third time.

By now Jivaka had become proud, thinking to himself, "There is no physician equal to me. The greatest healer of the body is me. The greatest healer of the mind is the Buddha." Therefore, he went to see the Buddha, and although he listened to him for some time, he did not see the truth. The Buddha saw the reason and took him to the Himalayas, the king of mountain ranges, where he told him to go and gather whatever medicine he wished.

"I am afraid," replied Jivaka, and so Buddha sent Vajrapāṇi with him.

After they had returned Buddha asked him to identify the medicines he had brought back. Although he knew most of them, there were many whose names he did not know, whereas Buddha was able to identify them and speak of their qualities. Jivaka asked, "Does the Buddha also know the science of healing?" [68]

"Jivaka," said the Buddha, "A doctor who possesses four qualities is fit to be in the company of a king, is essential to a king, is counted in the retinue of the king. What four are these? A pain-relieving doctor is one who knows about illness, who knows the origins of illness, who knows how to eradicate illness, and who knows how to ensure the illness does not return.

"What does it mean to know about illness? It means that the pain-relieving doctor recognizes illness, and is able to identify each illness. That is what it means to know about illness. What does it mean to know what causes illness? It means that the pain-relieving doctor knows the illness and is able to say that this illness is caused by wind, this by bile, this by phlegm, this by oneself, this by others, and this by a combination of these factors. That is what it means to know what causes illness. What does it mean to know how to eradicate illness? It means that the pain-relieving doctor knows the illness and knows that it will be eradicated by eye medicine, by massage, emetics, purgatives, nasal medication, fumigation, or enema. That is what it means to know how to eradicate illness. What does it mean to know how to ensure the illness does not return? It means that the doctor knows the illness and knows that following a particular regimen will ensure the illness does not return. That is what it means to know how to ensure the illness does not return. In this way a pain-relieving doctor who possesses these four qualities is fit to be in the company of a king, is essential to a king, is included in the retinue of the king.

"Likewise, the tathāgata, the arhat, the perfected buddha, possesses four qualities and is the supreme pain-relieving doctor. What are these four Jivaka? The tathāgata, the arhat, the perfected buddha, he knows that this is the truth of suffering, that this is the origin of suffering, that this is the cessation of suffering, and that this is the path of the noble ones that leads to the cessation of suffering. In this way he knows the truth exactly as it is.

"Jivaka, the doctor who relieves pain [69] does not know the medicine that eradicates the sufferings of birth. He does not know the medicine that eradicates the pains of old age, sickness, death, grief, anguish, distress, unhappiness, and disturbance. Jivaka, the tathāgata knows the medicine that puts an end to the sufferings of birth. He knows the medicine that ends all sufferings from aging to disturbance. Therefore, the tathāgata, the arhat, the perfected buddha, is the supreme pain-relieving doctor."

In this way Jivaka was taught different aspects of the Dharma, and then from the mouth of our Teacher came light that pervaded the medicine city of Sudarśana in the land of Oḍḍiyāna. The great Rishi Manasija appeared, and during the teaching of the tantra, Kumāra Jivaka was part of the audience. Therefore, although he did not need the transmission of the teachings, he was entrusted with the scripture. Our Teacher summoned King Bimbisāra, who had been reborn as the son of Vaiśravaṇa, and Jinarṣabha or Rājānaka Vajra Mārajit, and appointed them guardians of the tantra.

If you examine the above, thinking the three turnings of the wheel of Dharma were sequential events, discerning minds may raise some concerns regarding the discrepancies the narrative displays. However, from the highest perspective the three turnings were taught simultaneously, and in the inconceivable realm of perception that is the mystery of the Buddha the disorted perceptions of ordinary beings are no basis for argument.

At this time Kumāra Jivaka Bhṛtya developed the eye of Dharma, free of all obstruction, free of all taints, for all phenomena. Then Kumāra Jivaka saw the Dharma and heard the Dharma. He penetrated to the very depths of the Dharma and passed over all doubts and hesitancy. He no longer needed to rely on others, no longer needed to be guided by others. He gained the state of fearlessness toward the teachings given to him by the Buddha. He rose from his seat, draped his shawl over his shoulder, placed his hands together, bowed to the Buddha, and said, "I the monk have been elevated, truly elevated. I go for refuge to the Bhagavān, to the Dharma, and to the Sangha of monks. Please accept me as an *upāsaka*. From today for as long as I live, I go for refuge even if it should cost me my life." In this way he saw the truth. [70]

At that time the Himalayas were permanently covered in snow and very windy, and the Buddha became ill with a cold disorder. Jivaka thought to himself, "Like a universal emperor, I alone am here to perform service the Bhagavān."

He mixed purgative medicine with thirty-two *utpala* flowers and offered them to the Buddha to ingest as a nasal purgative. The Bhagavān accepted the medicine, and the purging was performed thirty-two times. Then Jivaka asked, "Has the purgative worked?"

The Buddha replied, "Jivaka, part of the disorder has been stirred without being purged, part has been purged without being stirred, part has been both purged and stirred, and part has been neither purged nor stirred. In that case, offer molasses and myrobalan and perform the purging once again." Jivaka did as he was asked and the illness subsided.

Jivaka's practice was that whoever he treated, be it kings, ministers, or anyone in need, he did it as work for the community or as an act of offering.

In chapters 23 and 24 of the *Short Vinaya* are the following accounts.[269] The son of Anantanemi, king of Avanti, was born at the same moment as the Bhagavān, and at that time the whole world shone with light owing to the Buddha's power. The king thought this was a sign brought on by his son's birth and so named him Pradyota, meaning "shining." Pradyota possessed the five forces, the five secondary forces, the elephant Nalagiri, which could cover a distance of a hundred leagues in one day, the she-elephant Bhadravat, which could cover eighty leagues in one day, the camel Samudrapada, which could cover seventy leagues in one day, the horse Ambarakaṇṭha, which could cover fifty leagues in one day, and the messenger Kāka, who could cover twenty leagues in one day. These were known as the *five limbs*. He had everything, but he suffered from insomnia, and he had an aversion to ghee and a liking for alcohol.

His doctors had prepared special medicine and mixed it with ghee, but when they tried to administer it, he refused to drink it, and even the word *ghee* was banished from his presence.

In the first part of the night he enjoyed himself with his queens, and in the second part he went to look at his horses and elephants. In the third part of the night he called to his night watchmen, and those who did not answer had their heads cut off. Therefore, he became known as Caṇḍapradyota, meaning Pradyota the Fearsome. [71]

Because of his insomnia, everybody had to take it in turns to act as night watchmen. One night it was the turn of a son of an incense seller. He was concerned that he might fall asleep, not hear the summons, and so lose his life. He therefore bribed a storyteller with five hundred *kārṣāpaṇa* to take his place. This storyteller was a clever man and kept the king amused with various stories, which are listed in the summary verse:

> The owl, crane, and *munjā* reed,
> the black-faced monkey and the partridge,
> a pot, salt, flour, and a corpse,
> a pit, a weaver, a potter, and a scorpion.

These stories concerned how an owl with feathers weighs the same as an owl without feathers; how a crane drinking water mixed with milk is able to drink the milk and discard the water; how *munjā* reed whether beaten or not beaten with a hammer weighs the same; how the tail of a black-faced monkey is the same length as its body; how the wings of the partridge have equal areas of color and non-color; how a pot full of water can be poured into a pot full of sand without overflowing; how a handful of water can be poured into a handful of salt and not increase; how a handful of water mixed with a handful of fine flour becomes neither thick nor thin; how a living body and its corpse do not weigh the same; how earth dug out of a pit does not fit back in again; how a weaver spent all day and night weaving cloth and a potter spent all day and night making pots, yet nobody knew where their products went. With these stories, backed up with reasons and evidence, he kept the king amused.

When the stories were over, the king said, "You seem to know everything; what is the cause of my insomnia?"

"Will you guarantee my safety if I tell you?"

"I will," replied the king.

"It is because you were born from a scorpion," said the storyteller.

"How do you know this? Prove it to me," demanded the king.

A pit was dug and filled with dry cow dung. On top of this was placed the king's mattress. As soon as he lay down he fell asleep. On waking he realized that what the storyteller had said was true.[270] Nevertheless, the king asked his mother about this.

"Will you guarantee my safety?" she asked.

"I will. Now tell me."

"Your father had a large harem of queens, and when he went away to other places, to them, during my menstruation periods, I would go to bathe. Once, while bathing, I saw a scorpion and thought, 'If only this were a man.' By the power of these lustful thoughts, the scorpion took the form of a man and we made love. This is how you were born."

The king thought to himself, "That storyteller is very clever. Even if he tells this to others, I can't kill him because I have promised him protection. However, I could send him elsewhere." Therefore, he gave the storyteller five hundred *kārṣāpaṇa* and sent him away. [72]

The insomnia became worse and he brought together his doctors and ordered them to cure it. They replied, "We are unable to treat this problem. However, in Rājagṛha, lives Kumāra Jivaka Bhṛtya, a master of medicine and the son of King Bimbisāra. He will be able to treat this illness."

A letter was sent to him, and just before he set out on his journey, Jivaka asked the messenger or servant about the nature of the illness. He then made up some ghee that had the smell, taste, and color of alcohol, and set off. On the way, in the district of Kanyakubja, he met a young doctor, who offered Jivaka myrobalan. "What is this illness of King Caṇḍapradyota?" asked Jivaka.

"He suffers from insomnia," replied the doctor. "Ghee would help him but he detests ghee and loves alcohol. Anyone who even mentions the word *ghee* in his presence is executed. Therefore, we dare not treat him."

"It is for that reason," said Jivaka, "that I boiled some ghee and mixed in it the color of alcohol, the smell of alcohol, and the taste of alcohol. When I give you the signal, give him this much of this ghee and then wait on him for a while."

Together they set off for Avanti. When they arrived Caṇḍapradyota received them with due ceremony, invited them inside, and then requested treatment from them. In order to familiarize himself with his plan of escape, Jivaka said that he needed to go out and search for some rare medicine. He mounted the she-elephant Bhadravat, which was able to travel eighty leagues in one day, and after an appropriate time returned to the king. He told the king first to bathe and then take his midday meal. Then giving the signal to the young doctor, he said, "Majesty, please drink what I have brought for you." With these words he left and fled the palace.

As soon as the king had drunk the medicine he fell asleep. He awoke in the middle of the night and belched up some ghee. He became angry and wanted to kill Jivaka. When he realized he had fled, this deceitful king sent the messenger Kāka, who could travel twenty leagues in a day, on the elephant Nalagiri, which could cover a hundred leagues in one day, in pursuit of Jivaka, saying, "Don't accept anything that trickster gives you, but bind him by the neck and bring him here."

As Kāka became closer, his elephant was somewhat held up by the smell of a she-elephant's urine. Finally, he caught up with Jivaka in a grove of emblic myrobalan. [73] As he was about to lead him away, Jivaka said, "Kāka, what's the hurry? Have some myrobalan."

"My master told me not to accept anything from you."

"Well, let's each eat half," suggested Jivaka.

Jivaka cut the fruit in half with his fingernail, which was harboring a purgative, and gave that half to Kāka, who took it and was thoroughly purged. He left him on a hillside and told the people living there, "These three are cherished by the king.[271] Do such and such practice and return them to him. Otherwise, you will seriously suffer." With these words he returned to Rājagṛha.

Meanwhile the ghee potion prepared by Jivaka had cured the king of insomnia. Kāka too had been cured of his leprosy. When he returned to the palace, the king questioned him about Jivaka.

"He escaped," said Kāka.

"That is not good," said the king.

"What was I supposed to do when I caught him?"

"Kill him, of course."

"But your majesty," protested Kāka, "hasn't he cured us both of our ailments?"

"So, what should we do?" asked the king.

"Surely, we should reward him," replied Kāka.

"That is good. I will do that," said the king.

The king therefore sent a large amount of money to Jivaka, who returned it, saying, "I have money. It would be better to give the money to the young doctor."

This the king did, and he sent Jivaka also a beautiful cloth worth one hundred thousand *kārṣāpaṇa*. Jivaka offered this cloth to the Bhagavān, and from it was made a set of the three robes for the Buddha, an upper and lower robe for Ānanda, and a small supplementary robe for Rāhula.

At that time there was a young monk suffering from a growth resulting from faulty diet and behavior. Jivaka pierced the growth, and the monk's suffering was relieved.

Once when the Bhagavān was residing in the Kalandaka Nivās bamboo grove, Ānanda developed an abscess on his head, and the Buddha asked Jivaka to treat him. While Ānanda was listening to the teachings of the Bhagavān, Jivaka applied ripening medicine to the abscess, and there, not having moved from his seat, he was cured without the slightest sensation of pain.

Once the Bhagavān himself was ill and told this to Jivaka, who thought to himself, "The Bhagavān's vajra body is large. The small amount of medicine needed to treat an ordinary being will not be sufficient."

Therefore, he prepared the medicine known as iron-arrow medicinal ghee using thirty-two measures of ghee and offered it to the Bhagavān, who accepted it and was cured. Devadatta thought to himself, "I, too, will take the same amount of medicine." He approached Jivaka: "Jivaka, how much ghee did you give to the monk Gautama?"

"I gave him thirty-two measures," replied Jivaka. [74]

"Well then, I will take the same," retorted Devadatta.

"The Bhagavān's vajra body is large," replied Jivaka. "Such a powerful body can digest that much. You would not be able to digest it."

Devadatta replied, "I also have a vajra body, so why can't I digest it?" With these words he drank thirty-two measures of the same medicine.

The next day Jivaka offered the Bhagavān some broth. Devadatta also took some broth on top of his undigested ghee, and as a result his stomach distended, reaching a precarious point and leaving him feeling wretched and in a sorry state. Ānanda spoke of this to the Bhagavān, who, like an elephant with his trunk, stretched out his right hand adorned with an auspicious wheel and laid it on Devadatta's head, saying, "I declare that the way I regard Rāhula, my beautiful and only son, is no more and no less than the way I regard Devadatta. By the truth of these words may this illness of Devadatta be cured." No sooner had he spoken these words than Devadatta was cured.

Devadatta, however, recognized Buddha's hand upon him and said, "Siddhartha, you have obviously become proficient in medicine, too, but I am not interested."

Once, a piece of stone fired by Devadatta in a catapult injured the large toe of the Bhagavān's foot. When the bleeding would not stop, Jivaka, the master physician, remained constantly by the Buddha's side in order to treat him. The people of Rājagṛha gathered. "This medicine is good," said some; "But this medicine is better," said others.

Jivaka said, "There is medicine that will help at once, but it is hard to find."

"What is it?" asked Ānanda.

"It is called *gośīrṣa* sandalwood," replied Jivaka.

After some time a merchant offered some *gośīrṣa* sandalwood to the Buddha. Accepting it the Buddha prophesized that as a result of his virtuous deed, he would become the pratyekabuddha Candandatta, "Giver of Sandalwood."

However, the bleeding did not stop. Jivaka said, "Now we must apply the milk of a young mother who has given birth to her first son."

In Rājagṛha was a young mother who had little milk and a thirsty child. However, she thought, "For me to be without my son is not important." She offered her milk to the Buddha, who prophesized that she would become the pratyekabuddha Kṣīradatta, "Giver of Milk." [75]

In Rājagṛha at that time lived a monk whose penis was very painful. He showed it to Jivaka. "Put it in the mouth of a woman," said Jivaka. This he did and was immediately cured.[272]

King Ajātaśatru had killed his father, a Dharma king who had insight into the nature of phenomena. Together with Devadatta he had spilled the blood of the Buddha with ill intent. He had caused a schism in the community of monks and had killed the nun Utpalavarṇī. In this way he had committed four heinous crimes, and as a result his body was plagued with burning sores, and moreover, the whole of Magadha was pervaded by a putrid smell. One day a voice came from the skies: "Great king, on the eighth day of the next month, the earth will open up, and you will be sucked down into the great hell."

Ajātaśatru went to the six non-Buddhist teachers and asked them how he could purify himself of his crimes, but they were unable to help. He was now overcome with remorse and regret, and he suffered relentlessly. Jivaka the master physician came to him and said, "The perfectly enlightened Buddha is residing in Mallavāstu. Go to him. Ask him what to do, and your sufferings will be ended."

The king replied, "Jivaka, Bhagavān Buddha is surrounded by arhats, immersed in the very heart of the Dharma. How can someone like me who belongs in the hell realms possibly go there?"

"Great king," said Jivaka, "Do not be so concerned. The Bhagavān Buddha does not only teach intelligent disciples like Śāriputra but also unintelligent disciples such as Kāpatha. He does not only accept alms from the rich, such as King Prasenajit, but also from the poor, such as Vasi. He has the same feelings for Devadatta, who has tried to hurt him many times, as he does for his only son, the good and beautiful Rāhula. He will definitely relieve your remorse."

"Jivaka, in that case, you and I shall mount an elephant and go before the Tathāgata. If on the way the earth opens up to take me to hell, hold me and prevent me falling," replied the king.

They mounted the elephant, and with a crowd of many thousands they traveled to Mallavāstu. [76] There the Bhagavān was sitting amid an ocean-like gathering of gods and men. Suddenly he called out twice, "Great king, great king!" Those in the gathering and even Ajātaśatru himself wondered whom among the assembly the Buddha was referring to. Was it Brahmā, or Indra, or a great emperor from another country?

The third time, the Buddha said, "Great king, Ajātaśatru!"

When he heard this Ajātaśatru fainted with joy. Water was sprinkled on his face to bring him round, and he said, "Bhagavān, I confess; I confess the wrong deeds of myself and of all living beings as vast in number as the realms of space." Three times he repeated this.

The Bhagavān said, "Noble one of the royal caste! Excellent! Excellent! As well as confessing your own wrong deeds, you confess those of all living beings. This is wonderful!"

Having purified himself of his wrong actions, he went on to gain forbearance in appropriate practice.[273]

Jivaka had skillfully turned Ajātaśatru away from wrong teachers. He himself had been honored three times as a master physician. He studied the basic principles of Āyurveda under the Takṣaśila doctor Ātreya, and yet the accounts of his knowledge from the very outset of his practice—his ability to recognize illness, his knowledge of medicine preparation, his skill in removing an insect safely from the brain—all indicate that he had become more learned than his master. Moreover, he is still alive today because he attained the *vidyādhara* of longevity.

6. Nāgārjuna, Pitṛceṭa, and Candranandana

The contribution of the glorious Nāgārjuna to the science of medicine

In the tradition of the science of medicine, Jivaka's disciple was Nāgārjuna. *Entering Laṅka Sutra* says:

> Mahāmati, you should know this:
> in the south, in the region of Vedalī,[274]
> will arise a monk of great renown.
> He will be known as Nāga,
> and he will destroy the extremes
> of existence and nonexistence.
> To the world he will teach my doctrine
> in the form of the sublime Mahayana,
> attaining the level known as Joyous,
> and be reborn in the land of Sukhāvatī.[275] [77]

And in the thirty-sixth chapter of the *Mañjuśrī Root Tantra:*

> Four hundred years after the Tathāgata passes away,
> the monk known as Nāga will appear,
> of great faith and benefit to the doctrine;
> he will attain the level known as Joyous
> and live for six hundred years.
> This great being will gain Mahāmayūrī knowledge[276]
> and will master the meanings of various teachings
> and the meaning of nonreality.
> When he leaves his mortal form,
> he will be reborn in Sukhāvatī.
> Finally, he will without doubt
> become a buddha.[277]

Furthermore, the *Great Cloud Sutra,*[278] the *Later Kālacakra Tantra,*[279] and many other texts prophesized the glorious guide and pioneer Nāgārjuna, famed as the second teacher of the Conqueror's precious doctrine.

His life is as follows. In the southern district of Vedalī lived a wealthy brahman who had no son. In a dream it was foretold that if he invited one hundred brahmans and made offerings to them, he would have a son. He did as the deity suggested and was rewarded with a beautiful son. The son was shown to a seer, who said that the child indeed had auspicious marks but that he would not live beyond seven days. His father asked what could be done. He was told that if he invited and made offerings to one hundred brahmans, the child would live for seven months, but if he did the same for one hundred monks, the child would live for seven years. The parents followed this advice.

As the seven years drew to a close the parents were unable to bear the thought of seeing their child as a corpse, and so, accompanied by an attendant, they sent the boy away. At the gates of Nālandā Monastery the child recited some verses from the *Sāmaveda.* Overhearing this, Brahman Saraha invited them inside, where they explained the reason for their journey. Saraha said that if the boy were to become ordained, he could avoid his fate. He therefore became a monk. He was initiated into the mandala of Amitāyus and told to recite mantras. As a result he received signs indicating that he had been released from the hold of the lord of death.

He studied and became learned in all fields of knowledge, especially the three baskets of scriptures, and the vast ocean-like collection of new and old tantras, including the vidyādhara tantras of the old translations.

Later on he again met his parents, who at first refused to believe it was their son, but he explained what had happened and dispelled their doubts.

He took the full ordination of a monk from Rāhula Śrībhadra, the abbot of Nālandā, and received the ordination name of Bhikṣu Śrīmata.

He propitiated deities such as Mahāmayūrī, Kurukullā, the nine yakṣī, and Mahākāla [78] and gained many attainments, including the power of the pill, eye ointment, sword, speed, essence medicine, and earth treasures, among others, as well as the power to kill and bring back to life. He brought under his control all kinds of nonhuman beings, such as nāgas and yakṣas. In particular he mastered the art of elixirs and gained the vajra body. He also developed clairvoyance and the power of miraculous display.

He thought that if he mastered the Mahākāla *vidyā* mantra, he could bring back the *Mahākāla Tantra* from Dhānyakaṭaka, where it resided. When he arrived there he invoked Acala and created an illusory display. While the ḍākinīs were distracted by his illusion, he carried off the tantra of goddess Kālī and the eight tantras of Mahākāla, the *Kurukulle kalpa,*[280] and others. He received teachings from the gnosis ḍākinīs and brought to this world 160 different sādhanas.

Once there was a twelve-year famine in the land of Magadha, and when the towns and cities had almost emptied, Nāgārjuna introduced a large number of monks to the alchemical production of gold. After the famine had ended, Rāhula Śrībhadra came to hear of it and remarked, "This was not good. When I have the power to bring about rains of food, you involve the monks in wrong livelihood. You are a man of little compassion. What you did goes against bodhisattva conduct. To purify this wrong you must construct 108 temples, one thousand shrines, and ten thousand stupas."

Nāgārjuna realized that one monk could not possibly accomplish these tasks alone. He begged the necessary money from the yakṣa Jambala and decided to entrust the actual work to the nāgas. With the *vidyā* mantra of Kurukullā, he summoned the two daughters of the nāga king Takṣaka with their attendants. When these two nāgas and their large retinues sat in human form amid the congregation at the teachings, the air around for a few leagues was permeated with the aroma of *gośīrṣa* sandalwood. Nāgārjuna asked the two nāgas for some sandalwood to construct a statue of Tārā and for some workers to help in the construction of the temples. "We will ask our father and give you our answer," they replied.

The next morning the young girls appeared again with a message from their father, who said that only if the Ācārya himself came to the land of the nāgas would he do as the Ācārya asks. Seeing the added advantage of bringing back the *One Hundred Thousand Perfection of Wisdom Sutra* and other texts, he traveled to the land of the nāgas. [79]

When he arrived there, he found many monks from the time of Buddha Kāśyapa, Buddha Kanakamuni, and others, whose bodies were larger than the others, as well as many arhats from our Teacher residing in the land of the nāgas as objects of reverence. They asked him, "We are arhats, whereas you are a human being possessed by the three poisons. How is it you were not harmed by the nāga poison in coming here?"

"By my attainment of the *vidyā* mantra of Mahāmayūrī," replied Nāgārjuna.

He satisfied the nāgas with Dharma and brought the *One Hundred Thousand Perfection of Wisdom Sutra* and many *dhāraṇī* and *kalpa* rituals back to this world.

He defeated in debate the monk Śaṅkara and others who had an aversion to the Mahayana. He buried in the ground many polemic texts written by the Saindhava[281] śrāvakas that argued against the Mahayana, which had become widespread.

In the south, in a place known as Jaṭāsaṃghāta, he defeated a gathering of about five hundred non-Buddhists and converted them to Buddhism.

On mountains such as Ghaṇṭa Rock and Dhīkoṭa in the north, he wanted to produce gold through alchemy. However, Tārā told him that this would lead to controversy in the future, and so he refrained.

On the way to the northern land of Uttarakuru, he came across a group of children playing. He picked out one of them and predicted that he would one day become a king. He stayed in Uttarakuru for twelve years working for the sake of humans and non-humans and then returned. The child had by then become King Udayibhadra and served and devoted himself to Nāgārjuna.

One time some baseless slander was leveled against the ācārya, but with the help of miraculous feats performed by Āryadeva, he was able to dispel them.

He had a vision of Tārā, who gave him a prophecy.

He is *Nāga* because, born into the dharmadhātu, he does not dwell in the extreme of existence or nonexistence, because he has control over the treasury of the jewels of the Buddha's teachings, and because he possesses a view that burns and illuminates.[282] *Arjuna* means "ruler," and he is called *Arjuna* because he governs the kingdom of Dharma and rules by subduing the foes of delusion. These two terms through the process of euphonic amalgamation *(sandhi)* become Nāgārjuna.

In his compositions on sutra and tantra, as illustrated by his six philosophical texts on the Madhyamaka free of extremes[283] and his *Compendium of Tantra,*[284] his contribution to the sciences has been enormous. Specifically, in the field of medicine:

> Taking the very essence of the countless tantras
> from the renowned science of medicine,
> here is compiled a hundred preparations
> praised by the masters of medicine.[285] [80]

This is from his *Hundred Medical Preparations.* Also:

> Having paid homage to the physician supreme,
> dispeller of the sicknesses of delusion,

I will write this *Sutra of Life*
not for those rishis of elevated conduct
but for those of intelligent minds,
who by living a healthy life of conscientious conduct
in accord with the humors of wind, bile, and phlegm
will give meaning to this human life.[286]

This is from his *Sutra of Life*. The following texts among others are also said to have been composed by Nāgārjuna: *Ritual of Ava Medicine, Secret Ambrosia: Preparation of Medicinal Plants, Precious Medicine, Jewel Garland Preparation of Mercury,* and *Treatment for the Four Kinds of Lhok and Infectious Fevers.*[287]

He founded many shrines and temples. He surrounded the vajra seat of Bodhgāya with stone mesh fencing and was instrumental in constructing edifices at Dhānyakaṭaka in the south.

It is generally accepted that Nāgārjuna lived and worked for the welfare of others for six hundred years, although the early translations talk of a thousand years. Kumāra Śaktimān, the son of king Udayibhadra, told his mother that he was in a hurry to ascend the throne. His mother replied, "The lifespan of your father is linked to that of Ācārya Nāgārjuna's by the elixir power of longevity. He will not die. Previous heirs to the throne have also died without becoming king." This made the son very upset. His mother said, "If you are so unhappy, go to the ācārya and ask for his head. He is a bodhisattva and will give it to you. If the ācārya dies, your father will also die, and you will surely become king."

Kumāra Śaktimān did as his mother suggested. The ācārya offered his head, but no sword could cut it off. "In the past I cut the head off an insect with a blade of grass. I have yet to experience the ripening of that act. Therefore, take some *kuśa* grass and cut off my head," suggested the ācārya. As the blow was struck, bodhicitta[288] flowed from the wound, and the ācārya said, "I am going to the world of Sukhāvatī. Later I shall again return to this body." With these words he died.

Since the ācārya had developed the elixir siddhi, the prince feared that the head and body would rejoin, and so he carried the severed head many leagues away, where some sources maintain it was taken by a yakṣī. However, the head was placed in the crevice of a boulder, which split apart, and a five-deity stone statue of Ārya Avalokiteśvara sprung forth naturally. The yakṣī funded the building of two temples, one for the head and one for the body.

Previously these temples were about four leagues apart. Now they are separated by less than a kilometer.[289] The walls of the temples have joined to look like a large rock, and it is a strange and frightening place. [81] It is said that looking through an opening, one sees the head and body as separate parts of a stone statue. Gradually the head is moving toward the body, and it is said that sometime in the future the ācārya will return to work for the welfare of living beings.

The contribution of Pitṛceṭa[290] *to the science of medicine*

According to the science of medicine's own system, the medical disciple of Nāgārjuna was Śrī Pitṛceṭa. In the thirty-sixth chapter of the *Mañjuśrī Root Tantra:*

> While I was happily residing
> with a group of disciples in the bamboo grove
> of the delightful city of Rājagṛha,
> a crow let his droppings fall upon me
> yet nevertheless developed faith in me,
> and as a result will be reborn into a higher realm.
>
> Moving on from the celestial realms,
> he will be reborn a human
> and become ordained into my doctrine.
> Possessed of great qualities and great ethics,
> he will be very learned and a preacher of Dharma,
> one of strict conduct known as Mātṛceṭa.
>
> At that time he will appear
> and will honor me by way of praise.
> By various means and to benefit all living beings,
> he will perform his practices well;
> and finally this intelligent being
> will come to the omniscience of enlightenment.[291]

His birthplace, according to Drukpa Pema Karpo,[292] was in the south, but I have not seen any authority for this. Most scholars, including Butön and the

Jonang tradition,[293] maintain it was in the east, and in a previous composition, *Cleaning the Beryl,*[294] I say the same. However, according to the early scholar Shangtön Shikpo in his *Compendium of Knowledge: Blazing from the Top of a Victory Banner,* this ācārya in his previous life was born in the east, where he took the eight-branched precepts from a forest monk. However, some outsiders from the west came and praised Mahādeva.[295] He became his follower and prayed to be cared for by Mahādeva. As a result his precepts waned, and he was reborn in the lower realms. When the coarse karma of his wrong deeds had expired, he was reborn in a Kashmiri city in the west. [82] Moreover, as will be made clear later, he was an ancestor of the Kashmiri Candranandana.

From these and other references we can say the following. He was born in the west, in Kashmir, near the palace of King Kaniṣka, where his father was a great physician who had mastered the eight branches of medicine in the brahman Vedic tradition. In Sanskrit he is known as Siṃhaguhya. Some translations render this Sengé Bepa (Siṃhagupta), others as Gendün Sangwa (Saṃghaguhya). These days it might be easier to refer to him as Sengé Sangwa (Siṃhaguhya). His mother was called Ratnasiddhi in Sanskrit, also known as Dedenma (Satyaśālinī) in Tibetan. In Tibetan the Sanskrit translates as Rinchen Ngödrup. While she was carrying her child, she received many auspicious omens, such as dreams of flying, and so she approached a brahman seer, who said:

> Beautiful, holding the medicine vase,
> looking with eyes of joy,
> of fragrant and glowing complexion,
> may he become the conqueror of pain.[296]

Because of this prediction the child at birth was named Pīyūṣa Kalaśa, "vase of ambrosia." He grew into a beautiful child, and because of his devotion to his parents he was known as Pitṛceṭa Mātṛceṭa, "obedient to father and mother." Before long he became learned in brahman philosophy, comprised of the four Vedas, the four subsidiary Vedas, the four branch Vedas, the six activities, and so on. He was henceforth known as Maticitra—"a beautiful mind." In particular, he studied medicine with his father, and because he mastered it with ease, his father said:

> Kaliṅga was the master of war,
> Trapuṣa the master of business,

> the beautiful Prabhāvatī was mistress of the grove,
> glorious Śūra is the master of medicine.[297]

Henceforth, he was known as Śūra.

His mother had great devotion for the teachings of the Buddha. Yet despite her urging he entered the non-Buddhist outsider doctrine because of the causal factor of the crow droppings falling on the Buddha's head and the power of his prayers made during his previous birth in the east. At that time he became known for his beautiful voice, and was henceforth also known as Aśvaghoṣa—"the song of the horse."

He became learned in the tradition of the outsiders with their philosophy of permanence. He decided to make a pilgrimage to the Maheśvara shrine of Liṅgaśvara Prasiddha in the western land of Oḍḍiyāna. As he was about to set off, his parents asked him to delay his journey, but he did not listen to them, and he became known as Pitṛceṭa Mātṛceṭa—one who is and who is not obedient to his father.[298]

Arriving at the shrine he bathed in the nearby bathing pool and sat on a seat of leaves and grass. He ate some rice and vowed that he would not rise from that place and not eat a single grain of rice nor drink a drop of water until he had invoked Maheśvara. Thus he practiced with great devotion, and after seven days he received a vision of Maheśvara. "What power do you seek?" asked Maheśvara.

"I want to be victorious everywhere," he replied. [83]

Maheśvara stated, "Be accompanied at all times by Brahmā, Viṣṇu, and Sarasvatī. Whenever they are unable to defeat others, I will enter your heart and debate. If your opponents cannot be conquered by any means, then the fire of anger will pour from your mouth and burn them up."

Granted, therefore, the siddhi of invincibility in debate with any womb-born human, he was accompanied by Sarasvatī in the form of his pandit sister, learned in language and logic, by Brahmā in the form of his pandit parrot, learned in language, and by Viṣṇu in the form of his "chalk" pandit, which could make the words of logic and language appear miraculously. He was told to destroy the doctrine of the Buddha until only its name remained. Consequently, he debated and defeated pandits in the west, causing the Buddha's doctrine to decline and forcing many to convert to the outsider doctrine. He thus became known as the black Durdharṣa—"difficult to conquer."

Once he was with his mother and saw her performing her devotions before a painting of Tārā. "Who is this?" he enquired.

"This is a Buddhist deity," she replied.

"Are there still Buddhists?" he asked.

"Son," replied his mother, "The doctrine of the Buddha is like the body of a horse. Those you have defeated in this uncivilized western land are only the ears of that horse. The rest of this country is filled with Buddhists."

On hearing this he prepared to travel to the south. However, his mother realized that there were none in the south who could defeat him and therefore urged him, "If you really desire fame in debate you should travel to the central Buddhist country itself. There, those with the power of wisdom shine like the multitude of stars in the nighttime sky. Go and beat the drum of victory in debate over them!"

He took his mother's advice and set out with his retinue. When he arrived in the vicinity of Nālandā Monastery, he met a girl carrying a pot of water on her head and her hands on her hips. "Where is the Nāgalandā Monastery?" he asked.

"Fool from some uncivilized land, you are ridiculed by your own words! What are you saying?" she retorted. "You should say, 'the glorious Nālandā Monastery, home of many a great scholar.'"

Chastened by these words he was suddenly plagued by doubt. Nevertheless, he traveled on to Nālandā, with its seven great *gaṇḍola* halls, its fourteen temples, and its fifteen hundred pandits. There he introduced himself to the monks, "I am the tīrthika, Durdharṣa the black. I have debated and defeated the Buddhists in the west. I have ousted all the identifying signs of the *śramaṇa* Gautama and replaced them with the outsider signs of longhair, deerskins, staffs, and drinking bottles colored with ash. [84] Such converts are in my retinue now. I will debate with you. If you win, I will jump and drown with my retinue in the Ganges. If I beat you, you will convert to the tīrthika doctrine."

He strung the letters of this proclamation onto a well-composed thread of words and pinned them to the four doors of the monastery and prepared to debate. The whole monastery knew they could not defeat him, and so they beat the *gaṇḍi* drum and convened a secret meeting. There they concluded, "This person is the outsider Aśvaghoṣa prophesized by the Bhagavān in his peerless sutras. Only the miraculously born Āryadeva can tame him. Therefore we must invite him here."

Some writers say that this was revealed to the monks in a dream. However it happened, the pandits of the central country planned to call Nāgārjuna and his disciple the lotus-born Āryadeva from Śrīparvata in the south.

However, Aśvaghoṣa came to hear of this plan, and so he lay down in front of the main gate to cut off the path saying, "Now, no one can enter and no one can leave."

The monks went to their midday meal and locked the door. Inside they realized that were they to send an invitation by foot, the ācārya and his disciple would arrive too late for the debate, and that this was a critical time for the doctrine of the Buddha. The crown jewel of the fifteen hundred pandits was Bhikṣu Mahāsthavirā Nagendra Gupta. Tears flowed from his eyes through his love for the doctrine of the Buddha as he hurriedly wrote:

> Alas, the chariot of the teachings
> sinks in the mud of tīrthika debate.
> Here we are powerless,
> our strength weakens.
> This burden lies with you,
> now is the time to shoulder it.

The letter was placed in a offering dish. From the heart of a statue of Mahākāla emerged a crow, which took the letter in its beak and in an instant was in Śrīparvata. Ācārya Nāgārjuna said, "Aśvaghoṣa is damaging the teachings. I will go and stop him."

Āryadeva replied, "The ācārya should not go. I will go instead."

"We will see if you can defeat him or not," said Nāgārjuna. The ācārya took the philosophical position of Aśvaghoṣa, debated with Āryadeva, and beat him. Some writers say that Āryadeva actually won the debate, but because of the ācārya's supreme skill in outsider philosophy, Āryadeva lost faith. How could that be correct? [85] Whatever happened, he threw his boots and accidentally struck the ācārya on the eye. He was at once filled with remorse and asked the ācārya to punish him. "At the time you saw me as an outsider," said Nāgārjuna, "so this is not a serious fault. However, if on the road a mendicant approaches you, do not be attached to whatever they ask for."

Before he set out, Āryadeva began to wonder, "What if I cannot defeat this tīrthika?"

"You need not have such doubts," said the ācārya. "Once, our Teacher was in the bamboo grove teaching the Dharma amid his disciples when a crow above let its droppings fall onto his head. The crow developed great faith in our Teacher in that moment. The disciples wondered at this occurrence and asked the Buddha what it foretold. Our Teacher replied, 'This crow will at some later time become the tīrthika Durdharṣa the black and will cause great harm to my doctrine. No womb-born human will have any chance of defeating him.'

"In the gathering of disciples was the young son of the Licchavi, Puṣpapaṇīkāra. He prayed, 'At that time, may I be born miraculously, defeat that tīrthika, and lead him to the Buddhist teachings.' Our Teacher concurred with this prayer. That young boy was you. Therefore, because of your prayer and because that crow subsequently developed faith, you will be able to defeat him and lead him to the Buddhist doctrine. Now go."

Āryadeva set off and traveled with the aid of miraculous power. On the road an earth goddess manifesting as a brahman appeared and asked him for an eye, which he promptly gave.

Outside the monastery he said to a Nālandā water bearer, "Tell them I have arrived." The message was relayed but not believed. Therefore, Āryadeva poured an amount of water sufficient only to fill a sheep's hoofprint onto a mirror and sent it inside the monastery. When the monks used it for bathing they found that the amount of water would not diminish but stayed the same. From this they recognized him and sent a message asking him to enter disguised as a water bearer, which he did.

When those appointed water bearers came and went from the monastery, they had to bow to the tīrthika guards at the door. However, Ācārya Āryadeva trampled on the head of the tīrthika, and by the power of the ācārya's inner *samādhi,* the tīrthika was unable to raise any protest. The ācārya took his place in the lower ranks of the monastic order. At the midday meal, Aśvaghoṣa counted the monks and found one extra. "Where is[299] this new bald head?" [86] He asked. Alternatively, the verb is "arise," meaning "Where does this new bald head come from?"

Another account of this event says that Aśvaghoṣa asked, "Who drinks vegetable soup and who drinks the meat soup?" Those who drank vegetable soup were hit on the head with a stick.

Āryadeva was hit and remarked, "Do not strike a bald head."

To which Aśvaghoṣa replied, "Where does this bald head come from?"

The answer from Āryadeva to either question was, "This bald head has come from its neck," to which Aśvaghoṣa had no response.

On another occasion Āryadeva went to where Aśvaghoṣa was making ancestor offerings. "What are you doing?" he asked.

"I am offering these to my ancestors," he replied.

"Oh, I too must water the flowers in my garden in Śrīparvata," said Āryadeva and began throwing water in the air.

"What use is it throwing water here for a garden far away in Śrīparvata?" asked Aśvaghoṣa.

"Well," replied Āryadeva, "What is the use making offerings now to ancestors who died long ago?" The tīrthika had no answer.

Another time Āryadeva filled a pot with excrement and began cleaning it from the outside. "When the filth is inside, what can you possibly achieve by cleaning the outside?" asked Aśvaghoṣa.

"If that is so, when the contamination is in the mind, what can possibly be achieved by cleaning the body?" he replied.

Aśvaghoṣa now realized that this was the man the monks had summoned to debate him. He took a bird in his hand and asked Āryadeva, "Is this bird going to die or not?"

"That depends on you," he replied.

Standing in a doorway, Aśvaghoṣa asked, "Am I outside or inside?"

"That depends on what you are doing," came the reply. Aśvaghoṣa could give no assured reply.

The monks told Āryadeva about the three helpers Maheśvara had granted as a siddhi to Aśvaghoṣa. To counteract these, Āryadeva brought in an immodest layman—although some assert it was a donkey's penis—to ward off the pandit sister, a cat for the parrot, and black oil for the chalk.

On the evening before the debate, three thrones were erected: one in the center of the debating area for King Hṛdayatilaka, who was responsible for banishing the loser and rewarding the victor; one on the right for Ācarya Āryadeva; and one on the left for the tīrthika Aśvaghoṣa. In order to prevent Īśvara coming near, the soles of old shoes and other dirty rags were placed under Aśvaghoṣa's throne. Analyzers along with summarizers were summoned, and on the following day all participants gathered for the contest.

Aśvaghoṣa lifted up his long hair and revealed an eye. Āryadeva lifted up his foot, revealing an eye on his sole, saying:

> Not seen by the three-eyed demon,
> hard to perceive by the thousand-eyed one, [87]
> yet Āryadeva with his single eye
> sees the nature of the three worlds.

This was the prologue to the debate. He then began the debate by presenting the greatness of the beautiful doctrine of the Buddha, its precepts, the great jewel of learning, and so on. Aśvaghoṣa said, "You cannot match my arguments," and called on the pandit sister to defeat Āryadeva. Beginning by using logic and language generally, and then specifically concentrating on the science of language, this beautiful and alluring woman began:

> As stains are washed away with stains,
> the desirous purify their minds with desire.
> You of introspective minds,
> the thirst borne of meditation on ugliness
> will only shrivel up your bodies.

The layman with no inhibitions or shame removed his lower garment and showed her his erect victory banner. Because the penis is an object of worship in the Maheśvara tradition, she immediately prostrated to it. Everybody was amused and the ground shook with laughter. She was unable to continue.

Durdharṣa, although a little embarrassed, nevertheless turned to the parrot pandit and commanded him likewise. The parrot began:

> Language as expressed in the mouths of the mundane
> lacks the grammatical authority of words, names, and letters.
> These inferior words uttered to clarify meanings
> are mere sounds; where is the teaching?

Because the sister pandit's contribution using the art of language had got off to an inauspicious start, the parrot rebutted language and began using logic. Suddenly a ferocious cat was let loose and with one jump seized the parrot in its sharp claws, sunk its fearsome teeth into its neck, and killed it.

Durdharṣa said, "You believe in cause and effect, and so you have committed a heinous act here."

Āryadeva replied, "My guru Nāgārjuna said he would purify me of this sin."

"How is it possible for Nāgārjuna to purify an action you have committed?" asked Durdharṣa.

"Well," replied Āryadeva, "How can the action of a cat killing a parrot rebound on me?"

Durdharṣa had no answer, but commanded the chalk pandit as he had the other two. The chalk jumped up and began to write using logic and language. But Āryadeva poured a pot of oil on the writing and erased it.

Durdharṣa recalled Īśvara's pledge to bless his mind and entered meditation to invoke him, but the dirty cloth under the throne meant that Īśvara could not come near. [88]

Three times Aśvaghoṣa was beaten in debates on language and logic, but his arrogance would not allow him to admit defeat. The summarizers could not summarize, the analyzers could not analyze, and so the king could not adjudicate.

"Ask a simpleton to decide," said Aśvaghoṣa, and so they went to ask some cowherds. The ācārya very cleverly came along playing a flute. The cowherds with their childlike nature loved the flute and declared the ācārya the winner.

They held a competition of miraculous powers. Aśvaghoṣa suggested, "Either you draw a circle in space and I will erase it, or I draw a circle and you erase it." Aśvaghoṣa was encouraged to draw the circle and Āryadeva was able to erase it.

"Either I fly into space or you fly into space," said Aśvaghoṣa.

"You do it," replied Āryadeva.

Since Aśvaghoṣa had the ability to fly far into space, Āryadeva manifested as a very large Mahāmātṛ goddess, placed his hands on Aśvaghoṣa's knees, and prevented him from flying.

Therefore, unable to prevail in debate and in miraculous powers, and unable to rely upon Īśvara entering his mind as pledged because of the dirty cloth under the throne, Aśvaghoṣa lamented:

> Great god, you have spoken false;
> in the midst of many we have been destroyed.
> As well as defeat in debate,
> we are betrayed by the gods.
> What suffering this is!

In another version, Aśvaghoṣa comes to know of the dirty rags under the throne and clears them away, and Maheśvara is able to enter his heart. In the first debate the assembled pandits are able to understand him. In the second debate all they hear is a tinkling sound but no comprehensible words, and Aśvaghoṣa loses all confidence. He assumes the form of the three-eyed

Maheśvara and tries to assume control over the ācārya, but the ācārya in turn manifests as thousand-eyed Prajñāpāramitā. Finally, Aśvaghoṣa issues the fires of anger from his mouth and tries to burn the ācārya, but Āryadeva enters the Stream of Water *samādhi* of Avalokiteśvara, holds his foot up to the fire, and extinguishes it.

Āryadeva said;

> Durdharṣa, come out of *samādhi,*
> the sun has set over the mountain,
> the people too are getting tired;
> apart from talk, what else is left?

The audience in unison cried:

> The many-eyed tīrthika with his sharp mind
> cannot see a single thing. [89]
> Āryadeva with his single eye
> sees even the subtle just as it is.[300]

With such pointed words coupled with the jeering and laughter, Aśvaghoṣa was ashamed of previous arrogance, and he decided to flee to the Brahmā realms. He flew off through the skies, but Āryadeva chased after him and closed in on him, saying, "Go no farther. A razor-like wind will cut your body to pieces."

"Who can possibly know such things?" retorted Aśvaghoṣa.

"Throw some of your hair and see," said Āryadeva.

He did and saw his hair shredded. Aśvaghoṣa was so scared he did not venture further. Āryadeva captured him and led him back. There he ordered Aśvaghoṣa to cut off his hair. Although he complained that he would rather drown in the Ganges than cut his hair, he nevertheless did as Āryadeva ordered. He was then locked inside a temple containing a collection of the Buddha's teachings. There he became bored and began reading the sutras, tantras, and commentaries. This made him realize that his views and behavior were wrong and that his disdain for the law of cause and effect would lead him to hell. He felt great remorse for his wrong actions. "This tongue has caused these problems," he lamented. "I will cut out this tongue." Because of this he was not allowed to possess anything sharp.

That night he had a dream in which he was told that although he had remorse for his previous actions, he was still not cleansed of them. However, now that he had entered the doctrine of the Buddha, if he were to write treatises that revealed the workings of the law of cause and effect, he would be cleansed of his past misdeeds.

Therefore, as prophesized by Tārā, he composed four medical texts in order to purify himself of past physical misdeeds. These are, *Extensive Exposition of Eight Branches; Engaging in Eight Branches; Essence of Eight Branches;* and his own commentary on *Essence of Eight Branches.*[301] In order to purify himself of past nonvirtuous speech, he composed the *Garland of Past Lives of the Buddha.* To purify himself of past nonvirtuous thought, he composed *Vajrayana Root Downfalls* and *Praise of the Praiseworthy* and over a hundred praises. In this way he composed many works on the five major sciences, and while he was composing the *Essence of Eight Branches,*

> Various auspicious signs occurred,
> auspicious for the three worlds.[302]

Three signs occurred in the subterranean world of the nāgas. Wisps of multicolored light formed a cloud, from this cloud fell a rain of ambrosia, and on trees fruits ripened out of season. Three signs occurred in the celestial world of the gods above. Banners and victory standards began to flutter, sending out rays of light pervading all directions, and rains of flowers fell. On the earth in the land of humans, the earth shook; a rain of *utpala* flowers fell; poison plants withered; golden parasols formed miraculously; [90] conch shells emitted sounds naturally; splits in wood issued milk and honey; Vasudhā, the blind king of Videha, regained his eyesight; an epidemic that had gripped the central region of Magadha suddenly subsided; the tīrthika master Ralapatra freed himself from his pride and threw himself to the ground; mantras were heard issuing from clay drums; Buddhist statues and shrines glowed; Buddhist pandits spoke words of auspiciousness. These eighteen miraculous signs accompanying the composition of *Essence of Eight Branches* and others were clearly observed in these three worlds.

The work itself is in six sections.[303] The first section or *sthāna* is the general or *sūtrasthāna* and has thirty chapters:

1. The eight branches as the main topic of this work, the nature of disease, doctor and medicine, nurse and patient, general principles, and an enumeration of the 120 chapters, much like the Root Tantra of *Four Medical Tantras.*

2. Daily behavior
3. Seasonal behavior
4. Prevention of disease
5. Drink
6. Characteristics of food
7. Protecting food
8. Food portions
9. Composition of medicine, and so on
10. Tastes
11. Understanding illness
12. Classification of illnesses
13. Treating illness
14. Two aspects of treatment
15. Purification therapies, and so on
16. Oil therapy
17. Compress therapy
18. Purgatives
19. Suppositories
20. Nasal purgative
21. Fumigation
22. Mouth gargles, and so on
23. Eye salves
24. Eye treatments
25. Instruments
26. Blunt surgical instruments
27. Bloodletting
28. Extraction of foreign bodies
29. Surgery
30. Alkali powders and cauterization procedures

The second section of *Essence of Eight Branches* is on the body and has six chapters:

1. Embryology
2. Prenatal illnesses
3. Parts of the body
4. Vital points on the body
5. Changes in the body
6. Messengers, and so on

The third section is on pathology. It has sixteen chapters:

1. Fundamentals of illness
2. Infectious fevers
3. Blood and bile disorder[304]
4. Respiratory ailments
5. Tuberculosis
6. Alcohol-related illness
7. Hemorrhoids
8. Dysentery and diarrhea
9. Urine retention [91]
10. Diabetes
11. Growths and tumors
12. Abdominal dropsy
13. First and second-stage edema and erysipelas
14. Leprosy, white leprosy, and worms
15. Wind-humor ailments
16. Arthritis and gout

The fourth section is on treatment. It has twenty-two chapters:

1. Treatment of infectious fever
2. Treatment of blood and bile
3. Treatment of cough with phlegm
4. Treatment of hiccups and breathing ailments
5. Treatment of tuberculosis
6. Treatment of vomiting, heart disease, and thirst
7. Treatment of alcohol-related illnesses
8. Treatment of hemorrhoids
9. Treatment of dysentery and diarrhea
10. Treatment of stomach disorder
11. Treatment of urine retention
12. Treatment of diabetes
13. Treatment of growths
14. Treatment of swellings
15. Treatment of abdominal dropsy
16. Treatment of first-stage edema
17. Treatment of second-stage edema
18. Treatment of erysipelas
19. Treatment of leprosy

20. Treatment of white leprosy and worms
21. Treatment of wind ailments
22. Treatment of gout and arthritis

The fifth section is on medicinal procedures and their administration. It has six chapters:

1. Emetic preparations
2. Purgative preparations
3. Complications in emetic and purgative therapies
4. Suppositories
5. Complications in suppository therapies
6. Pharmaceutical preparations

The sixth section is the concluding chapter. It has forty chapters. Three chapters are on pediatrics:

1. Pediatrics
2. Illnesses of infants
3. Demonic forces affecting infants

These are the four chapters on illnesses caused by spirits:

4. Spirits
5. Treatment of illnesses caused by spirits
6. Mental illness
7. Epilepsy

Nine chapters concentrate on the upper part of the body and deal with ailments affecting the eyes:

8. Diseases connected with the upper and lower eyelids
9. Treatment of the above
10. Diseases of the eyeball
11. Treatment of the above
12. Illnesses affecting vision
13. Partial blindness
14. Treatment of the above
15. Miscellaneous eye ailments
16. Treatment of the above

Eight chapters deal with ailments from other parts of the upper body and together with the previous nine chapters make up the seventeen chapters dealing with the upper part of the body:

17. Ear ailments
18. Treatment of ear ailments
19. Nose ailments
20. Treatment of nose ailments
21. Mouth ailments
22. Treatment of mouth ailments
23. Head ailments
24. Treatment of head ailments

Ten chapters are on various wounds, sores, and ulcerous growths:

25. Chronic sores, ulcers, and so on
26. Wounds [92]
27. Fractures
28. Rectal fistula
29. Glandular swellings, *kangbam,* growths, and so on
30. Treatment of the above
31. Minor sores and ulcers
32. Treatment of the above
33. Genital sores and ulcers
34. Treatment of the above

The final six chapters are:

35. Poisoning
36. Treatment of snake bites, and so on
37. Treatment of insect and spider bites
38. Treatment of rat and rabid dog bites
39. Elixirs
40. Rejuvenation therapies and aphrodisiacs

This work with its 120 chapters, which is the lifeblood of the medical tradition, and his other well-composed works are all on meaningful topics and his writing is graced with a host of beautiful thoughts and expressions, so much so that in reply to a question from King Saṃkusuma, the glorious Dharmakīrti praised Aśvaghoṣa's excellence in composition:

> Candragomin is pure in speech;
> poetry comes from Śūra, the skillful composer.[305]

In the beginning he sailed across the ocean of the tīrthika philosophy and later entered the Buddhist system, where he became a student of Nāgārjuna and his disciples. He was therefore a scholar of both Buddhist and non-Buddhist philosophies as well as of poetry and the other Vedas.

He was also known as Pīyūṣa Kalaśa, Pitṛceṭa, Mātṛceṭa, Saubhāgya-śubha, Aśvaghoṣa, Nandana, Maticitra, Aśvaka, and Durdharṣa. After he had embraced Buddhism he was known as Ratnaceṭa, Subhūtipālita, Bhavideva, Dīpaṃkara, Advayabhāva,[306] Gandharvadhara, Bhikṣu Śūra, Jitāri, Vajrā-yudha, Trideva, Bhāvabha, and Parahita Āryaśūra. He was known by many names, but these twenty-one are the most common.

The contribution of the Kashmiri Candranandana

Aśvaghoṣa's disciple was Candranandana. In his *Lexicon of Medical Terms from the Commentary on the Essence of Eight Branches,* he says:

> I, Candranandana, son of Kāmānandana, [93]
> prostrate to the omniscient one.
> From the teachings on the eight branches and...[307]

And in the fortieth chapter of his *Moonlight: A Commentary on the Essence of Eight Branches:*

> My grandfather Saubhāgyanandana,[308]
> forever hailed by the wise
> as one of untainted renown.
> His son was Kāmānandana,
> and I his son, Candranandana.
>
> Of great intelligence
> and with the wisdom of the tantras,[309]
> the ācārya known as Paramārtha,
> the supreme physician,
> was born in Kashmir.[310]

Concerning this "supreme physician," prior to the above quote the text says:

> The glorious Pitṛceṭa, the supreme physician,
> perfected in the science of Āyurveda.[311]

In the colophon of the *Essence of Eight Branches* it says, "Pitṛceṭa, son the master physician Saṃghaguhya."[312] This refers to Saubhāgyaśubha, who is Ācārya Śūra, whose son was Kāmānandana, who in turn was the father of Candranandana from Kashmir.

Candranandana devoted himself to countless works on Āyurveda, including the *Extensive Exposition of Eight Branches, Engaging in Eight Branches, Essence of Eight Branches,* the *Caraka Collections,* and so on. He himself, using sophisticated reasoning and analysis, composed an extensive commentary on *Essence of Eight Branches* called *Moonlight* and a separate lexicon of the medical terms found in *Moonlight,* among others. He became the crown jewel of those working to preserve and develop the science of healing in India at that time.

Others from India who made major contributions to medicine include the Oḍḍiyāna ācārya, Padmasambhava, who composed many medical texts, including *Vajra Armor Prevention, Sun and Moon Union, Ambrosia Vase Treatment, Precious Garland,* and *Ambrosia Essence.* Also included would be Sthiramati from east India who composed *Stainless Radiance;* the Oḍḍiyāna scholar Jinamitra, who composed *One Thousand and Ninety-One Treatments;* and the Nepalese Anara,[313] who composed *Three Translocations.*

Part 2

EARLIER DEVELOPMENT OF MEDICAL SCIENCE IN TIBET

7. Earliest Developments

[95] THE WAY that the science of healing arose in this land situated amid its white mountainous enclosure is as follows.

With the exception of a few barbaric and uncivilized tribes, most human races are reputed to have their own system of writing. This is something we can ascertain by observation, and *Stainless Light*—the Indian commentary on the *Kālacakra Tantra*—and other works also assert this to be the case. However, if it is true that a system of writing had not yet developed here in this land of Tibet up to and including the reign of Namri Songtsen, the father of Dharma king Songtsen Gampo (615–50 C.E.), then during those times there was no system of diagnosis nor treatment of disease through reliance on medical texts. People understood only what was good and bad to eat. Melted butter was put on wounds to stop the bleeding. Compresses of fermented grain were used as poultices, and so on. Some say these treatments had existed since humans evolved in Tibet and Lo.[314] However, general opinion is that it began in the reign of Lha Thothori Nyenshal.[315]

Three generations later King Dronyen Deu contracted a disease caused by an earth spirit, and in order to shield his royal line from the disease, he buried himself alive. As he did so he gave his final testament to his blind son, Könpa Tra:

> A good mind is like gold,
> good speech like ambrosia,
> so listen:
> Even the wicked are like your mother,
> so heal them;
> worldly dharma is all distracting thought,
> so throw it away.

The king then instructed his son to worship the Secret Signs,[316] to summon a doctor from the region of Asha[317] who could operate on his eyes, and to carry out the duties of a king. Therefore, Könpa Tra invited Ashajé, a wise doctor from the petty kingdom of Asha, who successfully operated on the prince's eyes with a golden surgical instrument. Looking with his new sight at the mountains of Kyishö Takri, he saw wild sheep and was henceforth known as Takri Nyensik—"he who sees wild sheep on Takri."

His son was Namri Songtsen, and in his time it is said that a few astrological and medical works were brought from China, but these cannot be identified.

His son was Songtsen Gampo, the noble Lokeśvara in the form of a king. During his reign the spoken word was rendered into writing. Therefore, the medical text known as the *Great Treatise on Medicine* brought by his Chinese wife, the princess Wen Cheng, was translated into Tibetan by Hvashang Mahādeva and Dharmakośa. [96]

Once when the king was ill, the Indian doctor Bharadhaja, the Chinese doctor Hsüan Yüan Huang, and the Taksik or Trom[318] doctor Galenos were invited to Tibet to cure him. There the Indian doctor translated a text called *Bushak Extensive and Short Exposition* and *Fresh Ghee Preparation.* The Chinese doctor translated a work called *Extensive and Short Expositions of Various Chinese Treatments.* The Taksik doctor translated a text called *Blue Head Collection* and one called *Dissection of Cockerels, Peacocks, and Parrots.* They held many discussions and jointly composed a medical text in seven chapters called *Weapons of Fearlessness,* which they offered to the king. A verse in this text reads:

> Without knowledge of the three great systems,
> one is not counted among the great physicians
> and is unable to benefit oneself or others,
> like the distance between thumb and finger
> hoping to measure the vast reaches of space.
> Bharadhaja, the great rishi,
> Galenos, the ambassador,
> Hsüan Yüan Huang, crowned lord of the land,
> these three great manifestations
> are praised as worthy vessels of ambrosia.[319]

Therefore, all medical science was compiled into these three main systems and propagated by them.

The king gave gifts to the Indian and Chinese doctors, and they traveled back to their own lands. Galenos stayed on as royal physician. It is said that he mostly resided in Lhasa, where he composed many texts. He married and had three sons. It is also said that the eldest was sent to upper Tsang province, where the lineages of Biji and others flourished, the middle son to the Yorpo region, where he developed the southern Lhorong medical tradition, while the youngest son stayed with his father, where he was known as Sogdian doctor.

Galenos was later known was Dzoro. Would-be students from upper-class families were discouraged from studying with him, whereas those from the four main lower classes, known as the Tuk, Jang, Nik, and Mong, were urged to take up the study of medicine, and Galenos was asked by the king not to differentiate between upper and lower classes as good or bad but to treat all equally. He was conferred with the title Physician Giver of Life[320] and was rewarded with nine great and three small royal commendations.

Jangtsa Lhabön,[321] the son of King Mé Aktsom,[322] took for his queen the princess Chin Cheng from China, who brought with her many medical and astrological texts. Many texts, exemplified by the work known as *Moon King,* or *Somarāja,* in 115 chapters, were translated by Hvashang Mahākyinda, the Chinese youth Garkhen, Khyungpo Tsetsé, Khyungpo Damtsuk, and Choklo Mönbar. [97]

Concerning this work, *Somarāja,* the *Chronicles of Ministers* says:

> *Somarāja, Drop of Ambrosia,*
> *Vase of Ambrosia,* by Nāgārjuna.[323]

This is a corruption indicating that this work was either composed or requested by Nāgārjuna, and because of this mistake there are one or two works in which medical scholars have added the prophecy of Nāgārjuna's coming, beginning "In the south in the region of Vidarbha...." However, the work was requested by Wang Té, or the Nāgarāja Gapa.

The later Chinese edition translated by Hvashang Mahāyāna and Vairocana has 112 chapters:

1. Development of the body
2. Bones of the body
3. Bones of the head
4. Bones of the limbs
5. Complete development and measurements
6. Fundamentals of illness

7. Vital points
8. Shape, nails, and tongue
9. Time, place, and age
10. Urine analysis in the Rishi tradition
11. Urine divination for spirits and illness
12. Urine divination according to the seasons
13. Teachings on urine divination
14. Teaching to Aśvinī on the nine diagrams
15. Pulse analysis: hot and cold, above and below
16. Heart pulse
17. Liver pulse
18. Kidney pulse
19. Lung pulse
20. Spleen pulse
21. Death pulse
22. Enemy pulse
23. Harmful demon pulse
24. Seasonal pulses
25. Characteristics of wind
26. Characteristics of bile
27. Characteristics of phlegm
28. Characteristics of heart disorder
29. Characteristics of the lung disorders
30. Characteristics of the liver
31. Characteristics of the spleen
32. Characteristics of the kidneys
33. Characteristics of the small intestine
34. Characteristics of the stomach disorders
35. Characteristics of the gallbladder
36. Characteristics of the large intestine disorders
37. Characteristics of the urinary bladder infection
38. Characteristics of disorders of the endocrine system
39. Characteristics of dysentery
40. Characteristics of nondigestion
41. Understanding swellings and tumors
42. Explaining growths and abscesses
43. Characteristics of smallpox
44. Characteristics of *gaklhok*

45. Characteristics of poisons
46. Characteristics of dropsy
47. Worms and other organisms
48. Shape and bones of the head
49. Nervous system and its ailments
50. Limbs and wounds
51. The abdomen and the organs
52. Prognostications
53. Sulphur preparations
54. The preparation of bitumen
55. Treatment of wind
56. Treatment of bile
57. Treatment of phlegm
58. Treatment of wind-bile-phlegm combination
59. Treatment of heart-wind ailments
60. Treatment of lung ailments
61. Treatment of liver ailments
62. Treatment of kidney ailments
63. Treatment of spleen ailments
64. Treatment of small intestine ailments
65. Treatment of stomach ailments
66. Treatment of bile dysentery
67. Treatment of large intestine ailments
68. Treatment of urinary bladder ailments
69. Treatment of ailments of the endocrine system
70. Treatment of digestive ailments
71. Treatment of dysentery
72. Treatment of swellings and tumors
73. Treatment of growths and abscesses
74. Treatment of smallpox
75. Treatment of *gaklhok*
76. Treatment of poisons
77. Treatment of dropsy
78. Treatment of worms
79. Powder preparations
80. Paste preparations
81. Decoction preparations
82. Decoction purgatives

83. Purgatives
84. Suppositories
85. Strong enema
86. Emetic purgatives
87. Nasal purgative
88. Channel cleansing
89. Reversal suppressants for the five therapies
90. Medicinal butter
91. *Daryakan*
92. Gems
93. Food and meat
94. Medicine and food
95. Internal and wound medicine
96. Bone treatments
97. Treatment of open wounds
98. Treatment of the channels
99. Channel flow
100. Treatment of the sides of the head
101. Medicine for wounds and internal medicines
102. Surgery on the head
103. Treatment of limbs
104. Treatments for the neck and face
105. General protection
106. Treatments for the upper body
107. Treatments for the lower body
108. Measurements of the body
109. Medicine and surgery for channels of the abdomen
110. Bloodletting
111. Cauterization
112. The powers of different medicines

The translation from Indian sources by the pandit Kṛṣṇa and Lotsāwa Bandé Chörap is similar to the above. [98]

During these times there was a doctor from Trom called Biji in his own language but whose actual name was Tsampashilaha.[324] He gathered many scholars together and translated and composed several medical works. Using his own *Crystal Mirror Tantra* in fifty chapters as a foundation, there followed *Red Ink Illuminating Beacon on the Abdomen Early Volume* in forty-two chapters, *Red Ink Magic Key to the Abdomen Later Volume* in twenty-five chapters, and *Teachings on Treatment of the Limbs* in forty-two chapters; a commentary, further commentary, and secret commentary on the above; the four mother-and-son medical works, namely, the large and small mother text *Heart-Like Network* and the black and red son commentaries. There are also four works—*Small Commentary, Lesser Network, The Beacon,* and *Lesser Treatise on Pacification*—known as the four son texts of the *Heart-drop Collection;* six works on treatments for arrow wounds, infected sores, burns, holding the drop, channels, and growths, known collectively as the six essential son texts. Together these make up the three mother texts and the seventeen son commentaries. Also included are *Essential Beacon for the Elimination of Hindrances, Four Conclusions from Examinations of Pus, Precious Base Emaciation Medicine,* and *Gentle Ambrosia Emetic for Pus,* known collectively as the four secret and exclusive son texts. These make up the extensive collection.

The intermediate collection consists of the *Essential and Quintessential Versions of Brown Compilation.* The abridged collection comprises the root, commentary, and essence of the *Lesser Red Ink Text.* Also included are the three chapters on the abdomen combined to form the work *Mirror of Ambrosia* in eight long and thirteen short chapters; *Clear Drop Treatise on the Threefold Classification of Wounds;* a combined treatment of head and abdomen called *Suspended Rope of Five Essentials; Precious Gem* in seventy chapters, written by a Chinese rishi, and *Feminine Gem* in seven chapters, which together make up twenty-five volumes; *Resolving Disputes Concerning the Head* composed by Vajrapāṇi; *Magic Almsbowl*[325] *of Daryakan Ambrosia,* composed by Trulpai Khyeu, and its commentaries by Hvashang Kyinda, these two known as *Great* and *Lesser Concise Annotations; Thirty-Five Faults; Magic Mirror of Anatomy* in twenty-six chapters; *Combining the Nine Anatomical Threads; Measurements of Living and Dead Bodies; Abdomen of Humans and Rishis* in ten chapters; *Structure of the Abdomen,* reputedly written by Ātreya. Secondary works include the greater and lesser *Bones of the Rishis; Thirteen Chapters; Restoring Joints; Treasure Mine: Ten Chapters of Beneficial Medicine; Four Chapters on Essentials for Physicians;* [99] *Precious Garland* in fifty chapters; and *Precious Gem* in seventy chapters.

All these texts were translated into Tibetan and offered to the king. They were then wrapped together in the best silk and became known collectively as *Collection on Health: Higher Texts on Medical Practice.*[326]

It is taught that Hvashang Mahādeva and Khyungpo Tsetsé also translated many medical works in these times.

Tsenpashilaha later became a ruler in Tibet for a while. The line of Biji was already established in Tibet but now was reputed to be even stronger. His lineage of disciples increased and was exemplified by Shang Lhamo Si, Tongsher Mepo, and Drangti Nyekhar. These three were appointed border protectors in Dokham for four years, and as a reward for their services the king presented them with the *Crystal Mirror Tantra* and the extensive, intermediate, and abridged commentaries, such as the seventeen mother and son texts on treatment of wounds, and the *Lesser Red Text.* It is said that they and their descendents were appointed as royal physicians and were taken out of the army.[327] Some accounts say that the king gave a text on the treatments of the head to Tongsher Mepo, treatments of the abdomen to Drangti Nyekhar, and a work on treatment of the limbs to Shang Lhamo Si.

After the passing of King Mé Aktsom, the noble Trisong Detsen,[328] known as "the celestial flower of Brahmā," became king. At the beginning of his reign three great scholars known as the three manifested sons appeared. They were the Indian physician Dharmarāja, Hvashang Mahākyinda, and Tsenpashilaha.[329] These three compiled many medical texts in accord with their own country's traditions and offered them to the king. They include:

1. *Calculation of the Orbits of the Sun and Moon: An Essential Root of Medicine*
2. *Commentary on the Healing of the Three Roots of Disease*
3. *Golden Mirror Analysis of Urine*
4. *Silver Mirror Charm Circle of Instruction*
5. *Iron Door Bolt of the Chinese Oral Tradition of Pulse Examination*
6. *Golden Door Bolt of Prognosis and Abridged Iron Axe of Prognosis*
7. *Secret Transmission of Precious Ambrosia*
8. *Golden Chisel: A Beacon on the Powers of Medicinal Substances*
9. *Precious Crystal Rosary Elixir*
10. *Bushak Copper Vase Medical Lexicon*
11. *Eye of the Conch Illustrations*
12. *Turquoise Network Compendium*
13. *Iron Garland of Tastes*
14. *Pearl Garland of Pacification Remedies*
15. *Conch Pus Cleanser*
16. *Precious Hook of Emetics*
17. *Silver Vase of Purgatives*

18. *Golden Sun Vase of Suppositories*
19. *Iron Cup of Strong Enemas*
20. *Turquoise Network: Entering the Forest of Medical Plants*
21. *Medical Baths: A Drop of the Sun and Moon*
22. *Fire and Water Needles of Massage*
23. *Iron Lotus of Bloodletting* [100]
24. *Ambrosia Drop of Cauterization*
25. *Weapon Wheel of Minor Surgery*
26. *From the Ocean of Dropsy to Dry Land*
27. *Compilation of Medicine Places*

These are known as the twenty-seven short commentaries and form the collection on internal diseases.

Works on minor surgery[330] include two general works on chronic wounds, twenty-three specific works, and a collection of treatments for head, abdomen, and limbs. This is the *Heap of Jewels* collection.

Other works offered to the king include *King of Khotan Treatment for the Neck.*

Several works attributed to Nāgārjuna were translated at this time. They include, *Curing Illnesses of the Five Aggregates, Secret Essence Beacon of Ambrosia Gem Medicine,* a treatise on precious stones, which is like a root treatise and has seventeen chapters. Also included are the seventy-six chapters of *Secret Commentary on the Precious Stones Treatise,* the twenty-five chapters of *Treatise on the Four Humors,* the sixteen chapters of *Descriptions of the Organs,* the thirty-seven chapters of *Short Gold Treatise;* the twenty-one chapters of *Treatise on the Head;* the forty-seven chapters of *Magic Black Key Treatise on the Abdomen;* and the forty chapters of *Treatise on the Four Limbs.* These works comprise 279 chapters.

Mitra Miwang Chandra[331] and Hvashang Devabodhi translated *Siddhi of Rishi Śūrya* and *Precious Beacon: A Magic Treasury of Medicine,* reputed to be the speech of Mañjuśrī to Kumāra Tapas. Using the seven types of myrobalan as illustrations, this work begins with seven sections: fundamentals of illness, symptoms, individual treatments, external therapies, reversal treatments, minor surgery, and treatment through charms. Just as *vijaya* myrobalan possesses all six tastes, the text continues with six sections on sudden onset of illness, sudden spread of the illness, elimination of mistakes in treatment, complications from other ailments, reversal treatments, miscellaneous instructions, and magical treatments. As there are eight powers found in medicines, the work has eight qualities. As there are three post-digestive tastes, so there are three sections on symptoms, treatment, and complete cure. In total these sections make up one complete volume.

Other translations include *Root Tantra,* reputedly by Vajrapāṇi, in forty-four chapters, its commentary by the eight main rishis and the thirteen lesser rishis in twenty-four chapters, *Twenty-Two Chapters on Treatments,* and the *Eight Verses.*

As Tsenpashilaha was about to return to his own country, he composed for his son *Black Compilation Collection with Units of Measurements; Three Collections on Clear Descriptions of the Head, Abdomen, and Limbs from Caraka's Rishi Essence Tantra;* [101] and seventy-eight root instructional works on treatments for disorders of the head, abdomen, limbs, and humors together with miscellaneous topics, known collectively as *Biji's Yellow Collection.* This last collection was also known as the *Radiant Exalted Documents of the King.* All these works were offered to the king.

Hvashang Penatseta composed the *Fundamental Treasury of the Five Collections* as advice to the king, ministers, and the people. The five collections are the head, abdomen, internal illnesses, supplements, and miscellaneous works. The collection on the head deals with surgery and head compresses, comprising seventeen scrolls. The abdomen collection comprises white phenomena, red phenomena, white purgative, and red purgative[332] and makes up forty-five scrolls. The collection on internal illnesses is made up of *Precious Cleanser for Dysentery, Precious Vase of Poison Treatments, Cloudless Sunrays for Meat Poisoning, Lifesaving Armor against Strong Poisons, Clear Mirror for Fevers,* and *Precious Meat Compound for Cold Diseases.*

The supplement collection consists of greater, intermediate, and lesser treasuries. The greater treasury has thirty-six chapters. The intermediate treasury consists of *Brilliant Jewel* in root text and commentary, an overview, and a section on dispelling immediate hindrances. The overview contains advice for ordinary people in accord with outer perceptions, advice for ministers in accord with the inner world, and advice for the king in accord with the hidden world. The outer version for the people contains the root-text work *Forty-Two Magic Keys* and *Large and Small Magic Keys of Instruction.* The inner version for ministers consists of root text, commentaries, aphorisms and short illustrations. The root text collection has seven commentaries, there are ten aphorisms and twenty-seven short illustrations.

The secret version for the king contains large grouped[333] treatments, lesser grouped treatments, and direct instruction treatments. The first of these consists of *Heart-Shaped Amulet* and *Heart-Peak Amulet. Heart-Shaped Amulet* is made up of five collections and *Heart Peak Amulet* has ten. Short lesser grouped treatments consist of supplements, essentials, rivets, and remedial therapy. There are eight supplements, four sections on essentials, six on rivets, and three on remedial therapy. Treatments according to direct instructions are made up of *Key Instructions* and *Quintessential Instructions.* There are twelve commentaries, including *Dispelling Immediate Hindrances* and *Beacon-Like Commentary on Difficult Points of the Root Text.*

The lesser treasury from the supplement collection is known as the *Hidden Treasury.* Miscellaneous works consists of 108 different works. He also translated *Key to Precious Titles* and many other mother-and-son documents.

On these times the precious *Book of Kadam* says:

> In the past they came together at Vajrāsana, [102]
> these days they are found in the land of Oḍḍiyāna,
> in the future they will come to the Land of Snow.[334]

Also:

> The glorious guru said, "To tame the demons I too will go there."[335]

Also:

> Although I am a monk without wisdom,
> to be your companion, lord among men,
> would be forever joy.[336]

As these citations indicate, the Dharma king Trisong Detsen, who was inseparable from the lotus-holding Avalokiteśvara and Mañjuśrī, and the Oḍḍiyāna knower of the three times,[337] who was inseparable from Buddha Amitābha, both appeared at the same time. They tamed the harmful demons of Tibet, blessed the foundations of the unchanging and spontaneous glorious red-rock Samyé Monastery and purified the building and their contents of hindrances. During the consecration, actual wisdom beings were absorbed into the commitment beings, evidenced by clay structures taking human form, speaking, and so forth. In this manner did its extraordinary temples and shrines arise.

8. From Vairocana to Shangtön Siji Bar

The contribution of Vairocana

MANY BRIGHT and intelligent young Tibetans were brought together and trained as translators, but they were unable to master spoken Sanskrit, and this distressed the king. However, the great ācārya prophesized:

> In the Tsang region of Nyemo Jekhar,[338]
> in a room in a house in a town,
> comes Genjak Thangta, son of father Pagor Hedö
> and mother Drönkyi from the Drenka clan.
> Having been asked, his parents will bring him here
> at the age of eight, to become without question
> a renowned incarnate translator.[339]

Therefore, this child was born to Pagor Hedö and Drönkyi in a place where the Nyangchap and Tsangchap rivers meet. At the age of eight he was brought before the king. For the next seven years he ate nothing but the three white foods and the three sweet foods.[340] In order to increase his knowledge, he was encouraged to practice wisdom-increasing mantra meditations. According to the *Great Mask*,[341] from the age of nine he served outer and inner ministers for three years, and from the age of twelve he served the king for three years. Whatever the truth, as it is said, "Then he became learned in grammar and translation,"[342] meaning that he studied language with the Oḍḍiyāna ācārya Padmasambhava and the Sahor master Śāntarakṣita until the age of fifteen and became a master scholar. In the bathing-house temple of Samyé, he took his monk vows in front of the great abbot Bodhisattva. [103]

At that time the king brought together ministers, scholars, monks, and representatives of the people for discussions. They agreed that the cause-and-effect teachings were complete in Tibet but that in India there were teachings beyond cause and effect and that these should be sought. In response Genjak

Thangta and Tsangön Lekdrup stood up in the assembly and pledged to fulfill the king's wishes. As preparation for their journey, gold leaf was molded to the shape of skulls, and the two young men wore them on their heads. Gold leaf, implements, and other strings of objects were hidden in their clothes. Gold dust, a pair of wild ox horns, gold nuggets, silver items,[343] claws from various wild animals, and so on, were all loaded onto white-foot, bird-face, and other types of pack horses, and they set off for the noble land of India.

On their travels they endured sixteen life-threatening hardships. Finally, however, they were able to study vast and profound Dharmas with twenty-five pandits, such as Ācārya Śrī Siṃha. Even in India at that time, the effortless Great Perfection was not widely promulgated, and so they received it secretly in Bodhgāya[344] from Ācārya Siṃha as a work doubly sealed by the Dharma kings and pandits, with Ācārya Siṃha disguised in the form of the Yakṣa Ulkāmukha, Vairocana[345] as the lion Susthira, and Lekdrup in the form of a swan. There they received the complete initiations and instructions.

Lekdrup sought fame and reputation, and he therefore succumbed to an earlier hindrance he had encountered on the journey.

Vairocana then cleared up all questions and doubts he had on the texts and instructions. He met with great beings that had attained the gnosis body, such as Garap Dorjé and Mañjuśrī Mitra. From them he heard various teachings, and their thoughts became as one. He gave the gold leaf to the Ācārya Kumāra, who possessed the fleet-foot siddhi, and became his companion. He said he himself needed the fleet-foot siddhi and having received the teachings on how to walk at the speed of a vulture flying from the mountains, he returned to Tibet.

At that time the pandits in India received bad signs in their dreams. They realized that these profound instructions had been taken to Tibet and set out in pursuit of Vairocana but could not catch him. Therefore, they sent a disruptive letter to Tibet saying, "This Tibetan monk has not found the true Dharma; he has taken the perverted dharma of the outsiders." The king read these letters and as a result did not immediately send a welcoming party out to meet Vairocana on his return. As a response Vairocana sent a letter to the king:

> Great king, sovereign of Tibet,
> casting off all concern for worldly dharmas [104]
> and yearning for the true and unmistaken Dharma,
> you dispatched gold dust and sent us off in search.

We traveled on paths that would purify hell,
and with fortunate karma I heard the words of many a scholar.
We bring texts on arts and crafts, the science of medicine, and others,
all works necessary for the happiness of this life;
texts on guardians of the doctrine, liberating those who break
commitments;
an armory of scripture of logic to defeat the outsiders;
and texts on all paths of practice according to faculty,
the complete path of the cause-and-effect vehicle.
Also the supreme vehicle, very essence of this wonderful doctrine,
the naturally perfected great bliss, mind of every buddha,
nonduality of cause and effect, the effortless Great Perfection—
all these, without omission, I have brought.
In your presence I will offer these for you to hear.
It is long since we met, I wonder if you are well?
To the mighty king I offer this letter in person.[346]

The king replied with a letter beginning, "Great navigator across the sea of samsara." Without delay this mighty king spread his hair across the threshold of his palace and invited the great translator to walk upon it. A speckled horse and a gold-flecked cream-colored horse with golden saddles studded with turquoise, gold, and silver, fine brocade, cloaks lined with lynx fur, fine drinking vessels, and much more were sent out to Vairocana, where the invitation was conveyed to him in verse.

In the daytime he translated the cause-and-effect teachings for the king, ministers, and people. At night he translated the secret-instruction teachings for the king. In return the king gave him the title Celestial Lord of the Ocean of Instructions.

Vairocana can be included in the twenty-five royal and commoner disciples of ācārya Padma as well as in those renowned as the nine great siddhas. He was responsible for the translation of so many texts into Tibetan that the *Lotus Chronicles* says:

Never has there been a translator like Vairocana,
and there never will be again.
In the future those who speak the languages of India
may be called translators,
but they will come nowhere near Vairocana.

He was called a translator,
in reality he was a pandit.
Generations hence will look on his work
with immense gratitude.[347]

Similarly, the later great translator Loden Sherap singled Vairocana out for praise while simultaneously humbling himself:

Vairocana was like the vast reaches of space;
Ka and Chok[348] are like the sun and moon;
Rinchen Sangpo is the great star of the morning; [105]
I am a mere firefly.[349]

Thus, unmatched in wisdom, compassion, and power, his true nature is the illusory dance of the gnosis of Buddha Vairocana. He is inseparable from Vajrapāṇi, the keeper of secrets. He is Ānanda, attendant of our Teacher and compiler of all his teachings, come again for the glory of living beings. This great manifested being, Vairocana, requested many medical texts from the Kashmiri Candranandana. In particular, as the fourth chapter of the *Crystal Rock Chronicle* says:

Vairocana translated Bön and Dharma;
Vairocana translated medicine and astronomy;
Vairocana translated sutra and tantra.
In the sutra translations he is written as Yeshé Dé;
in the tantra translations he is written as Vairocana;
in the Bön translations he is written as Genjak Thangta;
in the astronomy translations he is Indra Vairocana;
in the medical translations he is Chöbar Jawa—
he translated most of sutra and its commentaries.

As this quote indicates he translated various medical texts including *Instructions on Medicinal Plants,* also known as the *Hundred Thousand Medicinal Plants of Mañjuśrī,* and *Fungi Therapy for Poisons* by the ācārya Sūryasiṃha. More particularly, my lama the Great Fifth said:

In particular, the kindness of the great Trisong
in inviting the second Buddha from Oḍḍiyāna,

brought countless medical works to this snowy land,
nourishing the lives of living beings, objects of compassion.
Amid this galaxy of knowledge
shines the crystal moon of *Four Tantras,*
of few words but vast in meaning,
drawn by the wisdom wind chariot
of Vairocana, in reality a great pandit,
sole eye of the world.[350]

Therefore, as stated in this verse, he translated the *Essence of Ambrosia Secret Instruction Tantra on Eight Branches,*[351] the greatest, the best, the supreme of all medical scriptures and instructions. He is also credited with composing *Darkness-Dispelling Lamp of Explanation* and *Medical Dictionary in Five Parts.* The eighty-fifth chapter of *Lotus Chronicles* says:

The Chinese doctor Hvashang Deva,
court physician Nyangtsen Shila,[352] and others
translated the *Essence of Ambrosia Eight Branches*
and many works on preparation of elixirs.[353]

Here *Four Tantras* is said to be have also been translated from the Chinese. This exists, [106] but the transmission of the actual words of the Buddha together with the transmitted instructions came to Vairocana, and therefore, as the verses in his letter to the king made clear, he offered it to the king and to the ācārya second Buddha. Although the king saw that this work was vast as well as profound and that the meanings within were second to none, he understood that it would not be proper for the teachings of such a secret tantra to become corrupt. Therefore he did not disseminate it widely and kept it as the jewel of his own heart. Later, he decided to hide it as a treasure, because this would make the lineage shorter in the future, reducing the likelihood of the work becoming defiled, and so on. He approached the ācārya, who replied:

This supreme protector of life, this tantra of few words but vast meaning, this wish-fulfilling jewel: now is not the time for its dissemination. Protect it well by hiding it as a treasure for the duration of three days in the world of the desire gods.[354]

Thus the tantra was again entrusted to Vajra Mārajit, to the treasure guardian Yönten Gyalpo Shingja Chen, to the butcher-like Hapsé,[355] and to the red jackal-faced protector. The king prayed that in the future it would be unearthed by someone of great merit and would be of benefit to countless beings. The tantra was then hidden high in a pillar in the middle floor of Samyé Monastery. This is according to the Treasure tradition.

In the Transmission tradition, some assert different versions of events up to this point, and there are different traditions of the tantra, but I do not think they make any material difference. After this point it is generally accepted that the tantra was transmitted from the ācārya to whom it had been offered by the king and his son, who in turn had received it as a one-to-one transmission from Vairocana. However, in an old document from the Nya family line, it says that after the tantra was hidden as a treasure, the king's son Muné Tsenpo was certain that his father's beloved medical text had been offered to the king by the ācārya. He therefore approached the ācārya and requested it. "I did not offer the tantra to Trisong Detsen," he replied. "However, for the sake of the doctrine and living beings, I will teach it to the prince." Thus the ācārya made his own translation. The prince then offered this tantra to the father and Vairocana as transmission while receiving it from them as treasure. These days in the lineage of the tantra, the ācārya even precedes Vairocana. This is done either on the basis of it belonging to the Transmission tradition as recounted in this story or for special reasons, such as it being classified as a Treasure.

The nine royal physicians from surrounding countries

King Trisong Detsen thought to himself, [107] "In the past my ancestors—and now I, too—have been instrumental in founding and establishing the science of medicine in Tibet. Now is the time to bring together scholar doctors from other lands and to propagate all those works that are yet to be translated."

With gifts of gold, and so on, he sent messengers to different countries and invited Śāntigarbha from India; Guhyavajra from Kashmir; Tongsum Gangwa, Hvashang Bala, and Hangti Pata from China; Halaśānti from Taksik; Sengdo Öchen from Drugu;[356] Khyölma Rutsi from Dölpo; and Dharmaśīla from Nepal. These became known as the nine royal physicians from surrounding countries.

It was at this time that the king feigned illness in order to test these doctors, although Surkhar relates this as happening to Tsenpashilaha and others during the reign of King Mé Aktsom. The king remained inside Pangthang Kamé palace while the doctors stood outside the door. "You are wise and renowned in the science of healing," said the king, "Therefore, coming to a diagnosis from examining my wrist pulse in person would be nothing special. Examine this cord and make a diagnosis from it."

So saying, the king tied a thin cord to the leg of a cat and passed it through a small hole in the door for the doctors to examine. On examination the doctors replied, "Either the king is dying or we have failed in our diagnosis. Outside the pulse is slow, but inside it beats fast. It seems that the king has the pulse of that lowest of animals, the cat."

Then the king tied the cord to the leg of a chicken and gave it to the doctors to examine. "On the surface the pulse is active, but deep inside it has no essence. It appears to be none other than the pulse of that lowest of birds, the chicken," replied the doctors.

Then the king tied the cord to himself. On examination the doctors remarked, "On the surface the pulse is sunken, but inside it is firm and solid like a rock," and so on. Therefore, by relying on the clairvoyance of the medicine goddesses, the foreign doctors had correctly recognized each pulse. The king was pleased and bestowed the following honors on them:

> People of Tibet!
> Revere these great doctors, bringers of health,
> Why? Because they grant the gift of life.
> The god of men, the ruler, he reveres them,[357]
> therefore, they are to be known as divine physicians.
> They are the guardians of living beings;
> place them on the highest seat with cushions
> of the highest-quality Taksik brocade.
> Welcome them with horses;
> if on foot, offer them gold.
> Follow willingly whatever they say or do;
> do not disregard the physician's word.
> Though it may cost a royal kingdom,
> have no sense of loss—it is the price of life.
> Even though mistaken treatment
> or surgery may result in death,
> do not ask for blood money.

If they prescribe dust as medicine,
nevertheless send gold in payment. [108]
Offer them drinks, bring them meat.
Because you must rely upon them always,
leave behind any two-faced, deceitful words.
Offer them cloaks, brocade, and boots, complete sets of clothing.
Hold them in high regard, bow, and be courteous.
They show us great kindness in this life;
think long on how to repay them.
These thirteen honors I bestow upon them.
Those who disrespect them will be punished.

Inside the palace the best hospitality and service was arranged. With Ācārya Padma supervising and with translators, such as Ka Lotsāwa and Chok Lotsāwa, trained in their different languages, the king asked them to translate the medical texts.

The Indian doctor Śāntigarbha compiled and translated *Tantra of the Brown Casket, Four Collections of Verses,* great and lesser *Begging Bowl of Ambrosia,* and *Essence of Vase of Ambrosia,* all reputedly the word of the Buddha; *Five Collections,* reputedly the teachings of Avalokiteśvara; *Five Treatises,* reputedly composed by Nāgārjuna; and *One Hundred Thousand Medicinal Plants in 120 Chapters,* reputedly composed by Tārā.

The three Chinese doctors translated *Garland of Medicinal Compounds, Magic Mirror Exposition on Anatomy, Treatment of the Limbs: Five Jewel Treasuries from Arising from Gestures of the Hand, Untainted Jewel Remedial Treatment, Fire and Water Reversal, Wheel of Fire Treatment for Poisons, Specific Treatments for Miscellaneous Ailments, Urine Analysis, Magical Treatments,*[358] and *Beacon of Cauterization Practice,* all attributed to Mañjuśrī.

The Kashmir doctor compiled and translated *Beacon Dispelling the Darkness of the Difficulties of Medical Practice, Nine Works on Medicine,* and *Essential Prognostic Manuscript on Instruction.*

The Taksik doctor compiled and translated *Eight Outsider Root and Commentary Collections on Treatments for the Head, Greater and Lesser Tree of Instructions on Channel Treatment, Precious Wheel of Life Treatment for Humor Combination Disorders, Sogdian Tantra,* and *Saving the Life of the King of Garlok: Treatment for Poisoning.*

The Drugu doctor compiled and translated *Three Black Tantras, Greater and Lesser Annotations on the Three Black Tantras, Eye of the Conch Illustra-*

tions, Turquoise Network: Entering the Forest of Medical Plants, Guṇaśata in Five Hundred Chapters, and *Mirror of Equine Medicine in Three Collections.*

The Dölpo doctor compiled and translated *Weapons of the Eight Kinds of Fearlessness, Clarifying the Hidden, Chapter on Signs of Life and Death, Pulse Signs,* and *Bloodletting Therapy.*

The Nepalese doctor translated *Drampati, Yogaśataka, Illustrations of Precious Medicines, Minor Surgery, and Treatment of Lhokpa.*

Furthermore, Nup Sangyé Yeshé translated *Precious Compilation on Medicine and Treatment in Seven Fasicles,* reputedly composed by Nāgārjuna; *Ambrosia Drop Treatments of the Head in Seven Chapters,* [109] by Ketu Prajñā; *Ambrosia Mirror in Eight Chapters* by Vedura;[359] *Five Beacon Collection,* said to have been composed by Nāgārjuna; *Fire Wheel Treatments for Poison,* by Śuka, a manifestation of Mañjuśrī; *Fungi Treatment for Poisons,* by Rishi Sūryasiṃha; *Precious Belt of Liberation; Candraguhya Weapon Wheel Activity Tantra;* its commentary *Greater Fungi Treatment;* and various supplements. Works authored by Nup Sangyé Yeshé himself include *Precious Protection: The Light of Instruction, Precious Examination: Light Reflection,* and *Traveling Lamp of Good Remedies.*

Śrīvajra and Chökyi Wangchuk translated *Viramuni Tantra on Treatment for Poisons,* said to have been composed by Nāgārjuna, as well as *Rainbow Light Flash Tantra.*

Pandit Ratnavajra and Vairocana translated *Jewel Heap Planet Tantra,* in forty-six chapters, composed as a dialogue between Vajrapāṇi and Nāgārjuna.

The Chinese text *Bright Beacon Quintessential Treatment for Planetary Disorder; Extensive Question and Answer in Thirty-Four Chapters* between Nāgārjuna and the nāga king Takṣaka; the intermediate *Clear Mirror;* the lesser *Clear Insight; Beacon Illuminating the Meaning; Illuminating Beacon; Magic Mirror; Beacon of the Heart;* and the sixteen-part *Signs of Leprosy Manuscript,* reputedly spoken by Vetālaḍākinī, were all translated by Rishi Khadyota.

Precious Beacon Treasury, reputedly the speech of Mañjuśrī; *Pacification of Infectious Bile and Poisoning,* reputedly the words of Tārā, and *Precious Beacon of Materia Medica* in three chapters were all translated by Sāntigarbha.

Other works they translated include *Secret Body, Speech, and Mind Tantra of Ambrosia Preparation of Medicinal Plants,* written as a question-and-answer session between Ārya Mañjuśrī and four rishis; its commentary reputedly composed by the glorious Nāgārjuna; a twelve-chapter text on medical plant preparation known as *Brown Compilation* by Hvashang Mahākyinda; its commentary *Secret Quintessence;* Caraka's *Āyurveda Tantra: An Illuminated Treasury of Ten Thousand Jewels;* a work compiled from that tantra known as *Seventy Chapters*; *Ambrosia Tree: The Root Tantra on Meat Elixir Preparation* in seven chapters; *Treating Infectious Bile and Poisons,* taught by Avalokiteśvara to Tārā.

The king was satisfied with these works [110] and saw the benefits they were bringing to the people. He bestowed great honors upon the doctors and delivered a proclamation beginning:

> The doctor is the father,
> caring for the patient with compassion.
> The patient is the child,
> never replying with a bad word.

These great medical texts from the various traditions were bound together between acacia-wood covers and became known as the *King's Brown Medical Volumes.*

Nine bright Tibetan children were chosen and encouraged to study medicine. They were: Chejé Shikpo, Ukpa Chösang, and Baché Lekgön[360] from the upper regions; Yuthok Gönpo, Minyak Rongjé, and Drangti Gyalsang from the middle regions; Nyawa Chösang, Thazhi Darpo, and Tongpa Drakgyal from the lower regions. They became known as the nine wise Tibetan physicians.

The foreign physicians were laden with offerings given with great respect and returned to their countries. Not long after, the king became ill. Although the nine Tibetan doctors were available, in accord with the wishes of the ministers, invitations were sent out to the nine foreign doctors. Only the Chinese doctor Tongsum Gangwa accepted the invitation. He was learned in all sciences but was especially skilled in medicine and had received a vision of the venerable Mañjuśrī. On the way he composed a treatise known as *Traveling Lamp of Good Medicine* and one called *Four Refined Ingredients Compound from the Tradition of the Surrounding Countries,* among others, which he offered to the king as a visiting gift. With his treatment the king quickly recovered. Because he was said to encapsulate the doctors from all the borderlands, he was called Tongsum Gangwa of the Borderlands. As a reward he was granted land in Shung and Döl.[361] There he took a wife and became a local ruler, thereby establishing the borderlands tradition.

Therefore, it seems that the doctors from the borderlands were the actual royal physicians appointed by King Trisong Detsen and the other eight Tibetan doctors[362] were merely followers.

The destruction by King Langdarma of the *pratimokṣa* Vinaya code—the very foundation of the doctrine—divides the early and later disseminations of the Buddhist doctrine. [111] However, there has been no such break in the lineage of the medical tradition from the time of Songtsen Gampo up to the present day. Therefore, in terms of its development, I do not think there is any need to talk of early and later disseminations.

Earlier commentators talk of ten traditions: the Kashmir tradition with works such as *Stainless Radiance* by Sthiramati; the Oḍḍiyāna tradition with works such as *One Thousand and Ninety-Nine Treatments*[363] by Jinamitra; the central Indian tradition with works such as *Three Translocations* by Śrī Ānanda;[364] the Nepalese tradition with works such as *Three Preparations Compilation* by Sumatikīrti; the Taksik tradition with works such as *Six Accounts* by Urbaya;[365] the Dölpo tradition with works such as *Weapons of Fearlessness* by Vajrajvāla; the Hor tradition with works such as *Thirty-Five Methods of Bursting from Gagön*[366] by Lekpa Gyaltsen; the Minyak tradition with works such as *Sukhuk* by Tsöndrü Nyingpo; the Khotanese tradition with works such as *Seven Branches* by Gyalwa Dorjé; and the Trom tradition with works such as *Chasing Fever* by Tsenpashilaha. It is said that the texts, practices, and oral transmissions of these ten traditions gradually spread to Tibet, where their topics were compiled externally as texts of medical knowledge, internally as a collection of practical instructions, secretly as a direct-instruction collection for practice, and even more secretly as a collection of methods for direct experience.

During the time of Lha Lama Yeshé Ö,[367] the autocommentary to *Essence of Eight Branches*[368] was translated by Paṇḍita Dharmaśrī Varmā, Nyewo Lotsāwa Yikgi Rinchen, Mar Lotsāwa Rikpa Shönu, and Yikgu Gelong Shākya Lodrö.

The contribution of Lotsāwa Rinchen Sangpo

Later the great emanation and great translator Rinchen Sangpo (958–1055) was born in a part of Gugé called Chanyung Vaṃ Ratna. From the age of seventeen he spent ten years in India, where he devoted himself to seventy-five pandits, including the great Nāropa.[369] In the later dissemination of the doctrine he was unmatched, as illustrated by his taming of Sangyé Kargyal.[370]

He offered a hundred measures of gold to the Kashmir pandit Janarbha[371] and translated and established among others the *Essence of Eight Branches* in 120 chapters by Ācārya Śūra[372] and its extensive word commentary known as *Moonlight* written by the Kashmiri Candranandana. These became widespread in Tibet. [112]

During the time of the glorious Phakmo Drupa (1302–64), these works became widespread in China also, and during the reign of Huangti Huichi,[373] at the request of Yarlung Chikmen, these texts were edited and revised by Yeshé Pal (1350–1405) in the Taitung palace in China, and a Chinese woodblock edition was produced.

The great Rinchen Sangpo had many disciples who held medical lineages, but the most famous were Nyangdé Sengé Dra, Shaka Tri Yeshé Jungné, Ongmen Ané, and Mangmo Mentsün. These were known as the four doctors from Purang. Among them Mangmo Mentsün was very learned and very prolific in his activities, and most doctors from the central region of Tibet came to see him. In particular, he taught in its entirety *Essence of Eight Branches* and *Moonlight* to Chejé Tipang, who in turn taught them to his sons Jangchup Ö, Ulang Tashi Khar, and Dralé Gyalpo. Ulang was learned in the scriptures, commentaries, and practices and was said to be a manifestation of Kumāra Jivaka. He taught the medical texts to his eldest brother's sons Jotra, Yungdrung, and Jotsen, to his own sons Dawa and Nyingpo, and to his youngest brother's son Drotsa. They passed it on to Taktok Gyal, Jophen, and Jonak. Of these three, the first became the most famous, the second was the most familiar with the teachings, and the third was renowned for combining the scripture[374] and instruction into practice.

These three doctors were requested for teachings by Chejé Shangtön Shikpo, or Thukjé Triö, who was one of the ten doctors "likened to royal physicians of early times." He mastered the science of medicine and composed *Compendium of Knowledge Blazing from the Top of a Victory Banner, Outline: A Key to Open the Content, Meteor Destruction of the Hindrance of Difficulties and Doubts, The Pearl Garland: A Detailed and Extensive Word Commentary* in its abridged and full versions. For Shangtön Dülwa from Kyimé Khölma and others, he composed the *Drop of Ambrosia Direct Instruction on Practice in the Manner of an Old Woman Pointing Her Finger.* He also supplied excellent annotations to texts.

His many disciples included Dewa Pal, Yönten Gyatso, and the Tsang teacher Darma Gönpo. The last of these wrote down the oral transmissions: one for his disciples called *Essentials* and one for his son called *Quint-*

essentials. It is said that there many propagators of their lineages in the region of Bodong Roktso.

The master and sole protector Atiśa Dīpaṃkara and Naktso Lotsāwa translated *Daryakan Ambrosia Meat Preparations* [113] and compiled various medical instruction texts such as *Net of Treatments for the Head.*

Shangshungpa Sherap Ö, a disciple of Rinchen Sangpo, the sole eye of the world, taught the Chinese teacher Drakpa Sherap. There is an old medical manuscript in accord with the Explanatory Tantra of *Four Tantras,* and a *Golden Treasury History of the Buddha* composed by someone known as Khorlo Gyalpo, who could be Sherap Ö under another name. He passed the teachings to Yuthok Gyagar Dorjé, who composed an outline, wrote out all difficult points as a small text, made a compilation of the main points, made clarifications, and wrote down the practices, thereby greatly facilitating their understanding.

Then the lineages gradually passed to Yuthok Jipo, Yuthok Khyungpo, Yuthok Gönpo, and others. It seems that Shangshung Sherap Ö also passed the lineages on to Dokgyön Men, Yuthok Draksé, Gönpo, and others.

The contribution of Shangtön Siji Bar and others

Shang Siji Bar (b. eleventh century) was born on Yarlung Cliffs to father Geshé Sönam Wangchuk and mother Merza Bumkyi. He was ordained by Nyak Nyingpo Gyaltsen and became very learned, especially in the five treatises of Maitreya. Once while he was in a park, he threw a stone at a rabbit and broke its leg. Using the slingshot as a splint, he was able to heal it, and he became known as the rabbit doctor. Like a man discovering a new taste, he developed the desire to study medicine but was unable to find a teacher worthy of the name. Therefore, he studied with those who held the lineages of the nine learned doctors and vowed to find answers to his queries. In the beginning he studied with the lower-region doctor Ya Gyongpo of Yoru, Lhajé Sumen from the upper region of Tölung, and Thazhi from the central region. However, apart from receiving teachings on one or two small texts, he was not completely satisfied and had not resolved his doubts. He approached Tongmen, but because Shangtön was so much cleverer, Tongmen did not give him the teachings for fear of being superseded by him. He also studied with this master's disciple Gyalwa Darmen Dütsi of Phenyül.

He studied *Limbs: Wheels of the Great Chariot* with Gyagar Dorjé, *Great*

Exposition on Medicinal Plant Preparation and so forth with Dawa Drakpa of Minyak, and *Special Treatments for the Head* with Drangti Gyalpo but still remained unsatisfied. He studied with Biji Lhuné of Tö, Ukpa Chösang, and Chejé Taklaga [114] and realized that they possessed much supplementary material but little real practical instruction. Therefore, he saved up much gold and set off for India. On the way he met Loden Sherap of Ngok,[375] with whom he studied and became proficient in Sanskrit.

Finally he arrived at glorious Nālandā.[376] "Who is the most learned doctor?" he asked. All were agreed that the rishi Candravi[377] was the wisest. He approached the rishi, who was living in a grass hut, and sat outside his door for seven days.

"What are you doing this for?" asked the rishi.

"Because I want to learn medicine," Shang Siji Bar replied. Thereupon, the rishi gave a single explanation of the eight branches from memory without using a text. As Shang Siji Bar was about to leave, the rishi asked, "Have you understood it all?" Again he beseeched the rishi with a gold mandala, and Candravi gave him a single explanation using a text. He also gave him the history, the instructions, and the practices. The rishi told him to write books on medicine and to be of great help to living beings.

With that he returned to Tibet, where he nurtured disciples. For Buktön Gyagar Rāja and the Nepalese teacher Sherap Tribum, he composed *Stainless Radiance* in four chapters, its commentary *Sun Rays,* and *Rosary of Illustration and Meaning. Thirty Instructions* and the two commentaries to its first and later sections were left unfinished and reputedly taken up by Buktön Gyagar Rāja.

For his disciple Balchung of Lhasa, Shang composed *Outer and Inner Collections.* For Trangchung from Ölkha he wrote *Three Heart-Like Continuous Writings.* For Rokchung from Nyal he wrote *Thirty Instructions.* For his disciple Sherap Tribum from Kyok he composed *Mother and Son Stainless Radiance.*

Dölpa Ringmo requested teachings from the above four disciples and from Darmen, the disciple of Tongmen, and subsequently composed *Essential Transmission of the Thirty Instructions; Thirteen Paths of Fever;* other miscellaneous instructions; a handwritten commentary, word commentary, and overview of the main points on *Stainless Radiance; Important Rivets for Fever;* and many others.

Minyak Mikyö Dorjé composed a medical history, *Pearl Necklace; Supplement to Scriptural Explanation; Accounts from History; Main Point Overviews;*

Nine Treatments; Fifteen Difficult Paths of Illness; and *Golden Garland Word Commentary.*

Tötön Könchok Kyap from Tsalung traveled to India, where he met the later Śāntipa, known as the omniscient one of these degenerate times. From him he learned the eight branches of medicine in their entirety and returned to Tibet. [115] There he composed *Jeweled Net Outline.* He annotated the scripture and gave it to Yuthok Yönten Gönpo.

The *Hundred Medical Preparations* by Nāgārjuna and *Lexicon of Medical Terms from the Commentary on the Essence of Eight Branches* by the Kashmiri Candranandana were translated by Thar Lotsāwa Nyima Gyaltsen. The translator himself wrote *Instructions on Calcite.*

9. The Treasure Tradition and Drapa Ngönshé

The Treasure tradition

YESHÉ KHADRO'S *Instructions on Curing Illness,* translated by Jalipa and Tropu Lotsāwa, and the Nepali Devacandra's *Ambrosia Drop Oral Transmission* are said to be unearthed treasures. On the subject of treasures Ācārya Padmasambhava said:

> For the sake of those in the future
> the precious Dharma is hidden as treasure.
> For as long as the teachings of the Buddha exist,
> for so long will the treasure teachings exist.
> The treasures, therefore, will guide countless beings.[378]

As this prophecy states, there are countless profound treasures in existence, as is well illustrated by those of Oḍḍiyāna Ācārya Padmasambhava. They comprise Dharma treasures, medicine treasures, astrology treasures, Bön treasures, and many more.

Bönpo Draktsal recovered the Dharma text *Four Great Perfection Gurus* and the extensive medical collection *Ambrosia Vase of Healing* from Tsilung temple in Bumthang. *Lotus Chronicles* says:

> When the people of the stronghold of Tsenyül
> use their weapons for farming[379]
> and descendents of the king of the world
> are suppressed by their subjects,
> signs will appear for unearthing
> the southern treasures and others,
> and the treasure finder Kusa Menpa will manifest.[380]

The treasure finder known as the Kusa doctor discovered many profound treasures on Dharma, medicine, and Bön at Padrochal and other places. Of these treasures, the medical texts were of greatest benefit to living beings.

A verse in the *Lotus Chronicles* begins: "In the northern region of Chigong, households will be carried away by a fierce storm,"[381] This is a prediction of signs foretelling the coming of Aya Bönpo Lhabum, so called because he was born in the region of Tölung and was of Bönpo stock. He discovered treasures of medicine, astrology, Dharma, and Bön from Rutsam in the central region. The *Lotus Chronicle* says:

> Even those not traveled to India are claimed as translators;
> the wise and holy of Tibet wander to the ends of the earth;
> a new law of patronage is made with the Mongolians;
> black inside, white outside, like whirls of smoke,[382]
> the merits of Tibet decline and decline—
> these signs will appear when it is time to unearth
> this hidden treasure of Lotus Crystal Cave,
> and the treasure finder will be Ramo Shelmen.[383] [116]

This treasure finder was born in Ramo Menchu in Yartö when the teacher-patron relationship between the glorious Sakya and the Mongolian king was first established. From a cave near the Menchu mountain hermitage, he recovered the Guru, Great Perfection, and Enlightened Mind collections and many collections on medicine and astrology. However, in the beginning, because he practiced medicine together with other practices of help and hindrance, he was not greatly beneficial to people in terms of the Dharma. Moreover, regarding his secret medicines, apart from a collection on dropsy treatment, white radish, and black pepper preparations for elephantiasis-like disorders, and treatments for urinary stones, most of the treasure could not be transcribed from the yellow scroll and remained unread. The treatments for dropsy and elephantiasis-like disorders have remained in unbroken transmission to this day.

Once in Damtrok Khar in Gugé, many children were falling sick, and this was causing great anxiety. One child, however, was never ill and his parents asked him why.

"In the middle of the village is a stone cairn. I moved it and took a stone pot out from inside. I opened the pot and inside was a folded scroll. I wear it day and night and never get sick."

His parents invited a lama learned in the ways of the old tantra schools. They gave the yellow scroll to him to study. It read:

> In the future, in this Damtrok district of Gugé,
> when the children are threatened by disease,
> may this treasure be discovered by a blessed child,
> and may it be of benefit to living beings.

The scroll continued with complete instructions for treating children's diseases and for taking preventative measures. These were copied from the yellow scroll and were of great benefit to the population.

The Indian treasure finder Vajramati unearthed the *Extraordinary and Profound Ḍākinī Treasures* in Liśānti in Nepal. Among the works of Shönu Samten from Tsalgung plains is *Treatment and Prevention of Epidemics from Guru Padma's Journey to Wild Boar Mountain,* which he received from a treasure finder while in Nepal. There are many medical works in Rikzin Gödem's (1337–1408) Northern Treasure collection as supplements to the practices known as the accomplishment of the enlightened mind *(thugs sgrub)*. These include medical collections on white, yellow, and blue scrolls, *Brilliant Lamp,* and *Small Vase of Ambrosia.* The Vajra Armor collection includes *Essential Instruction for the Treatment of Infectious Fevers,* and the Khyungnak collection includes treatments for *lhok*. There are countless other treasures. [117]

Treasure finder Dorbum Chökyi Drakpa

The emanated treasure finder Dorbum Chökyi Drakpa is listed in *Stream of the Ganges: An Account of Teachings Received* by my lama, Ngawang Losang Gyatso, in reality the omniscient one. Dorbum's *Great Vase of Ambrosia* yellow scrolls, so called because it can be compared to one's own heart or to a wish-fulfilling jewel, he most likely received in northern Tradüntsé from the heart of Hayagrīva who Eclipses the Arrogant. He also recovered some supplementary material hidden separately under the stone statue in Jamtrin temple. This work is comprised of four collections:

1. The root, or mother collection; outwardly a catalog of contents;
2. The inner, son documents, which are presented as an intermediate step[384] and which include the arrowhead teachings among other teachings;

3. The no-step collection, dealing with topics not clearly listed in the contents chapter and the stepped collection;
4. The mind-treasure collection on the essentials for the practice of the other three.

In the first collection, the treasure text's catalog of contents, it says:

> In this *Ambrosia Vase* teaching,
> three tantras, five forces,
> the life-treasure force,
> five keys to open the secret treasure house,
> secret ḍākinī heart blood.[385]

These are classified into six main headings: (1) the tantras, (2) the five forces, (3) life treasure, (4) treasure-house keys, (5) heart blood of the secret ḍākinī, and (6) supplementary material.

Tantras

The first of the three tantras in the first group is the *Ambrosia Vase of Immortality Root Tantra* on the eight branches, which is in ten chapters. It is also known as the *Three Collections.* The second root tantra is the *Essence of the Mind of Mañjuśrī,* which consists of a general examination and a specific teaching on the three signs. Its explanatory tantra is *Illuminating Mandala of the Sun,* in which the points are explained generally and specifically under the headings of preliminary, actual, and subsequent practices. These two tantras are counted as one. The third of the three tantras is the *Vajra Armor of Thunderbolt Iron Explanatory Tantra* on the essence of the mind of Vajrapāṇi, dealing with outer, inner, and secret mantra protection and with fire offerings and seals of entrustment.

Five forces

The first force[386] of the five forces is the initiation of suitable vessels, which is a root compilation on torma arrangement, deity visualization of self and assembly in front, initiations, the offering of the assembly torma, and dedications and their benefits. This is a force that supports the ambrosia vase.

The second force comprises the sections known as "the son exceeding the mother." It has seven sections:[387]

1. Victory over *jinlok* with sections on protection and five treatments. [118]

2. Pacification and cleansing combination victory over *sertung* with sections on protection (in which you are referred to the *Vajra Armor Explanatory Tantra*), two types of examinations, and four kinds of treatment.
3. Pacification and cleansing combination victory over *lhok* by eliminating the swellings with sections on the specifics of three protective measures, three examinations, treatment, medicine, therapies, diet, and behavior.
4. Pacification and cleansing victory over *gakpa,* with sections on protection by ordinary substances, general examination, specific examinations, divisions according to location in the body and type, treatment, diet, behavior, and mantras.
5. Pacification and cleansing victory over *gyuser,* with sections on the three kinds of the illness; outer, inner, and secret methods of protection; the ten colors of the diarrhea; four examinations; three treatments; and nourishing bodily tissue.
6. Curing and cleansing victory over smallpox, with sections on conditions, symptoms, types, treatment, reversal suppressants, protection, drying up of the pustules, convalescent treatment, complete cure to ensure the disease does not return, and bloodletting treatments.
7. Victory over *beké,* with sections on recognition and treatment.

These seven sections have the name of "son texts," but actually their subject matter is included in the more fundamental mother literature.

The third force is the utterly secret hidden treasure. This is the elixir essence of the mind of Avalokiteśvara, "the essence of the vase of ambrosia, a bright lamp illuminating the practices." It is a compilation of treatments for the three types of the black infectious *chokgyal* treated as one, an effective medical therapy, as well as instructions on administering the medicine.

The fourth is the force of life, the ambrosia attainment. This concerns the demonic illness *hala chokgyal.* Its treatment is "the great treasure of life medical compound spoken of in the songs of the lotus lord and master Padmasambhava." It deals with the immediate causes and conditions of the illness, examination of pulse and urine, observation, questioning, the magic mirror for recognizing the six secret signs. Treatment consists of "gathering, killing, and cleansing" and "killing the companions."

The fifth force is the secret heart-blood instruction. This is the consecration of medicine as ambrosia, consisting of the preparatory rites of offerings, and so forth; the actual practice of meditation on the crushed herbs, powders, pills, and so on; and the subsequent practices of treatment, protection, and benefits of the practices.

Life treasure

The third main section is that of the life-treasure force. The text here says:

> This great life pillar of reversal suppressants
> is written as a separate work.

This is a scroll on reversal suppressants, containing a ḍākinī prophecy, the very secret great pillar of life, the three black forces as one, "riding the horses,"[388] entrances, pathways, regions and households, protection, examinations, treatments, signs of life and death, [119] along with a final prayer that the scroll will be revealed to each lineage holder.

Treasure-house keys

The fourth section listed in the list of contents is the five keys to open the secret treasure house. The first is the entrustment instruction to the guardian of this secret treasure. The second is a compendium of the eighteen fundamentals and nine mantras. The third is "efficient transformation[389] to break the intestinal pain of *gyuser*." The fourth is a "short text of essential instructions; the key to open the secret door," describing "a great charm circle if one does not wish the mucus to change." The fifth is the mandala key, taught by ten essential instructions.

Secret ḍākinī heart blood

This concerns "accretion" *daryakan,* the blood of the ambrosia goddess.[390] It is in twelve chapters, namely, introduction, causes, conditions, types, examination, treatments, racing through the channels,[391] hot bile, cold bile, bodily tissue bile, remedies for the three types of bile, and *kṣaya,*[392] ending with a summary. It is a "force that holds up the ambrosia vase." Also taught in this section are "the six heart bloods of the ḍākinī, a precious and quintessential teaching," comprising "the key to unlock the heart blood of the goddess."

Supplementary material

Here the contents list reads:

In the utterly secret hidden treasure
is the heroic-force sword collection.

This is a supplement to the third of the five forces mentioned above. These are reversal suppressants in the form of protections of the bodily entrances. They act as counteracting forces to wind, bile, phlegm, hot and cold disorders, organisms, complex disorders, and so on. A panacea entrusted as a treasure by the "blood-drinking lotus king" to his consort, sealed as a profound work together with a prayer, this "thunderbolt-force sword collection" was to be guarded, with the appropriate prayers, by the four kings and by Yangleber.[393]

The list of contents says, "There is the ambrosia garland practice." This is a supplement to the fourth of the five forces mentioned above. It teaches treatments for *hala chokgyal,* comprising single-ingredient treatment, three-method and wisdom combined treatments, the four-hero preparation, the five-garuda preparation, the six whites preparation, the seven types of animal bile, the eight aromatic medicines, the nine-yellow-ingredients preparation, the eight general principles, and finally "the garland of ambrosia pills as taught to the lady of Kharchen."[394]

This completes the mother text as documented in the list of contents.

The inner, son documents presented as an intermediate step

The second collection includes the arrowhead teachings[395] and other teachings. [120] This has a general section and a specific section. The general teaching consists of a commentary written by the Lady Yeshé Tsokgyal on ten lines of the explanatory tantra dealing with the fire offering; a section in extensive and abridged forms on protection against *gyuser,* consisting of an outer protection using urine and a charm circle, an inner protection using medicine and mantra, and a secret protection using deity and mantra; and treatment interspersed with root text, followed by "victory over *gyuser:* a pacification and cleansing commentary."

Son text on five forces

The precious-scroll son literature is divided into five forces:

1. Advice to the treasure finder, together with a teaching on self-initiation
2. A treatment of *jinchung* called the arrowhead of refining

3. The reversal suppressant *zedoary,* the great life-treasure ambrosia, deceiver of death
4. Examination of urine, preparatory tests, together with teachings on the identification of demons
5. The essential scroll on the nine-deity medicinal preparation, pills, massage, and medicinal incense

The armor of the hero consecration is the great pillar-of-life arrowhead that gives power to substances. It has nine sections:

1. The penetrating arrowhead of internal medicine
2. Arrowhead protection of medicinal incense
3. Arrowhead protection by healing with ointments
4. The special arrowhead known as essence of the illuminating sun, for symptoms, prognosis, and treatment of *leser*
5. The arrowhead treatment of *töser,* known as the cooling moon ambrosia
6. The arrowhead treatment of the foreign illness[396] *gyuser*
7. The arrowhead treatment of blood-vomiting *gakpa*
8. The arrowhead treatment and "killing" of *lhokpa,* under fourteen headings
9. The valley fire and skull arrowhead protection

Eight son texts similar to the mother literature

1. The protection arrowhead of the life mantra of the mistress[397] of infectious fever and colds
2. The protection arrowhead of the life mantra of the mistress of foreign *gyuser*
3. The protection arrowhead of the life mantra of the mistress of four-way *jinchung*
4. The protection arrowhead of the life mantra of the mistress of the foreign illness *mikser*
5. The protection arrowhead of the life mantra of the mistress of *sané gaklok*
6. The protection arrowhead of the life mantra of the mistress of black *goshöl* smallpox
7. The protection arrowhead of writing on the method-and-wisdom sun and moon circle
8. The arrowhead instructions to Yeshé Tsokgyal [121]

Refinement of a hidden treasure with reference to heart-blood daryakan

This is the bone *daryakan* section divided into four chapters: introduction, general summary, characteristics, and treatments. The flesh *daryakan* section is in six chapters: introduction, the three nourishments when little,[398] protecting one's body, opening the doors of the senses, curing the illness, and purging.[399] The bright-moon *daryakan* section comprises six chapters, in which its qualities are taught by way of introduction, presentation of the body,[400] channel cleansing, protection, elimination of illness, and longevity.

The next section is a supplement to the sword collection:

1. The very secret hidden treasure, gathering of restorative medicine for the solid and hollow organs
2. Tetanus: treatment, examination, cure, and behavior; the ambrosia essence of the teachings
3. Basic outline

The next section consists of the ambrosia waves instructions giving intensity to the four ambrosia garlands:

1. Compound that tames all fierce disorders
2. The seven-hero preparation, a life-sustaining deathless compound, "ambrosia conquering all serious disease"
3. Examination and treatment for cold-related infectious phlegm disorder, "a life-restoring ambrosia"
4. "Horse and rider together" restorative mercury preparation
5. A special jewel for treatment of "bile becoming wind" infectious disorder
6. Examination, treatment, reversal suppressants, causes, and conditions of black *lhok* and *chokgyel;* ending with the prayer for the treasure to be recovered and the entrustment to the Kaṇḍagauma, or "the eight classes of protector"

The special, or hidden, collection consists of root and branch teachings. The root teaching is that of the great being of Oḍḍiyāna teaching the king and begins with an introduction commencing, "Having built Samyé...." The following branch section is divided into general, specific, and special sections on examination. This is followed by the branches of outer, inner, and secret methods of protection, treatments, restorative medicine for the organs, reversal suppressants, and a prayer for recovery of the treasure.

No-threshold collection, dealing with topics not clearly dealt with in the contents chapter and intermediate step collection

- The force known as the self-sustaining charm circle, the minister of four forces acting as armor for protecting the body
- The instruction known as the key penetrating the inner secrets, comprised of the essential diagnoses of the early, later, and intermediate spies and the three wise men riding the four fast horses
- "The rays of the sun guarding against infectious disease, a force that supports the vase," comprised of the six kings, the six citizens, the two ministers, and spreading and development[401]

Thirteen[402] core scrolls, the essence of the ambrosia vase: [122]

1. Scroll on the killing of *lhokpa*
2. Scroll on the destruction of infectious fevers
3. Scroll on emetics for *gakpa*
4. Scroll on eliminating throat constriction
5. Scroll on curing red diarrhea
6. Scroll on curing *jinlok*
7. Scroll on curing *lhokpa* with mercury
8. Scroll on curing *töser* and bronchial fever
9. Scroll on curing *gaklhok* by being "chased by a warrior"
10. Scroll on purifying wrong treatments given by others
11. Scroll on the reversal suppressants that directly eliminate *lhokpa,* known as "sucked by Black Vārāhī"

These are followed by:

- The cleansing ambrosia stream that washes away all serious illness, exclusive instructions lifting one away from death
- Self-protection, essential oral instruction on purification, supplementary instructions on the four-warrior preparation, protection in dependence on the intermediate-stage urine
- The arrowhead of instruction on medicine measurements
- Arrowhead treatment of *yumo:* recognizing its three types, their cures, and post-illness behavior
- Heart-like arrowhead instructions on the treatment of children's infectious diseases: diagnosis from the five kinds of diarrhea, five types of treatment, total elimination of the disease, and protection of intestinal juices

- The clear silver mirror: practices for the treatment of children's infectious diseases
- The great cooling medicinal compound, antidote to the fever that rages like a fire: an exclusive arrowhead precious heart-like scroll
- Vajra armor protection practice of meditating on a swastika between the eyebrows, and so on: a *hala chokgyal* taught by way of causes, conditions, examinations, treatments, and antidotes; a death-destroying ambrosia definitely reviving even from the brink of death
- Instructions on recognizing the jackals[403] of eating, behavior, and medicine.

This list continues and the text concludes with sealing prayers for the dissemination of these works.

There is also a manuscript on resinous *daryakan,* compiled by Chögyal Tashi Topgyal, describing "the extremely rare resinous *daryakan*"[404] and various other documents.

The essential mind-treasure collection for the practice of the above

This collection was compiled from various manuscripts by Chögyal Tashi Topgyal. It includes: Dorbum Chökyi Drakpa's *Deity Meditation: A Wish-Fulfilling Tree Ornament, Pāñcalika-Necklace Mind Recitation,* [123] *Peacock-Feather Fire-Offering Ornament,* verses on the protection of individuals and the country through substances and charm circles, and texts on how the treasures were unearthed. Other works compiled from the eighteen fundamentals acting as supplementary teachings to the scrolls unearthed separately from Mangyül Jamtrin temple include:

- *Bright Lamp of Oral Instruction Teachings* on the *Vajra Armor Explanatory Tantra, Charm-Circle Force, Garuḍa, Twenty Essences of Charm-Circle Mudra, The Arrowhead Essence,* and so on
- *Three-Garuḍa Self-Sustaining Wheel Collection on the Practices of the Root Forces*
- *Ambrosia Vase Secret Magic: Mantra Fulfilling to Behold*
- *Stream of the Pure Initiations: The Vase-Elixir Initiation Rituals,* which is my lama the Great Fifth's *Illuminating Ambrosia Moonlight Initiation Rituals*

Trülku Dampa Marpo revealed the *Great Ambrosia Elixir Collection: Root of All Siddhis* from the foot of Scorpion Rock[405] at Lion Cliff in Padrochal. It included:

1. *Blessings of Ambrosia*
2. *Tantra on Ambrosia-Producing Teachings* in twenty-one chapters
3. *Ambrosia Practice of Precious Garland Preparations,* beginning with the different names of the great Ācārya
4. *Excrement Ambrosia Accomplishment,* ending with the words "This concludes these teachings on longevity, an exclusive transmission, an abridged but essential practice for liberation from the ravine of ignorance."
5. *Ambrosia Teachings,* with an incidental section on offering substances, sections on types of ascetic practices and meditation on substances to be purified, and ending with a prayer that the finder is able to comprehend the meaning
6. *Instructions on the Use of Elixirs,* covering ascetic practices, types of protections, and ways to dispel hindrances to protection, and ending with the words, "This concludes the instructions of the sacred lama."
7. *Instructions on Ambrosia in the Form of Butter,* which includes teachings on protective substances and the making of elixirs from the *Mañjuśrī Secret Moon;* incidental teachings on their benefits; instructions on using fumigation, ointments, pills, and medicinal incense in dependence on the nine-powerful-black-ingredients compound in order to change the direction of an illness; a text on liquid-butter ambrosia known as the *Vairocana Method of Producing Elixir from Liquid Butter;* instructions on changing the direction of a disorder by using substances blessed by mantra; sections on substances to be purified, diet, and the benefits of improved complexion; and a conclusion that ends with the words "This concludes a short manuscript on instructions concerning ambrosia liquid butter, taught under seven headings, a force for the wise."
8. *Clearing the Difficult Paths of Medicine,* a text on eliminating hindrances by examining demonic influences, illnesses, and so on, that ends with a colophon [124]
9. Incidental teachings on immediate and ultimate benefits and on modes of liberation into the three bodies; ending with the words, "composed by the guru"

In the *Three Warrior Deities* profound treasure collection of the king-like Nyang Ralpachen, in the section on the eight groups of activities, it only talks about:

> Controlling insanity, averting infant mortality,
> curing leprosy, and averting hail.

The section on wrathful activities has practices for averting epidemics, infant mortality, planetary demonic illness, leprosy, *lhok,* and other serious conditions; treatments for counteracting poison, controlling insanity, and curing infant diseases; treatments for *leser,* the Nepali illness, rabies, liver illness, and tumors; cures for urine-retention disorders, illnesses caused by spirits, and *lingtok* and other eye diseases; and ways to destroy *lhog.* He also revealed *Tantra on Shining Ambrosia in Sixty Chapters.*

Guru Chökyi Wangchuk discovered eighteen treasures. The first was found at Namkechen[406] and contains one work on medical examination; three instructional teachings; and *Ambrosia-Vase Heartdrop Treatise in Twenty Chapters: A Storehouse of Jewels and Compilation of the Thoughts of the Twenty-One Rishis.* These can be found in *Stream of the Ganges: An Account of Teachings Received.*[407]

His *Sealed Vase Producing Ambrosia Medicine* includes setting out the meaning of names[408] of the instructions, a list of medical mantras, instructions on creating medicine, and explanations of the mantras, all under one section. A supplement to the above work contains a list of peaceful ritual activities. Practices and activities concerning medicines are grouped in nine sections:

1. What the teachings are based upon
2. Compounds from the general production of the five ambrosias, whose controlling powers will eliminate the poison of infectious illnesses, disturbed blood, diseases of the liver, lungs, heart, kidneys, gallbladder, spleen, and intestines, and leprosy; encourage the growth of hair and eyebrows; cure smallpox; develop the ability to go without clothes; develop the power of fleetness of foot; prevent cracked feet; and cause thunder and hail
3. Individual preparations for ripening and completing bodily development; strengthening the bones; ensuring the teeth grow close together; promoting healthy growth of infants; future development

into the vajra family; producing the best elixirs; dispelling leprosy wind; developing muscle tissue; bringing later development into the jewel family; enhancing clarity of mind; preventing bodily cold power; combatting smallpox; overcoming infectious diseases of the intestines; future development into the lotus family; creating a good complexion; [125] overcoming poisons; and future development into the activity family

4. The king, minister, and people excrement preparation:[409] the root preparation is like a king, while the disorder-changing preparation is like the minister. Taking them for twenty-one days will cure nāga-created illnesses, *gaklhok,* chronic and acute bronchial illnesses, smallpox, eye diseases, *sakong,* and natural and synthetic poisons. The people preparation is known as the *ambrosia emanation*. It is for taming, increasing, and dispelling; eliminating cold disorders caused by wind; improving sight; preserving essential nutriments; acting on the channel openings; generating heat; and for making pills, pastes, gruels, noodle soups, alcohol, medicinal butter, hot barley cake, milk noodle soups, and other everyday foods.
5. Outer, inner, and secret preparations: the outer is prepared using the excrement preparation, the inner in dependence on the seven-births compound, the secret in dependence on a consort
6. Individual rituals: for pacifying eye diseases, synthetic poisons, throat constriction, *gakpa,* leprosy, and disorders of the four constituents; for increasing bodily tissues; for pacifying bile, heart winds, mental confusion, meat poisoning, poisoning of unknown origin, all disorders arising from poisoning, *shazer,* growths, *polok, sharo,* spasms, abscesses, bone disease, cold disorders, fevers, *lhokpa,* male and female spirits and demons, local rulers, and nāgas; for increasing one's lifespan, merit, wealth, and youthful appearance; for bringing men, women, and land under one's control; for enabling the three controlling activities of subduing, burning, and torma throwing; for protecting against poisons; for becoming like a little child; for becoming young; for curing liver disease; for attaining the fleet-foot superpower and the ability to fly through the sky; for granting the ability to give sons to a hundred women; for curing the upper cold and wind disorder, scabies, and blood disorders; for restoring sight; and for completely curing leprosy
7. Pledges

8. Remedial treatment
9. Qualities

Furthermore, Gyaben Dorjé Ö discovered the *Elixir of Sadāprarudita Collection* from the Dadrochen cave in Karchu Pal. Thangmen Drangsong Döndrup discovered the *Tarima Death-Defying Ambrosia* from Dadro Black Rocks in Lower Nyal. Ratna Lingpa (1403–79) discovered *Creation of Medicine: The Complete Secrets* from Kongpo Sangwa Yangzö. Kusa Menpa discovered *Pile of Jewels* from the thigh of Palden Lhamo in Chimpu. Pönsé Khyungö discovered the *Intermediate Ambrosia Vase* from Lhodrak. Latö Marpo discovered *Liquid Butter Ambrosia Treasure Collection.* Guru Jotsé discovered the *Liquid Butter Collection.* [126] Sangyé Lingpa discovered *Eye Medicine.* Rinchen Lingpa discovered *Ambrosia Mercury Elixir* and *Eye Medicine.*

The work *Lotus Precious Garland: A Short Work on Medical Treatments* and supplementary texts were first taught by Oḍḍiyāna ācārya Padmasambhava for the benefit of Kashmiri Bönpo[410] and hidden as treasure between Elephant Nose Rock and Mireng Drawa in Tsarong. There it was discovered by Sihara, king of Tsami. He offered it to Muné Tsenpo, son of Trisong Detsen, who decided the time was not right for it to be of benefit to others and so hid it at Rinchen Ené in Bumthang. There it was discovered by Tsangtön Chöbar.

King of Khotan Treatment for the Neck, which was offered to Trisong Detsen, was discovered by the Mongolian Menpa Jangchup. *Fungi Therapy for Poisons* by the ācārya Sūryasiṃha, translated by Vairocana, and offered to the king and his son, was hidden by Muné Tsenpo and discovered by Nanam Thupa Gyalpo. The *Brown Casket Branch Treasure* was hidden by Muné Tsenpo at Padro Kyerchu and discovered by Cheyu Sher. *Treatment for Bird Demons*[411] was discovered by Nuptön.

In this way countless medical texts were drawn from the great wealth of treasures.

The contribution of Drapa Ngönshé

In the *Lotus Chronicle* it says:

> When the wall built by Tai Tu[412] is complete,
> and Jing[413] and the Chinese are like an ants' nest disturbed,
> signs will appear for the unearthing

of medical treasures from the central pillar
and from the three Jomo places;
the revealer will be Drapa Ngönshé.[414]

This is the prophesy of Drapa Ngönshé (1012–90), an incarnation of Vairocana whose actual name was Wangchuk Bar. I will say a little of his life, beginning with his lineage.

Dharma king Trisong Detsen had a minister from Chimpu known as Dorjé Drechung. He was not wealthy, but he was very intelligent and a good speaker. Consequently, he became a favorite of the king, and he was made supervisor of the construction of the blue reliquary[415] and other projects at Samyé. He had three sons. The middle son, Lhajé, governed Dra Dakpo Drong, or Kyilru. [127] He in turn had a son called Nyané, whose descendents were Nyachung, Palek, Tsenö, Shang Setsa, Lekten, and so on. The last of these, Lekten, had a son called Joga. He in turn had three sons called Shangtön Chöbar, Shangtak Karwa, and Shangten. The eldest entered the doctrine of the Buddha as a monk and became a great geshé in tantra and sutra. Shangtak Karwa had four sons—Taktsap, Takchung, Shenpa, and Yang—and two daughters. The eldest, Taktsap, was born in the male water rat year (1012), the same year as the translator Lhodrak Marpa. In the biography of Marpa there are a few mistakes, such as confusing Taktsap's birthplace, Dra Dakpo Drong, with the Dakpo in Edak.

In his early years Taktsap was a goatherd for about five years in the region of Ba. Then he became ordained by Geshé Yapshü Gyalwa Ö, disciple of the preceptor Lumé, and received the name Sherap Gyalwa. For five years he studied Vinaya. It is also said that from his uncle, Shangtön Chöbar, he learned sutra and tantra, and from Sü[416] he learned medicine. By meditating on minister Vajra Mārajit, he gained an actual vision of this protector, who vowed to work on his behalf.

After Shangtön Chöbar had passed away, one of his disciples invited Drapa Ngönshé to teach. Because of his attainment of a fearless confidence in the sutras and tantras, his teachings gave great pleasure to the scholars attending, and he was given the name Geshé Drapa. Moreover, because he was learned in the Abhidharma, he became known as Drapa Ngönshé—the "one from Dra who knows the Abhidharma."

He mastered completely the instructions on the nine *Lantern of Pacification* collections from Phadampa Sangyé and the instructions on the six yogas of Kālacakra from the Kashmiri pandit Somanātha.

A family from Phodrang Bukpachen who had no son came to him for help. He performed a fertility rite using Glorious Cakrasaṃvara, and a son was born within a year. For this he was presented with a tasseled gold-handled knife, a silver ladle embossed with a deer, a sword with an ornamented hilt, and armor embossed with a scorpion.

In Thangpoché, there was a person called Khutön Tsöndrü Yungdrung[417] who had been a disciple of Drapa Ngönshé but had become envious of his wealth and now regarded him as an enemy. In order to discover if Drapa Ngönshé had clairvoyance or not, he faked an illness and invited him to his house. There he wrapped himself in clothes in such a way that it was not possible to know the back of the person from the front and lay down on a carpet. Drapa addressed him from the rear, [128] "Great geshé, how are you feeling? Please give your hand so that I can read your pulse."

Khutön jumped up and mocked him, "You are renowned as Drapa Ngönshé—the one from Dra with clairvoyance.[418] What a strange kind of clairvoyance it is that does not know the back of a patient from his front!" In response, Drapa Ngönshé initiated the yoga of increasing fire on the outskirts of town, and Thangpoché was burned down. This illustrates the great powers he possessed.

Apart from being a disciple of Yapshü Gyalwa Ö, the identity of Sü remains in doubt. However in some accounts he is referred to as Drapa Ngönshé's lama, who became ill with fluid accumulated in the heart. Medicine did not affect the fluid. Therefore, Drapa, according to tradition, splashed water on him, causing the patient to gasp, and at the same time began to remove the water from his heart with a surgical spoon. However, due to the ripening of karma, the surgical treatment had an adverse effect and the lama died.

To atone for his misdeed he constructed 108 monasteries and temples, including Drathang Monastery on the border of Nashu, which was modeled upon Mingyur Lhündrup of Senyang, as well as Chenyé, Kyilru, Küngara, Serkhang, Khangpo, and Dragya. Of these the most important was built at Dünphü and so was called Dünphü Ganden Chökhor.

His disciples included Dratön Bumlhé Bar, who founded Nekor, Dönchung Tönpa, who founded Droga Dra, Geshé Lhap, who founded Sothang, and Bhandha Jangchup Sempa who founded Riphuk.

In accordance with the prophecy of Rājānaka Vajra Mārajit he revealed the treasure of the *Four Medical Tantras: Essence of Ambrosia Secret Instruction Tantra on Eight Branches* from the upper reaches of the middle story at Samyé. My lama, the Great Fifth, says:

The pure-milk words of the medicine guru
were sealed as a secret mudra
to prevent adulteration by the water of self-creation
and revealed by Drapa Ngönshé,
the incarnate treasure finder.[419]

He composed many treatises, including *Essence of the Tantra,* and spent his life in extensive service to others. The karma for the failed operation on his master ripened and was purified in his lifetime when at the age of seventy-nine, while being operated on by a disciple, the heart surgery was excessive and he passed away.

He passed on his medical works and their oral teachings to his disciple Üpa Dardrak. He in turn gave them to Tönchen Könchok Kyap, who was born in Mangkhar Tsalung and was of the Rok family. Roktön came to the central region to study the sutra vehicle and while there was cured of *kang-bam* by Yuthok Yönten Gönpo. Later he became ill with abdominal dropsy and was cured by Üpa Dardrak. [129] He offered red-cornered turquoise[420] as clear as the sky and worth thousands of *khal* of barley[421] to Üpa Dardrak and received the complete teachings on *Four Tantras*.

10. The Earlier and Later Yuthok Yönten Gönpo

The contribution of the early Yuthok Yönten Gönpo

IN GRATITUDE for curing him of *kangbam,* Roktön Könchok Kyap entrusted the teachings to Yuthok Yönten Gönpo, of whom my lama the Great Fifth said:

> Through his extraordinary illusory works, Yuthok Gönpo
> brought the Ganges stream of teachings of this flawless tradition
> down from the study and contemplation valleys of the hair of
> Brahmā;
> he is truly one who emanated and withdrew the mandalas
> of the gathered enlightened families.[422]

As this verse says, Yuthok Yönten Gönpo was a manifestation of the extraordinary illusion-like play of the gnosis of the all-pervading medicine guru and the receiver of all the different commentarial traditions. I will say a little of his life beginning from his early ancestry.

According to medical tradition, in Padmagarbha, the central city of the nine cities in the land of Padmadvīpa in India, the celestial youth Śvetaketu fell to earth. There a wish-granting cow offered him milk, and by accepting it he became known as Banu, "he who drinks cows' milk." He met with a brahman woman called Dharmamati, and they produced two sons called Brahman Paṭala and Prajñā Khaḍga. Their father gave them a pot of gold each as their inheritance and returned to the god realms by way of the celestial rope ladder.

Prajñā Khaḍga met a beer seller's daughter named Manohara, who was a manifestation of a medicine goddess, and they slept together on the hearth of the inn. A son was born to them called Nandamati. With her supernormal powers, Manohara was able to procure from the monastic community a calf that produced a measure of gold each day. She was also granted various siddhis, including the following. The rishi Gupta Agupta gave her the charm circle that, among other things, binds kings, expels ministers, stupefies generals, and brings all beings under one's dominion. He also gave her a noose, made from his own hair, that binds whoever it touches. A rishi who was a manifestation of Mañjuśrī gave her the charm circles for victory in all battles, for control of the five elements, and for protection against the poison of nāgas. From the nāga teacher Tiṣya she gained a wheel that granted all her wishes. [130] From Acara she received the charm circle for planting all seeds of medicinal plants and bringing them to fruition.

With these powers she was able to bring others under her control, including a wealthy man known as Bahu Hiraṇya—"he with much gold"—and the king, Utpalamukha. Nandamati became king and Prajñā Khaḍga became minister. The celestial *gośīrṣa* sandalwood tree was brought from the god realms. Mahāta, the king of the *rākṣas* was subdued. The doctrine of the outsiders was destroyed. Many corpses were brought back to life with death-defying ambrosia. These and many other stories are recounted in great detail.[423]

In accordance with the dying testament of the calf that produced gold, the rishi Gupta Agupta, the brahman Aṅga Vāṇādirghya, Ācārya Kṛṣna Garuḍa, Pandit Snānamukha or Padmasambhava, King Utpalamukha, Queen Śaṃkara, Minister Mahāmati, and King Nandamati all gathered at Vajrāsana. There Manohara cast a thousand pieces of gold into the air like flowers and prayed:

> In India east and west, in the lands of China,
> in Khotan, Nepal, Tibet, and in other lands,
> for the sake of future generations,
> may the seeds of these medicinal plants
> that cure the diseases of the three poisons
> take root as they are planted,
> blossom with full leaves and petals,
> and ripen with fruit.[424]

With the planting of the seeds and the prayer, they returned home.

A short time later Manohara invited Pandit Padmasambhava and asked him if the seeds and prayer had taken root or not. In reply he said:

Ambrosia goddess in the form of Manohara,
your simultaneous planting of seeds and prayer,
for the benefit of future generations,
ripened by blessings of buddhas and bodhisattvas,
empowered by the common karma of living beings—
this planting of prayer and seeds I will describe.

One league and half a *krośa* west of Vajrāsana in India
are the medicinal mountains of Gandhamārdana,
on which only the rare snake-heart sandalwood grows
and whose aroma can be smelt ten leagues away.
There are varieties of medicines, such as myrobalan forests,
none not growing, none incomplete,
curing every variety of illness and disease;
there are smooth slate mountains, rocky mountains, grassy mountains,
all magically manifest and made from precious stones.
There is found the medicine guru mind manifestation,
formed from sandalwood, of the color white, [131]
brilliant with the marks and features of enlightenment,
an entourage solely of bodhisattva sons of buddhas,
not a place reached by ordinary beings or by Hinayana adepts,
but a place only enjoyed by noble ones of the Mahayana.

West from there at a distance of one league,
formed entirely of precious stones and jewels,
is the medical city of Sudarśana,
its beautiful and well-structured celestial mansion,
sixteen thousand pillars, built of precious stones,
crisscross jeweled beams, four doors, eight-story portals,
five-layered walls embossed with friezes of sensory objects,
garlands, half garlands, jeweled guttering, and parapets,
and in the midst of this celestial mansion,
on a throne of beryl, the king of medicine,
the Buddha, manifest enlightened form,
radiant with the marks and features of enlightenment,
an entourage of Buddhist and outsider gods,
with vidyādhara-lineage rishis and goddesses,

teachers, the sun and moon, the three family guardians,
Ānanda, Kumāra Jivaka, and many others in rishi vidyādhara form.
The entire entourage is bodhisattva,
the place filled with emanated birds and animals,
no trace of gravel, dirt, or mud,
a supreme and magic place of total purity,
not to be enjoyed by the śrāvaka and pratyekabuddha,
a place for noble ones of awakened Mahayana lineage.

There the body manifestation of Medicine Buddha spoke:
"The seeds planted by goddess Manohara,
as you have seen Snānamukha, have taken root
and without doubt will bear their fruits.
One league east from this place
are the medicine mountains of Gandhamārdana;
the qualities of these mountains of medicinal plants
are as you have seen with your own eyes;
remember these qualities and make prayers.

"Two leagues south of this place
are the medicine mountains of Vindhya.
There forests of red sandalwood grow,
with pomegranate, long pepper, and so on;
there is no kind of medicinal plant for cold disorders
that does not grow there.
On those mountains blessed with these qualities
is the medicine guru, formed from fire crystal,
a manifestation of enlightened qualities,
of no fixed color, ornaments, or implements,
radiant with the marks and features of enlightenment,
his entourage are all emanations.
Remember such qualities and make prayers. [132]

"West of here, six thousand leagues away,
are the medicinal mountains of Malaya.
There forests of *gośīrṣa* sandalwood grow,
the six excellent plants, the medicinal plant *sukha,*
grassy meadows of saffron, various salts,

medicine from stones and from the earth,
medicinal jewels, extracts, medicinal trees,
decoctions, medicinal plants, and animal medicines;
in short, no medicine not growing and none incomplete.
There, formed from precious stones and jewels,
is the manifestation of enlightened speech,
the king of medicine, dispeller of the ills of the three poisons,
radiant with the marks and features of enlightenment,
his entourage all ḍākas and ḍākinīs.
Remember such qualities and make prayers.

"Five hundred leagues north of here
are the medicinal mountains of Himavat.
There one finds forests of white sandalwood,
forests of chiretta, *neem,* and aloe wood,
every medicine for relieving heat disorders,
none not growing or incomplete.
There, formed from water crystal,
is found the manifestation of my enlightened deeds,
the medicine guru, king of medicine,
radiant with marks and features of enlightenment,
skilled in working for living beings,
with an entourage solely of gods and goddesses.
Remember such qualities and make prayers."[425]

And further on:

"Now, Snānamukha, hold me in your mind,
go to the four medicinal mountains,
see that the wishes of Manohara are realized."
I, Pandit Snānamukha, went to the four medicinal mountains,
the words of the Buddha were not false;
remembering these qualities
I was moved by profound faith;
without doubt future generations will be free of disease;
the wishes of Manohara will be realized.
Rejoice![426]

Manohara was filled with joy.

King Nandamati took Śrī Suśīla as queen and they produced a son, Padmaśrī. He took Śrī Pradīpa as his queen, and they produced a son called Śrī Saṃpanna. He took Svaradevi as his queen, and they produced a son, Gaṇiḍa. He took Sītā as his queen, and they produced sons called Dundubhi and Sādhumati. Dundubhi befriended the daughter of a drum maker called Gaṇgadevi, and together they had a son, Biji Rāma. A liaison with the daughter of a bell maker produced a daughter, Amaranandi. [133] These two became childhood friends and studied medicine together. They received many teachings from Ātreya and Kumāra Jivaka. Having mastered the ability to produce ambrosia medicine, they achieved the ambrosia siddhi of longevity. Noble Tārā told them:

> By the power of prayers in former lives,
> you and your descendents will preserve
> the teachings of the science of medicine.
> Rejoice, and set off for Tibet.

Urged by this prophecy, brother and sister traveled to Tibet. King Lha Thothori Nyenshal invited them to his palace, Yumbu Lagang. There he presented them with much gold, and to Biji Rāma he gave his daughter, Yikyi Rölcha, as a wife. They produced a son named Dungi Torchok Chen. When he grew up, his father gave him the five *Jīva* sutras, the commentaries, histories, outlines, and practices. Brother and sister then returned to India.

Dungi Torchok Chen's son was Lodrö Chenpo. His son was Lodrö Tsungmé. His son was Lodrö Gyalzö. His son was Lodrö Shenyen. It is said that they became the physicians of kings Trinyen Sungtsen, Drongnyen Deru, Takri Nyensik, Namri Songtsen, and Songtsen Gampo, respectively. The list continues with further descendents of physicians and kings.

In these various histories, the account of Śvetaketu coming to the human realm, the statement that Tibet was in existence during the era of Buddha Kanaka, that the rākṣa king has twenty-one heads, and so on, do not accord with the teachings in general. Also, to say that one league and one *krośa* from Vajrāsana the city of Sudarśana meets the mountains of Gandhamārdana, and that the mountains of the four directions are about five hundred leagues away, contradicts the *Root Tantra*. The concept of a celestial rope connecting the human and god realms is a notion of the Yungdrung Bön, while charm circles such as those that grant all wishes seem Vedic in origin and are difficult to accept. However, the history from Dungi Torchok Chen onward is factual.

The son of Lodrö Shenyen, mentioned above, was Drejé Gyagar Dorjé. One day, while he was staying at Tölung Kyina working and caring for the sick, he met a strange woman near a bridge. "Please come to my country," she insisted. [134]

He stepped onto a white cloth she had unfurled and immediately found himself on a large black cliff shrouded continuously in dark mists. Before him lay a city he had never seen before filled with people. In the middle of the city sat a large castle decorated with exalted sensory objects. On going inside, he found the lord of the castle, dressed as a black tantric practitioner with his hair tied up on his head; he was the size of three ordinary men. Surrounded by his servants, he lay there struck down by illness, groaning with pain. At the head of his bed was a high seat draped with the best cloth to which the doctor was invited. "What brought about your illness?" The doctor asked.

"I brought about hail in a particular country, and so I was hit with mustard seeds empowered by a powerful tantric practitioner."

"Show me," said Drejé Gyagar Dorjé. The lord of the castle took off his clothes and revealed the places where the mustard seeds had penetrated flesh, bones, and veins. The doctor treated him internally with the five-garuḍa compound and mercury, and externally with an ornamented wheel massage. Immediately the demonic nāga in the form of a tantric practitioner was cured. As reward the nāga presented him with many gifts and enjoyments and, as a sign of his gratitude, offered his life to the doctor.

The woman again unfurled the cloth for him to step onto, and immediately he was back at the bridge. "I too wish to offer you a gift," she said. "Come here tomorrow at this time." With that she disappeared into a whirlwind.

The next day he returned to the bridge, and amid rain, thunder, lightning, and darkness, he saw under the bridge, being carried along in the river, the corpse of a woman ornamented from the waist upward with gold and turquoise. He understood this to be the gift promised by the messenger. He took the gold and turquoise, casting the body back into the river. These he spread on the roof of his house to dry. Local shepherds and others, on seeing this, exclaimed that he had a turquoise roof. From then on he was known as Yuthok—"roof of turquoise."

Then the great Drejé went to India to master the practice of ambrosia medicine. In the south, on Śrīparvata, he offered the glorious protector, Ārya Nāgārjuna, a thousand pieces of gold and requested *Precious Essential Points*

Commentary on the Anatomy of the Head, together with all auxiliary and supplementary material. He then traveled to Padmavīpa and in a marketplace met a radiant brahman. After some questions the brahman introduced himself as Biji Rāma. [135]

"Go down south to the sandalwood forest and pray to me and the king of medicine as inseparable," said Biji.

Drejé followed this command, and there the medicine guru, the eight goddesses, the three rishi brothers, and Kumāra Jivaka all appeared and bestowed upon him the practice of achieving ambrosia medicine, together with all auxiliary material. He then returned to Tibet.

There he married Gakyongma, the daughter of a local governor, and they produced a son called Yuthok Khyungpo Dorjé. Blessed with faith, perseverance, and intelligence, he became wise at an early age. With the attainment of ambrosia medicine, he received visions of the goddesses and the rishis. With these powers he could see any illness in a patient's body as clearly as a berry in the palm of one's hand. His father was delighted:

> Son, you being born is a father's glory,
> and from the son of the father the joyous gift of a son,
> one whose name will be Yönten Gönpo,
> shining like the sun of the medical teachings.[427]

Just as he had prophesized, Khyungpo Dorjé married Gyasa Chödrön, who gave birth to the son, Yuthok Yönten Gönpo.[428] At his conception and birth, indescribable and wonderful omens were observed. From the age of three onward, he had visions of the king of medicine, rishis, and male and female vidyādharas. For the most part he did not need to study medicine or learn how to read and write, as it came to him naturally. His father gave him the student Gewa Dorjé as a servant, and he was encouraged to work for living beings.

Once in Tölung, on Poisonous to Touch Rock in Drelung Nakpo, while performing a *gaṇacakra* offering feast, he had a vision of the Medicine Buddha mandala. His heart leapt, and as a result he left footprints on the rock as if it were made of mud.

When he was five he requested from his father the ambrosia medicine practice and the practice permission and sādhanas for the practice of Medicine Buddha, goddesses, and the vidyādhara lineage. During his prayer requests Medicine Buddha came in person and gave him blessings.

At the age of ten he was invited to Samyé Monastery by King Mé Aktsom. As a test, the king asked him to debate with the other doctors, such as Drangti Nyekhar. He defeated them all and became foremost among the nine wise Tibetan physicians.

In Samyé was a patient no doctor could cure. Yuthok saw that his rib had attached itself to his lung and cured him by tying him behind a trotting horse.

A doctor called Küngyuk was very jealous of and competitive with Yuthok. He had a daughter who had watched a pair of donkeys and a pair of pigs mating. [136] This had made her mad with desire, and so she had fashioned a radish into the shape of a penis and inserted it into her vagina. However, the back-and-forth movement broke the radish, and it was lodged inside. This disturbed her genital organisms, bringing her close to death. After all else had failed, Yuthok prepared fumigating salt and burned it under her nose, causing her to sneeze repeatedly until the radish emerged.

He cured the king, who had problems with his eyes and teeth, using hardly any medicine or surgery, and in this way his methods were comparable with those of Kumāra Jivaka Bhṛtya.

In Chimpu he met a manifestation of Vajravārāhī called Tokpai Rang Drölma. He sang a song of his meditation experience, and she sang a song of praise. At the end he had a vision of Medicine Buddha, who bestowed upon him the *Garland of Ambrosia Medicine, Ambrosia Medicine Practice,* and the *Medical Teachings on Practices of the Five Sword Collections.*

As predicted by a ḍākinī, he set out for India at twenty-five years old, having first requested Ācārya Padmasambhava for protective substances and mantras to dispel hindrances. He met the Nepalese doctor Dhanaśīlaha,[429] from whom he received teachings on treatments for specific heat disorders and the practice of cupping. On the Nepal-India border at Parivrājaka Mountain, he met the translator Vairocana. They discussed many topics in great detail, and Yuthok asked him not to hide *Four Tantras* as treasure until he, Yuthok, had returned to Tibet.

In India he met the great pandit Candrabhīra,[430] who bestowed upon him the *Pearl Garland Supplement to the Four Glorious Tantras* with its *Bright Beacon Table of Contents.* From the scholar Agniśa he received the *Outer, Inner, and Secret Stone-Removal Collection; One Thousand and One Commentaries on the Tantra; One Hundred and Eighteen Clear Instructions on Chasing Disease; Magic Mirror of Anatomy; Pointing Out Secret Divisions of the Torso; Essential Key to Surgery; Essential Charm Circle; Secret Measurements;* and countless minor teachings on various eliminative and beneficial methods. With such a treasury of teachings he returned to Tibet to a delighted king.

Again Yuthok returned to India, and from the pandits Candrabhīra and Agniśa he again received many medical texts and instructions, such as the *Hundred Manuals.* Using various magical powers he tamed King Mitsa Yokhur, who had wanted to kill him. He then returned to Tibet, where he worked extensively in the service of others.

Once more he went to India. There he received teachings on Great Perfection from Ācārya Pravahasti; the whispered transmission from the *ḍākinī* Siṃavaktā; from Agniśa *Collection on the Science of Healing,* [137] *Crystal Mirror Tantra,*[431] and the *Somarāja* with supplements. From the pandit Candrabhīra he received *Whispered Transmission of the Rishis* and *Eight Branches.* These are listed in his *Sealed Manuscript Biography.*[432]

In Vajrāsana in India a girl holding a mirror and carrying a medicine bag on her shoulder addressed him, "Great scholar Yuthok, if you wish to go to the medicine city of Sudarśana, single-pointedly pray to the medicine guru and the vidyādhara lineage." He did this, and there in Sudarśana he saw the Buddha, the king of medicine, as well as the palace, the surrounding environment, all the features of the city of Sudarśana. There he met Jivaka Kumāra and his ancestors. The Medicine Buddha addressed him:

> The medical city of Sudarśana
> has outer, inner, and secret locations.
> This outer Sudarśana is in the land of India,
> in the western land of Oḍḍiyāna,
> in Akaniṣṭha, on the summit of Meru, and elsewhere.
> It will be seen by the fortunate who pray
> to the supreme emanation dwelling there.
>
> The inner Sudarśana is wherever one dwells,
> with oneself as the *vaidūrya.*
> Secret Sudarśana is found within one's body.
> At the great-bliss cakra at the crown,
> see your mind as beryl light,
> see the enjoyment cakra at your throat as Malaya,
> see the dharma cakra at the heart as Gandhamārdana,
> see the emanation cakra at the navel as Vindhya,
> and see the nourishing-bliss cakra at the secret area as Himavat.

Go to these four mountains,
see the qualities of these places of medicine,
take the essence of the instructions from India,
and light the lamp of medicine in the center of Tibet.
So that you may care for many people of Tibet,
you will live for 125 human years;
then without doubt you will come to Sudarśana
as lord of the *ḍāka* vidyādhara warriors.[433]

This was followed by more prophecy, reassurance, and praise. Consequently, he went and saw in great detail the four medicine mountains and the emanations of Medicine Buddha that lived there.

In a border land of India populated by women, he exhibited magical powers and flew into the sky.[434] Using language and logic, scripture and reasoning, he tamed the non-Buddhist teacher Advitīyavada. After these and other adventures, he returned to this land surrounded by its white ring of snowy mountains.

Once he was invited to the land of the nāgas because Darśanīya, the eldest of the three queens of the nāga king Anavatapta, had fallen ill. [138] While there he asked them why they were putting so much effort into making various offerings. They replied that they were making offerings to the buddha Nāgeśvara Rāja, who dwelt in their realm, in order to suppress the more unruly nāgas. In answer to the queen's plea to him to cure her of the illness, Yuthok manifested as the king of medicine, washed the patient's body with saffron water, offered a water torma and a nāga torma, performed a nāga treasure ritual, conferred the initiation for the achievement of ambrosia medicine, gave her the precious mercury compound, and she recovered at once. As a gift they presented him with a statue they had made from vajra nāga clay of Medicine Buddha under a turquoise parasol, which came to be known as the statue with the turquoise parasol. Then they cast these flowers of praise:

Outwardly, an emanated form,
supreme siddha of the five sciences,
inwardly, the king of medicine,
eliminating the three poisons inside:
Samantrabhadra, all secrets gathered as one,
these qualities indivisible, to you we bow.

This very special statue was brought by Yuthok to the land of Tibet and eventually came to this capital. Once my revered lama, crown jewel of samsara and nirvana, appeared, in the eyes of ordinary beings, to be suffering from poor sight. He called for this statue, made prayers to it, and without resorting to a great deal of medical treatment was cured of his ailment. Because of this and other incidents it is held in great esteem. It radiates blessings, such as granting the successful consecration of precious pills, and therefore remains to this day a repository of death-destroying ambrosia for living beings tormented by illness.

After the noble Yuthok had been to India and to the land of the nāgas, his fame spread far and wide, and he amassed countless disciples, such as Jangchup Dorjé. When he came to the glorious Dharma wheel that is Lhasa, he ornamented Jowo Śākyamuni and the fivefold self-arisen statue with silk robes embroidered with pearls. He put on a month of festivities for about five thousand people.[435]

Then he went to Yerpa where he stayed in Moon Cave for five days. The medicine goddess Amṛtā came to him and spoke of future events, such as the coming of a later Yuthok, how he would appear in the world, and so on.

The Nepalese king Hadharu was ill with a disorder known as descending cold. His doctor, Śrī Siṃha, said that salt was poison to the bones, alcohol was poison to the flesh, the sun was poison to the skin, and women were poison to bodily tissue, and predicted that if the king abandoned these, his life would be as long as the sun and moon. The king had followed this advice, but it had not helped him at all. [139] Yuthok told the king of the brahman Ulkāmukha, who had abandoned these four—his flesh and eyes had sunk into his bones, and his limbs were swollen, his skin was rough and troubled with wind disorders, his semen had solidified and had stopped flowing, and any physical movement gave him a pain, as though his bones were breaking. The medicine goddess told the brahman, "Because you have given up alcohol, you are emaciated, and the dropsy brought on by the cold and the wind element have made your limbs swell. Because you have given up sunlight, you are troubled by wind disorders. Because you no longer take salt, your bones are weak. Because you have given up women, your semen has stopped flowing." The story continues with an account of how Yuthok cured the Nepalese king of his illness. In reply to questions put to him by his son Bumseng and others, Yuthok replied with details of his past and future lives:

> I the wise Yönten Gönpo
> was Tāravimala early on;

in between I was known as Kumāra Jivaka;
and now I am Yuthok Yönten Gönpo.
From here I will go to Sudarśana
as head of the rishi vidyādharas.
Again in India I will be Agnideva of amputated hand,
and in Tibet, the land of snow, I will be Yuthok Gönpo,
a son born of the Yuthok lineage.

As prophesized by the medicine guru, he identified the medicinal spring of the seven hundred thousand qualities, and by the side of the spring he built a stone pillar inscribed with a list of the qualities.

He went to Ārya Vati Sangpo, where he offered butter lamps and gold leaf to adorn the faces.[436] In the month of miracles[437] he had visions of countless medicine buddhas and rishi vidyādharas. The great rishi Rāhula came to him in person and offered him the profound treatment for planetary diseases. In Lhasa the Jowo Rinpoché statue gave him teachings. From a gnosis ḍākinī he received teachings on how to treat rabies, and so forth. He traveled to Mount Wutai in China, where the noble Mañjuśrī gave him many teachings, such as *Garland of Medical Compunds* and *Exposition on the Abdomen.* In Jayül he saw Medicine Buddha amid a swirl of rainbow light in the sky granting him many gifts with his speech, such as:

In the beginning you were Tāravimala,
then you became Kumāra Abhayakīrti,
now you are known as Yuthok Yönten Gönpo.
From here you will go to Sudarśana,
as head of the rishi vidyādharas.
Then in times of the five degenerations,
great being and incarnation of my speech, [140]
you Yönten Gönpo will come again
to be known as the new Yuthok
and spread the *Garland of Ambrosia Medicine*
and *Ambrosia Medicine Practice.*[438]

As the ḍākinīs prophesied, he had three sons, Bumseng, Palbum, and Gagang. He brought huge benefits to others, working tirelessly until he was one hundred and twenty-five years old. Finally, he was summoned by Yeshé Khadro[439] and, without leaving his bodily form, went to the pure land of Medicine Buddha.

The contribution of the later Yuthok Yönten Gyatso

Those accounts of the coming of the later Yuthok that talk of the demon of Brass Pillar path granting Drejé Gyagar a siddhi using the corpse of a woman laden with turquoise, and so on—similar to accounts found in the biography of the earlier Yuthok—are words of the fool who uses a hat as a boot and are not correct.

In the thirteenth generation of the Tölung Kyina family, in Goshi Rethang in the upper Nyang River region of Tsang, he was born to father Yuthok Khyungpo Dorjé and mother Pema Ödenma amid wondrous and unimaginable signs. He was blessed by the vidyādhara rishis and washed by the medicine goddesses.

Virtuous karma awoke in him from an early age, and he was able to recognize various medicines and so on without mistake. As he himself said:

> At the age of eight I, Yuthok Gönpo,
> nurtured the science of medicine.[440]

From the age of eight onward, he was cared for by the noble guide Mañjuśrī and became wise in the sciences, especially in the science of medicine, and nurtured and developed an attitude of working for others. At the age of ten a longevity goddess prophesized that in two years he would meet the *Essence of Ambrosia Secret Instruction Tantra on Eight Branches.* Accordingly, Roktön Könchok Kyap from Mangkhar Tsalung came to Goshi Rethang. There Yuthok made him a grand offering of the *Hundred Thousand Verse Perfection of Wisdom Sutra* as well as smaller offerings, including a saddle and bridle, and in return he received *Four Tantras* in its entirety. For a while he did not release this work from its seal of being a one-to-one transmission and kept it for his own practice.

At the age of eighteen he went to India. In the land of Kuda he received the *Tantra of the Black Lock of Hair* from Śrīmālā, head of the gnosis ḍākinīs. [141] In Vārāṇasī he received *Essence of Ambrosia Eight Branches,* the *Somarāja,* the *Sutra of Help,* the *Heap of Jewels,*[441] the *Kumuda Flower,* the *Sutra on Pulse,* and the *Commentary on Protecting Life.* In the country of Singhal[442] he received black and white editions of Candranandana's *Moonlight,* the extensive, intermediate, and short exposition of the *Ambrosia Vase.* In Rājagṛha he received Śūra's treatise on the eight branches, the extensive and short *Illustrations of Medical Plants,* and the *Secret Preparations of Minerals.* In Suvarṇadvīpa[443] from the rishi Kanakavarman he received *Four Tantras* and the following tantras: the *Union of Sun and Moon,* the *Nourishing Flesh and Blood,* the *Liberation of Beings,* the *Arising of Tārā,* the *Craft of Precious Stones and Metals Such as Gold,* the *Leaves of the Birch Tree,* the *Mañjuśrī Mother and Father,* the *Hide Casket,* the *Ḍāka Liberation,* the *Chapter on Anatomy,* the *Fragment Transmission,* the *Individual Elements,* the *Great Treatise on the Pulse,* the *Teaching of the Essence,* the *Ambrosia Inscriptions on Presentation of the Body,* the *Examination of the Pulse,* the *Brief Indian Work,* the *Guṇaśāstra,* and the *Three Hundred Fasicles.*

In the middle of a forest called Kala he met goddess Amṛtā. She took care of him and gave him *Three Collections of Question and Answer,* and *Ambrosia Preparation for Healing Wounds.* Later, in the region of Vedha, he met the goddess again, and she bestowed upon him many ordinary and supreme siddhis and gave him the three collections on the *Beacon Medical Texts,* and on his journeys he was not harmed for a moment by the punishments of rulers, poisonous snakes, elephants, tigers, leopards, bears, robbers, and so forth. He arrived in the Shang Palkyé region of Tibet, and there he made many prayers for gathering disciples and bearing sons, working and caring for others mainly in the field of medicine.

Then in accordance with the prophecy of the goddess Amṛta he again set off for India. Over time he met with many pandits and siddhas there. Śrīmālā, chief of the gnosis ḍākinīs, gave him the *Sixty-Five Classes of Moonbeam Essential Tantras on the Eight Branches* and teachings on the more-profound-than-profound secret Vajrayana path, such as *Heart Blood of the Ḍākinī.*

It is said that he traveled to India six times. On those journeys he gave indescribable displays of his magic powers. In particular he defeated five hundred non-Buddhist teachers using language and logic and converted them to the Buddhist path. In Śrīparvata, in the south of the country, he was accosted by a group of wild bandits on the road, but he gave them a wrathful stare that paralyzed them on the spot. In Oḍḍiyāna angry *gandharva* ḍākinīs hurled a thunderbolt at him, [142] but with his fingers in the threatening gesture, he caught it and threw it back. Once when he was in a boat off the country of Singhal, a outsider black magician caused the boat to sink, but he flew up into the sky like a bird. When a snake in the forest of Kala caused the air to become thick and dense with its poisonous exhalations, he meditated on great compassion and immediately pacified the snake. He traveled unimpeded through Meru and the lesser mountains. He could see all animate and inanimate phenomena as clear as a berry in the palm of his hand. In Nepal, in a competition of magical powers with followers of Bön, he sat in the sky for half a day. He could recite from heart all the precious teachings of the Buddha and the commentaries, and he became supreme among the hundreds of pandits in Vajrāsana. He traveled from India to Tibet in one day and was able to bring as gifts fresh myrobalan with its leaves and *soma* flowers. In his own words:

> Flying through the sky I am like a bird,
> moving through the water I am like a fish,
> penetrating mountains I am a thunderbolt,
> amid fire I am the fire god.
> In these degenerate times beings have little merit,
> few have seen me, few hear my name.
> Those who see, hear, remember, and touch me with faith
> will soon come to unsurpassed enlightenment
> and purify the unwholesome deeds of an eon.[444]

Also:

> I travel at one time to a hundred worlds,
> meet at one time a hundred buddhas,
> send out at one time a hundred emanations,
> bring in at one time a hundred sentient beings;
> I have attained every eclipsing samādhi.[445]

Because he had achieved the bases of the totally eclipsing meditative concentrations,[446] his host of emanations were beyond description.

In the early part of his life he worked solely with the eight branches. Later he composed *Naturally Illuminating Knowledge of Pulse Examination* in five sections, *Small Volume on Practice,* the *Ambrosia Essence Short Tantra,* the *Three Scroll Collections,* the *Six Key Collections,* and many more. [143]

11. The Word of the Buddha

YUTHOK YÖNTEN GÖNPO realized that the glorious *Four Tantras* were the very pinnacle of medical science, and so for the sake of future generations, he released them from the seal of being purely a one-to-one transmission and propagated them as crown jewels to be venerated by all living beings. He revised the translation and, as I describe later, made additions to accord with time, place, and conditions. He also composed *Golden Annotations* for his sons, and *Copper*[447] *Annotations* for his disciples.

These deeds have given rise to various positions on whether *Four Tantras* is the actual word of Buddha or not, and consequently on whether the actual teachings of the Buddha and the later commentaries are mutually exclusive or not. These points have been dealt with extensively elsewhere. However, on the subject of what constitutes the word of Buddha, or the sacred Dharma, the highest yoga father tantra *Vajra Essence Ornament* states in its ninth chapter:

> The meanings of the 84,000 collections of Dharma
> I have condensed as this.[448]

Also, in the first chapter of the *Vajra Garland Tantra* it says:

> In brief, in the glorious Guhyasamāja,
> the 84,000 collections of Dharma of the Buddha
> in the form of the highest of yoga tantras.

Also, in the *Sutra of Limitless Life and Gnosis,* which can be classified as either a Mahayana sutra or an action tantra:

> By copying or encouraging someone to copy this sutra, one encourages the copying of the 84,000 collections of Dharma.[449]

In the second summary of the nondual tantra, *Stainless Light Great Commentary to the Kālacakra,* it says:

> Therefore, because of the dispositions of sentient beings, all tathāgatas teach the three vehicles and teach the 84,000 collections of Dharma.[450]

These and other citations belong to the category of passages that talk of the Dharma in general terms as a collection of 84,000 categories or collections.

In the *Understanding Highest Yoga Tantras* by Ācārya Śraddhakara Varman and translated by Lotsāwa Rinchen Sangpo it says:

> The Bhagavān taught 84,000 collections of Dharma. These are also included in the one resultant vehicle. Thus it is the great vehicle.[451]

Also:

> The great vehicle is of two kinds: the vehicle of the levels and perfections, and the resultant secret-mantra vajra vehicle.[452]

The term "vehicle" comes from the Sanskrit *yāna* meaning "mount,"[453] and that can be great or small when applied to the size of the vehicle of the minds of disciples. In this connection, the term "basket" is *piṭaka* in Sanskrit and means a "collection" or "compilation." The three baskets apply to the great vehicle as well as to the small vehicle, as in the three baskets of the śrāvakas for example. So, although they are different in terms of their names, in actuality "vehicle" and "basket" are not mutually exclusive. Therefore, secret mantra too is included in the 84,000 collections of Dharma. Furthermore, the same text says:

> The secret mantra vehicle is explained as being included in the three baskets. [144] This is because the nine categories of scripture are the basket of the great vehicle, and the basket of the secret-mantra vehicle is included in the nine categories of scripture. Secret mantra is also included in the three baskets because it teaches the three trainings.[454]

The above citations belong to the category of passages that clearly teach secret mantra as being included in the collections of Dharma.

Concerning the early translations, the twenty-seventh verse of the *Crystal Rock Lotus Chronicle* states:

> As an antidote to cure the affliction of desire
> he taught the 21,000 baskets of Vinaya.
> As an antidote to cure the affliction of anger
> he taught the 21,000 baskets of Sutra.
> As an antidote to cure the affliction of ignorance
> he taught the 21,000 baskets of Abhidharma.
> As an antidote to cure the three poisons equally,
> he taught 21,000 baskets of secret mantra.
> These are the 84,000 gateways to Dharma,
> compiled to form the twelve categories of scripture,
> condensed as Sutra, Abhidharma, and Vinaya.[455]

The *Tantra of the Self-Appearing Mind* says:

> The vehicle divisions are as follows:
> the sutras, the vast and great,
> and the even vaster and greater.
>
> The even vaster and greater
> is the 84,000 beyond conception,
> vast, numerous, and great,
> beyond conception, immeasurable,
> indescribable, and beyond thought.
>
> The vast and great is divided into nine:
> those of the śrāvaka, pratyekabuddha, the bodhisattva,
> the vehicles of *kriya, upa,* and *yoga,*
> *mahāyoga, anuyoga,* and Great Perfection *ati.*
> This is the great doctrine of Dharma
> explained in nine aspects.[456]

Longchenpa explains these verses in his *Treasury of the Supreme Vehicle,* where he says:

Generally speaking, the different Dharmas of the Buddha are beyond number. When they are compiled into vehicles, however, we can make an abridged classification into great and small vehicles, or causal vehicle and resultant vajra vehicle. To expand on these, the śrāvaka, pratyekabuddha, and bodhisattva vehicles are the three types of beings with lesser faculties. The *kriya, upa,* and *yoga* vehicles are for those of middling faculties, while the *mahā, anu,* and *ati* are for those of the sharpest faculties. In the *Great Presentation of Atiyoga* it says:

> The doctrine I have taught is of two levels,
> characterized as lesser or great [145]
> according to levels of sentient beings' minds,
> each possessing their own particular views.
>
> Each is of two levels: of wrong views and of right.
> Those of wrong views dwell in samsara,
> those of right views are of three levels:
> those taught for lesser minds, those for middling minds,
> and those for great minds.
>
> Those of lesser minds are three,
> and the doctrines taught according to their minds
> are that of the śrāvaka taught to those tainted by concepts,
> that of the pratyekabuddha taught to those with discernment,
> that of the bodhisattva taught to those who penetrate
> concepts.
>
> Those of middling minds are also three,
> and the doctrines taught to them
> are *kriya* to the very low, *carya* to the low,
> and *yoga* to those of higher consciousness.
>
> For those three of the sharpest minds,
> there is generation for those beyond mind,
> completion for those with the essence of mind,
> the Great Perfection for those of the supreme and
> most secret.[457]

For the even vaster and greater vehicle, all the teachings of the Buddha are included in the three baskets, and mantra is in the basket of great Abhidharma. With 21,000 categories each in the baskets of Sutra, Vinaya, and Abhidharma and 21,000 more distributed among all three baskets equally, there are generally speaking 84,000 collections of Dharma. However, on the basis of individual antidotes for pacifying the hosts of conceptions found in sentient beings, these can be expanded even further to become "vast and numerous, inconceivable and indescribable."

The three divisions of the Great Perfection—namely the mind, sphere, and precept divisions—also have further divisions. The *Consequence* says:

> From the natural great perfection appear the specifics
> of words;
> from the three divisions come the nine spheres.
> From the compilation of words come verses
> numbering 6,400,000,
> in chapters numbering 35,000,
> in categories numbering 21,000,
> of content equal to the reaches of space,
> severing the conceptions of sentient beings.
> From these come the compilations of topics:
> in 180 rivets are 1,500 hindrances[458]
> and 3,000 essential points.
> On the 400,000 mistakes are 20,000 name-bearing
> tantras,
> word and content clearly arranged.[459]

In terms of the three baskets, these passages place secret mantra in the basket of great Abhidharma. Therefore, even the early translations include both sutra and tantra in the 84,000 collections of Dharma. [146]

Furthermore, the *Stainless Light Commentary on the Mañjuśrī Saṃgīti* by Kalkī Puṇḍarīka says:

> "Arising by way of three vehicles" refers to the vehicles of the pratyekabuddha, śrāvaka, and bodhisattva. "Dwelling in the one resultant vehicle" refers to the three vehicles included in the indivisible secret-mantra vajra vehicle.[460]

The great scholar Butön says in his *General Presentation of the Tantras:*

> "The baskets of scripture number three or two" means that the baskets of scripture may be divided into the smaller-vehicle basket and the great-vehicle basket. The basket of the great vehicle in turn can be divided into the causal sutra vehicle and the resultant vajra vehicle.[461]

The great Tsongkhapa, Mañjuśrī incarnate, says in his *Stages of Mantra:*

> In *Understanding Highest Yoga Tantras* it says that there are two traditions: one of not including the vidyādhara vehicle in the three baskets of scripture but according it the status of a fourth basket, and another tradition that does include it in the three baskets. However, in the *Questions of Subahu Tantra* it says, "Listen I will explain secret mantra in the manner of the sutras."[462] Also, many tantras are explained as being sutras and are mentioned in the categories of sutra. Therefore, Ratnakaraśānti's assertion is correct that because these tantras explain the profound in an abridged form, they are classified as sutra. However, in terms of the internal divisions of scripture, they also teach topics from the other baskets, and so Abhayakara's assertion that they belong in all three baskets is also correct.[463]

Khedrup Gelek Palsangpo in his extensive commentary on the Kālacakra, *Illuminating Reality,* explains this point in accord with Jetsün Tsongkhapa and states:

> To include them in the basket of sutra, and to assert that in terms of their own internal divisions, parts can be included in the basket of Vinaya and parts in the basket of Abhidharma is not contradictory.[464]

These and other passages talk of secret mantra being included in the three baskets of scripture without particular reference to the 84,000 collections of Dharma.

In *General Aspects of the Classes of Tantra* it says:

> All the teachings of the conquering Buddha are included in the 84,000 collections of Dharma. 21,000 are for disciples whose minds are predominantly affected by desire, 21,000 for those predominantly affected by anger, 21,000 for those predominantly affected by ignorance, and 21,000 for those affected by all three equally. These were taught, therefore, as antidotes for the 84,000 afflictions.[465]

This passage follows the thinking of *Lotus Chronicle* cited earlier. Bodong[466] in his *Compendium of Reality* says:

> However, some might wonder, if the four classes of tantra are included in the three baskets, [147] then they become part of that categorization. If they are not included, then they are no longer the word of Buddha. There is no problem here. They are mostly included in the basket known as the very vast scriptural basket of the bodhisattva and are special components of the sutra division of the three baskets.[467]

Therefore, although there is no clear reference here to the 84,000 gateways of Dharma, he asserts that secret mantra is included in the three baskets and so actually is not in contradiction with the position of those mentioned previously—the early translation school, and so on. However, in the third fascicle of the *Jewel Lamp Dhāraṇī* it says:

> Ānanda said, "Bhagavān, I have heard the 84,000 collections of Dharma from the Tathāgata, but I have not heard such a Dharma before."[468]

Taking into account the vagaries of translation, the verses from this sutra are identical to those of chapter 17, the Śrībhadra chapter, of the *Avataṃsaka Sutra.* Therefore, when this chapter of the *Avataṃsaka* was being taught, the 84,000 categories had already been delivered. Also, even though there are many who assert the *Jewel Lamp* to be action tantra, scholars of tantra tend to leave this work unclassified.

These and other points are the bases for doubt and query, and so the scholars of the past have not been clear on this. However, Taktsang Lotsāwa Sherap Rinchen in his *Knowledge of All Sciences* says:

> The glorious Guhyasamāja root tantra is taught to be
> the scriptural basket holding 84,000 categories of sutra
> and the root of 33,000 categories of tantra.
> Basket and root are therefore differentiated,
> and so a fourth, called the vidyādhara category,
> is validly asserted by the scholars of India and Tibet.[469]

Here, he is asserting the existence of a fourth category and also differentiating between "root" and "basket." In his *Ocean Overview of Kālacakra* he says:

> Therefore, some so-called scholars say that sutra and tantra are not mutually exclusive, because of passages such as "Listen I will explain secret mantra in the manner of the sutras" or "If you listen to this sutra" or because the *Tatvasaṃgraha Root Tantra* is described as a great-vehicle sutra, or that the category of sutra is taught in the root and explanatory Guhyasamāja in terms of sādhanas being mixed within sutras, and so on. Some even more pretentious scholars maintain that sutra and tantra may be mutually exclusive but that these citations teach that secret mantra is included in the basket of sutras from the three scriptural divisions. To them I say, in that case there are works called the *Kalāpa Sutra,* the *Candravyākaraṇa Sutra,* [148] the *Pramāṇa Sutra,* the *Caraka Sutra,* and so on, and you would have to include them in the basket of sutra regardless of whether they contradict Buddhist sutras or not.[470]

He is using overly intellectual reasoning here to establish his point, the essence of which is a refutation of Jé Tsongkhapa's position. The authority for his position on the three baskets of 84,000 categories of Dharma and his asssertion that the 33,000 categories of tantra are not included in them, is found in the *Ocean of Wealth:*

> That the 33,000 categories of tantra are not included within the 84,000 categories of sutra is described in the *Vajra Gnosis Compendium Tantra.*[471]

The actual text is from the second part of the tantra entitled *Chapter on Great Bliss:*

> "Bhagavān, what are the numbers of great yoga tantras, dual tantras, conduct tantras, action tantras, and conceptual tantras?"
>
> The Bhagavān replied, "There are 12,000 with the name of great yoga tantras. Expanded further they would be beyond number. There are 6,000 dual tantras, 8,000 conduct tantras, 4,000 action tantras, and 4,000 conceptual tantras. This comes to 34,000 tantras."[472]

In this tantra, and in the *Vajravarāhyabhibhava Tantra*[473] and others, we find this division into five classes of tantra. However, this tantra makes no mention at all of the 84,000 categories of sutra. Also, maybe he has not noticed that this tantra talks of 34,000 tantras. Whatever the reason, it is as false as a headless ant.[474] Furthermore, in the commentary to *Knowledge of All Sciences,* the verses quoted above are not commented upon but have had to be left as they are.

My lama, the Great Fifth, in his *Stream of the Ganges: An Account of Teachings Received,* asserts that the tantras are included in the basket of sutras when he says:

> Concerning the collection of tantras, the very pinnacle of all vehicles, the *Questions of Subahu Tantra* says, "Listen I will explain secret mantra in the manner of the sutras."[475]

Therefore, to include all the tantras of the old and new schools in the three baskets described earlier is not unacceptable. However, in *Stream of the Ganges,* at the back of the *kha* volume, my lama, the Great Fifth, says there is a citation from the early-translation work *Compilation of the Enlightened Mind,* under a different translation, that is also quoted as being from the *Sutra of Secret Prophecies* in the Tengyur work *Eliminating the Two Extremes* by Jñānaśrī, [149] and that is identical in thought to a citation from *King of Teachings on the Sutras.* It runs:

> Having turned the wheel of causal phenomena
> for those predisposed to the causal path,
> the result vehicle—a swifter path—
> will appear at a future time.[476]

As a general truth, the tantras were taught by the Buddha. However, in the eyes of ordinary disciples, he first turned the Dharma wheel of the three baskets of scripture and then the result vehicle only began to appear about one hundred and twelve years after his passing. Therefore, says my lama, the three baskets and the four classes of tantra were said to be separate divisions of scripture.

The *Vairocana Enlightenment Tantra* was taught on the summit of Mount Meru, and the Yamāri collection was taught while taming the māras. Nāropa in his *Commentary on a Short Teaching on Initiation* quotes a verse from the *Kālacakra Root Tantra:*

> On Vulture's Peak our Teacher gave
> the perfection of wisdom teachings,
> and likewise on Śrī Dhānyakaṭaka
> he taught the secret mantra.[477]

Also in Anupamarakṣita's commentary to the *Saṃgīti:*

> In the shrine of Śrī Dhānyakaṭaka...

up to:

> The initiations were bestowed
> on all the gods and other beings,
> and the four classes of tantra,
> and, to make five, the essence tantras
> were extensively taught by Vajradhara.[478]

Therefore, in the Kālacakra tradition all the tantras were taught in the year of Buddha's passing.[479] The fifty-first chapter of the *Ḍākārṇava Tantra* states:

> Tantras spoken by the lion of the Śākya
> travel to the perfection of yoga.[480]

This refers to the *Saṃvara* collection and also the *Guhyasamāja* being taught before the passing of the Buddha. These assertions make up the various common positions on tantra. Other more exclusive positions, I think, are based on the prophecy made in the *King of Teachings on the Sutras,* also known as the *Sutra of Secret Prophecies:*

> After I have gone from here
> in years numbering 112,
> the quintessential teachings
> renowned in the three celestial realms,
> augured by auspicious signs appearing
> to the king known as Ja
> in the eastern region of Jampudvīpa,
> and of a lineage of glorious human merit
> will be given by Vajrapāṇi in Ugra
> in the company of the king of Lanka and other
> great beings of a lower lineage.[481] [150]

Concerning the number of new translation tantras, the twenty-second chapter of the *Cakrasaṃvara Tantra* states:

> The number of yoga tantras
> is ascertained at 60 million;
> Likewise, the number of yoginī tantras
> is said to be 160 million.
> Sutras other than those of the great vehicle
> number 800 million,
> while those of the perfection vehicle
> number 500 million times a million;
> all of them taught by the Munīndra,
> embodiment of the three bodies.[482]

Also, the *Buddha Skull Tantra* says:

> There are 60 million yoga tantras and 160 million yoginī tantras. Individual sutras number 800 million. Likewise those of the perfection vehicle number 500,000 times 100 million. All of these were taught by the Munīndra.[483]

Therefore, unless they are talking about the number of verses, the sutra count mentioned in this tantra and the *Cakrasaṃvara* is far greater than 84,000.

With the line "There are 12,000 with the name of great yoga tantras" from the *Vajra Gnosis Compendium Tantra* citation quoted previously, it is as if it is counting the names of individual tantras such as *Cakrasaṃvara* and *Guhyasamāja*. Also the *Vajra Essence Ornament Tantra* says:

> Goddess, these 507 treatises
> I have taught them perfectly for particular reasons.[484]

Therefore, in the *Guhyasamāja* category of tantras alone, there are 507 treatises, or tantras, and each of these also contains related tantras. For example:

> Of the *Krodhacandratilaka*,
> there are 500,000.[485]

Therefore, this comes to an enormous amount.

There are also many subcategories of action tantras. The tenth chapter of *Tantra Requested by Subāhu* says:[486]

> For the benefit of gods, demigods, and humans,
> 30,500,00 different *vidyā* mantras—secret mantras[487]—
> were taught by the conquering Buddha
> to form the vidyādhara basket of scripture.
>
> To alleviate the sufferings of poverty
> and to destroy the secret ones,[488]
> I have taught 70 million tantras
> with mandalas and mudrās.
> To the ten messengers, the seven *vidyā* kings,
> likewise the sixty-four attendants,
> and eight supreme deities of my essence, [151]
> *Amṛtakuṇḍalī,* and so forth, of the wrathful guardians,
> *Vidyottama,* and so forth, the powerful ones,
> the *vidyā* lords, and other followers of mantra:
> to these of the vajra lineage, I teach extensively.
>
> I have taught 30,500,000 tantras of Avalokiteśvara;
> their *vidyā* lord is Hayagrīva.

Mandalas bearing his name
are those of the three supreme ones,
the twelve-armed, the six-armed,[489]
the Crown Protrusion Fulfilling Desires,
and the four-faced Amoghapāśa—
seven secret mantras shining above the earth like seven suns;
these are the secret-mantra mandalas of Hayagrīva,
granting the supreme to humans
and worshipped in the three worlds.

White Tārā, Pāṇḍarā, Vipaśyin,
white Ekajaṭa, Yaśovatī, and Bhṛkuṭi,
the great mantra queens of the lotus lineage.
These have mandalas of different forms
and mudrās of different designs.

In the vast lineage, Mekhalāvat,[490]
mistress of knowledge, queen of mantra,
her mantra granting the supreme siddhi
adored by Pañcaka, lord of the lineage,
always in accord with the powerful lords of the *yakṣa,*
with her words a host of tantras are taught.
In the Pañcaka tantra, twenty thousand verses,
and in that of his wife, half that number.

The lord of wealth (Pūrṇa) has thirty thousand verses,
the father of Pūrṇa,[491] one hundred thousand.
Limitless tantras have been explained by those
gods and demigods who have faith in the Conqueror.

These passages give some idea of the number of tantras.

The Hinayana position

In the first chapter of the *Treasury of Abhidharma* it says:

Eighty thousand collections of Dharma
taught by the mighty Buddha

> are either word forms or names included in
> form and compositional factors. [152]
>
> Some say it has the measure of a treatise,[492]
> that it refers to each teaching of the aggregates, and so on.
> It is taught that the Dharma collections
> correspond to practices to counteract particular behaviors.[493]

In the *Bodhisattva Abhidharma Commentary,* a work more extensive than the auto-commentary and other commentaries, it says:

> Just after that it says,[494] "What is this Dharma known as the speech of the Buddha? It is a collection of names, word forms, and syllables that were set down in order, formed in order, joined in order." According to followers of the Abhidharma, the eighty thousand collections of Dharma belong to the category of form and compositional factors. A sutra says: "I have held all at once[495] the eighty thousand categories of Dharma heard directly from the Bhagavān." Other types of sutra talk of 84,000 categories.
>
> "Some say it has the measure of a treatise." On this some say "This *Sutra of Collection of Dharma (Dharmaskandhasūtra)*[496] is about the length of a treatise." "That has six thousand verses" means that a treatise has a textual length of six thousand verses. The eighty-thousand collection has diminished, and this is all that is left."
>
> "Others say that the eighty thousand refers to each teaching on the aggregates and so on," meaning that each teaching on the aggregates and so on is one Dharma collection *(dharmaskandha).* These are explained as making up the eighty thousand collections.
>
> "It is taught that the Dharma collections correspond to practices to counteract particular behaviors." This is said either to refute the previous point or as a definitive statement. "Differentiated by behaviors such as desire, anger, ignorance, pride, and so forth." The phrase "and so forth" includes doubt and wrong views. The behavior of some beings is desire....

And so on, up to:

> Some abandon anger but pursue desire. As practices to counteract these behaviors, the Bhagavān taught these Dharmas.[497] [153]

The Mahayana position

In the *Clear Words Commentary to Ornament of Realization* by Mādhyamika Dharmamitra it says:

> "As practices to counteract particular behaviors" refers to the four main kinds of behaviors—desire and so forth—which when subdivided become the 84,000 types of behaviors. Every wheel of Dharma of the mighty Buddha exists as practices to counteract these behaviors. "Dharma" here mainly refers to the Dharma that is taught. "Wheel" is used to portray the image of something moving toward the mind of the disciple. It also means "collection" or "gathering."[498] These two meanings of the word closely reflect its use here. "Every" means all 84,000 heaps of Dharma. So, what is the measure of one heap of Dharma? It is one thousand verses of thirty-two syllables each. Therefore, the collections of Dharma in their entirety consist of 84 million verses.
>
> This is the shared position. The position of the peerless vehicle is, "One Dharma collection is the amount that can be written with a load of ink that can be suitably carried by Indra's powerful elephant." If that is so, the statement from a sutra that talks of Lord Devadatta reciting the number of volumes able to be carried by five thousand elephants also makes sense.

Further on the text says:

> These collections of Dharma are presented as the three baskets of scripture.[499]

"Statement from a sutra" in the above passage refers to the *Sutra of Repaying the Kindness of the Skillful Buddha,*[500] and the three baskets are those of Vinaya, Abhidharma, and Sutra.

The uncommon Mahayana position

The thirty-seventh chapter of the *Great Cloud Sutra,* entitled "Collection of Sacred Dharma Mandalas," says:

> As much Dharma has been spoken,
> and therefore definitely taught,
> as the number of sutras multiplied by
> the number of grains of sands in the Ganges.[501]

The meaning of this verse has already been explained elsewhere. The *Samādhi of Śūraṅgama Sutra* states:

> Celestial son, of the Dharma of the Tathāgatha, I have not taught a ten millionth part, a ten thousand millionth part, a million millionth part of the Dharma of the fully enlightened Buddha. [154] Of what I have taught, the monk Ānanda does not hold even a million millionth part.[502]

In the sixty-sixth fascicle of the *Avataṃsaka Sutra,* it says in the chapter called the "Inconceivability of the Dharmas of the Buddha":

> With a single body the bhagavān buddhas can grant blessings with as many heads as the number of very subtle particles in an indescribable-beyond-indescribable number of buddha realms.[503] In each head they can grant blessings with as many tongues as the number of particles in an indescribable-beyond-indescribable number of buddha realms. With each tongue they can speak with as many voices and languages as the number of very subtle particles in an indescribable-beyond-indescribable number of buddha realms, and be understood by every living being of every realm possessed of every conceivable disposition. Each voice and each language teaches as many sutras as the number of very subtle particles in an indescribable-beyond-indescribable number of buddha realms.[504]

This passage expresses the inconceivable range of activity of the buddhas.

Chomden Raldri (1227–1305), in his *Commentary to the Compendium of Knowledge,* says:

> The etymological explanation is that because it moves, severs, and paves the way like a precious wheel, we talk of the wheel of Dharma. Alternatively, because it is a collection of spoken Dharma, we talk of collections of Dharma or the collection of teachings.[505]

These teachings of the Buddha inscribed on paper made from birchbark,[506] dyed or not dyed, are known as "volumes." Concerning the etymology of this word in the celestial language of Sanskrit,[507] "*Pūla* and *pustaviḍi* mean 'collection.'" Therefore the root is *pusta.* The affix *vu* is added because the second *kṛta* rule says, "*tṛ, vu,* and *ṇ*" (the affixes *tṛ, vu* and *ṇ* can be added to roots). The *vu* becomes *aka* because the sixth *kṛta* rule says "*yu* and *vu* become *ana* and *aka*" (when affixes *yuṭ* and *vuṇ* shed their *anubandha, yu* becomes *ana* and *vu* becomes *aka*). The final *a* of the letter *ta* on the root is for pronunciation purposes and is elided. The letter *t* without its life-giving vowel is brought to the *a* of *aka.* The first case ending *si,* which merely expresses the nominative, is added. This ending becomes a *visarga* because "*s* and *r, visarga*" (affixes *s* and *r* on nouns and word forms become *visarga.* The *i* of the first case *si* is elided because it is for pronunciation purposes). This results in the formulation *pustakaḥ.* These days we use the corruption *po ti,* which means "volume."

Concerning the meaning of the term,[508] in the twenty-first fasicle of *Ascertainment from Stages of the Yogacaryā* by Ārya Asaṇga it says:

> Of the five sciences, the inner science is the supreme and most important of all the sciences, [155] all treatises, and all scripture.[509]

Also:

> In brief, the words of the Buddha should be understood in six ways: in terms of the truth of reality, in terms of attainment, in terms of explanation, in terms of abandoning the two extremes, in terms of inconceivability, and in terms of the Buddha's intention.[510]

Better known is the description given by the great scholar Vasubandhu in the first chapter of his *Science of Explanation:*

> *Dharma* means objects of knowledge, path,
> nirvana, object of mind, merit, life,
> teachings, arising, certainty, and traditions.[511]

To paraphrase and quote briefly from the same text: the term *dharma* refers to objects of knowledge because "a dharma can be a composite or non-composite phenomena." It is the path because "the right view is Dharma." In terms of going for refuge to the Dharma, it is nirvana. As a mental phenomenon, *dharma* refers to an object of the mind. It is merit in the sense of your lifestyle and social circle.[512] It is life in terms of cherishing the experiences of this life. *Dharma* as the category of sutras, and so on, refers to the teachings. *Dharma* refers to arising phenomena as in, for example, "this body has the dharma of aging." "Certainty" refers to the *four dharmas.*[513] *Dharma* as "traditions" refers to the dharmas of different countries and the dharmas of different races. These are ten etymologies of the word *dharma.*

Concerning the defining characteristics of the Dharma, or word of the Buddha, it has been said:

> The sacred Dharma:
> dispelling all suffering,
> dispelling all obscuration.[514]

In terms of its nature, it can be divided into scripture and knowledge. The eighth chapter of the *Treasury of Abhidharma* says:

> The sacred Dharma of our Teacher has two divisions:
> that of scripture and that of knowledge.[515]

Division in terms of the type of disciple is spoken of in the *Ornament of Mahayana Sutras:*

> The baskets of scripture can be three or two.[516]

The words of Buddha can be categorized into the three baskets of Vinaya, Sutra, and Abhidharma, or into the two baskets of the Small Vehicle of the śrāvakas, whose predilection is for the lesser, and of the Great Vehicle, whose predilection is for the vast.

Division in terms of cause and effect is described by a passage asserted by Butön, Lotsāwa Rinchen Sangpo, and others to be from the *King of Teachings* and which is actually quoted by Jñānaśrī in his *Eliminating the Two Extremes in the Vajrayana* as being from the *Sutra of Secret Prophecies:*

> If the three guiding vehicles
> are definitely taught by the Bhagavān,
> why has he not spoken of the definitive vehicle,
> in which cause and effect are spontaneous
> and which will not be taught by other buddhas?

The answer: [156]

> Having turned the wheel of causal phenomena
> for those predisposed to the causal path,
> the result vehicle—a swifter path—
> will appear at a future time.[517]

Those of lesser faculties are attracted to the process of causality, and so that is taken as the path and known as the causal vehicle. Those of higher faculties are attracted to the spontaneous accomplishment of cause and effect, and so they take the result as their path, which is known as the path of mantra.

Divisions in terms of subject matter are two: that which is taught as non-abiding through conventional perception and that taught as valid through ultimate perception:[518]

> The doctrine taught by the buddhas
> is well founded on two truths.[519]

Divisions of the words of Buddha in terms of their antidotal practices is dealt under many headings: reasons for the three-scriptural-basket categorization, the etymological explanation of the term *basket,* how the teachings fit into the twelve branches of scripture, their individual etymologies, and so on.

Dividing the words of the Buddha in terms of the time of teaching results in the initial teachings known as the *Dharma wheel of the four truths,* the intermediate teachings known as *Dharma wheel of no sign,* and the final teachings known as the *Dharma wheel of ascertaining the ultimate.* In general terms this is explained in the *Sutra of the Definitive Explanation of the Buddha's Thought.*

Divisions on a textual basis are recorded in Ācārya Śāntipa's *Supreme Essence Commentary to the Eight Thousand Perfection of Wisdom Sutra:*

> Sutra prose, occasional verse, and prophecies,
> versed teachings, specific expressions of joy,
> introductions, parables,
> teaching through past events, past-life stories, vast teachings,
> wondrous deeds, teachings on ascertainment:
> these are the twelve branches of scripture.[520]

Alternatively, Puṇḍarīka's *Kālacakra Great Commentary* has another list with different numbering.

In terms of their determining causes[521] there are three divisions: teachings actually spoken by the Buddha, blessed teachings, and the words of the Buddha by permission. An example of a sutra actually spoken by the Buddha would be the *Dharma Compendium.* Blessed teachings are of three types. The *Sutra of the Ten Levels* is a teaching blessed by the enlightened body. The *Sutra Dispelling the Remorse of Ajātaśatru* is a sutra blessed by enlightened speech. The "Meditative Activities of Samantrabhadra" chapter from the *Avataṃsaka Sutra* is an example of a teaching blessed by enlightened mind.

This third category can be divided into three further categories. The *Heart Sutra* is an example of a teaching blessed by the *samādhi* of the enlightened mind. Mantras uttered by the gods, nāgas, yakṣas, and so on, to produce particular results are examples of teachings blessed by the compassion of the enlightened mind. Teachings blessed by the power of truth of the enlightened mind are, [157] for example, those issuing from mountains, trees, and so forth, with the invocation, "By the power of truth of the Bhagavān's enlightened mind."

Words of the Buddha by permission are introductions to the teachings and sentences to link the narrative, inserted under the instructions "Compile the teachings" and "Do it in this way."

12. The Meaning of "Treatise"

THOSE WHO HAVE sought to preserve the teaching have commented on these teachings by composing treatises. This section has three headings: definition, etymological explanation, and types.

The definition of "treatise" (śāstra)

The conqueror Maitreya says in the fifth chapter of *Uttaratantra*:

> Whatever is based upon the Conqueror, the sole Teacher,
> explained by those with undistracted mind
> in accord with the path attaining liberation,
> should be raised to the head
> as one would the words of the Sage.[522]

This indicates the vast difference between a teaching of the Buddha and a treatise. There are various interpretations of this verse among early scholars such as Künkhyen Rongpo and Gö Lotsāwa. Later scholars, too, who have cited this verse have not examined the words closely, leading to variations such as "teachings of the Conqueror" and "Teacher, the Conqueror," and so on. The Indian text is in *indravajra* meter,[523] and I will explain this verse in detail using the method of forming nominal stems from the roots by adding *kṛt* suffixes and word forms constructed through the addition of *ti, si,* and so forth.[524]

"*Yatī* means 'offering' or 'great effort.'"[525] This is the root. "To the root *kvip*" (the *kvip* affix can be added to all roots to create nominal stems). Therefore *kvip* is added to the root. *Ī* at the end of the root is for pronunciation purposes. Moreover, "That which has the name of *it* is elided." (*Kṛt* affixes and case endings that have no particular meaning and *anubandha* particles are known collectively as *it*. When they meet other affixes, their work is finished and they are elided.) Therefore *ī* is elided. The sutra says that the affix *kvip* is also to be elided. This leaves *yat.*

"*As* means 'to be.'" This is the root. The *parasmaipad* first-person singular of the potential tense, *yāt,* is added. In-between *ap* is added, because, "For the agent, *ap*" (for expressing the agent from roots such as *bhū,* the in-between affix *ap* is added when followed by any of the eighteen affixes from *tip* to *mahe*). The *ap* is then elided because "with *ad,* and so on, it is destroyed." *(Karaṇa* affixes such as *ap* are omitted from roots such as *ad.)* "*Nam* and *a* of *as*" or "for *nam* and *as*" [158] (when meeting affixes without *guṇa,* the in-between affix *nam* is elided, and the root *as* loses its initial vowel *a*). Therefore the *a* of the root is elided. "That without a vowel carries over to the next," and so the *s* without the vowel is brought forward to make *syāt.* "The *ca* to *pa* group becomes the *ja* to *ba* group with *ava*" (when word forms ending in consonant forms from the *ca* to the *pa* group meets *ava,* meaning a vowel or voiced consonant, they become by euphony equivalent forms from the *ja* to *ba* group). Therefore the *t* is changed to *d* to become *syād.* With the previous syllable *yat,* this means "whatever." *Nak* is a negating particle. "*Na, a*" (in the process of compressing word forms, the negating particle *na* becomes *a*). Therefore *nak* becomes *a* and is brought to the preceding *d* without its vowel *a.* This leaves *syāda.*

"*Vī* means 'to be created, beautiful,' 'to be in a place,' 'to eat.'" This is the root. "*Uṇ ḍi,* and so forth, always." (The special category of affixes like *uṇ* can always be added to roots regardless of tense and case considerations), therefore the affix *ḍi* is added. "For *ḍit, ṭi*" (*ḍi,* or vowel endings, meeting affixes with *anubandha* are elided). Therefore the vowel of the root is elided. *Ḍ* follows the same rule and is also elided. The *i* is brought to the remaining *v* to create *vi,* meaning "having the aspect of."

The next root: "*kṣipa* means 'to take away.'" "*Kta, ktavatu*" (to indicate the *bhāva* of the past tense, add *kta;* to indicate the agent in the past, add *ktavu*), and so the affix *kta* is added. "Except for *us, kit,* and *dit*" (the *guṇa* is blocked when *k* and *d* follow a root except when following an *us* affix). Therefore the letter *ka* has the meaning of blocking the *guṇa* of the root and is elided. The final *a* of the root is for pronunciation and is elided. This makes *kṣipta,* meaning "distraction."

"*Mana* means 'to know.'" This is the root. "On *vac,* and so forth, *as*" (*vac,* which means "speech," and other roots such as *mana* take the affix *as*). Therefore the affix *as* is added. The final *a* of the root is for pronunciation and is elided, and the affix is joined on to form *manas.* "*S* and *r* become *visarga.*"

Therefore, the *s* without its life-giving vowel becomes *visarga.* "To *hava, u*" (when a *visarga* is on a short vowel and meets *hava,* meaning a voiced consonant, that *visarga* becomes *u*). Also, "*a* and *u* become *o.*" Therefore, the *a* and the *u* join to become *o,* resulting in *mano,* meaning "with mind."

To that is added the plural of the third-person *bhis.* The *s* becomes a *visarga.* "From *nāmi, ra*" (when a *nāmin* vowel takes a *visarga* and meets a following *a,* the *visarga* becomes *r*). Therefore, the *visarga* becomes *r* to make *bhir,* which indicates the instrumental case.

"*Vac* means *talk.*" This is the root. "*Kta ktavatu*" (to indicate the *bhāva* of the past tense, add *kta;* to indicate the agent in the past, add *ktavu*), and so the affix *kta* is added. "The *ya, va, ra* of *yaj,* and so on, to *ka anubandha* take *samprasāraṇa* into *i, u, ṛt*" (when roots such as *yaj* meet *anubandha* affixes such as *ka,* the *ya, va,* and *ra* of those roots perform a vowel interchange, or *samprasāraṇa,* with *i, u,* and *ṛ*). Therefore the *va* becomes *u.* The affix *ka* follows the same rule and is elided. "*Cu* becomes *ku*" (the consonants of the *ca* group can become those of the *ka* group). Therefore the *c* becomes *k,* which is moved to the following consonant to form *ukta.* To that is added the first case *si.* "From *at, am*" (on neuter genders ending with short vowel *a,* both *si* and *am* become *am*). Therefore the *si* becomes *am.* "The *a* of *am* and *śas*" (with an *a* ending, the following *a* of *am* and *as* is elided). Therefore the *a* is elided, and the *m* takes an *anusvāra* to become *uktaṃ,* which means "explain." The *visarga* that became *r* above is brought to this word form.

"*Śāsu* means 'to teach.'" This is the root. The affix *tṛn* is added because "for being of that nature, *tṛn*" (the affix *tṛn* is added to a root to give the meaning of "having the nature of" or being in the state of that particular root). The letter *n* is a marker or is there for the vowel, and is elided. The final *u* of the root is for pronunciation purposes and is elided. This forms *śāstṛ.* "*Si* and so forth always" (the endings of the seven cases and the three persons beginning with *si* are added as terminations). Therefore the *am* of the second case is added. "The *ār* of *stṛ*" (when a preceding vowel *ṛ* is followed by a different vowel it becomes *ar*). Therefore the final *ṛ* becomes *ār,* which is brought to the *am* to make *śāstāram.* The *m* is left as it is, or "*ma* can become an *anusvāra,*" and therefore a zero is added to form *śāstāraṃ,* meaning "teacher."

"*Ik* means 'remember.'" This is the root. "*A* and *ṭa*" [159] (when a root has a previous noun and an action is applied to this noun via the root, the affix *a* or *ṭa* is added). To this *a* is added as an affix. "The *upadhā* letter is short" (when the penultimate or *upadhā* vowel is a short *nāmin* vowel, it becomes its *guṇa*). Therefore the *upadhā i* of the root becomes *e.* With the sixth case, *ṅas* is added and "from *at, am*" (a neuter gender with a short vowel *a* termination becomes *am* when preceding a subsequent *si* or *am* of the first and second case, although here this rule is taken to apply to the sixth case also), resulting in *ekaṃ,* meaning "sole."

"*Ji* means 'Conqueror.'" This is the root. "*Naṭ* and *ki*" (to express the *bhāva* from the root, *naṭ* or *ki* is added), therefore the affix *naṭ* is added. The *ṭ* is an *anubandha* and so is elided. To that is added the third-case instrumental ending *ṭā.* "From *at* the *ātmanepada* ending *am,*" therefore *tā* becomes *am.* "The *a* of *am* and *śas*" (when the previous gender ending of a non-root is the same letter as the following *am* and *śas,* the *a* of those two is elided), and so the *a* is elided. "*M* becomes *anusvāra,*" therefore a small zero is added to the *m,* and the result is *jinaṃ,* meaning "Conqueror."

"*Vad* means 'clarify.'" This is the root. "The affix *kvip*" is added. "The *ya, va, ra,* of *yaj,* and so on, to *ka anubandha* take *samprasāraṇa* into *i, u, ṛt*" (when roots such as *yaj* meet affixes devoid of meaning such as *ka,* the *ya, va,* and *ra* of those roots perform a vowel interchange, or *samprasāraṇa,* with *i, u,* and *ṛ).* Therefore the *va* becomes *u.* The *kvip* is elided to leave *ud,* for which "this also applies to completion" (when the consonants from *jha* group to the *sa* group engage word forms complete with case endings they can become consonants from the *ja* group). Therefore, alternatively, the *d* becomes a *t* to leave *ut,* and then the term means "well."

"*Diśa* means 'to expel utterly.'" This is the root. "From *at, śatu; īp* also" (roots having the short vowel *a* ending take the affix *śatu* and the feminine affix *ip* also). Therefore the affix *śatu* is added. The *śa* behaves according to "the *śa anubandha* is like the four" (the affix *śa* as an *anubandha* marker and when in the position of a following particle behaves like the four affixes—*tip,* and so on—from the all-encompassing affix section). Therefore the *śa* of the affix is elided. The *u* of the *tu* is for pronunciation purposes and is also elided. The final *a* of the root is elided (although this seems to eliminate all vowels), and the two syllables are brought together to form *diśat.* "The *ca* to *pa* group become the *ja* to *ba* group." Therefore the *ta* changes into *da* to become *diśad,* meaning "taught." The *s* of the case ending *bhis* becomes a *visarga* to become *bhiḥ,* giving the instrumental case. Beginning from *jinaṃ,* the *anusvāra* becomes *m,* and by the euphonic rules of the *ca* to *pa* group and the *ja* to *va* group, the result is *muddiśadbhiḥ.*

"*Mucḷ* means 'liberation.'" This is the root. "*Uṇ* and so forth always" (the special category of affixes like *uṇ* can always be added to roots regardless of tense and case considerations). Therefore the affix *sap* is added. The *anubandha ḷ* in the root is elided because, "The *anubandha ḷ* from *puṣ* and so forth, *ṅ*" (the *anubandha ḷ* on roots such as *puṣ* changes to *ṅ*, which is then elided because it is a marker indicating the blocking of the *guṇa*). The *u* of the root takes its *guṇa* to *o* because "The *upadhā* is short" (when the penultimate or *upadhā* vowel is a short *nāmin* vowel, it becomes its *guṇa*). The *p* of the affix *sap* has a similar meaning and is therefore elided. "*Cu* becomes *ku*" (the consonants of the *ca* group can become those of the *ka* group), therefore the *c* of the root becomes *k*. "From *ku, i,* and *la, sa* becomes *ṣa*" (when gender endings of the consonants in the *ka* group, the eight vowels beginning with *i,* and the five consonants *ha, ya, wa, ra,* and *la* take a subsequent *sa,* it becomes *ṣa*). Therefore the *sa* of the affix becomes *ṣa. Ka* and *ṣa* are joined to form *kṣa,* which when put together becomes *mokṣa* ("liberation").

"*Āpḷ* means 'pervading' and 'focus.'" This is the root. The *anubandha ḷ* is elided, as was done previously. "*Kti*" (the *kṛt* affix *kti* can be added to roots to give the *bhāva* form), therefore *kti* is added. *K* blocks the *guṇa* and so is elided. This results in *āpti,* meaning "causes to attain."

"*Ṣama* means 'disturb.'" This is the root. "*Kvip*" (the *kṛt* affix *kvip* can be added to all roots to create nominal stems), therefore the affix *kvip* is added. The final *a* of the root is for pronunciation purposes and is elided. "Initial *ṣa* and *ṇa* become *sa* and *na*" (to create the agent, the initial *ṣa* and *ṇa* of a root become *sa* and *na*), therefore *ṣa* becomes *sa.* The affix *kvip* is elided. This results in *sam,* which means "perfect" or "complete."

"*Bhṛñ* means 'to hold.'" This is the root. The affix *ghañ* is added because "for the *bhāva, ghañ*" (the affix *ghañ* is added to create the *bhāva* of the root). "Both from the *anubandha ñ* and the *svarita*" [160] (from a root with an *anubandha ñ* and a middle tone *svarita* vowel, both *parasmaipāda* and *ātmanepada* word forms are made). Therefore the *ñ* of the root is elided. "The *nāmin* vowels of the root" means that the *ṛ* in the root is strengthened to *ār* by the *vṛddhi* process. The *ñ* of the affix follows the same rule and is elided. The *gha* of the affix is also elided because "*ca* and *ja* with *anubandha gha* become *ka* and *ga*" (the *gha* is an *anubandha* and is elided). A life-giving vowel *a* is brought to the *bhār* to form *bhāra.* Putting this together with the previous word-form results in *sambhāra,* which means "gathering" or "to hold perfectly."

Anything that is a method to bring about the attainment of liberation is a path. Such a path elevates one to the level of freedom, and for those seeking the glories of fulfilling the wishes of oneself and others, it becomes the ground on which the vehicle of method and wisdom travels. Therefore, because it is the foundation of all the wonderful qualities of the paths and levels, it "holds perfectly." Because it is universally praised by all traditions as the path of the conquerors of the past, present, and future and their bodhisattva princes, it is the journey to be commonly undertaken by living beings, and therefore it also means "gathering" or "accumulated."[526]

"*Yat* means 'harm.'" This is the root. "*Kvip*" (the *kṛt* affix *kvip* can be added to all roots to create nominal stems) can be added as an affix, and with the construction of a nominal stem it can be elided. On *yat* the *Kalāpa Treatise* says, "For vocal expression, *thā.*" Therefore *thā* is added. The affix and case share a common basis, and so, "The *si, ṭi,* and so forth of *tyad* and so on becomes *a*" (when *tyad* and other pronouns take endings *si, ṭi,* and so forth, they become *a* before a following form). Therefore, the *t* is elided, and the subsequent *ṭi* becomes *a.* This results in *yathā,* meaning "exactly as it is" or "like that."

"*Śvas* means 'life,' as does *ana.*" Therefore, *ana* is a root meaning "life." "*Ṣaka, u, ukaṇ*" (the affixes *ṣaka, u,* and *ukaṇ* are added to show that the root possesses that nature), therefore the affix *u* is added. The final *a* of the root is for pronunciation purposes and is elided. The two parts are brought together to form *anu.*

Added to this, the root "*kūla* means 'obstruction.'" "From *nāmi upadhā, ka*" (when the *upadhā,* or penultimate, is a *nāmin* vowel, the affix *ka* can be added), therefore the affix *ka* is added. The final *a* of the root is for pronunciation purposes and is elided. "Except for *us, kit* and *dit*" (the *guṇa* is blocked when *k* and *d* follow a root, except when following an *uṣ* affix). Therefore the *k* of the affix has the function of blocking the *guṇa* of the root and is elided. This gives *kūla. Si* is added. "From *at, am*" (on neuter genders ending with short vowel *a,* both *si* and *am* become *am*), therefore *si* becomes *am.* "The *a* of *am* and *śas*" (with an *a* termination, the following *a* of *am* and *as* is elided), therefore the *a* is elided. "*M* can become *anusvāra,*" which produces *kūlaṃ.* This is joined to *anu* to form *anukūlaṃ,* meaning "in accord with."

The root "*mṛdhu* means 'perfection.'" "*Naṭ* and *ki*" means that the affix *ki* is added (to express the *bhāva* from the root, *naṭ* or *ki* is added). The *u* of the root is elided because, "from *ut anubandha, ktvā; iṭ* also." (From roots with short *u* ending the affix *ktvā* or the *āgama it* can be added. This *sutra* is found in some editions only.) The *ṛ* becomes *ur* because "the *ṛ* of *su* becomes *ur*" (untraced). The *k* of the affix follows the same rule and so is elided. This leaves the vowel *i.* "*I* and *u* to *r* and *v* to *ha* and *sa*" (the vowels *i* and *u* as *upadhā* or penultimate letters added to the letters *r* and *v* become long vowels when succeeded by any consonant). Therefore the *upadhā* of the *r* in the root becomes a long *ū*. Brought together this forms *mūrdhi.* To this is added the singular of the third case, *ṭā.* "From *nāmin* a vowel, *num*" [161] (neuter genders with *nāmin* vowel endings, when meeting case endings beginning with a vowel, include the affix *num*), therefore *num* is added. The *u* is for pronunciation purposes, and the *m* is an *anubandha* particle, therefore they are both elided. "For *śas* and so forth, the *at* of *asṭhi,* and so on." (Alternatively, "for the *ṭā* and so on with *asthi* and so on, *at.*" For case endings like *śas,* the *āgama num* is included in words like *asṭhi,* and the letter *i* becomes *a,* from *ṭā* onward.) Therefore the *i* of the gender ending becomes *at.* "For *śas* and so on, when *ma* and *va* are not connected to a vowel, the *at* can be elided" (when case endings such as those from second case *śas* onward, which do not include *ma* and *va,* begin with a vowel, the *upadhā a* is elided). Therefore the *at* is elided. The case ending *ṭā* is a distinguishing marker and can be elided. The life-giving *ā* is added and brought up, resulting in the construction *mūrdhnā* meaning "crown of the head."

The root "*tamu* means 'desire.'" "*Uṇ* and so forth always" (the special category of affixes like *uṇ* can always be added to roots regardless of tense and case considerations), therefore the affix *daka* is added. "Except for *uṣ, kit* and *dit*" (the *guṇa* is blocked when *k* and *d* follow a root, except when following an *uṣ* affix), therefore the *ka* is elided. The *a* is for pronunciation purposes and is elided. The *u* of the root is elided because "from *ut anubandha, ktvā; iṭ* also" (from roots with short *u* ending, the affix *ktvā* or the *āgama it* can be added). Or, "Whatever has the name of *it* is to be elided" (*kṛt* affixes and case endings that have no meaning and *anubandha* particles are known collectively as *it.* When they meet other affixes, their work is finished and they are elided). The final *m* of the root is also elided because "the *anudātta* are elided" (the *ñ* and *ma* low-tone letters are elided). "This also applies to completion" (when the consonants from the *jha* group to the *sa* group engage word forms complete with case endings, they can become consonants from the *ja* group), therefore *da* becomes *ta.* This leaves *tat,* which means "that."

The root "*avi* means 'sound.'" "*Naṭ* and *ki*" means that the affix *ki* is added (to express the *bhāva* from the root, *naṭ* or *ki* is added). The final *i* of the root is elided because "from *anubandha i, mum*" (when roots with an *anubandha* particle *i* meet *tip* and *ap,* the final vowel takes the *āgama mum*). The *v* becomes *p* because "the *atiśaya* letters change" (untraced). The *k* of the affix blocks the *guṇa* and so is elided. This leaves *api,* meaning "also."

The root "*ṛṣi* means 'go.'" "*A* and *ṭ*" (when a root has a previous nominal stem and an action is applied to it via the root, the affix *a* or *ṭ* is added), therefore the affix *a* is added. The *i* of the root is elided because "whatever has the name of *it* is to be elided." (*Kṛt* affixes and case endings that have no meaning and *anubandha* particles are known collectively as *it*. When they meet other affixes, their work is finished and they are elided.) "The *upadhā* is short" (when the penultimate or *upadhā* vowel is a short *nāmin* vowel, it becomes its *guṇa*), therefore the *ṛ* of the root becomes its *guṇa*—*ar*—to form *arṣa*. To this *si* is added. "From *at, am*" (on neuter genders ending with short vowel *a*, both *si* and *am* become *am*), therefore *si* becomes *am*. "The *a* of *am* and *śas*" (with an *a* ending the following *a* of *am* and *as* is elided). Therefore the *a* is elided, and the *m* takes an *anusvāra* to become *arṣaṃ*, which means "scripture," "the words of the Sage."

The root "*iṇ* means 'to go.'" "*Uṇ* and so forth always" (the special category of affixes like *uṇ* can always be added to roots regardless of tense and case considerations) and like the previous roots "*kta, ktavatu* are suitable" (to indicate the *bhāva* of the past tense, add *kta;* to indicate the agent in the past, add *ktavu*), and so the affix *kta* is added. The *k* is elided because "Except for *uṣ, kit* and *dit*" (the *guṇa* is blocked when *k* and *d* follow a root, except when following an *uṣ* affix). "From the *anudātta* and *ṅit*, the *āt*" (the *anudātta* or low tone acting as an *anubandha* at the end of roots and the *anubandha ṅ* take the *ātmanepada* form). Therefore the connecting consonant *ṇ* on the root is elided because it is a particle indicating the *ātmanpada*. The *ta* of the affix *kta* becomes *va* because "from *paca, va*" (from the root *paca*, a *ta* letter conjoined with the *anubandha* particle *k* becomes *va*). Because *va* is *anubandha ka* and *ṅ*, the root is not strengthened by *guṇa*. This results in *iva*, meaning "like."

The root "*prā* means 'to perfect' or 'to complete.'" The affix *kti* is added because "*kti*" (the *kṛt* affix *kti* can be added to roots to give the *bhāva* form). *K* is *it* and "whatever has the name of *it* can be elided." (*Kṛt* affixes, case endings that have no meaning, and *anubandha* particles are known collectively as *it*. When they meet other affixes, their work is finished and they are elided.) Therefore the *k* is elided. The long *ā* of the root weakens because "from ascertained word forms, the letters weaken." This leaves *prati*, meaning "renowned."

The root "*iṣu* means 'desire.'" [162] The potential-tense particle *yāt* is added. "For the agent, *ap*" (for expressing the agent from roots such as *bhū*, the in-between affix *ap* is added when followed by any of the eighteen affixes from *tip* to *mahe*), and so *ap* is placed in between. The *p* of *ap* is elided because of the meaning of "*pa* of *nu* and *u*"; alternatively, "*nu* and *up*" (when the *vikāraṇa* affixes *nu* and *up* meet certain case endings, they strengthen into *guṇa*) and also "from roots with two syllables with *anubandha pa,* the *upadhā*" (when certain roots of two syllables meet endings and affixes beginning with consonants and forms of *anubandha pa* beginning with a vowel, the root *upadhā* is strengthened). Here a *guṇa* is not necessary because of the endings from *ha* to *sa* (an ending in any consonant). "Whatever has the name of *it* can be elided." (*Kṛt* affixes, case endings that have no meaning, and *anubandha* particles are known collectively as *it.* When they meet other affixes, their work is finished and they are elided.) Therefore the final *u* of the root is elided. The *ṣ* becomes *cha* because "the *cha* of *gam,* and so on" (individual parts of roots such as *gam, iṣu,* and *yamu* transform into *cha* before certain affixes). The *cha* is doubled because "of *cha*" (when a short vowel *upadhā* or ending meets *cha,* the *cha* is doubled). The first *cha* becomes *c* because "the *jha* and *sa* to *kha* and *sa* groups become *ca* and *pa*" (when consonant endings from groups beginning with the fourth or *jha* group up to *sa* meet consonants beginning from the second or *kha* group up to *sa,* the former consonant becomes a consonant from the first or *ca* group). The *yā* of the *yāt* becomes *ī* because "to *a, ya*" (untraced). The *a* and *ī* merge to become *e* because "*a* and *i* become *e*" (euphonic rule that short- or long-vowel *a* meeting vowel merges to become *e*). This forms *icchet.* This is put together with the former *prati* to form *pratīcchet,* meaning "lift up" in the imperative tense. Alternatively, *iccha* means "desire" and *yāt* means "type."

Therefore a direct literal translation would be:

> That explained by those without a distracted mind,
> in line with the great gathering
> for the attainment of liberation, exactly as it is,
> well taught by the Conqueror, the sole Teacher,
> should be lifted like a scripture to one's head.

This is a rendering of:

> *yatsyadavikṣiptamanobhiruktaṃ*
> *śāstāraṃekaṃ jinamuddiśadbhiḥ*
> *mokṣāptisambhārayathānukūlaṃ*
> *mūrdhān tatapyarṣaṃiva pratīcchet.*

The translation of the meaning becomes:

> Whatever is based on the Conqueror, the sole Teacher,
> explained by those with undistracted minds
> in accord with the path attaining liberation,
> should be raised to the head
> as one would with the words of the Sage.

The usual explanation of this verse is as follows. A treatise presents its subject matter based solely on the transmissions of the teachings or words of the Conqueror and not based on the composer's own self-belief derived from his own reasoning. It is to be explained with a mind undistracted by thoughts of the outsider traditions, wondering, "Does this accord with our Teacher's tradition or does it accord with an outsider tradition, such as the Īśvara school?" Alternatively, the composer presents his work with a mind undistracted by aspects of motivation with regard to others, and by worldly thoughts of honor, personal gain, and reputation with regard to himself. [163] Moreover, it is not taught merely for the things of this life, nor for the glories of a higher rebirth, but in accord with the path of attaining nirvana. Such a work should be raised and held above your head as you would revere a work containing the words of the Sage, our fully enlightened Teacher.

Etymological explanation of "treatise"

In terms of its formation from the root: "*Śāsu* means 'to teach.'" *Tra* is added to the root because "*iman, tra, asuka*" (the affixes *iman, tra,* and *asuka* may be added to any root). The *u* of the root is for articulation only and is elided. This leaves *śāstra,* which has been rendered as "treatise" *(bstan bcos).*

In terms of how the term is used in this context, "*śāsu* means 'to teach.'" *Yu* is added to the root because "*yuṭ*" (*yuṭ* can be added to all roots to express the *bhāva*). "*Yu, vu* become *ana, aka*" (when affixes *yuṭ* and *vuṇ* shed their *anubandha, yu* becomes *ana* and *vu* becomes *aka*). Therefore, *yu* becomes *ana.* The *u* of the *su* is an *anubandha* particle and is elided. The *s* is brought to the following letters, and the result is *śāsana,* meaning "teaching." It also means "transforms" because the mind is transformed from the three poisonous afflictions to become endowed with the three trainings.

Concerning the explanation that *traya* also means "protect": The root "*tṛ* means 'conquer' and 'save.'" As explained above *yu* is added to the root and is changed to *ana*. By *guṇa* strengthening, the *ṛ* becomes *ar* because "*guṇa*" (as long as it does not have the function of blocking the *guṇa*, affixes and endings that prompt the *guṇa* will strengthen the *nāmin* vowel of the root with its *guṇa*). *Tar* is joined to the *ana*. "From *ṣa*, *ṛ*, and *ra*, no-ending *na* becomes *ṇa*" (when *ṣa*, *ṛ*, and *ra* meet *na* not ending with a non-vowel—in other words, ending with a vowel—the *na* becomes *ṇa*). Therefore the *na* becomes *ṇa*. This results in *taraṇa*, meaning "to protect or save from the resultant sufferings of samsara." The vowels and the *ṇa* are elided, and the life-vowel *a* is added because, concerning the endings of roots, "it is explained here that the remainder are from the world and other works" (all noun and word forms not taught in this text but which can be known from worldly usage and from other easy-to-understand treatises can be used as supplements to this treatise); "furthermore, there are two: letters change and become corrupted." This leaves *śās* and *tr* with the life-vowel *a*. "That without a vowel is carried over to the next," which leaves the formation *śāstra*.

In the fifth chapter of the *Science of Explanation* it says:

> It is correct to call the teachings of the Buddha treatises because the etymology of the term is "transform" and "protect":
>
> > Transforming all the foe-like afflictions,
> > protecting from existences in the lower realms,
> > a treatise has the qualities of transforming and protecting,
> > two qualities not found in other traditions.
>
> Therefore, only the words of the Buddha are true scriptural treatise [164] and so possess these qualities of transforming and protecting. Therefore, you should strive to retain their meanings.[527]

Also, it says in *Commentary on the Five Aggregates*, translated by Yeshé Dé and composed by a disciple of Vasubandhu, Guṇaprabha, who in Vinaya was wiser than his own teacher:

> What is it that is asserted as being a scriptural treatise? It is the forms of letters that represent its meaning, and the generality of their sounds classified as non-associated phenomena.[528] In terms of its etymology it is a treatise because it transforms the affliction enemies and protects from the fears of the lower realms and

> samsara. Therefore, "it teaches higher birth and definite happiness." Because it protects you from the lower realms, it teaches higher birth. Because it transforms the affliction enemies and protects you from the fears of samsara, it teaches definite happiness. Ācārya Āryadeva also says:
>
> > Transforming all the foe-like afflictions,
> > protecting from existences in the lower realms,
> > a treatise has the qualities of transforming and protecting,
> > two qualities not found in other traditions.[529]

The citation in this passage is a duplication of the *Science of Explanation* citation above, which means that either Vasubandhu was quoting Āryadeva or that there is some error in the translation or scripting of the latter citation.

Nevertheless, these passages indicate that the words of Buddha and a treatise are not necessarily mutually exclusive.

Types of treatise

Treatises are divided into types according to their status, function, subject matter, the teaching of Buddha that is being explained, and classification.

Status

Ācārya Asaṅga says in the twenty-second chapter of his *Ascertainment from Stages of the Yogacarya:*

> There are three kinds of scriptural treatise: those that concentrate on learning, those that concentrate on debate, and those that concentrate on practice. Examples of those that concentrate on learning would be the secret texts of the brahmans. [165] Those that concentrate on debate are the logic treatises of the outsiders. Those that concentrate on practice are the words of the Buddha.
>
> Again, treatises can be divided into three: meaningless treatises, perverse treatises, and ultimate treatises. These three can be included, where appropriate, in the previous three types. Treatises can also be treatises of harmful distractions, treatises devoid of essence, and treatises that lift one out of suffering. These three too can be included, where appropriate, in the first three.[530]

These divisions have been compiled and written on by great scholars of the past and in Tibetan compositions are usually presented as follows:

> Meaningless, perverse, and meaningful,
> distracting, of no essence, eliminating suffering,
> concentrating on learning, on debate, and on practice,
> six that lack and three that do not.

The treatise that investigates whether a crow has teeth is an example of a meaningless treatise. A treatise on the performing of sacrifice in order to gain a high rebirth would be a perverse treatise. [Vasubandhu's] *Abhidharmakośa,* which comprehensively teaches on the aggregates, spheres, and sources is a meaningful treatise. Those treatises that teach how to create magic and illusions are examples of distracting treatises. Treatises that promote the hardships of putting the body through the ritual of the five fires are those that lack essence. The five treatises of Maitreya are treatises that eliminate suffering. The treatise of the Saindhava śrāvakas is a treatise that concentrates on learning. Treatises that teach the eight topics of logic are treatises that concentrate on debate. [Śāntideva's] *Engaging in the Practices of the Bodhisattva* is an example of a treatise that concentrates on practice.

Treatises classified as meaningful, eliminating suffering, and concentrating on practice are said to be superior treatises, while the remaining six are inferior and only seemingly treatises.

Division according to function

There are those that bring together large areas of Buddha's teachings, such as *Vinaya Sutra* by Guṇaprabha; those that lay out the profound meanings, such as *Ornament of Realization* by the conqueror Maitreya, and those that are essentially compilations, such as [Maitreya's] *Ornament of Mahayana Sutras* or [Śāntideva's] *Compendium of Practice.*

Division according to subject matter

These are of three types: those that teach varieties of conventional phenomena, those that teach the nature of phenomena, and those that teach liberation and omniscience. The first of these is again divided into ordinary and exclusive. Ordinary treatises of this type are worldly treatises, such as works on the eight or eighteen areas of investigations.[531] [166] Exclusive treatises are those that teach the five sciences. Treatises that teach the nature of phenomena are those that teach the four truths in sixteen aspects, such as [Dharmakīrti's] *Ascertaining Valid Cognition,* or those that teach the nonduality of subject consciousness and object of consciousness, such as [Vasubandhu's] *Thirty Verses,* or those that teach the truth of no-nature, such as [Śāntirakṣita's] *Ornament of the Middle Way*. An example of those that teach liberation and omniscience would be *Engaging in the Practices of the Bodhisattva.*

Division according to the teaching of Buddha being explained

There are two divisions: commentaries on the teachings in general and commentaries on specific teachings. The first of these is said to be of two kinds: grammatical commentaries that clarify the words of the teachings in general, and logic-based commentaries that clarify the meanings of the commentaries. However, such a division is rendered uncertain by the grammar and logic texts of the outsiders.

Commentaries on specific teachings of the Buddha are of three types corresponding to the three turnings of the wheel of Dharma. Treatises of the first turning are divided according to view and practice. An example of a treatise that clarifies the view of the first turning would be the seven Abhidharma texts, which the Kashmiri Vaibhāṣikas assert to be the words of Buddha while the Sautrāntikas maintain they are treatises. These texts were compiled into the *Great Treasury of Detailed Explanation,* which in turn was compiled by Vasubandhu into the *Abhidharmakośa.*

A treatise that clarifies the practices or conduct of the first turning would be [Guṇaprabha's] *Vinaya Sutra,* which first deals with the topic of ordination from the seventeen Vinaya bases[532] found in the *Basic Vinaya* and then deals with the *Detailed Vinaya* and the remaining sixteen bases, thereby forming the basis of the text. Explanations of the discipline of requesting and so on from the *Later Vinaya* and the discipline for specific occasions from the *Short Vinaya* are inserted where appropriate. Other such treatises would be [Viśākhadeva's] *Vinaya Flower Garland* and [Vinītadeva's] *Three Hundred Verses,* which take the *Detailed Vinaya* as their basis and comment on the others where appropriate.

Treatises that clarify the middle turning are also divided into those of view and those of practice. Those of the view include the following works from among the four great founders of traditions: *Fundamental Stanzas on the Middle Way,* which explains the meaning, or the essential meaning, of the actual content of the sutras; *Refutation of Arguments,* which is an expansion of the first chapter of the previous work; *Seventy Verses on Emptiness,* which expands on the seventh chapter of the previous work; *Sixty Verses of Reasoning,* which specifically refutes those of our own insider tradition; and *Finely Woven,* which refutes sixteen logical positions. These are accepted by all as [Nāgārjuna's] Five Collections of Reasoning.

On top of these five texts, earlier scholars also included one of the following: *Establishing the Conventional, Precious Garland,* or *No Fear from Anywhere: Commentary on Fundamental Stanzas on the Middle Way.* This made varying sets of six collections of reasoning. By including all three works, they must have asserted eight collections also. [167] Dharma king and Mañjuśrī incarnate, Tsongkhapa, in his earlier work, *Golden Rosary of Eloquence,* agrees with these earlier scholars, but in his later work, *Ocean of Reasoning,* he adds *Precious Garland* to make the now established Six Collections of Reasoning.

Another example of this type of treatise would be [Maitreya's] *Ornament of Realization,* which teaches the view of the middle turning only indirectly or through its realization primarily by way of the eight phenomena.[533]

Treatises that clarify the practices of the middle turning would be [Nāgārjuna's] *Compendium of Sutra* and [Kamalaśīla's] *Stages of Meditation.*

Treatises that clarify the view of the last turning include the following: *Commentary to the Sutra Unraveling the Intent of the Buddha* by Asaṅga; *Commentary to the Sutra Requested by Akṣayamati* by Vasubandhu; *Presentation of the Levels to Enlightenment* by Sīlabhadra; *Explanation of the Kāśyapa Chapter from the Heap of Jewels Sutra* by Sthiramati; and *Commentary to the King of Meditative Concentrations Sutra* by Mañjuśrīkīrti.

Treatises that specifically clarify the practices of the last turning include *Ornament of Mahayana Sutras,* the five treatises on the levels, *Compendium of Abhidharma,* and *Compendium of the Mahayana.* Of the works of Maitreya, the two works, *Differentiation of the Middle Way and Extremes* and *Examination of Phenomena and the Nature of Phenomena,* only teach the view of the third-turning teachings. The superficial view that the works connected with Maitreya comment on all Mahayana thought while primarily teaching the message of the third turning has produced some confusing explanations. However, from a more precise view, the *Ornament of Realization* never moves beyond the middle turning.

Classification of treatises

This has three headings:

1. Those reliant upon the words of the Buddha
2. Those not reliant upon the words of the Buddha
3. Differences between the words of the Buddha and a treatise

Those reliant upon the words of the Buddha

This is under two headings: commentaries based around the actual words of the Buddha and autonomous compositions on the meaning of the words of the Buddha.

The first is of five kinds. A commentary on the words of the Buddha focuses on the words of the text and explains those parts difficult to understand. Examples would be the two Collected Verse commentaries.[534] A word commentary focuses on the words of the text and explains by expanding upon them. An example would be [Prajñāvarman's] *Commentary to Collection of Aphorisms*. A concise commentary takes the essential meaning of the teaching and explains it. An example would be Synthesis of the Sañcayagāthā.[535] A commentary on the speech summarizes what has been said. An extensive commentary expounds on both text and meaning—the fifty-fasicle *Extensive Commentary on the Sutra of Liberation,* for example. [168]

Autonomous compositions on the meaning of the words of the Buddha include those that explain fully one particular genre of teaching, such as [Maitreya's] *Ornament of Realization* and [Guṇaprabha's] *Vinaya Sutra;* those that teach parts of a teaching, such as [Kamalaśīla's] *Fifty Verses for the Monk;* those that explain the meanings of many teachings, such as [Śāntideva's] *Compendium of Practice* and [Nāgārjuna's] *Friendly Letter.*

Generally, treatises go under many names: commentary, explanation, presentation, root and commentary combined, compilation, word commentary, extensive commentary, composition,[536] analysis, and so on, but within these it is important to distinguish between genuine and false treatises.

Those not reliant upon the words of the Buddha

Ordinarily, treatises on logic and language are said to be examples of this particular kind of treatise. However, with respect to *pramāṇa*[537] in an exclusive sense, it is difficult to say that the thinking of the Dharma king and Mañjuśrī incarnate, Tsongkhapa, and others is that the words of Buddha are not actually found in treatises on both logic and language. Therefore, texts such as [Daṇḍin's] *Mirror of Poetics* and [Candragomin's] *Drama* are given merely to illustrate this classification of treatise.

Differences between the words of the Buddha and a treatise

It goes without saying that "word of the Buddha" refers to teachings actually spoken by the Buddha, but it also refers to teachings where the determining cause is set by the Buddha, a member of the entourage is inspired and proceeds to teach, and ends with the Buddha's instruction to "do as has been explained." All else is treatise.

The way to compose a treatise according to the Mahayana is explained in the twenty-second fascicle of *Ascertainment from Stages of the Yogacaryā* by Ārya Asaṇga:

> Those who wish to compose a treatise should do so with the following six causes: the thought that the treatise will deal with many points of Dharma; the thought that the dispositions of living beings are wide and varied and that some will respond to this work; the thought that it will lay out clearly those points that have become confused; the thought that it will bring together points that have become scattered; the thought that it will throw light on the profound points; and the thought that it will create beauty with beautiful words.[538]

Here, "causes" refer to intentions. The text continues:

> Those who wish to compose a treatise should do so possessed of four qualities: an absence of pride in the face of one's former teachers; compassion for living beings; affection for those in the Dharma; a absence of self-proclamation.[539] [169]

A composer of a treatise should possess all four qualities.

For those who have pretensions of being an author, Daṇḍin says:

> A natural self-belief,
> much learning, free of taints,
> not lacking in application,
> the cause of perfect poetics.[540]

In terms of it being a superior work as opposed to an inferior one or of it using a wide range of language as opposed to a narrow and restricted range, "a natural self-belief" refers to an innate and deep wisdom produced from the complete awakening in this life of potential developed in previous lives by accomplishing great familiarity with the teachings of the Buddha and with Buddhist and non-Buddhist sciences. More specifically, "much learning" means that one has studied many well-composed works, both generally, as explained above, and in particular the scriptures and texts of that particular field of knowledge, as well as the history, tradition, terminology, and so on, connected with it. Moreover, by never being satisfied by this learning, one will be "free of the taints" of doubt. "Not lacking in application" refers to perseverance, in terms of dedicated application and constant application to the mental engagement and familiarization with the above. These three qualities are the causes for producing within oneself a perfect knowledge of, in this context, poetics, but of any literary field.

In terms of the science of medicine and of highest yoga tantra, the Kashmiri pandit Candranandana says in his *Moonlight:*

> I venture into this composition,
> having clearly understood the truth
> and the transmission from the guru.[541]

Therefore, the best qualification for composing is having perceived the nature of reality. Then:

> Because the deity, glorious and pure,
> has taken hold of my mind...[542]

The next best qualification is to have gained permission from the meditation deity, and so on. The minimum qualification is to be in receipt of the unbroken stream of initiations, transmissions, and explanatory teachings, and so forth, to be learned in the knowledge of what is to be established and what is to be refuted, and being familiar with the teaching and accomplished in the sciences of logic, language, and poetics, one is said to be qualified to compose a treatise. [171]

13. Yuthok's Legacy

How Four Tantras *is the word of the Buddha*

If this great tantra, the work in question, is considered in terms of its inner meaning, then the secret places and so on taught by the medicine guru to the great Yuthok are factual. However, if you consider the various assertions on the outer, inner, and secret locations, then it can be said of the outer location that the various designations of "place of the sages" mentioned previously are not that contradictory, no matter which one you prefer. Nevertheless, to give an appearance of definitiveness, my lama the Great Fifth asserts that the tantra was taught outwardly in the western land of Oḍḍiyāna. The inner and secret locations are as described by the medicine guru in the biography of the earlier Yuthok.

In tantras taught in the Heaven of Thirty-Three and elsewhere, our Teacher also explained various methods for taming human disciples. Likewise, although this tantra was taught in the land of Oḍḍiyāna, it undoubtedly contains many elements that accord with conditions of time and place prevalent in Tibet. However, in order to make it easier for discerning masters, these elements were not originally included. To accord with the time and place of Tibet, the great Yuthok added to the chapter count in the Root Tantra, and in the Explanatory Tantra he added sections on tea and made miscellaneous additions to the chapters on medicines and diet. In the Final Tantra he inserted sections on pulse and urine diagnosis, the mother-son and friend-enemy cycles that follow the thinking of the *Somarāja,* and passages on the use of white-china tea bowls, and so on.[543] In the Instruction Tantra, too, he makes similar additions. He also conducted an excellent revision of the text. For all this work, not only did the great Yuthok arise in his definitive form of the medicine king, the synthesis of all lineages, but in his outward aspect he possessed all the necessary causes for composition explained above. In the Dzemakhang *History of the Heartdrop: Hook of Virtue* it says:

> Because the master Yuthok in a single form achieved the two types of siddhi in this life, and because of the prophecies and permissions given by the meditation deities, there is not the slightest distinction in terms of their blessings between these tantras and the highest yoga tantras.

Also:

> Surrounded by the buddhas and bodhisattvas of the ten directions, gods and goddesses with countless offerings came to the space in front and said to the protector, synthesis of the three buddha families, "Ah! In the future this great tantra will become the supreme refuge for living beings. [172] The country in which it dwells will have good fortune, happiness, and all that is good in all its quarters. Those who preserve it, hold it, read it, hear it, master it, and teach it widely to others will become the main disciples of the conquerors. At the very least, those that commit the verses of this scripture to memory will not fall within samsara again, and all wrongs and obstructions accumulated since beginningless time will be washed away."[544]

Making these additions so that they become indistinguishable from the words of the Buddha was done to guide the minds of those beings of these degenerate times that do not think about meanings but simply read the words. It is not wrong to do this. As my lama the Great Fifth has said, it is similar to the *Sixteen Drops of the Kadampa* appearing from the illusory play that was the gnosis of Atiśa and his main disciple but whose lineage in reality has to come from Vajradhara.

Concerning the auxiliary texts for aiding the understanding of *Four Tantras,* some old manuscripts say:

> For this wish-fulfilling jewel of a tantra,
> essential and treasured son texts
> numbering thirteen have been taught;
> these are the sunlight expositions
> shining on the exposition of this tantra.[545]

Therefore, with the reasons for their composition given in the above verse, the thirteen are then taught in verse as follows:

1. *Sunlight of Wisdom Outline*
2. *Son Manuscript Supplement on the Body*
3. *Complete Heart-Teachings Collection*
4. *Hidden Document on Names*
5. *Way of Compiling the 404 Diseases*
6. *Word Commentary on Causes of Excess and Deficiency*
7. *Word Commentary of the Three Humors*
8. *Page on Compress Treatment for Head Injury*
9. *Three Treatments for Lhok*
10. *Rishi Treatment for Planetary Illness*
11. *Investigation of Bezoar*
12. *Collection of Beneficial Mantras*
13. *Inventory without Fault*

Eighteen auxiliary texts are also asserted:

1. *Great Garuḍa History of Medicine*
2. *Beautiful Rainbow Overview*
3. *Outline: Wrathful Pose of the Tigress*
4. *Darkness-Dispelling Lamp of Explanation*
5. *Illuminating Beacon: Black Commentary Collection*
6. *Refutation of Arguments: Hindrance-Destroying Wheel*
7. *Eleven Sectional Overviews*
8. *Lexicon in Five Parts*
9. *Precious Jewel Heap of Medical Practice*
10. *Precious Heap of Miscellany*
11. *Short Works on Incisive Medical Practices*
12. *Three Indispensables*
13. *Eighteen Secrets* [173]
14. *Three Profound Instructions*
15. *Four Wondrous Superior Features*
16. *Ambrosia Essence Short Tantra*
17. *Pearl Garland Medical Practice*
18. *White Collection of Beneficial Mantras*

Of these two sets, the eighteen auxiliary texts are better known. Concerning those that survive in print to the present day, the *Illuminating Beacon:*

Black Commentary Collection was never received and has been substituted by the *Illuminating Beacon Small Collection Commentary.* Other works with similar titles regardless of content are simply the result of overzealous supplicants for the printing of texts at a time when only various corrupt mother texts were available. Two other texts not included in the original publication, but which have since appeared in print, are definitely included in the auxiliary texts. They are Yuthok's *Teachings on Medicinal Plants: Lamp Dispelling Error* and *Three Scroll Collections.* Of those in the original publication, *Eleven Sectional Overviews, Short Works on Incisive Medical Practices, Eighteen Secrets, Three Indispensables, Precious Heap of Miscellany, Three Profound Instructions, Four Wondrous Superior Features, Ambrosia Essence Short Tantra,* and *Pearl Garland Medical Practice* are mostly accepted as being Yuthok's own work. However, some verses of the first part of *History of the Lineage,* which is one of the *Three Indispensables,* could be seen as being the work of Yuthok, but on the whole, lines such as "that great sage Yuthok Gönpo" and "I, the son of Rutsam Sumpa" indicate without doubt that this is the work of Sumtön Yeshé Sung.[546] The printed work *Small Commentary Collection,* over which there was some doubt for a while as to whether it was composed by Sumtön, and which is listed in the original inventory as *Illuminating Beacon: Black Commentary Collection,* is now established as the work of Sumtön. These works are all are part of the auxiliary collection. Of the other works in the publication, *Darkness-Dispelling Lamp of Explanation* and *Lexicon in Five Parts* may or may not be the similarly named texts reputedly composed by Vairocana. Nevertheless, as the above they are included in the auxiliary collection. I think that the remaining works were composed by earlier Tibetan scholars of varying degrees of knowledge, such as Dza Yeshé Sung, Shakrampa Nyima Pal, Balmen, Drangti, Rok Könchok Kyab, and others.

Yuthok's compositions

Yuthok Yönten Gönpo, the king of medicine, also composed the following works: *Great Collection on Medicinal Plants; Fistful Collection on the Gathered Essence of Instruction; Heat Lancing of Boiḷs and so Forth; Illustrations of Bandages, Ties, and Splints; Clear Depiction of the Channels of the Abdomen; Stream of Instructions on Treatment of Brown Phlegm Disorders; Small Volume on Practice; Urine Charm Circle; Mirror of Clear Image; Texts for My Sons; Eliminating Physical Disturbance Caused by the Elements; Pacifying Poisoning; Fourteen Works on Women's Diseases;* [174] *Five-Ingredient Pain*

Medicine; Brief Document on the Work of the Doctor. With these and other compositions he shone the bright beacon of medicine in this dark land of Tibet. My lama the Great Fifth said of him:

> Fusion of all buddha families of the three enlightened bodies,
> the lord of medicine, Vajradhara,
> in the dance performed according to the minds of disciples,
> appears the one renowned as Yuthok Yönten Gönpo,
> in reality the naturally arising lord of myriad mandalas.[547]

As this verse indicates, Yuthok Yönten Gönpo, a prince of the Conqueror, a support and protector for the beings of these hugely degenerate times, came in the form of the medicine guru, synthesis of all buddha families, performing inconceivable and wondrous deeds that burst forth from the valley of the thoughts of his mind in the form of direct vision teachings.

In the *Clarifying Lamp Inventory* it says:

> Sunrays of compassion in thirty-five chapters,
> the very souls of the three sources rolled into one,
> ultimate life practices of the conquerors of all times.[548]

This refers to the most profound *Heartdrop Collection.* The text continues:

> Common to all, first the history,
> a hook to seize disciples' conviction.

This refers to the teachings on the *Heartdrop* history.

> Great sphere of bliss, ripening of the fortunate.[549]

This refers to the prerequisite ripening process of entering a cloth drawn mandala, a process that includes the following: the ceremonies of the crown, vase, head, and clothing ornaments, the medicine and alcohol torma collection, the great drum, the volume of *Four Tantras,* the skull, the mirror, and the medicine; the surgical-instruments initiation comprising the instruments for draining blood and cauterizing and for using forceps, surgical hammer, and surgical spoon; the external initiations of the hand implements of the five buddha families—the begging bowl, curved knife, and blood-filled skull cup; the inner initiations of the buddha families deity initiation; the five gnosis initiations together with the initiation of the rishi protector; the bodhicitta secret initiation; the wisdom-conduct initiation into the mandala of the mudra; the knowledge-gnosis initiation taken by way of vajra, bell, mirror, water crystal, and so forth; the reality initiation by way of glance meditation, conduct, and introduction to the result; the ambrosia-longevity initiation; the permission of the goddess; and the knowledge entrustment of Rishi Kapila. The text continues:

> Generation-stage practices combining outer, inner, and secret.

This refers to the collection on the profound guru practices of the supreme path.

> Outer torma and the activities,
> medicine torma, and supplements.

This refers to satisfying the invited guests and the section on the urging of activities for the production of siddhis. [175]

> The very profound completion stage,
> life essence of the ḍākinī.

This is the completion-stage collection on attaining enlightenment in one life.

> Eliminating hindrances, clarifying the signs on the path, and making the requests.

This is the supplementary collection that completes what is incomplete.

> Destroying the demon of death,
> the supplement fire offerings.

This is the collection on the long-life practice of obstacle elimination, longevity, protection, and fire offering.

> Prognostication practice, permissions,
> and suppression of hidden demons.

This is the medical-prognostication collection on curing illness without relying on others.

> Insight, radiance, satisfaction for the protector,
> the list of mantras, like a knife,
> like powerful poison, and like a thunderbolt,
> weapons to destroy the enemies hindering the doctrine.

This refers to the tantra-protector collection on annihilating enemies and the profound ninefold Dharma collection.

The Great Fifth said:

> The master Yuthok, the medicine king,
> guru with all buddha families combined,
> venerable Sumtön, in the class of mighty manifestations,
> with the glory of Ānanda, keeper of the treasury of instruction and scripture;
> the very essence of the speech of glorious Vajradhara,
> the ambrosia of those elixirs of immortality,
> endowed with the power to lead to enlightenment,
> profound vehicle bringing omniscience in a single life;
> is there an illustration worthy of this supreme vehicle?

As this verse indicates, my lama the Fifth, in reality an omniscient one, Ngawang Losang Gyatso, received the initiations, transmissions, and teachings of the *Heartdrop* in their entirety and propagated them widely, as illustrated by his *Wish-Fulfilling Tree: List of Practices from the Yuthok Heartdrop.*

Once, the chieftain Jodar and his family invited Yuthok, attended by a great number of masters and disciples, to a gathering in the Tsang market town of Gurmo. There he composed a commentary to *Fundamental Stanzas on the Middle Way.* He gave teachings on *atiyoga* Great Perfection for five months. During the customary celebrations at the end of the teachings, the chieftain sponsored the great gathering feast and made many offerings to him. Yuthok conferred, among others, the initiation for the secret accomplishment of the medicine guru, bestowed initiation permissions, and conferred blessings to many participants. One day at the end of the ceremonies, he prevented the sun from moving and performed miraculous physical displays. In the clear sky a rainbow of five distinct colors formed a canopy. A delightful aroma never before experienced pervaded the air. Flowers of sixteen petals fell from the skies. Around the chieftain's house fell a rain of fresh, golden myrobalan. A myrobalan fruit, the size of a fist and of a yellow color that eclipsed the golden color of the Jambu River, fell into the hands of Yuthok. [176] The assembly gathered the myrobalan together and distributed them, and it is said that each person received fifteen *dré* and half a *phül*[550] of myrobalan.

In the sense of being of the same mind lineage, Yuthok declared that in India he was Kumāra Jivaka, Guru Padma, Śūra, Śreṣṭha, Virūpa, and Puruṣa Agnideva, and here in Tibet he was the elder Yuthok Yönten Gönpo and Dakpo Lharjé.[551] To summarize:

> Hey! Listen! All you fortunate ones, listen well!
> People of this world, and you gods and humans gathered here,
> whatever you have heard or not heard in the past
> is but meaningless and flawed talk, of no significance,
> but what you hear today is of great importance.
> Whatever you have witnessed or not witnessed in the past
> are but misleading appearances, false pictures;
> look today and you will be free of obstacles.
>
> If you do not know my name,
> I am the messenger of all tathāgatas,
> the guardian and protector of all beings.
> Wherever animate and inanimate existence may be,
> there my body, speech, and mind will be too.
>
> This illusory body, this aggregate of form,
> is in the nature of the meditation deities;
> its material residue purified in its own abode.
> Like the rainbow it cannot be found;
> like the dance of the moon reflected in water,
> it appears where it will.
>
> My speech, the melody of an echo in an empty cave,
> proclaims the sounds of the 84,000 Dharmas,
> causing the rain of Dharma to fall

> whenever and wherever beings are to be tamed,
> ripening them and bringing them to freedom.
>
> My mind of clarity and emptiness is free of fabrication,
> the primordial state, and pervaded by great bliss, a continuum unending,
> an indivisibility of emptiness and compassion,
> with all signs and fabrications vanishing within its own abode.[552]

Also:

> I, Yuthok Gönpo, have for seventy-six years
> cherished the precious science of healing
> as I would my life.[553]

Thus, for seventy-six years he dedicated himself to the welfare of others and then traveled to the land of the ḍākinīs without abandoning of his own body:

> Those present and those to come,
> sons and disciples, understand this:
> now my work in this realm is complete,
> and now I go to the land of the ḍākinīs.[554] [177]

Yuthok's disciple lineage

Were every disciple of this great being counted, they would equal the number of stars in the sky or specks of dust on the earth. That said, his most well-known disciples were Jangmen Lepsé, Balmen Nyima Pal, Jé Yeshé Sung, Tönpa Atsé, Shakrampa Nyima Pal, Yuthok Bumseng, Yuthok Söseng, Sumtön Yeshé Sung, and Geshé Rokchung.

Among these disciples was Sumtön Yeshé Sung, who is counted in the garland of births of my lama the Great Fifth, and who worked unceasingly for the welfare of others through the manifested play of the seven lotus-holding conquerors.[555] He was born the son of Rutsam from Darsumpa in Nyemo. He trained in the other sciences until he had perfected them, and then one day he heard the life story of the master Yuthok. His mind was captivated. He decided to seek out teachings in medicine, and for twelve years he lived in the service of the master. *Four Tantras: The Essence of Ambrosia Secret Instruction Tantra,* a king among tantras because of its profound nature, was at that time expounded only to Yeshé Sung, and so he was truly the main heart-disciple of master Yuthok. In his *Sunlight of Compassion Clearing the Darkness of Suffering* he says:

> In the presence of the great Yuthok, whose name is hard to say, whose nature is the very gnosis inseparable from every deed, quality, body, speech, and mind of every buddha of every direction and of every time, through the kindness of the compassion of this great being, I, the physician Sumtön Yeshé Sung born of Rutsam, served him and delighted him for many years with the three ways of pleasing: through devotion in action, speech, and thought. Because of this I received the profound essence of the scriptures and instructions, the transmissions and practices in their entirety, in the manner of one full vase poured into another, and like a son receiving his inheritance from his father. Every profound and essential point was taught without error, and all arose from the churning stick of guidance through experience. I was appointed as his main heart-disciple. I can state, not with mere words but from my heart, that this unparalleled and venerable guru is truly the great sixth Buddha Vajradhara. Through his blessings I have also developed without difficulty the unmistaken, profound, and subtle view—exactly as it is—of that special state of emptiness and compassion combined, [178] and so all auspicious conditions for effortlessly fulfilling the needs of oneself and others are in place. In particular, the transmission of *Four Tantras,* the very king of all medical scriptures, and all the auxiliary texts has been entrusted to no one else but me.
>
> As for the extent of my future lineage, he delightedly prophesized, "Having taken the firm ground of working for living beings until samsara has been emptied, you will be of inconceivable and indescribable help to others through the science of healing."[556]

In his *Effortless Accomplishment of the Five Bodies,* he also says:

> A person such as I, Jñānadhara,[557]
> son of Rutsam Sumpa,

heard of the fame of my master from afar,
and merely hearing his name filled me with joy.

Enduring the journey's hardships, I came into his presence,
and merely seeing his face bestowed on me his blessings.
Although I had no wealth with which to offer,
I exchanged land for horses and made offerings.

Although I did not serve him physically,
whatever he commanded I never disobeyed.
Although my practice of the texts was not great,
I studied for three years without distraction.

While staying in Gyaché Nyendrong,
though I had not ascertained the fundamentals of his teachings,
I made a single prayer, and by his great compassion
he gave me this tantra on the science of healing.
He made the pledge to grant without omission or excess,
the blessings of the Rishi lineage, and said,

"So that the one-to-one transmission remains unbroken,
I now entrust it to you.
For the time being, do not expound it
but keep it as secret hidden treasure,
and unseen by your companions,
write it down secretly as a manuscript.
Keep it secret for one yearly cycle,[558]
the power of which will bring you siddhi."

As he commanded, so I followed.
Sometimes I wrote in secret on mountaintops,
sometimes in the deepest valleys,
sometimes in the deepest forest.

Thirteen years later, in the *jina* horse year[559]
in the Palkhor temple of Yeru,
I put the writing into print.
A scripture never before seen, heard, or experienced

now shines like the sun in the sky.
May it shine in glory for all living beings.

The master Yuthok Gönpo is like Vidyājñāna,
and I feel as if I am truly Manasija;[560]
I think that surely he was my lama in lives gone by.
His kindness was immense, and I never forget [179]
to place him upon on my head.
Grant me constantly your blessings.

This master had so many disciples,
but in the early part of his life
Jangmen Pelé of Tsida was the most renowned.
He was very competitive with the master
and did not penetrate to the root of these teachings.
These days what has his fame accomplished?

In the middle part of his life,
Tönpa Atsé of Kham was the most renowned.
Constantly collating and comparing
root texts and commentaries of the eight branches,
he did not penetrate to the root of these teachings.
These days what has his explaining of texts accomplished?

In the latter part of his life,
Geshé Rokchung of the west was the most renowned.
Constantly attached to his family line,
he did not penetrate to the root of these teachings.
These days who looks after his family?

At all times the two sons and two sons-in-law
were over-familiar in the master-disciple relationship,
and they did not penetrate to the root of these teachings.
These days who looks after the son disciples?

Of the disciples that came from afar,
some only learned one important thing,
some valued everything they saw,
some concentrated on investigation,

some wrote on whatever arose,
some went away empty handed,
some watched the practices and then left,
some spent their time singing and dancing,
some were content with meaningless things.
Not penetrating to the root of these teachings,
these days how will they heal the sick?

The one who truly gained the teachings
of the master Yuthok Gönpo was me alone.
The stream of his words flowed into me;
and if even Kumāra Jivaka himself were here,
I think I would have nothing to ask of him.

I do not need fame and fortune—
I have truly met the guru rishi;
there is no way I can be deficient in the teachings.[561]

Therefore, the heart-disciple of Yuthok Yönten Gönpo, master of manifesting and withdrawing an ocean of mandalas, was Sumtön Yeshé Sung. As an author he composed a variety of works, such as the life story of Yuthok entitled *Effortless Accomplishment of the Five Bodies* or *Sealed Biography of Yuthok; Secret Biography; Illuminating Beacon Small Collection: Commentary on the Explanatory Tantra;* and *Treatment of Kangbam: Notes from the Whispered Tradition.* He concentrated primarily on spreading the teachings of the glorious *Four Tantras.*

His main disciple was Shönu Yeshé. In the *Effortless Accomplishment of the Five Bodies* it says:

Vidyājñāna was Yuthok Gönpo,
Manasija was the divine master, [180]
I am Tsojé Shönu Yeshé.[562]
He was my master in births without beginning;
I have been held by the compassion of the lama;
How kind the lama to this worthy vessel![563]

Moreover, during the reign of the ruler Tsedé,[564] a doctor from Oḍḍiyāna came to Tibet. A specialist in eye treatments and so forth, he was a son of Jinamitra. He had so perfected his knowledge of medicine that he was appointed royal physician. Once while treating the queen, he committed a sexual indiscretion. The king thought it too great a loss to have him put to death, however, and so he was punished by having one of his hands amputated. Because of this he became known as Bharo of Amputated Hand. His other name was Puruṣa Agnideva. He composed many instructional works, such as *Whispered Tradition Black Compilation; Blue Compilation of Children's Disorders; Fistful Collection; Outer, Inner, and Secret Stone-Removal Collection.* His closest disciples were Thazhi, Gön, Tong, and Seu Menpa. He had several other disciples, such as Nyang, Ya, and Bé.

There were many other miscellaneous works during those times. They include the following: *Instructions on the Four Categories of Chong Diseases* handed down from Virūpa and written down in note form by Tharpa Lotsāwa; *Opening the Eyes: A Lamp Dispelling Darkness,* in the tradition of Mitrayogi; a cure for rabies received by Jowo Atiśa from his guru Avadhūtipa in the land of Kampoché;[565] a medical work based on *Four Tantras* that was extant from the time of the later Yuthok; *Jewel Garland Biography of Zé Yönten Gönpo* by Yuthok Kharak Lhajé; *Brilliant Jewel Treasury Biography* by Kongpo Degyal; *Sunlight Clarity of Meaning* by Phaktön Śākya Gönpo; *Three Collections on Mercury* and *Precious Pill Collection* by Panchen Jaliwa from Droding[566] in the west, translated by Orgyenpa Rinchen Pal from Changlung Pütra, who was one of the "ten physicians manifested to work for others"; *White, Black, and Multicolored Magic Treatments* and *Charm Collections,* and so on, by Phadampa Sangyé, famed for his stick treatment;[567] *Ocean of Medicine Names* and *Brief Essence of Eight Branches* and *Bezoars,* and so on, by Karmapa Rangjung Dorjé; *Miscellaneous Knowledge Collection* by Bari Lotsāwa; *Compilation of Essentials* by Lotsāwa Drakpa Sengé; *Pearl Garland Instructions* or *Fist Collection* together with a list of contents, compiled by Chakmen Rinchen Gyaltsen and Shakya Yeshé; *Thirty-Two Instructions of the Fist Collection* compiled from the previous work and composed by Changmen Sangyé Gönpo; the work known as the *Drongtsé Compilation,* which includes *Black Exposition on Medicine* and so on, by Lhatsün Drong Tsewa; [181] *Great Commentary to the Root Medical Tantra* by Dongnak Chemen Dargyé; many instructional works known as *Bag of Instructions for Entering* by Barmenpa; and *Commentary to the Explanatory Medical Tantra: Light Rays of Validity Radiating Afar* by Chipa Palgön Dorjé.

14. The Drangti Lineage and a Summary

THE DRANGTI LINEAGE began with Drangti Gyalnyé Kharphuk, reputed to be royal physician and minister to Dharma king Tridé Tsukten Mé Aktsom. It continued in an unbroken lineage of appointed royal physicians and ordinary trained physicians through Drangti Darma Nyingpo, Drangti Drakphuk Sumpa, Drangti Dartsün,[568] Drangti Palden Bum, and so forth. The lineage was also responsible for maintaining one-to-one lineages of profound instructions, such as "channeling the ambrosia," that were eventually written down and became known as the *Drangti Multicolored Works* and *Drangti Red Works.*

Among the lineage was Drangti Sönam Bum. His son was Jampal Sangpo who from an early age showed exceptional intelligence and compassion. Karma Pakshi[569] proclaimed that he was a bodhisattva and prophesized that he would be of great service to others. From his father he received teachings, collections, instructions, and practices, including the root text and commentaries to the *Treatise of Eight Branches,* the *Red Ink Son and Mother Texts,* and the *Three Ācārya Medical Collections.* In Goshi Rethang he met with Yuthok Jampal, from whom he learned and mastered *Four Tantras* and its auxiliary works, along with Yuthok's oral teachings and practices. In Tsiphu Jangmo Khyü he studied for a long time under the Jang doctor Yeshé Sangpo and became so learned in the eight branches and so on that he became renowned in Tibet as the master of nearly all of medical science. A great lama invited him to his monastic seat, and there he initiated classes in the study of the eight branches. He was given the position of governor of half a hundred[570] and became the principal of the senior physicians. He was constantly teaching the tantra, the eight branches, the practices, and the canonical scriptures. In this way his time was spent solely in the service of others.

Jampal Sangpo composed the *Five-Section Commentary,* also known as the *Small Volume on Practice,* containing measurements and amounts for the medicinal preparation from the Final Tantra. This serves as an authoritative source for measurements in medicinal preparations and is probably confused with Yuthok's *Small Volume on Practice*. He also composed *Treatment of Bird-Like Demons*.

His eldest son was Drangti Shingkang, or Gyalwa Sangpo. [182] He studied with his father and Biji Palgön among others and learned the scriptures, the oral teachings, and the practices. He came to Yuthok Tsojé,[571] from whom he received many teachings, such as *Four Tantras,* its auxiliary texts, and *Small Volume on Practice*. He came to give new teachings at Goshi Rethang, and whereas others had to teach from small side thrones, the physician in charge said to him, "You are a lineage physician like no other. Please teach from the throne of Yuthok."

He maintained his father's dynastic seat and nurtured the uncle-nephew lineage[572] as senior physicians of the past had done. He passed on the texts, oral teachings, and practices to students all over the country and made an immense contribution to the welfare of living beings.

Gyalwa Sangpo's younger son became ordained at an early age and was known as Palden Tsojé. He studied for a long time under his elder brother as well as Phaktön Śākya Gönpo, where he received complete teachings on *Four Tantras,* its auxiliary texts, the commentaries, the essential commentaries, and the practices. This was not just superficial learning but a thorough understanding. For many years he propagated the teachings of the *Treatise of Eight Branches* using Yuthok's commentary, Jangmo Khyüpa's commentary, the teachings passed down from his father, Chejé, and Minyak,[573] and annotations made by the great scholar and great upholder of the baskets of scripture, Nedrukpa Lodrö Tsungmé. Altogether he composed about eighteen works of various lengths, and his contribution to the welfare of others is inconceivable. His compositions include:

- *History of Medicine: Illumination of Knowledge*
- Commentary to the Root Tantra called *Illumination of the Meaning of the Tantra*
- Commentary to the Final Tantra called *Illumination of the Three Ways*
- Commentary to the pulse section of the *Four Tantras* called *Rays of the Sun*
- *Exposition of Eight Branches*
- *Rishi Chronicles*
- *Commentary on Difficult Points on the Malaya*
- *Illustrations of Medicinal Preparations from the Final Tantra*
- *Sādhana of the Pulse Goddess*

- Commentary to the urine section of the *Four Tantras* called *Wish-Fulfilling Jewel Clarifying the Text*
- *Commentary on Decoctions and Powder*
- *Lamp Illuminating the Structure of the Torso*
- *Compilation of Essentials*
- *Thirty-Chapter Wooden-Board Commentary to the Compilations and Sections of the Tantra*[574]

Drangti Palden Gyaltsen was a nephew of Drangti Palden Tsojé. He produced a compilation consisting of the commentary to the first chapter of the Root Tantra, the thoughts of his paternal predecessors, and particularly those of Palden Tsojé, as well as the teachings given to him by his meditation deity Mañjuśrī, such as *Compound of the Six White Ingredients.* This compilation was given to his son, Namgyal Sangpo, and is known as *Golden Measuring Dish of Instructions.* [183] I have not seen any documents setting out his family line, but according to the lineage of the instructions on treatment for dropsy from the *Shorter Golden Measuring Dish of Instructions,* the line passed from Palden Gyaltsen to Drangti Künga Sangpo, to Drangti Takla Pal, and then to Drangti Dorjé Palsang, who composed *Illuminating Commentary to the Explanatory Tantra.* He passed the texts, instructions, and oral teachings to Drangti Paljor Döndrup and composed the *Shorter Golden Measuring Dish,* compiling it from the longer version. This he passed to his son, who in turn propagated the *Silver Measuring Dish of Instructions,* which is shorter than the versions of *Golden Measuring Dish* and seems to be inferior in content. In the Sakya Mendrong medical tradition, he maintained the medical tradition as his fathers had done before him.[575]

There are two physicians called Palgön Dorjé and Chögyal Tashi, also prefixed with the title Drangti, but whether they are sons of the above is difficult to say.

Other medical works of those times mostly based on the eight branches include the following: *Revealing Mirror Commentary* by Mara Gomchen, manuscripts such as *Brief Work on the Number of Chapters, Increase and Diminution, Taste Preparations, Stages of Niruha Enema Therapy,* and *Twenty Characteristics,* and so on, composed by Yuthok Tashi Gön; *Scripture Count: Essence of the Sun* and *Great Compilation* by Yuthok Gyaltsa. Balmen Nyima Pal, a disciple of Yuthok Bumseng, composed *Wish-Fulfilling Jewel of Essentials* and taught it to Yuthok Jampal. He in turn taught it to Palden Sangpo, who passed it on to Gyalwa Sangpo, who in turn passed it to his son Palden

Tsojé. Palden Tsojé handed it down to Palden Gyaltsen, thereby forming an unbroken lineage of transmission and teaching.

Elsewhere, other works include: *Moonlight Flower Commentary to the First Chapter* by Chejé Śākya Pal; *Clarifying Explanation: Essence of the Sun* by Jangmo Khyüpa Yeshé Sangmo; *Stream of Ambrosia Medical History* by Thazhi Śīlasaṃgha; *Profound Commentary* and its outline by Minyak Dorjé Bum; *Clear Overview* by Dzajo Sung; *Sunlight Commentary* by Shakrampa Nyima Pal; *Clarifying the Meaning of the Text* by Geshé Roktön; *Sun Circle Commentary on the Shorter Eight Branches* by Palchen Öpo; *Essence of Eight Branches* by the great Sakya Paṇḍita; *Flower Ornament Medical Text* by Chomden Raldri; *Exposition on the History of Medicine* and *Essence of Medical Practices* by Taktsang Lotsāwa; *Compilation of Essentials of the Eight Branches* and *Treatise on Mercury Preparation* by Tongmen Tsojé Shönu; [184] *Treasury of the King* by Jetsün Drakpa Gyaltsen; *Golden Measuring Dish* and *Silver Measuring Dish* from the Sakya medical tradition, and so on.[576]

Summary of Tibetan medical traditions

In short, the works of Tibetan medical scholars are listed in an old manuscript:

> Point seven: the tradition of Tibetan scholars,
> of which there are nine principal scholars:
> Tong, Nyah, and Thazhi,
> Minyak, Drangti, and Yuthok,
> Biji, Chejé, and Ukpo.
>
> The first of these, the tradition of Tongmen, includes
> Commentary to *Differentiating the Middle Way and the Extremes* and other works by translator Jñānamitra;
> *Collection on Knowledge* by Dharmapāla;
> *Magic Mirror Compilation on Pulse and Urine* by Künga Wangchuk;
> Gyaltsen Jungné's *Stream of Ambrosia Compilation on Fevers;*
> *Magic Draining of Dropsy Instructions* taught by Jñānadhara;
> *Treatment of Growths* by Tsojé Drupa;
> *Structure of the Torso* by Shāka Lodrö;
> Yeshé Wangchuk's *Ambrosia Drops Collection on Gaklhok Treatments,* and so on;

Treatments for Women's Diseases: Fulfilling to Behold composed by Palgön Sherap;
Thirty Chapters on Examination by Charms by Gönpo Dorjé that teaches the supreme attainment treatment of *gakser* and the oral transmission on all-knowing eye;
Treatment for Urinary Stones and so forth by Jangchup Pal;
Magic Circle of Water Surgical Removal by Samten Sherap;
Elixirs by Öser Gönpo;
Commentaries to the Root, Explanatory, and Final Tantras, with annotations to the Instruction Tantra, and so forth, by Tongla Takchung;
Types of Elixir by Künga Nyingpo;
Essence of Eight Branches by Palshé;
Treatment of Infectious Diseases by Dondrup Gönpo;
Treatments for Poisoning by Lekden Gönpo;
Compilation of Miscellaneous Treatments by Jamyang;
Secret Commentary to the Heart Tantra by Sherap Öser;
Commentary on *Differentiating the Middle Way and the Extremes* and so on, translated by Jñāna Śākyaśrī;[577]
Essence of Somarāja by Shönu Wangchuk;
Arrowhead Treatment for Eyes and Urinary Stones by Tsojé Drupa;
Chapters and Commentary to Eight Branches by Könchok Gyaltsen;
and commentaries on the Root, Explanatory, and Final Tantras, on *Essence of Eight Branches,* and on others by Tsojé Namkha Gyaltsen. [185]

Texts composed by Nya and his followers include:
True Illumination Commentary on the Heart Tantra
and *Six Sections Explaining Reversal Treatment;*
Refutation of Arguments by Jangchup Sherap;
and *Essence of Differentiating the Middle Way and the Extremes* and so on, by Tsöndrü Sengé.

Thazhi Rinchen composed *Matted-Hair Core Meaning,*
and Darseng Gönpo composed *Treatments.*

Minyak Rongjé Gaga composed *Mountain Stack Commentary* and so forth.

Drangti Dréu composed *History* and others;
Trikhu composed *Six Chapters on Fever;*
and Drangti Gyalnyé wrote *Secret Treasury of Ambrosia* among others.

Yuthok Gönpo composed *Annotations and Accounts from the Golden Jewel Tantra Golden Jewel Tantra;*
Yuthok Gönpo Drupa composed *Commentary Clarifying the Meaning* and others;
Yuthok Gönpo Sherap composed *Ambrosia Essence Instructions* and so on;
Gönpo Rinchen composed *Son Teachings in Ninety-Four Chapters;*
Yuthok Gönpo Dorjé had *Auxiliary Texts for the Tantra,* among others;
Khyungwo composed *Commentary on Eight Branches;*
and Gönpo Drakpa compiled *Collection on Practice.*

Biji Leklo composed *Essentials of Knowledge* and others;
Palchen composed *Three Fundamentals Collections;*
Lhuné composed *Ocean Garland Treatments for the Head;*
Marlo composed the *Peacock* and *Parrot* collections;
and Sherap Lodrö composed *Treatments for Naga Illness* and *Essential Instructions.*

Chejé Gyalwa wrote *Charms* and *Essentials of Knowledge;*[578]
Lhasé composed *Ambrosia Essence;*
Gönseng composed *Brief Work on the Abdomen;*
Takla Gah composed *Laying Out the Keys to Eight Branches,* among others;
Tisang composed *Essentials of Eight Branches;*
Ulang composed *History of Medicine;*
and Shikpo composed *Fourfold Exposition Collection.*

Ukpa Chösang taught *Crystal Jewel Commentary* and so on;
Wangchuk taught *Commentary on the Causes of Purification;*
Rinchen Gyalpo taught *Collections;*
and Chösé composed *Jewel Heap of Miscellany.*
These were taught by the traditions
known as those of the nine wise Tibetans.

Various works taught by other scholars include:

- *Eight Ambrosia Chapters* by Yiwong Lekpa [186]
- *Six Illuminating Lamps* by Shangtön Siji Bar
- *Drop of Ambrosia* by Chejé Shangtön Shikpo
- *Stainless Brilliance* by Phenné
- *Six Beneficial Clarifications* by Drakpa Dorjé
- *Precious Garland* by Tashi Dorjé
- *Extensive Work on Medical Plant Preparation* by Chikmen Gawo
- *Mercury Preparation* by Jampa Tsönseng
- *Short Essential Work on Fevers* by Tashi Dar
- Small collection by Geshé Marpo called *Fire Circle*
- *Fever Collection* by Dorjé Bum
- Gyalbum's *Treatments for the Head*
- Gadè's *Teachings in the Field of Knowledge*
- *Compilation of Essential Miscellaneous Treatments* by Takgom Ngönshé Chen
- *Collection on Stone Removal* by Mönlam Gyaltsen
- *Cauterization* by Nyima Pal
- *Treatments for Stones* by Balmen Karnak
- *Treatments for Poisoning* by Yeshé Lodrö
- *Essence of Eight Branches* by Dawa Shönu
- *History of Medicine* by Lodrö
- *Essence of the Tantra* and so on by Drapa Ngönshé
- *Collection on Urine and Pulse* by Darma Drak
- *Compilation on Hot and Cold Disorders* by Tsojé Könchok Kyap
- *Five Bodies Biography, Divisions of the Tantra Auxiliary,* and others, by Josung
- *Compilation of Various Teachings* by Bönlep
- *Treatment of Wounds of the Head* and so forth by Achö
- *Draining and Drying Dropsy Procedure* by Rokchung
- *Compilation of Essential Profound Treasures* by Tertön Gyashang Trom
- *Padma Transmission Holder Compendium* taught by Rakshak Tertön
- *Essence of the Enlightened Mind* by Khyung Tri
- *Commentary on Meanings of Treasure Writing* unearthed by Lhabar
- *Lamp Illuminating the Four Points* and so on by Nyemo Chökyi Wangchuk
- *Eighty Charms* by Dampa

- *Small Collection on Knowledge* and so forth by Bari
- *Medical Treasury of the King* by Jetsün Drakpa Gyaltsen
- *Sun Circle Short Commentary on Eight Branches* by Palpoché
- *Essence of Eight Branches* by the great Sakya Paṇḍita
- *Black Medicine Text* by Orgyenpa
- *Flower Ornament Medical Text* by Chomden Raldri
- *Head Compresses without Surgery* by Jangmo Khyüpa and Melingpa
- *Annotations on Eight Branches* by Lodrö Tsungmé

This sections ends, "This has been just a rough listing."

Physicians coming from other lands as well as resident physicians were responsible for the propagation of fifty-six medical traditions. [187] The text continues:

1. Śāntigarbha propagated medicine and treatment for leprosy;
2. Hvashang Mahāyāna propagated cauterization and stick treatment;
3. Tsenpashila propagated cupping treatment, dietary rules, behavior, and other practices;
4. Drugu Sengdo's treatments for horses;
5. Khyölma Rutsé's treatment of broken limbs;
6. Dharmaśīla's special treatment for poisoning;
7. Lotsāwa Rinchen Sangpo's teaching tradition of the eight branches;
8. Puruṣa Agnideva's extensive teachings on practice;
9. Purang Nyangmen's extensive use of the surgical spoon;
10. Tongmen Takchung's special treatments for fevers;
11. Ukpa Chösang's splints for limbs;
12. Biji Yorwo's reversal treatment;
13. Chejé Nagu's special treatments for women;
14. Drangti Sekhyung's clear anatomy of the torso;
15. Minyak Dawa Drakpa's *Great Compilation;*
16. Thazhi Śākya Dar's explicit treatments on stone disorders;
17. Nyenak Köntön's treatments for ligaments and joints;
18. Sumen Tashi's treatment for chest illnesses;
19. Chejé Draksö's removal of arrowheads;
20. Thekar Gyalwa Rinchen's surgical treatment for opening the eyes;
21. Gyimjang Gokar's cauterization of growths;
22. Jomo Namo's compress treatment of arrow wounds;
23. Dartön Gendün's commentary on the essentials of hot and cold disorders;

24. Drupchen Orgyen's preparation of mercury;
25. Rongtön Chösang's compilation of practices;
26. Rongtön Shewang's extensive medical plant preparation;
27. Geshé Rokchung's extensive and concise works on remedies for poisoning;
28. Bamen Tsönwang's treatments for limb bones;
29. Limen Sizin's surgery for the head;
30. Gongjé Mentsün's examination of signs;
31. Tratsang Druklha's teachings on charms and illness-causing spirits;
32. Drapa Ngönshé's explicit teachings on symptoms;
33. Shangtön Siji's main points;
34. Geshé Suktön's practice by reference to texts;
35. Purang Zemen's compress treatments for the head;
36. Sumen Josö's Chinese magical cures;
37. Chemen Jodor's treatment for limb wounds;
38. Bamen Jothok's complete treatment for fevers;
39. Sokgong Merin's practices of the eight branches;
40. Dromen Tashi's head and eye surgery;
41. Chuktsam Darsö's magical treatments for the abdomen;
42. Dokmen Samten's special treatment for *gaklhok;*
43. Bhenak Mebar's the use of the substitution pulse;[579]
44. Shangdrung Lodrö's tinder cauterization instructions;
45. Kukpa Gotum's arrowhead instructions;
46. Khyungpo Gyina's extensive teachings on remedies for poisons;
47. Rakshak Tertön's miscellaneous treatments; [188]
48. Bamen Chenmo's removal and drying up of pus;
49. Jemen Shalu's structure of the abdomen;
50. Tongmen Sengdrak's teaching tradition on urinary stones;
51. Chikmen Gawo's *Words of a Simpleton* teachings;
52. Nupmen Josö's general treatments for poisoning;
53. Kharak Tsangmen's extensive teachings on the treatises;
54. Chejé Triö's commentary on the eight branches; and
55. Lhajé Gebum's union of Dharma and medicine.[580]

Therefore, throughout the past, in this land of the nine regions of Purgyal,[581] countless spiritual-friend physicians transmitted and propagated the science of medicine.

Renowned Tibetan physicians

The most renowned Tibetan physicians are classified under fifteen categories:

1. One whose wisdom was that of a paṇḍita
2. One as pervasive as the sky
3. Two as renowned as the sun and moon
4. Nine trained and lineage physicians of the king
5. Ten who manifested to work for others
6. Six who developed great qualities through training
7. Ten renowned physicians like medicine buddhas
8. Nine whose qualities came from training in previous lives
9. Ten whose traditions arose individually
10. Six whose renown arose naturally
11. Five whose renown was promoted by the Mongolians
12. Two who specialized in surgery
13. One as famous as a king
14. Nine central pillars
15. Fifty-eight renowned propagators

These are identified as follows:

1. Rinchen Sangpo
2. Puruṣa Agnideva
3. Nyangmen Lotsāwa and Tongmen Takchung
4. Biji, Chejé, and Ukpa from the upper regions; Yuthok, Drangti, and Minyak from the central regions; and Nyawa, Tongpa, and Thazhi from the lower regions
5. Druptop Orgyenpa from Changlung Pütra, Dartön Gendün from Jangna Ngön, Gochen Mentsün from Khulung, Tongtön Chösang, Tratsang Druklha, Sumen Josö from Urtö, Drapa Ngönshé, Shangtön Siji Bar from Yarnga, Purtong from Nyal, and Öchen Trülku from Kham
6. Könchok Kyap from Mangkhar Chelung, Gyatsa Chakdor from Nyangtö, Gyatön Josung from Rutsam, Tsangmen Dorjé from Kharek, [189] Bomen Japé, and Tongmen Sengdrak
7. Yuthok Yönten Gönpo, Thazhi Śākya Dar, Minyak Sakyong from Gyangkhar, Jangmen Lepsé, Rokchung from Nyangtö, Shangpa Bamen, Jemen Shalu from Langdro, Chemen Jodor, Chejé Triö from Gungthang Menlung, and Lhajé Gebum from Kyishö

8. Jomo Namo from Latö, Toknyi from Latö, Mebar from Kham, Lhündrup Lodrö from Samyé, Gyina from Bumthang, Kuktsal from Lhodrak, Rakshak Tertön from Lhakhang, Gyalwa of Tradruk, and Künga Döndrup from Dranyé Do
9. Purang Zemen, Öser Phendar from Latö, Ngokmen Gyongpo from Gyangkhar, Shershak from Nyangtö, Phenpo Dzongdöl, Gyokmen Tashi from Dromtö, Darsö from Urtö, Palsang from Nyal, Sengé from Yarlung, and Chökyi Gyaltsen from Shangro
10. Drakpa Dorjé from Nyangro, Tashi Dorjé from Tölung Nyen, Chikmen Gawo from Yartö Gyewo, Menkhap Tseseng (Tsasang), Nyalmen Tashi, and Marwa from Yarlung
11. Shangmen Karpo, Shangmen Nakpo, Shakrampa Nyima Pal from Nyemo, Gönthang Pakṣi from Yarlung, and Lotön Yönten from Gyeré
12. Tsöndrü Sengé, who was a specialist on the abdomen, and Baré Lhajé, who specialized in using the surgical spoon
13. Drangti Gyalnyé Kharphuk
14. Shentön Yeshé Lodrö from Darding, and so on
15. Lotsāwa Shaser Chen, and so on

PART 3

LATER DEVELOPMENT OF MEDICAL SCIENCE IN TIBET

15. The Jang Tradition

In the benefits they brought to others, the renowned physicians listed above can be compared to the waxing of the moon. However, in later times[582] there arose two great scholars—Jangpa Namgyal Draksang (b. 1395) and Surkhar Nyamnyi Dorjé (1439–75)—who loosened the knots of the difficult points of medicine in general and of the four glorious tantras in particular, and in doing so were like masters of doctrine of this highest of sciences.

Jangpa Namgyal Draksang

His father was Guigung Chödrak Palsang, who was a seventh-generation descendent of the Seu king of Minyak[583] and who was ordained by the writ of heaven as emperor on the Chinese throne, a position produced by the glories of extraordinary merit. [190] The Sechen emperor[584] had presented to him a jeweled seal and appointed him to the position of Situ, greatly elevating his status. His mother was Bumkyong Gyalmo, the daughter of Situ Chörin, and Jangpa was born as their son in the wood-pig year of the seventh sixty-year cycle[585] in the great kingdom of Ngamring, a place to which the great capital of the northern land of Shambhala had seemingly moved.

From an early age instincts of the past awoke within him, and he spent his days displaying the behavior of a noble being. From the great master of study and practice, Lochen Jangchup Tsemo, from Tenpa Gyaltsen of his own blood line, and from the high-ranking Dagön Sherap he received, on more than one occasion, the ambrosia gift from the great feast of the sacred Dharma. When he was four or five he lived in Kyema palace in the south. There, without any difficulty, he mastered subjects such as reading, writing, and spelling. Later he settled back in Ngamring.

At the age of ten he had a pure-vision dream in which he met Orgyen Padma. From then on he had visions and received the gift of teachings from the Bhagavān Munīndra, from kings Bimbisāra and Sucandra, from Asaṇga and Vasubandhu, from Milarepa, and from many other deities and lamas. Under many qualified guardians,[586] such as the master of the five disciplines Paljor Sherap, Rinchen Palsang, Sengé Gyaltsen, Bodhgāya abbot Śāriputra, pandit Vanaratna,[587] and Bodong Choklé Namgyal, he studied to perfection the sutras, tantras, and the sciences. From the Mongolian master of four disciplines, Sengé Gyaltsen, he took the vows of a layman and was given the name Chögyal Namgyal Draksang. Until then he had been known as Gyaruk Darma Rikzin.

The glorious Sakya lama Künga Tashi Gyaltsen Palsang had visited by invitation the great Chinese Tai Ming emperor, who bestowed upon him the title of Mahayana Dharma king and other tokens of respect. Following this precedent, the emperor also presented this high-lineage Dharma king with a silver seal and the position of Tai Situ.[588] [191]

When he was almost thirty-one he took as a bride Namkha Palbum, the daughter of Sengé Tsewa, and eventually they produced sons and daughters.

His fame spread throughout the land, and soon Drenwang Dorjé Gyaltsen, Minyak Chödrak Sangpo, Sangyé Lhündrup from Tsedong, and many others crushed their mountains of pride and came to worship at his feet. Even Panchen Jampa Lingpa offered flowers of praise. He engaged in question-and-answer communication with the omniscient Gendün Drup and was recognized as an incarnation of the Dharma king Sucandra.[589]

From the age of forty onward, he created many representations of the enlightened body, speech, and mind. These include the construction of very special and complete three-dimensional body, speech, and mind mandala of Kālacakra—the supreme tantra among the vast ocean of the highly secret tantras—made almost entirely from gold and silver and adorned with precious stones. He also erected statues of Maitreya and Kālacakra and produced the Jangtsek Kangyur and Tengyur.

Using his high position he chose people from the local community to become monks and founded the Jamtruk monastic community.

He developed qualities of insight beyond measure. For example, by visualizing Sakya Paṇḍita on his head and dissolving him into his body, all the profound and essential points of Sakya thought dawned in his mind.

As an author he composed thirty-five works on general aspects of the doctrine, such as a work on the lineage of the Tathāgata, various praises, and many compilations drawn from the Kangyur and Tengyur. From the outer, inner, and "other" divisions of the glorious Kālacakra, he wrote, based on the first two chapters of the tantra, forty-two explanatory works, such as the *Easy to Understand Astronomical Treatise;* based on the Initiation and Methods of Accomplishment chapters, he wrote fifty-four explanatory works, such as *Stream of Great Bliss Initiation Procedure;* he wrote twelve explanatory works on the Gnosis chapter, such as *Body Mandala Completion Stage of the Path;* and he wrote six general summarizing commentaries, such as *Clarification of Phenomena* and *Explanation of the First Summary.* On the essence of grammar he wrote *Ornament to the Kalāpa Sutra.* On crafts he composed *Measurements of the Form of the Tathāgata.* He wrote no works on logic, but in the company of logicians he would pose consequences, and so forth, and became known as the pandit king, spending his time teaching, debating, and composing. [192]

He excelled in the science of medicine in particular, and his medical compositions include the following:

- *Essence of All Eight Branches: A Precious Wish-Fulfilling Jewel* in 120 chapters
- *Beacon Illuminating the Meaning of the Tantra: Explanation of the Root Tantra*
- *Stream of Ambrosia: Extensive Commentary on the Explanatory Tantra*
- *Short Commentary Illuminating the Meaning of the Explanatory Tantra*
- *Fulfilling All Needs and Wishes: Commentary on the Final Tantra*
- *Word Commentary on the Text of the Entrustment Section*
- *Precious Casket Medical Text*
- *Short Text Dispelling the Darkness on the Difficult Path of Four Tantras*
- *Identifying the 360 Healing Methods*
- *Beacon Illuminating the Root and Explanatory Tantras*
- *Categories of the Nine Fatal Illnesses*
- *Heartfelt Magical Manuscript for Doctors*
- *Response to the Physician Sengé Tsé*

With these and other works his teaching, debating, and compositions began a renaissance within medical science.

He revealed many indications of siddhi. For example, a thunderbolt once struck the palace, rendering most people inside unconscious or terrified, but it had no effect on him whatsoever. Also, one time when the wife of a local governor was possessed by a demon, he was able to exorcise it merely by posing with a ritual dagger.

In this way, until the age of eighty-one, he accomplished much for the doctrine and for living beings. Finally, having retired to Salachöpa Ögmin Lhündrup Ding he showed signs of being slightly ill for about a month, and during that time a continuous shower of coral tree flowers fell each day, cast by the lotus hand of deathlessness. In the wood-sheep year,[590] during the sixth day of the *Jyeṣṭha* month, the union of the *saṃbhogakāya* and the illusory gnosis body arose from the container of his coarse *nirmāṇakāya* form and merged into the heart of Kālacakra.[591] Rainbow light, a rain of flowers exuding a beautiful aroma, and countless other wondrous signs were seen.

Jé Drölchok says:

> In the sciences, from ultimate-vehicle Kālacakra
> to medicine and astronomy,
> he led each disciple according to disposition,
> bringing them all to levels of scholarship and attainment.[592]

The list of his disciples is beyond number. However, his main disciples were headed by the great being Palden Chökyong. Others include Jamyang Namkha Chökyong of Jonang Monastery, Tsanawa Samten Gyatso, and Shangtön Künga Palden. [193] These were among his main disciples maintaining the tantra tradition.

Minyima Thongwa Dönden

Among the above was the medical disciple, and also court physician, Minyima Thongwa Dönden or Jampa Könchok Rinchen. He was born the son of Sönam Dorjé, who was of the pure lineage of the great Tibetan kings, which included the lotus-holding conqueror in noble human form, the lord of the black-haired people, and the emanated celestial emperor, known collectively as the three noble ancestors.[593]

From an early age he held the Three Jewels as his lama and was blessed with great faith and perseverance. His behavior, such as his tendency to look after the poor and the wretched with compassion, was beyond the ordinary. He mastered reading, writing, and so on without any difficulty. In his youth he served under many masters of great scholarship and attainment, such as the Indian pandit Vanaratna, Lotsāwa Sönam Gyatso, the Jang master Rikden Namgyal Draksang, and Drangti Palden Tsojé, and built a solid foundation of the three scriptural baskets, the four classes of tantra, and the commentarial treatises. He mastered the sciences and, being particularly proficient in the science of medicine, he taught *Four Tantras,* the root text and commentaries to *Eight Branches,* the great commentaries of the Oral Tradition, commentaries on the inner, outer, and secret, and the twenty-five sealed works, all explained using the six limits and the four methods.[594] He maintained the teaching traditions of the Eighteen Auxiliary Texts to the Treasure tradition form of the tantra, and so forth. Specifically, from Rikden Namgyal Draksang he learned most medical works, including *Somarāja, Moonlight Commentary on Eight Branches, Vase of Ambrosia, Hundred Medical Preparations,* and the five sutras. From his father Sönam Dorjé he received the initiation for the entrustment of the tantra, the collection of goddess practices for urine divination, and the complete blessings of the oral transmission. From Drangti he received the urine divination goddess practices and the rishi practices.

In short, with his eyes of wisdom as open as the sky, alighting upon the whole range of medical science that had spread throughout this snow-mountain land, the banner of his fame flew in all ten directions. Even Jé Surkhar Nyamnyi Dorjé was captivated by him, and under the pretext of wanting to know about his family, lineage, name, and so on, Surkhar composed a letter to Minyima Thongwa Dönden. In reality Surkhar himself was unable to go to central Tibet to meet him and was in fact requesting teachings like a good disciple. The master replied as follows: [194]

Svasti siddhaṃ
I prostrate to the glorious Vajrasattva.
To the great friend of the sun, Gautama,
son of the Ikṣu[595] lineage, Munīndra, god of gods,
to him with countless names,
king of the Śākya race, I prostrate;
and I will now explain my name.

I was born into a **noble** *(jowo)* family of **celestial** *(lha)* lineage
and came into the well-trained Rishi lineage of medicine.
Moreover, I was born into a lineage wise in the sciences;
I am known as Lhatsün José.

Not lacking in the **glory** *(pal)* of wholesome deeds,
I have attained this form of leisure and opportunity.

Endowed *(den)* with faith, perseverance, and compassion,
I have great joy in the teachings.
Holding the **vajra** *(dorjé)* of unshakeable faith in the Teacher,
I am known as Palden Dorjé.

Because I have developed to the fullest the joyful **love** *(jampa)*
that cares for all living beings,
not seeking a refuge other than the Three **Jewels** *(könchok),*
holding spiritual friends as my crown **jewel** *(rinchen),*
I am known as Jampa Könchok Rinchen.

With the full-moon mandala of learning complete,
satiated with ambrosia of nondiscriminating compassion,
producing the *kairava* flower[596] in the dark night of the *kaliyuga,*
I am known as Rishi Dawa Özer (Moonlight).

Opening the petals of the medical tradition lotus grove,
giving light to the inner eyes of those who wish to learn,
ripening a bountiful harvest of health and long life,
I am known as Minyima (Sun of Humanity).

Reflecting the colors of the various sciences,
drinking without satiation thousands of rivers of knowledge,
supported by the golden foundation of mindfulness and awareness,
I am known as Rishi Tsojé Gyatso (Ocean).

For those struck by karma-caused illness, I teach the gathering of
merit, the purifying of obstruction.
For those greatly disturbed by spirits, I am equally the great
hindrance destroyer.[597]
Even to those who will die from their illness, I teach the Dharma,
providing relief from the pain.
I am known, therefore, as Rishi Thongwa Dönden (Beneficial
to See).

Seeing my own faults and doing what I can to eliminate them,
seeing the faults of others and doing what I can to remedy them,
I am **without pretension** *(drang)* and **honest** *(song).*

I am of the lineage that **holds** *(zin)* the great Rishi **tradition** *(gyü).*
I am known, therefore, as Rishi[598] Gyüzin.

Holding those who work for the doctrine dearer than my life,
nurturing with kindness those of evil disposition and bringing
them to happiness,
helping as best I can even those who would harm me,
I am known as Rishi Küngyi Shenyen (Spiritual Friend to All).

Healing the exhaustion in those sent by others,
showing particular love to the destitute and friendless,
taking care of visitors in unfamiliar surroundings,
I am known as Tsojé Kyegü Pal (Supreme among Living Beings).

Feted by the great, I have abandoned all pride; [195]
mistreated for the sake of others, I am not disheartened;
having given up all thoughts of praise and respect,
I am known as Rishi Mipaksam (Wish-Granting Tree for
Humanity).

Now I protect human beings from the ripened fruits of disease.
For the future I yearn to dispel the three poisons in all beings.
At all times my thoughts and deeds are for helping all.
I am known, therefore, as Rishi Shenphen Thayé (Of Boundless
Help to Others).

The translated sutras and tantras on medicine,
the many treatises of the four traditions,
the medical practices in this snowy land,
I understand most of them;
I am known, therefore, as Rishi Sorik Rabjam (Of Vast Medical
Knowledge).

Difficult to obtain medicines I have produced with hardship
and effort;
those easy to produce I have cast off laziness and gathered them;
fulfilling the hopes and wishes of all those to be cured,
I am known as Rishi Menjin (Giver of Medicine).

Unattached to power and impartial;
holding as equal those who like me and those who loathe me,
the high and the low, the rich and the poor;
not working in search of gratitude,
I am known as Genyen Tsojé (*Upāsaka*[599] Doctor).

Toward the wise physicians I give praise and respect;
toward the inexperienced I have no disdain and instead rejoice;
toward my peers I surrender all thoughts of jealousy;
I am known as Rishi Sempa Leksem (Brave One of Good Mind).

Reducing to shreds the net cast by the lord of death;
forcing out the fearsome and poisonous arrows of pain;
transforming old age, brought on by bodily deterioration, into youth;
I am known as Rishi Mijik Sokjin (Giver of Life and Fearlessness).

I cure the sick and produce a great festival of joy
for their friends and loved ones
unable to bear the thought of separation;
I am known, therefore, as Rishi Nya Ngenmé (No Sorrow).

Illnesses easy to cure are treated with medicine, diet, and behavior;
for more difficult ones, reversal treatments and swift magical remedies
 are recommended;
for neither of the above, charm circles and mantras are taught;
I am known, therefore, as Rishi Thaptsül Pakmé (Of Limitless
 Methods).

I compose works illuminating the thoughts of Medicine Buddha;
I give teachings to open the wisdom eyes of my followers;
I wield the sword that cleaves the arguments of wrong ideas;
I am known as Rishi Sorik Tenzin (Preserver of the Doctrine of
 Medicine).

I nourish the healthy with protections and suitable elixirs;
I nourish the sick, their humors disturbed, back to health;
I nourish future lives with virtues to be cultivated and wrongs to be
 discarded;

I am known, therefore, as Rishi Taktu Tsojé (Constantly
Nourishing).

Honored and feted by kings of celestial lineage,
praised by those gods devoted to the doctrine,
and acclaimed with great joy by many a scholar, [196]
I am known as Rishi Lhayi Jewo (Lord of the Gods).

A refuge for the wretched, wherever and whoever they be;
an affectionate mind, like a mother or father, toward all strangers;
all activities of body, speech, and mind given solely to helping
others,
I am known as Rishi Drowai Phama (Mother and Father of
Sentient Beings).

For those lost day and night in the land of darkness,
I open the bubble of their eyes with the golden surgical spoon,
causing them to see at once this world of forms;
I am known therefore as Rishi Saljé Drönma (Illuminating Beacon).

I pray that all who see, hear, remember, or touch me
be free of all adversity and misfortune
be endowed with wholesome conditions,
and attain the state of the great rishi.
I am known, therefore, as Rishi Mönlam Thayé (Limitless Prayers).

Toward pus, blood, excrement, and urine I am like a dog or a pig;
doing everything for the sick, I am like their servant;
to their relatives I am the wish-fulfilling cow;
I am known as Rishi Drowai Khölpo (Servant of Living Beings).

Perceiving ultimate reality as being free from mental fabrication,
knowing conventional dependent arising to be like dreams,
seeing method and wisdom combined as the sole path,
I am known as Rishi Gyalsé Shönu (Young Prince of the Buddha).

Eschewing alcohol, the cause of a hundred faults,
refraining from eating meat, the enemy of compassion,

holding the *kumuda* flower of bodhicitta, root of virtue and
goodness,
I am known as Rishi Drimé Tülshuk (Of Pure Spiritual Conduct).

Having found conviction in the pure view of the world and its beings;
understanding that initiations are to be received, pledges to be
guarded;
seeing the two stages as the life channel of Vajrayana;
I am known as Rishi Chimé Nyingpo (Essence of Deathlessness).

Seeing the lama as the sole incorporation of the refuge objects,
seeing that my master sentient beings are the incorporation of those
worthy of offerings,
realizing that all Dharma traditions are as one as samsara and nirvana,
I am known as Rishi Sangwai Dzözin (Keeper of Treasury of Secrets).

Many lives I have trained in the tradition of medicine;
in India and Tibet I have helped sentient beings.
In this way I have pledged to guide living beings;
I am known, therefore, as a rishi of many names.

Joyfully teaching all those who wish to learn medicine,
laboring to heal all the sick in this land of snow,
staying wherever I will be of greatest help to others,
I am known as Gyalkham Lhajé (Lord of the Land).

But I jest! Among living beings close and distant,
where is the witness to say that I possess such qualities?
This is a prayer that from now on, I may have such qualities,
and also an encouragement to motivate my followers. [197]

In a faraway land, yet with yearning heart so close,
you who have such great hopes in me,
asking this nameless one about his name;
be free of doubts, free of hesitation.

These longed-for supposed names of mine
I have written as a letter to please the wise.

> By its power may all beings in the not-too-distant future
> receive their prophesized names from the great rishi.

In this way he writes of his lineage and his qualities.

The perfect teachings born from his mind include the treatise known as *King of Medical Practice;* commentaries on *Four Tantras* called *Four Presentations* and *Four Streams; Realization Requests; Ascertainment of Four Tantras* also known as *Established as Enlightened Speech; Large and Small Wish-Granting Cow Commentary on the Difficult Points of the Mālaya; Exalted General Medicine; Extraordinary General Medicine; Treatments of Infectious Diseases: Giving Life to Mankind; Illumination of the Truth: A Commentary on the Fourth Chapter of the Explanatory Tantra; Vajra Verse Oral Transmission Commentary on the Pulse Section;* and *Precious Garland Quintessence.*

He was responsible for spreading the works and oral teachings of medical science generally and, in particular, the doctrine of Jangpa Namgyal Draksang, holder of the spiritual discipline of a pandit king and recognized by the lotus holder Gendün Drup and many other holy beings as an incarnation of *Kalkī*[600] Sucandra.

Lhatsün Tashi Palsang

His son was Lhatsün Tashi Palsang. From an early age he was lovingly cared for by his grandfather Sönam Dorjé, and he pursued his studies extensively in disciplines such as writing and reading. Later on, with his grandfather and father, he studied the vast ocean of medical literature in its entirety. In particular, he received the initiation for the entrustment of the tantra, the urine divination goddess practices, the great commentaries on the inner, outer, and secret from the oral tradition, teachings on the twenty-five seals, and so on. He developed the teaching tradition of medical practice for future fortunate disciples.

He sat at the lotus feet of many a great master and drank without satiation the nectar of sutra, tantra, and the sciences. These masters included Pandit Vanaratna, Lochen Sönam Gyatso, the great being Shönu Gyalchok, Müchen Könchok Gyaltsen, Drupwang Thangtongpa, Khedrup Dönyö Palwa, Lekshé Sangpo, and the omniscient Chak Lotsāwa. [198]

Developing a renunciation of samsara, he took the full ordination of a monk from Panchen Śākya Chokden and became a worthy recipient of offerings for the gods and mankind.

He brought great relief to sentient beings with his use of profound methods such as mantras, swift magical remedies, and reversal treatments.

His compositions include *Jewel of Excellent Explanation: A Commentary on the Explanatory Tantra; Treasury of Jewels Fulfilling All Needs: A Commentary on the Final Tantra,* also known as *All-Knowing When Studied; White Smile of the Sun: A History of Medicine;* and *Wish-Granting Tree: Verses on the Ascertainment of Four Tantras.*

Finally, from within the state of total absorption in the yoga of the two profound stages, he recited verses beginning, "I am going to Sukhāvatī," and having issued many last instructions, he passed beyond sorrow with full mindfulness and awareness. A rain of flowers fell and the area was covered by a rainbow arc. Sounds of music came from the sky, and many other wonderful signs were seen.

There are many important biographical details about him such as the prophesy by venerable Tārā that he would become a buddha in a world known as Śuddhilocana.

Early in his life he had a son, who became known as Rishi Sönam Yeshé Gyaltsen and sat at his father's lotus feet for many years to learn medicine. There he learned the texts, the oral instructions, and in particular the oral teachings on *Four Tantras* from the two rivers of Treasure and Transmission merged into one. Like a vase overflowing, he received the entrustment initiation, the collections of urine divination goddess practices and rishi accomplishment practices, the practices of the oral tradition, the commentaries, and so on.

Through the circumstances of the troubles between Jang and Rong[601] he later became the chief Rinpung physician. In Tsangrong Ralnga he composed the medical history called *Sun that Nourishes the White Lotus*. In Jakthang he withdrew from this life.

Lekdrup Pal and the Nya lineage

One of the main medical disciples of the Dharma king and lineage holder Namgyal Draksang was the trained doctor Lekdrup Pal of Lhünding, who was also of royal physician lineage. I will begin with a brief account of the origins of his lineage.

Once (ca. eighth century), the province of Gesar in the northern part of Dokham was ruled by a Dharma king called Gewazin, [199] who had a vast knowledge of the two traditions and who looked upon each living being with love and gentleness as if he or she were his only child. Because of this he became to everyone like ambrosia for their eyes, and all agreed that he deserved to be carried on their shoulders. In this way he became known as Nya ("back of the neck").

The eldest of his five children was Nyawa Chökyi Sangpo. He was good-looking, his senses were bright, and he was renowned as one of great faith and intelligence. The noble emperor Trisong Detsen heard of him and summoned him from Dokham to central Tibet. He was given a great amount of gold leaf, provided with many companions, and sent to India to study and to invite translators and pandits back to Tibet. He stayed for many years in India, where he mastered most of the sciences and became a great scholar, and then he returned to Tibet. The king was delighted with him and conferred upon him the status of a lama worthy of offering and as a master physician. Under the Oḍḍiyāna second Buddha, Padmasambhava, he studied many Vajrayana practices of ripening and liberating the mind and became the foremost of the nine wise Tibetans.

Several generations later Nyawa Namkha Shönu came to northern Yeru. There the Jangdak Tawen[602] or Jangdak Tenpa presented him with the communities of Yarong and Tsang Olung, local hermitages, and so on. Nyawa Dorjé Bum, the son of Nyawa Namkha Shönu, became the chief physician and personal attendant to Jangdak. His son, Lhai Gyaltsen, had a vast understanding of sutra and tantra and became an abbot at Pal Ngamring Monastery. There, with his fame and youth, he furthered the science of medicine and administered the affairs of the district.

His son Könchok Shönu was a master of medicine and Nyingma tantra. He had great compassion for all beings and was renowned as a bodhisattva. He went to the Thekchen Chöjé, lama to the Chinese,[603] and became his chief physician, whereupon he received a royal proclamation and was conferred great honor.

His son was Lekdrup Pal. He mastered most of the sciences, particularly the science of medicine. He sat meditation retreats on venerable Tārā and studied at the feet of Tertön Ngödrup Gyaltsen. From having received so many teachings on the vast and profound, many wonderful events occurred. Once while he was concentrating on offering a torma to Dark Blue Guru,[604] the torma actually traveled toward the deity, and the enemies were destroyed. From Rikden Namgyal Draksang he received many teachings and instructions on the medical texts and was conferred as his chief disciple. [200]

His son was Sherap Palden. Many wonderful omens were observed at his birth, and so Rikden Namgyal Draksang was asked to name the child. The master gave the name Tsojé Pema Sithar. When Pandit Vanaratna came to Tibet on his third and last visit, Sherap Palden met him on the way,[605] and the pandit gave him the transmission of the *Heart Sutra* in Sanskrit and the complete initiation of the glorious Kālacakra.

When he was twenty-six he came into the presence of the powerful siddha Thangtong Gyalpo[606] and immediately received a very special blessing. For sixteen years he lived close to this yogi. By receiving and practicing countless teachings he became Thangtong Gyalpo's chief disciple. After this great siddha passed away, Sherap Palden secretly acted as his replacement for thirty-two years, during which time he brought immeasurable benefit to living beings, comparable to that of his master himself.

His son Lhünding Gema, who was born before the master Sherap Palden met Siddha Tongthang Gyalpo, preserved and developed the medical tradition and became chief physician to the Yeru Jangpa.[607]

His son in turn was Tenpa Dargyé, whose virtuous imprints were awoken at an early age, and who soon became endowed with faith, enthusiasm, wisdom, and compassion. He had such a great capacity for memorizing that in the time it took to put on the monastic robes, he was able to memorize one page the length of an arrow. To the Jangdak he offered a memorization test of *Four Tantras,* its commentaries, and its synthesis.

Rishi Sönam Yeshé Gyaltsen, the son of Jang physician Lhatsün Tashi Palsang, withdrew from his life in the Rinpung settlement in Jakthang. Because of his fondness for the Jang hierarchy and concern that his own transmission of teachings would dry up and vanish, Lhatsün Tashi Palsang sent a messenger to the Jangdak. It read, "My son, successor to my family and my Dharma lineage, has died, and I offer the one-to-one lineage to your trustworthy and intelligent chief physician. Therefore, I request you to send him to me."

Accordingly, Tenpa Dargyé, with his chief-physician lineage and his great intelligence, was sent to Lhatsün Tashi Palsang, at whose lotus feet he studied for a long time. He received like a vase full to overflowing the sutras, tantras, the sciences, and in particular the literature and instructions on medicine, including the transmission and teachings of the Oral tradition, which since the time of Rishi Manasija had never been written down. Although the previous masters of this Nya family line were all great scholars who had served at the feet of many noble dynasties, it is said that up to this time the profound teachings of the Jang one-to-one lineage of Treasure and Transmission had not appeared in their tradition. [201]

Tenpa Dargyé's son was Sönam Chöphel, who became a master of the Oral tradition, the oral teachings, and instructions. He had mastered fully the seven extraordinary pulses,[608] and so in diagnosis he was as if clairvoyant.

His son was Dütsi Gyurmé. He became supreme in his knowledge of the science of healing and consequently became chief physician to the Jonang incarnation Künga Nyingpo.[609] He also oversaw and was editor of a new publication of *Four Tantras.* He composed a work called *Practices of the Science of Medicine: Fulfilling All Needs and Wishes.*

His son was Namgyal Dorjé. He mastered knowledge in general and specifically *Four Tantras,* supreme among the works of healing.[610] He examined minutely the commentaries and oral instructions, and practiced the one-to-one lineages passed from the wise to the wise, such as those of his father, Dütsi Gyurmé. Up to the age of almost sixty, he could still memorize one verse a day. He was unhindered in his ability to thoroughly undertake word-for-word memorization tests on the tantra, and so forth.

However, as the *Treasury of Wise Sayings* states:

> As long as the wise are not thoroughly questioned,
> their depths have not been measured.
> As long as a drum is not struck,
> its difference from others remains unknown.[611]

Because of his writings affixed to the Lhasa stone pillar and other reasons, he came to the notice of the Great Fifth in the latter part of his life, who presented him with grain coupons, and so forth. He then ignored a request by the Great Fifth to give teachings to the local residents on measurements of the body and the allegorical tree of medicine. After that I set out with many questions designed to stump him and break his pride. Namling Panchen, too, was encouraged to ask him various questions in the upper courtyard. As a result it became clear that—his arrogance, great pride, and disrespect aside—there is none these days in this science of caring for others who can match his abilities to explain texts, identify medicinal plants, or reveal knowledge of the channels, the body, the medicine tree, and so on. Therefore I, too, received from him many oral teachings in one-to-one transmission on the measurements of the body, the allegorical tree of medicine, and so on.

His lineage, the Ganden Medicine Guru lineage, survives merely in the form of its study of the tantra and in identification of medicine. However, because of indolence, laziness, lack of effort, one has to wonder if Sakya Paṇḍita's example of the cuckoo and the hawk is not applicable here.[612]

Therefore the two lineages of Transmission and Treasure appeared within the Jang medical tradition. Their transmission of each is as follows.

Treasure lineage: [202]

The Medicine Buddha
Speech-manifestation Manasija
Ārya Ānanda
Jivaka Kumāra
Orgyen Padma
The master scholar Nāgārjuna
Ācārya Śūra
Kashmiri Candranandana
The great translator Vairocana
Dharma king Trisong Detsen
Manifested treasure finder Drapa Ngönshé
Üpa Dardrak
Roktön Könchok Kyap
Biji Menshön
Daö Shönu
Shang Menak
The king of medicine, combiner of lineages, Yuthok Yönten Gönpo

Yuthok Yönten Gönpo also received a lineage directly from Roktön Könchok Kyap that was passed down[613] through Biji and so on. Concerning the son lineage and disciple lineage that came from Yuthok, on which Surkhar has a different assertion, the disciple lineage runs as follows:

Dza or Sumtön Yeshé Sung
Sumtön Yeshé Künga
Sumtön Bumé
Lungmar Gönpo Rinchen
Takdé Phaktön Śākya Gönpo
Takdé Bukmawa

The Yuthok son lineage:

Yuthok Bumseng
Yuthok Jampal
Drangti Jampal Sangpo[614]
His son Drangti Gyalsang
His youngest son Drangti Palden Tsojé
Jangmen Sangyé Rinchen
The royal physician Sönam Dorjé
Jampa Könchok Rinchen, also known as Minyima Thongwa Dönden
Tashi Palsang

The transmission lineage runs as follows. The great Oḍḍiyāna master received it from Kumāra Jivaka and Nāgārjuna. He then passed on his own translation to the divine prince Muné Tsenpo, which continues:

Trisong Detsen
Ralpachen Tsangma
Gyalpo Dorjé
Lhajé Lhündrup
Ralpachen
the two Lhalungpas
Ösung
Pal Khartsen
Kyidé Nyima Gön
Tashi Tsekpai Pal
Tashi Paldé
Detsuk Dé
Yeshé Ö
Jangchup Ö
Tsedé
Dawa Ö
Nyima Ö
Drakden
Sönam Dorjé
Dharma king Namgyal Draksang
Minyima Thongwa Dönden
Tashi Palsangpo

From here on it is asserted that the two streams of the Treasure and Transmission lineages combine as one. The lineages continue: Nya Tenpa Dargyé, Sönam Chöphel, Dütsi Gyurmé, up to the master orator Namgyal Dorjé.

In the twenty-fourth chapter of the *Crystal Rock Lotus Chronicles* it says:

> Then Padmasambhava went to the land of Padmavati,
> where he met with the son of Kumāra Jivaka.
> "What do you know?" he asked.
> "Medicine," he replied.
> "Teach me medicine," he asked. [203]
> "I am old, my body shakes;[615] I am no longer a scholar.
> The ācārya did not come. If you had, I would have taught."[616]

Orgyen Padma actually studied with Kumāra Jivaka himself, and although the verse is written this way, I think there must have been some corruption with the sixth grammatical case, resulting in "son *of* Kumāra Jivaka."[617]

16. The Sur Tradition

Surkhar Nyamnyi Dorjé

THE MASTER LAMA, the Great Fifth said:

> In those times, in the dance of the magic net of beryl light,
> many intelligent beings, masters of the science of healing—
> Surkhar Nyamnyi Dorjé and the nephew-based succession,
> and so on—
> smiled from within the joy of help and happiness for living beings.[618]

The glorious Surkhar Nyamnyi Dorjé was renowned with names such as Tsojé Drupa, Könchok Rinchen, Yuthok Bang, Pawö Kyang, Künla Jampai Lodrö, Lhündrup Gyaltsen, and Dharmaswami—*Dharma* in Tibetan is *Chö,* and *Swami* is *Jé,* making Awo Chöjé. He was born in Latok Surkhar in Dakpo in the east, in the earth-sheep *siddhārtha* year of the seventh sixty-year cycle.[619] His father was Rikzin Phüntsok of the Gyerkar medical lineage, which included Bangrimpa and Gyama Rinchen Gangwa and is said to be of celestial descent. His mother was the daughter of the omniscient Tashi Namgyal.

At the age of ten he stayed for three days on Dharmadhātu Peak, where he made single-pointed requests to Yuthok Yönten Gönpo. As a result Yuthok actually appeared and gave him the transmission on the oral instructions, as well as the interpretations and textual meanings of the *Heartdrop Collection, Four Tantras,* and the scroll collections. Yuthok also pointed out where previous generations had unknowingly corrupted the supplements to the *Heartdrop* and *Four Tantras* and told him to correct the mistakes. As it is written:

> On the waves of your faith-filled requests,
> Mañjuśrī Guṇa[620]—in reality or in dreams—

gave you continuous teachings in great delight;
to you, physician dispeller of errors, crown jewel of all...[621]

Therefore, in reality or in dreams, [204] the venerable Yuthok gave him teachings, and a flawless understanding of the meaning of profound emptiness was born within him, enabling him to dispel all errors.

From his father, from Trükhang Lotsāwa (1424–82), from Heruka-attired Shara Rapjampa—who initially was at Sera Monastery but later became a disciple of Taklung Ngawang Drakpa (1418–96)—from the medical teacher Wangchuk Sangpo, and from many other great beings, he learned and mastered the sciences, excelling above all in the science of medicine.

When he was fourteen he composed a letter with questions for the Jang physician Minyima Thongwa Dönden:

> *Śrī Vajrasattva nāmamī*
>
> We sent a scholar physician and Dharma teacher from Erong[622] to learn more about you. Hearing his report filled my mind with joy. However, the distance makes it difficult for me to come to meet you myself.
>
> In which particular sciences are you learned and to whose kindness do you owe that to? What is your family, your lineage? Which of the great texts do you rely upon? Whose oral instructions are you familiar with—those of the nine scholars or those of others? Which special medical practices do you perform? For your experience which collections do you have confidence in? In Buddhism, for your deity practice, which Oral traditions and Treasure traditions do you hold as the essence of your meditations? Do you have a fixed residence? If some who are connected with me were made known to you by way of messengers or letters, would it be acceptable for them to gain an audience with you? If you were entreated to travel here for the sake of others, would you consider coming? How many works have you composed? By what name should I address you? I have on many occasions been convinced that you and I are linked by virtuous past karma. Please send me a genuine reply that is neither distant nor disapproving and bring my hopes to fulfillment.

The reply he received did not respond directly to the questions asked but instead consisted of verses on the meanings of his names, lineage, and so forth, as is clear from the life story of Jang Thongwa Dönden above.

From around the age of sixteen he thought of composing a supplement, based on oral instructions, to *Meditation on the Guru: Sunlight of Compassion Clearing the Darkness of Ignorance,*[623] as well as four works on dispelling obstacles to its practice. These four were an external work on elemental disturbances to the body, an inner work on disturbances to meditative concentration, a secret work on types of hindering demons, and a work on all four in common. [205] He first composed, as a single book with many sections, the work on the disturbances to the body, using both prose and verse. From this one small volume, the size of a holy relic, comes millions of oral teachings. It is therefore known as *Relic of Millions.* It consists of the following sections.[624]

1. Sunlight illumination pulse examination
2. Mirror of the moon urine examination
3. Rain of ambrosia: yantra of *manu* medicine
4. Ocean of elixir: general treatment for wind ailments
5. Generating happiness in the mind: treatment for life-wind ailments
6. Wish-fulfilling ambrosia: curing specific types of *tötsang*
7. Waves of ambrosia: specific treatments for *tötsang*
8. Gathering of the elements: vajra that destroys life-wind ailments
9. Warrior's advice on *gojé*
10. Pure moonlight: tales of the seven female relatives[625]
11. Drops of ambrosia: preparation of medicinal plants
12. General relief of fever: using a camphor decoction
13. General relief of fever: preparation of camphor
14. Ambrosia mirror: treatment of black-skin bile disorder
15. Ambrosia of strong taste and potency: treatment for heart fevers
16. Moon drop: instantaneous treatment for new fevers
17. *Loma* ambrosia: general medicine
18. Delaying death: the treatment of pain
19. Short-work revelatory instructions on "Delaying death: the treatment of pain"
20. Armor of love: specific treatments for the pains of serious ailments
21. Mending the breaks in life: treatment of *gakser*
22. A few words of experience: curing infectious humor disorders
23. Elixir from the vase of ambrosia: destroying cold disorders
24. Treasure of ambrosia: preparation of the king of mineral exudates

25. Brief but essential advice on mineral exudates
26. Profound point of practice: powder preparation of calcite
27. Mirror of ambrosia: creating salts
28. Preparation from lymph: putting an end to goiters
29. Ambrosia jewel: instructions for eliminating the three dual-type disorders
30. The practice of applying medicinal butter
31. Twelve medical preparations
32. The ultimate practice: instructions on the four-color, five-ingredient garuḍa compound
33. Verses of instructions on the four-colored, five-ingredient garuḍa compound
34. Teachings on the five garuḍas and a few words on the beak, claws, and wings
35. Garuḍa with wings compound
36. Stream of ambrosia dew: the three-family general medicine
37. Instructions on preparation of the three-ingredient Nāropa preparation
38. Quintessence of *Vase of Ambrosia:* treatment of serious fevers, dual wind disorders, and *lhokser*
39. Treatment of *nyenkhamé*
40. Notes of the practice of compounding the precious heat medicine
41. Jewel of immortality: clarifying the mysteries of the great, intermediate, and lesser black pills
42. The practice of refining mercury
43. A short work on translation of essential terms
44. Profound binding of mercury
45. Preparation of powdered copper [206]
46. A method for refining sulphur and a heart-like technique for extracting poison
47. Secret swift path: preparation of precious mercury
48. Preparation of the four types of mercury
49. The practice of drying mercury
50. Special treatment of the seven precious gems
51. Secret extraordinary treatment of *kangbam*
52. Instructions from the oral tradition on curing rheumatic gout
53. Preparation of hot gruel to relieve *sinlang* and indigestion
54. Granting life: brief work on treating worm disorders

55. Medicine for worms: the seven-goddess preparation
56. Wonderful protection of life: brief section on preparation of white *datura*
57. Treatment of bowel worms
58. Teachings on bringing health and well-being to the five organs
59. Secret scroll annotation on the five kinds of eyes according to the tradition of Mitrayogi
60. Chinese water treatment for clearing obstructions to the eyes
61. Eye medicine for curing blindness
62. Purging the eyes: an illumination bringing about sight
63. Essence of the sense power: a profound purging of the eyes
64. The six-ingredient *vindhya* preparation: internal medicine for the eyes
65. Instruction for the eyes: total elimination of *lingtok*
66. Precious compound of seven ingredients: medicine for the eyes
67. Compound of nine bile medicines: medicine for the eyes
68. Using a decoction of Indian barberry eye medicine
69. Teachings on mud-horn cupping: final elimination of eye disorders
70. Eye medicine to cure *lingtok*
71. Eye medicine from the Mitrayogi tradition for *lingro* horned cataracts together with the practice of mud-horn cupping
72. An unfailing and guaranteed treatment for stopping bleeding even that of a decapitated body
73. The sound of Utta: teachings on purging the ears
74. Drum of Brahmā: treatment for the voice
75. Gathering the melodies of Brahmā: treatment for the voice
76. Roar of the lion treatment for the voice
77. Essence of many texts and teachings: treatment for the voice
78. Compound outshining all others: medicine for the lungs
79. Illuminating lamp: layout of the torso
80. Magic explanation: sour mash treatment
81. Five-ingredient secret compound: head medicine
82. *Beldungma:* medicine for the head
83. Garland of ambrosia drops: treatment of wounds
84. Clarifying the obscure points of the "Garland of ambrosia drops" section
85. Collection of every ambrosia: medicine for wounds

86. Text on compounding black *mingchen*
87. Instructions for preparing the class of compounds on the owl-hand plant
88. Teachings from Dumabu: precious epaulette wound treatment
89. Precious refined ambrosia
90. The king of single remedies wound medicine
91. Brief work based on experience: internal medicine for wounds
92. Eliminating the torment of the flesh, bones, and channels: treatment for growths
93. Penetrating secret treatment for growths
94. Powdered conch shell treatment for growths
95. Treating bones according to the tradition of the scholar Thazhi
96. Instructions on removing splinters and thorns
97. Diagram of the soles of the feet in connection with "Instructions on splinters and thorns"
98. Swift path of the rishis: expelling and drying up mucus from the respiratory system
99. Eliminating pain: treatment for *sūrya* ulcerated lungs
100. Secret ambrosia preparation: drying up mucus [207]
101. Account of the secret and sealed *Kāñcavati Dhāraṇī*
102. Written reminders on the *Kāñcavati Dhāraṇī*
103. Sound of the celestial drum, the famous emanation: definitive account of white radish medicine
104. Ambrosia festival: treatment for poisoning
105. Revelatory oral teachings on the ambrosia-festival treatment for poisoning: a clarification and key to release the main points
106. Wonderful vase of ambrosia: curing and protecting against poisoning
107. Ambrosia heartdrop: guarding against poisons
108. Jé Rangjung Dorjé's *Vajra Diamond Expelling and Protecting against Poison*
109. Uncovering the hidden: commentary to *Key Opening the Lock of Deep-Seated Poison*
110. Specific treatments for poisons affecting bodily tissue
111. Light of the path: white cure
112. Instructions on four-ingredient rhino preparation
113. Secret teachings: instructions on rabies
114. Very profound treatment for rabid dog bites

115. Oral tradition on head purging
116. Head purging and specific treatment for purging serum
117. Magic purgative: instructions for ridding the head of all disorder
118. Dispelling all ailments: stomach purging
119. General balancing of the humors: preparation of the plant known as ambrosia holder of milk
120. Profound aspects of the secret purging of blood in the abdomen
121. Magic purgative: the castor oil plant
122. Hook of knowledge: the magical drawing out of dropsy
123. Stream of ambrosia: the magical purgative *gatik*
124. The magical purgative called "old woman holding a walking stick"
125a. Words for the ears: instructions on cleansing the channels and stomach
125b. Cleansing faults purging instructions
126. Jewel purification of the channels
127. Demon-purging iron thunderbolt
128. Extreme action of wrathful Vajrapāṇi: Teachings on the purging flame
129. Magical ambrosia rivet: instructions on putting an end to dysentery
130. Quick development of happiness: treatment for *gyugen*
131. Treatment of *gyugen* in brief
132. Teachings on extracting red stones
133. Explicit teaching on extracting red stones
134. Ambrosia lotus garland: specific treatments for women's ailments
135. Purging of women's ailments by mantra
136. Method to bring on the red ambrosia of joy
137. Bringing on the red lotus
138. Wish-fulfilling tree of bliss: elixirs
139. Rejuvenation: ocean of qualities
140. Seven lists of miscellany
141. Instruction on protecting the seminal drop
142. *Dali* elixir: a shoot of ambrosia
143. Words of experience on treating *gyazer*
144. Treatment for black *lhok* serious worm ailments: drops of death-cheating ambrosia
145. Nonconceptual wheel of weapons: protection for black *lhok*
146. Diagram of the nonconceptual wheel of weapons: the black-pig union cakra

147. Profound substance protection for infectious diseases: vajra armor guarding life and granting fearlessness
148. Door-opening ambrosia key [208]

Up to here is the main table of contents. What follows is the "son" or "short-arrowhead" table of contents containing a statement of intent.

149. Oral teachings on purging from the crown to eliminate head ailments
150. Treating organisms in the head: expelling sinus disorders
151. Oral teachings on cupping
152. Magic knot of plaster
153. The iron-drumstick method for finding arrow heads
154. Goiter treatment: swift removal of excess flesh
155. Expelling sinus disorders
156. Black bdellium ultimate preparation for wind disorders of the head
157. A treatment for excessive fluid disorder
158. A small work on itching disorders
159. Saving the life of horses and donkeys
160. General medicine for infectious fevers: the great application
161. The parting-gift teaching on medicinal water application for wounds
162. *Pakabheta* ambrosia preparation
163. Oral teachings on *gamsé* preparation
164. The shoot of moon crystal preparation
165. Notes on the great fire-like preparation
166. Stream of the moon ambrosia
167. An application to reduce swelling
168. Oral teachings on preparing brown sulphur
169. Eliminating worms
170. Great preparation of black medicine
171. Clear mirror for the examination of pus
172. Caring for horses
173. The magic purgative of borax
174. Golden bile purgative
175. The four wrathful ingredients preparation
176. Preparation of *mingchen* ambrosia
177. Treatment for wind disorders in the head: essence of the ambrosia vase
178. A preparation for smallpox: a hook holding on to life

179. Oral teaching on medicine for *kheldrum*
180. Aconite concoction
181. Refined sunlight ambrosia preparation
182. Heat rays: oral teachings on treatment for bones
183. Little gold pill: protection against infectious fever
184. Heat application for lymph swellings
185. Pain relief: treatment of lung abscesses
186. Ambrosia *phala* eye medicine
187. Oral teaching on *kramuka* nine-ingredient preparation
188. Preparation for stiffening the organ
189. Medicine for the voice: a dragon roar of the world

The "no-step" section

190. Indra's bow: various oral teachings
191. The preparation of *siddhimūla*
192. Profound treatment for white, black, and multicolored *kangbam*
193. A small work on treatment for kidneys
194. A small work on increasing essential plasma
195. Curing with fire
196. Bringing relief to the knees: treatment of wolf-face wind
197. Four-ingredient preparation of mercury
198. Four-ingredient black pill preparation
199. Protection against intestinal disorder
200. Close lineage of the lama lineage
201. Dispelling the illnesses of all beings: special and extensive treatment for respiratory mucus
202. Ambrosia moonlight: instructions on wind-induced diarrhea
203. Treatment for lactation problems
204. Mirror of jewels bringing great benefit
205. Oral teachings on sulphur: the destruction of all demon-caused disorders
206. The ambrosia pool: wonderful oral teachings on various jewels
207. Indra's rainbow: various oral teachings [209]
208. Long pepper black medicine: essence of the enlightened mind
209. Black medicine fifteen-ingredient wrathful preparation
210. Great fire-like preparation
211. Unfailing remedy to stop bleeding
212. Unfailing remedy to stop bleeding, or "cutting the brown flow"

213. Blood purgative: seeking deeply for the fault
214. Magic mustard purgative: the purifying essence
215. Profound skin purgative
216. Refined essence surgery: instructions on splinters
217. Relief on contact: the removal of swellings
218. Instructions on swellings
219. Cakravartin treatment for sinus disorders
220. Emetic treatment for *nyalhok:* release from the ropes of the lord of death
221. Five-ingredient powerful preparation for treating pain
222. Jewel of joyful immortality: a teaching on a single-ingredient secret treatment for the head
223. Head medicine: happiness on contact
224. A wonderful medicine: mineral wax for head injuries
225. *Udumbara* secret medicine
226. Preparation of hematite as head medicine
227. Uses of white radish
228. Teachings on mercury taken from a letter of instructions to the bodhisattva Puṇya
229. Ambrosia dewdrop general medicine
230. The black valley plant: the sliver ambrosia general medication
231. The crown jewel general medication
232. The vajra of immortality general medication
233. A definite cure for *gyaser*
234. The treatment of *gyaser,* abbreviated
235. Cutting the continuum of blindness: a cure for eye disease
236. Ear treatment: the *utta* roar
237. The light-radiating ambrosia elixir: the ambrosia vase to give the body strength
238. The garuḍa accomplishing *lukmur* elixir
239. The diamond purging of demons
240. Wrathful fire-substance yantra, the roar of thousands of dragons
241. The diamond internal protection
242. Food and drink to avoid and partake: detailed and correct
243. The vine of unmistaken teaching: identifying the four kinds of chronic degenerative disorders
244. The unmistaken jasmine smile: identifying the five kinds of calcite, and so on

245. Potencies of the three kinds of the *jangwa*[626] flying beetle, prepared according to the tantra and oral tradition
246. Identifying the nine channels that carry plasma
247. Light of scripture and reasoning: resolving doubts about camphor
248. From the work on making precious crystal: the alluring, smiling lotus that is meaningful to behold
249. Treatment of poxes
250. A jewel garland of miscellany
251. Profound heartdrop medical preparation for treating *lhok*
252. Preparing the six-leafed plant
253. Satisfying on application: an ointment for relieving swelling
254. Poultice for growths: relieving the pain of swellings
255. Relief on contact: treatment for *semok*
256. Fire yantra for the eliminating indigestion
257. Putting an end to diarrhea: the elimination of intestinal fever
258. Putting an end to diarrhea: the clasping hook
259. Preparation of the brown-phlegm balancing compound
260. Putting an end to the diarrhea that is like water falling down a steep mountainside
261. Putting an end to diarrhea: five-ingredient mother of pearl preparation [210]
262. Putting an end to diarrhea: myrobalan four-ingredient medicine
263. Great liberation from all diarrhea
264. Oral teachings on the powerful method for treating advanced leprosy
265. The four wrathful ingredients preparation
266. The practice of channel cleansing
267. A gently flowing stream: the practice of purging
268. Magical purging of edema serum
269. Magic mirror of channel cleansing
270. Massage ointment for treating growths and skin sores
271. Twenty-five ingredient rhinoceros preparation
272. Five-ingredient garuḍa preparation for halting seepage
273. Thunderbolt blood purgative
274. Blood purgative oral transmission
275. Snow frog ambrosia preparation
276. Teeth elixir

277. Treatment of *semok:* the teachings of Mahāguṇa
278. Teachings on *semok*
279. Blue poppy preparation: a treatment for *tötsang*
280. Treatment for *tötsang*
281. Secret jewel treatment for wind disorders
282. Preparation for pulling down *tötsang*
283. The eight-bandit preparation
284. Thunderbolt-dew magic purgative
285. Teachings on the red seal
286. Preparation of the moon king of elixirs
287. Preparation of the wish-fulfilling compound
288. Short reminder of Samdé Nangso
289. Vajra armor: garuḍa profound points
290. Superior, middling, and lesser iron pills
291. Preparation of powdered copper
292. The cure for all blood ailments
293. The shoot of happiness: a general medicine for hot and cold stomach disorders
294. Vajra-diamond salt beer
295. Lake salt beer preparation
296. Amazing pills: medicine for emaciation
297. Eye medicine: louse horse, louse-egg sheep[627]
298. Clearing the eyes
299. Teachings on the eyes: curing all disorders
300. Purging the eyes through the channels and stomach
301. A preparation beneficial in curing all eye diseases
302. Seven-ingredient mantra and *carex* preparation for cataracts
303. Instructions on using the *yumo* plant for expelling arrowheads
304. Profound protection medicine of Yuthok
305. Aroma captivating the minds of all: eliminating body odor
306. Methods for inducing labor and expelling the placenta
307. The twenty-one-ingredient preparation with beer as the conveyor[628]
308. Seven-ingredient preparation for purging severe disorders
309. Thunderbolt yantra for purging demons
310. Using bezoars
311. A short work on the practices of the siddha Orgyenpa
312. Medical collection on treating poisons from the *Treatise on Mercury Preparation*

313. Treatment of fang poisoning: the ambrosia called good vase of immortality
314. Ambrosia vase: specific treatment for fang poisoning
315. Oral teachings on treating fang poisoning
316. Oral teachings on the medical plant preparation known as the "three brothers ambrosia"
317. Comment on the insight in the words of the siddha: the song of Vatāki
318. Vajra lines
319. Commentary on the vajra lines arranged as practice
320. *Treatise on Mercury* as arranged by the scholar Shönu Gyatso
321. The practice of making magic ink
322. Essence of *caṇḍālī* wrathful fire yantra, with reliance upon substances [211]
323. The elixir of the five ambrosia substances: the great benefactor and life sustainer

The no-seal collection, which I organized subsequently:

324. Vajra-diamond general medicine, oral teachings on the treatment of smallpox, and benefits for almost all disorders: offered to the Yargyap Drungchen
325. Instructions on preventing lice
326. The four *ka* eye treatment
327. Treatment for the gored-by-bull stomach pain that is caused by intestinal worms
328. An instruction on the magic destruction of stones
329. Ambrosia tree elixir
330. Table of causal processes of potencies, tastes, and post-digestive tastes
331. Profound and special treatment for tongue diseases
332. Grass in summer, insect in winter preparation
333. Seven-ingredient mercury preparation
334. Twenty-six-ingredient powdered copper preparation
335. Praise of the five medicine gurus: the all-virtuous Brahmā-like roar
336. In praise of the guide Yuthok: the dance of the cool moonbeams of faith
337. Various preparations of the king of minerals

338. Treatment of disturbance and accumulation in the stomach brought on by the poison of indigestion
339. A treatment for fever: the cream of butter
340. A treatment for the eyes
341. A treatment for the ears: bringing hearing and gladdening the mind
342. Six-ingredient wolf preparation: oral tradition on treating a swollen tongue
343. Tiger-lion confrontation preparation
344. Instructions on tooth powders
345. Various instructions from Yeshé Khadro: *caṇḍāli* inner heat in reliance upon substances
346. Questions: a portion of white silver mirror
347. Rays of sunlight: well-uttered questions and answers
348. Various aromatic preparations
349. Songs
350. A few words on Surkhar's previous births
351. Refined heartdrop: the whip of enthusiasm

The above are included in the works of Surkhar. The following include those works that are probably not the works of Surkhar himself but have been attributed to him:

352. The quintessence of a secret wrathful manuscript
353. Incense-stick cleansing of the eyes
354. Incense-stick cleansing
355. Tarima arrowhead
356. Writings on working with precious stones
357. A treatment for swollen tongue
358. Mantra treatment for *kangbam*
359. Betel nut remedy: instructions on the brown phlegm
360. Medical manuscript of various oral teachings
361. Brief oral-tradition teachings on preparing torn-mouth rhododendron, and so on
362. Different cures for warts
363. Instructions on the Bālāhaka ḍākinī medicine for the head
364. *Lado* preparation of the six excellent plants
365. Shredded ambrosia preparation
366. Profound and special treatment for rabies
367. Very profound specific treatment for *kangbam*

368. Brief teaching from the oral tradition on smallpox, and so on
369. Preparation of the red pill
370. The ambrosia six-white-ingredient preparation
371. Practices from the oral tradition using female stones
372. Precious hundred-tongues preparation for protection on difficult paths
373. Stamping seals on the tongue [212]
374. Precious heart purgative
375. Seven-ingredient saffron preparation
376. A specific treatment for meat poisoning
377. Treatment for tongue swelling
378. Mercury preparation
379. Ambrosia stream: cure for heart-wind disorder
380. Explicit instructions on the magical yantra of fire substances
381. Practical application of Nāropa's three-ingredient preparations
382. The red pill general medicine
383. *Tsadik* preparation
384. The swift and secret path: curing *kangbam*
385. Directions for preparing the little red pill
386. Seven-branch solidified animal bile preparation
387. Preparation of the eight aromatic ingredients
388. Preparation of the nine yellow ingredients
389. Preparation of the six hero ingredients
390. Preparation of the six ingredients of the powerful class
391. A medical preparation to sever the blood-vessel webbing of the eyes
392. Black aconite medicinal butter preparation
393. Black aconite medicinal butter
394. A medical preparation for smallpox
395. Medical preparations for smallpox: a hook holding on to life
396. Ambrosia vase elixir: medicines for wind disorders in the head
397. Various *phala* preparation eye medicines
398. Four-ingredient rhinoceros preparations
399. Brown sulphur preparations
400. Secret notes on the extraordinary treatments of *kangbam*
401. A brief instruction tantra: cures for the 101 disorders that need treatment as taught in the Final Tantra
402. Treatment of rheumatoid disorders
403. Healing the mind: medicine that encourages the mind

404. Red skull pill: protection against infectious fever
405. Origins of the white single powerful medicine, its transmission, and protection against poisons
406. Life armor: protection against weapons, with illustrations
407. An instruction on treating leprosy transmitted from the unparalleled master of speech
408. Aphrodisiac known as "treatment for the tree"
409. Treatment for white and yellow jaundice
410. Losing weight by fasting
411. Sewing the disfigured lip
412. A treatment for intestinal worms
413. A treatment for stones
414. A treatment for miscellaneous disorders

Together with a table of contents and an account of how the work is set out, there are 416 sections to this work. Other works of Surkhar Nyamnyi Dorjé include:

- *A Work of Fine Crystal: Extensive Commentary on the Four Glorious Tantras*
- *Mirror of White Mercury: Questions on the Difficult Points of the Tantra.* Also known as *Overview*
- *Sunrays: A Well-Composed Work*
- *A Letter to Far-Flung Physicians*
- *Advice Beneficial for Others and Myself*
- *Vajra Songs of Experience and Collection of Praises*
- *Commentary on the Kālacakra Tantra*
- *Guidance on Mahamudra and on Places for Cutting-Off Practice*
- Sixteen small works on Great Perfection called *Golden Spoon of Excellent Explanation*

In Ngönga in the east he gathered all the physicians of Nyal, Lor, and Jar, together with those of E, Nyang, and Kong[629] [213] where he taught definitive reference works on the tastes, powers, post-digestive tastes, natures, etymologies, and functions of medicines, works such as *Precious Illustrations* or *Identification and Clarification of Medicines; Iron Garland Collection on Tastes; Ambrosia Pool; Ambrosia Treasury; Fundamentals of Medicines.* He also taught the identification of medicinal plants and so forth. Therefore, in composition, discussion, and teaching, he added to the development of the science of medicine.

Although he did not actually take monastic vows, he outwardly maintained the aspect of a monk, with no wife or children. Moreover, from the age of twenty onward, after he had met with Shara Rapjampa, it is said he went naked from the waist up and made use of meditation straps. As a way to remove obstacles on the path, he secretly used a consort endowed with the proper signs. He also gained mastery over tantric powers and tantric behavior and clairvoyance.

The biography *Irrefutable and Extensive Written Account* compiled by Lodrö Gyalpo says though Nyamnyi Dorjé's compositions on the Great Perfection cycles are undeniably prolific, his main practice was in fact Mahāmudrā, noting also that he rooted out false treasure scriptures, and so on. Such assertions were made by the compiler in order to discredit the Nyingma and the Treasure traditions. In reality, this great master did no such thing, and he simultaneously practiced the profound heartdrop and other practices of the Great Perfection. This is the assertion of my lama the Great Fifth.

At the age of thirty-seven, in the wood-sheep year, on the fifteenth of the *srāvana* month (in 1475), he withdrew his physical formation. His younger brother Pön Jetsün, his nephew Migyur Tseten, and his disciples Trakpön Sönam Tashi, Tsebum Dorjé, and others took the body to the cremation ground. As they approached the site, the body shrunk and became very small, causing consternation all round. Suddenly, from an array of lights in the corners of the sky came the sounds of the Sanskrit vowels and consonants. This was heard by everyone present, bringing great joy and a deep faith. In order to ensure that the body burned without remain, the disciples offered the body swiftly to the fire. In the course of the cremation, rainbow lights and many other perfect signs appeared.

Disciples of Surkhar Nyamnyi Dorjé

It is said that this great master had four disciples who were accomplished in medicine: Migyur Tseten was accomplished in the transmitted instructions, Trakbön Sönam Tashi was accomplished in his medical activities, [214] Tsebum Dorjé was accomplished in the practices, and Lichung Pema Kyap was accomplished in teaching. He had many other disciples: eight in whose minds blessings had entered, sixteen disciples of great wisdom, twenty disciples who found great fame, and sixteen disciples known by their titles.

Kyempa Tsewang

Of his many disciples, Kyempa Tsewang,[630] who was a direct disciple of Tsebum Dorjé, composed a commentary on the Root Tantra called *Arising of the Essence,* a commentary on the Explanatory Tantra called *Sun Word Commentary,* a commentary on the Instruction Tantra called *Granting Wishes of Happiness,* a commentary on the Final Tantra called *Clarification of Practice,* and a work known as *Medical Practices: Hundreds of Life-Granting Empowerments.*

Kawa Śākya Wangchuk or Tsomé Khenchen

Kawa Śākya Wangchuk was born of the Kawa lineage in Langdrong in Tölung, a line that included those rich in scholasticism and practice, such as the great being Kawa Paltsek, and many brave, wise, and noble beings such as the attendants[631] of early Tibetan kings. He himself said that he clearly remembered his birth as Lhajé Gewa Bum. He became abbot of Tsomé temple and lived in the hermitage of Tiné Ngowo Yaphu Pal. Relying upon Trakbön Sönam Tashi and other masters, he became learned in the sciences and especially in medicine. Because he was a descendant of the Kawa Śākya Wangchuk who lived at the time of Atiśa, he too named himself Kawa Śākya Wangchuk. He was also known as Tsomé Khenchen.

His compositions include: *Mirror of White Silver: A Well-Composed History of Medicine; Commentary on the Final Tantra: An Illuminating Lamp on Its Difficult Points; Flower Garland: Clarification of the Five Families;* and *Explicit and Essential Compilation of Practices.* He had many disciples, such as Langbu Chöjé.

Jarpo Panchen

Jarpo Panchen[632] was an adherent of the Kagyü tradition, a disciple of Dakpo Mengom[633] Dorjé Gyaltsen, and a third-generation descendant of Döndrup Dar, revealer of early-translation treasure scriptures. He was born the son of Pema Karpo, Karmapa Chödrak Gyatso's[634] chief physician, who had been appointed minister of medicine and had founded a center of learning.[635] Jarpo Panchen was also honored by the Karmapa by being appointed ācārya of medicine. He trained in his own family medical tradition and in the Surkhar tradition under Kyempa Tsebum Dorjé. He was known, therefore, as Jarpo Panchen.[636]

He contributed to the spread of the science of medicine in the south and composed commentaries on all four tantras, as well as *Golden Sheaves: A Well-Composed History of Medicine; Table of Contents for "Relic of Millions"*; and other works. [215]

Surkhar Lodrö Gyalpo

Lodrö Gyalpo of the Surkhar family was a disciple of Langbu Chöjé. At first he was named Tseten Gyalwa. Karma Trinlepa (1456–1539) then gave him the name Palden Döndrup Namgyal at the hair-cutting ceremony. The Eighth Karmapa Mikyö Dorjé (1507–54) named him Lekshé Tsöl and Shamarpa[637] named him Lodrö Gyalpo. He took his ancestral name because, as mentioned above, he was born into the Surkhar family in the *śukla* earth-snake year of the ninth sixty-year cycle (1509).

From an early age he followed the medical tradition of his predecessors, although at times he immersed himself in Mahāmudrā and other practices. He was ordained by Karma Trinlepa and trained himself in the causal Sutra Vehicle at the Lekshé Ling Dharma center. Under Kyok Lotsāwa [Rinchen Tashi], also known as Möndrup Lotsāwa, he studied poetry. On the advice of the Karmapa he went back to Langbu Chöjé, the student of Tsomé Khenchen, and received the initiations and transmissions of Yuthok's *Heartdrop, Four Tantras, Relic of Millions,* and others.

He received the transmissions of [Candranandana's] *Eight Branches* and its autocommentary, *Moonlight;* the Eighteen Auxiliary Texts; [Drangti Palden Gyaltsen's] *Golden Measuring Dish of Instructions;* and *Silver Measuring Dish of Instructions* from Drungné Jangpa Kuché; Pöntsang Phendarwa; the nephew of Chakmen Ringyal of Ngari; Apa Tsering from Gugé; the nephew of Biji; the grandson of Ukpa; Jang Taktse Tsojé; and particularly from the Drangti family lineage within the Sakya medical tradition. I think that he received these Jang transmissions from a later lineage stemming from Jangpa Tashi Palsang[638] because the Jang lineage founder Namgyal Draksang and his disciple Minyima were of a different time, and there is nothing about this transmission in the Jang literature from those times, but this list does occur in Lodrö Gyalpo's *Testament of an Old Man.*

Examining carefully the words of *Heartdrop,* he came to understand that he should concentrate solely on the teachings of Yuthok. To this end he came to the area of Lower Nyang, and it is said that after much searching he discovered the work on *Four Tantras* by Yuthok called *Golden Annotations,* which became known as the "well-worn copy." There the local king Wangyal Drakpa provided for all his requirements, and over four years he composed a commentary on the root and explanatory tantras called *Oral Transmission of Our Ancestors.*

He came to central Tibet, and on a Lhasa stone pillar he attached a manuscript of questions concerning practices of the basis, path, and result.[639] Though he did this three times and the document consequently became widely known, still no one came up with answers. Therefore, Nangso Dönyö and other disciples requested an explanation of the questions. Accordingly Lodrö Gyalpo wrote his own commentary known as *Golden Ornament,* but apparently most did not understand it. [216] Medical scholars of the time included Dölda Nyang Khangpa, Chongyé Röl Khongpa, Depa Lhasa Dzongwa, Nangso Dönyö from Yarlung Chedrong, Lata Tsewang from Kyem, Lodrö Tenpa from Kyishö Nawo, and Korap Gelawa. The *Testament of an Old Man* also mentions someone called "the great Jangdak Dharma king from Latö." Since these events did not occur during the era of the lineage founder Jangdak Namgyal Draksang and so on, only the father of Dharma king Tashi Topgyal fits the description at that time. Moreover, a good knowledge of medicine was not so prevalent during that time. Whatever the reason, these scholars advanced some responses to the manuscript that did not please Lodrö Gyalpo, and consequently he composed *My Own Response: The Testament of an Old Man, a Flash of Lightning on a Dark Night.*

He asked the Rinpung ruler[640] to sponsor the printing of the edition of *Four Tantras* that he himself had revised and edited, and although the ruler initially agreed, the sponsorship was not forthcoming. Therefore, in the present Drathang[641] edition of *Four Tantras,* in the colophon after the praises to the Yargyap,[642] he says in a mocking or biting tone:

> In the beginning promising, "I will do this,"
> they willingly take on a host of difficulties,
> but like the crow that died,
> they never achieve their crowning glory.[643]

Finally the Yargyap sponsored the publication himself, and these days it can found in Drathang.

Lodrö Gyalpo's other works include:

- *Irrefutable and Extensive Written Account of the Life and Liberation of Rishi Nyamnyi Dorjé*

- *Requests Based on Biography: A New Enjoyment Ocean of Faith*
- *Dispelling the Torment of Sorrow: Entreating the Compassion of the Two Rishis*
- *An Outline to Captivate the Minds of the Wise: Contents of Relic of Millions—Great Dispeller of Hindrances*
- A supplement to *Relic of Millions* called *Flower in the Cupped Palms of the Faithful*
- *White Singly Powerful Medicine, or the Vajra of Indra: Reply to Jang Position on Establishing the Tantra as the Word of the Buddha*

In order to resolve the debate over whether *Four Tantras* is the word of the Buddha or a later treatise, he asserts that it is outwardly the word of the Buddha, inwardly a treatise composed by Indian pandits, and secretly a Tibetan treatise. The position of a succession of great scholars of the past is that it is the word of the Buddha. In particular, it is possible to understand that Jé Dharmaswami, Lodrö Gyalpo's own ancestor, was also of this view because of the following. I have only seen one small section of his *Mirror of White Mercury Overview* up to now and have not seen his *Work of Fine Crystal: Extensive Commentary on the Four Glorious Tantras* and other works. However, in that small section of *Mirror of White Mercury,* the words of Buddha in *Four Tantras* have been left as they are. [217] Also, there is a reference to this in a manuscript by Lata Tsewang[644] cited in *Stream of Beryl* by Drö Tsoknyi Gyatso.

Moreover, his shout of blatant disregard for the very clear assertions in *Well-Composed History of Medicine* by Tsomé Khenchen, the master of his own teacher, could be explained by Sakya Paṇḍita's verse:

> Having lost all sense of shame,
> holding their own wicked words in high esteem,
> those of royal caste in Kāñci
> beat the drum of victory
> at the murder of their father.[645]

Alternatively, it may be a case of vulgar language breaking the helmet of his own medical tradition from the inside.[646]

Other compositions besides that one include:

- A collection of praises to Yuthok, Nyamnyi Dorjé, and other holy masters

- *Table of the Powers, Tastes, and Post-Digestive Tastes of Medicines.* The previous work on this topic by Dharmaswami can be compared to holing a diamond, while this work is like threading that diamond.
- *The Cuta Vine: Questions Put to Gongmen Könchok Phendar* (1511–77)
- *Ford for Those of Bright Minds: Questions to the Panam Physician Künga Lekpa*
- *Questions and Answers: A Well-Composed Emetic*
- *Moondrops: An Ocean of Light*
- *Thunder: The Rousing Drum of Summer*
- *Eliminating the Impurities of Camphor, Saffron, Eaglewood, Sandalwood, and the Like*
- *Eliminating Mistakes: Comments after the Printing of Four Tantras*
- *Boiling Water*
- *Refined Drop of Summer Sun: Answers to Questions from a Phenyül Doctor on the Rising of the Wind Element*
- *Questions and Answers on Manu*

With these and other works he contributed much to the medical collection. It seems that he also composed various works on the other sciences, such as a treatise on *Mirror of the Mirror of Poetics.*

However, in all the above works, apart from Jé Yuthok, Nyamnyi Dorjé, and Karmapa Mikyö Dorjé, nowhere does he praise or pay homage to those with the status of lama, such as his actual medical teacher Langbu Chöje, or to his poetry teacher Möndrup Lotsāwa, also known as Kyok Lotsāwa Rinchen Tashi. This seems to be a perfect illustration of the line from the Final Tantra: "Keeping the master secret while promoting oneself."[647] In this connection, the Final Tantra section of his *Oral Transmission of Our Ancestors* commentary on *Four Tantras,* and his *General Knowledge History: A Presentation on the External, Internal, and Other, Indispensable for Physicians Wishing to Engage in the Practices of the Bodhisattvas, the Wide-Open Door to the Unending Ceremonial Offering, a Dance Delighting the Rishis*[648] were both left unfinished as he was afflicted by a stroke. [218]

If the status of one's birth is not authenticated by valid prophecy, such as that found in the Treasure and Transmission traditions, and if from one's own side one does not display evidence of conduct that is a direct awakening of imprints from previous lives, then there can be no reliability from merely making claims. However, he himself stated that he was the rebirth of Dharmaswami, and it is said that this was recognized by the Shamarpa. Moreover, the sounds emanating from his rather superficial training in other disciplines such as poetry and sutra-mahāmudrā philosophy are merely those of the blue dragon,[649] while in medicine far from being the successor to Surkhar, it is clear he does not even measure up to Kyempa Tsewang.

His fundamental disregard of the words of Tsomé Khenchen, who is within his own teaching lineage, his over-intellectual attacks on authoritative medical works of the past such as those from the Jang tradition, and his refutations of standard poetical wisdom are a wound inflicted upon medical science. He makes the claim that the Rinpung ruler at first promised to sponsor a publication of *Four Tantras* but then failed to deliver on his promise. However, this ruler, Ngawang Jikten Drakpa, was someone who did not mistake brass for gold, and he was clearly aware of the errors of the other's twisted interpretations of the text. His corpus of medical literature, including his commentary on *Four Tantras* called *Oral Transmission of Our Ancestors,* are illustrations of his own words, "like the crow that died, they never achieved their crowning glory."[650]

In *Testament of an Old Man* he writes, "When I was approaching the age of sixty-three" and "When I was weakened by the harms of the great rishi." I can find no authoritative references to his life and activities beyond this age, and he probably died soon after.

Other physicians of the Sur tradition

Of the many other physicians of the Sur tradition, Tashi Dargyé of Jayül composed a commentary on the powers of individual medicines taught in the Explanatory Tantra in connection with a materia medica and other works. Dru Sengé or Drangsong Thutop Dorjé wrote *Ambrosia Treasury of Medical Practice.* Pawo Tsuklak Trengwa composed *Quintessential Notes on Medical Practice, Illuminating Beacon on Mineral Exudates,* and so on, which seem to have been copied from *Relic of Millions.* The Kyishö Nao physician, Lodrö Tenpa, also known as Bodhisattva Losang Gyatso, composed *Clear Mirror: A Word Commentary to the Final Tantra* and *Ornament to the Thoughts of the Rishis: A History of Medicine.* The Dakpo physician Karma Künphen composed a commentary to *Relic of Millions* together with orally transmitted instructions, *Golden Rosary of Ambrosia: Quintessence of All the Profound Points of the Instruction Collections,* [219] *Treatment of Kangbam,* and others.

The Sur lineage, therefore, runs as follows:

Our Teacher the buddha of medicine
The speaker of the tantra, Rishi Vidyājñāna
The compiler, Rishi Manasija
Kumāra Jivaka
The master Nāgārjuna
Śrī Ācārya Śūra
The Kashmiri Pandit Candranandana
The great translator Vairocana
King Trisong Detsen
The treasure finder Drapa Ngönshé
Üpa Dardrak
Roktön Könchok Kyap
The king of medicine, combiner of lineages,
  Yuthok Yönten Gönpo
Sumtön Yeshé Sung
Tsojé Shönu Yeshé
The Yuthok scholar Bumseng
The Tsang teacher Sangyé Rinchen
The scholar Döndrup Rinchen
Tenzin Döndrup Gyaltsen
Drangti Könchok Gyaltsen
Drangti Palden Tsojé

Up to this point, apart from the extension to their list to include Ānanda, Ācarya Padma, and others, this lineage is similar to the Jang Treasure lineage. It continues:

The monk Tsalpa Wangdrak
The great scholar Phüntsok Sangpo
Surkhar Nyamnyi Dorjé
Kyempa Tsewang
Jarpo Panchen
His direct and chief disciple, Dawa Wangpo

He is followed by the Chushöl Nao physician Lodrö Tenpa, who served as physician to the Kyishö governor and, because he practiced the graduated path to enlightenment and lived in Rinding, was also known as Rinchen Ding Bodhisattva Losang Gyatso. He also composed several works, as mentioned above.

He is followed by Rishi Tenzin Gyalpo. He was driven out of the northern or Jang region of Tölung—which is divided into the regions of Mön, Jang, and Gé—by the local community. He came to Rinding Bodhisattva to seek relief and studied medicine there for seven years. On the night before he met Tsojé Karma Künphen, he dreamed of an extraordinary turquoise stupa. "This reflects the auspiciousness of our meeting today," said Tsojé, who predicted that Tenzin Gyalpo would be of great benefit to those beings living on the Lhasa side of Kyishö and would contribute greatly to the preservation of the lineage of medical teachings.

From Drosa Neten, Tenzin Gyalpo received teachings on the use of surgical spoons in the treatment of the heart, kidneys, eyes, and so on. From Panchen Losang Chökyi Gyaltsen (1567–1662) he took the vows of a novice monk and received the name Rishi Tenzin Gyalpo.

When he was caring for the health of the omniscient Yönten Gyatso,[651] who had displayed some illness, it is said that Tenzin Gyalpo received the extraordinary prophecy that he would always be cared for by Medicine Buddha. [220]

From the Dharma king Jangpa Tashi Topgyal he received, among other teachings, the initiations and transmissions of Yuthok's *Heartdrop* and Dharma works. He became a great master much learned and practiced in the science of medicine. He was also praised by Tsangpa Dung Töchen. The date and month of his passing coincides with that of Yuthokpa. He was said to be an incarnation of Sumtön Yeshé Sung.

His son disciples were Jang Ngö Nangso Dargyé and his younger son, Shenphen Wangpo. His main disciple was Lingtö Chöjé Losang Gyatso.

My teacher, the Great Fifth, in his *Stream of the Ganges: An Account of Teachings Received,* in the *ka* volume, in the section on the explanation, outline, stone layout, and introduction to the practices from the three shorter tantras,[652] talks of the lineage passing from Rishi Tenzin Gyalpo to his son Rishi Dargyé and in turn to his younger brother Khechok Shenphen Wangpo.[653] The younger son had a short life and so his contribution to the welfare of others was small. His brother, the elder son, was appointed physician to the great patronized lamas, as exemplified by my great lama, and was also hugely beneficial to many beings in his capacity of teacher in the medical school in Lhawang Chok.[654] He consequently had many disciples that he took over from his younger brother, Khechok Shenphen Wangpo. These include

Drak Jukpa, who gave recitation examinations on *Four Tantras,* Lhaksam or Sumga, who rose from being like a personal servant to the younger brother to being a chief physician, and Darmo Losang Chödrak, who began as a monastic entrant of the medical school and later, under the direction of the Great fifth, took over the revision classes.

The tantra transmission lineage together with the Instruction Tantra passes from Rishi Tenzin Gyalpo to Lingtö Chöjé Losang Gyatso, who received Yuthok's *Heartdrop* from Jangdak Tashi Topgyal. While Surchen Chöying Rangdröl was receiving teaching from Lingtö Chöjé, Yerpa became filled with the aroma of medicine. It is clear from the list of teachings received that there was a prophecy predicting him as an incarnation of Tsomé Khenchen. His own unmistaken incarnation lives on today as a being with a combination of the wise, noble, and good qualities. His details can be found elsewhere.

From Lingtö Chöjé Losang Gyatso, the transmission lineage, together with the early translation *Heartdrop,* passed to Mengom Drangyé Garwang, the maintainer of the biographies of the siddhas. He passed it to Khyapdak Lochok Dorjé, an incarnation of Vimalamitra,[655] whose extensive life and deeds are found in the collected works of my great lama. [221] Like a thirsty man wishing for water, I yearned to acquire all the transmissions, teachings, and practices of this Sur tradition as listed in the precious *Account of Teachings Received* in order to correct any corruption, errors, and omissions it might have had by comparing it with the Jang tradition. However, although I requested from my great lama the oral transmission of *Four Tantras,* due to his advanced age and his illnesses such as eye ailments, I had not the merit to receive it, receiving only the Yuthok *Heartdrop* and *Vase of Ambrosia.*[656]

However, the lineage I received of this Sur tradition, which accords with the accounts of teachings received, and therefore differs somewhat in the latter stages from that found in the precious *Account of Teachings Received,* runs from Jé Nyamnyi Dorjé to Tashi Wangchuk of the Gyer family, Sönam Sangpo, the Dzokchen practitioner Sönam Rinchen, Trinlé Dönyö, Rikzin Nyingpo of Nying Phu, Sungtrül Tsültrim Dorjé, Rikzin Trinlé Lhündrup, up to the Vairocana incarnation Khyapdak Gyurmé Dorjé

17. The Gongmen Tradition

IN THE WORK known as *Red Works of Drangti* it states:

> I, Drangti Chögyal Tashi,
> in the two-story Sakya medical school,
> to the suitable vessel Könchok Delek...

Therefore, although Könchok Delek practiced medicine in a branch of the Upper tradition under Gongkhawa Chökyi Dorjé, he became a follower of the Drangti tradition and rose to a very prominent position as scholar, and he became the most prominent figure of the medical lineage known as Gongmen.[657] Könchok Delek studied most of the well-known medical books in this land of snow. Moreover, he brought out the hidden oral traditions of many Chinese and Tibetan scholars, and for the sake of self and others composed several compilations. These include the following seven volumes:

1. *Red Volume of Instructions*
2. *Black Volume of Instructions*
3. *Multicolored Volume of Instructions*
4. *Beacon Illuminating All Places: Commentary on the Difficult Points of the Final Tantra*
5. *Biographies of the Lineage*
6. *Medical Lexicon*
7. *Yellow Scroll that Disentangles the Precipice Path of the Difficult Points of the Tantra*

Other shorter works include *Direct Teachings on Disentangling the Main Points of Pulse and Urine Analysis, Brief Illustrative Descriptions of Medical Plants,* and *Compilation of Tastes and Powers.* A particular noteworthy composition is his extensive annotations and corrections to the tantra known as *Khadira Tree Multicolored Compilation on the Great Tantra*, for which it is claimed that merely looking at this work will bring about a liberation, without the need to rely upon a master. [222]

Gongmen Könchok Phendar

Gongmen Könchok Phendar's compositions include:

- *Caturyoga Requests to the Rishi Lineage*
- *Consecration Ritual for Calling Down Blessings for Medicine*
- *Collection on Medicine Goddess Practices*
- *Table of Contents for the Extensive, Intermediate, and Abridged Preparation of the Great Black Medicine*
- *Treatise on Preparing Mercury*
- *Clear Mirror: Commentary on the Root Tantra*

His collection on transmitted instructions and charms is a very extensive and fully comprehensive collection in three volumes known as *Jeweled Garland Fulfilling All Needs within the Science of Medicine.* A more abridged composition is *Summarizing the Thoughts.* An even more abridged work is *Compilation of the Essentials.* There is also a summary of the main points of these works known as *Hundred Works of Experience.*

Gongmen Könchok Phendar had disciples known as the four pillars and the eight beams. The four pillar-like disciples were Apa Dechen from Ngari, the scholar from the upper regions; Gongkar Sertokpa, the scholar from the lower regions; Surtsé Drangsong Lhashakpa, the scholar from the middle regions; and the renowned Tsarong Chöjé. The eight pillars were Nyima Drak from Mangkhar Deling, Samten Palsang, Namkha Tashi from Thangring, his nephew Künga Tashi, Döndrup Gyal from Ngari, Palden Lekpa, Lodrö Phakpa, and Samdrup Sangpo.

Among these disciples Tsarong Chöjé Palden Gyaltsen composed *Overview of Medicine* or *Lamp Dispelling the Darkness: A New Tradition of Teaching* and more, all of which became known as the Tsarong Oral tradition compilation. His nephew Namkha Delek's compositions include:

- *Light of Excellent Explanation: An Overview of Four Tantras*
- *Abridged Outline of the Pulse Compendium from Four Tantras*
- *Divisions and Abridgements of the Ailments, Remedies, and Healing Methods of the Final Tantra*
- *Ambrosia Garland;* a collection of miscellaneous instructions
- *Identification of the Four Classes of Chronic Degenerative Disorders*
- *Diamonds;* remedies for the above chronic disorders

His son was Rishi Tsewang Rikzin, and at that time local governor Lhünpo Tsewa sent Porkhawa to study the practices of the Upper tradition, while Tsarong Tsewang Rikzin was sent to the place of Jarpo Panchen to study the Lower tradition and thereby became a follower of that system. On his contribution to medicine, he extended Surkhar's work on history and composed *Swift Path Traveled by the Fortunate.* [223] The lineage up to Tsewang Namgyal maintained a succession of physicians to the Lhünpo Tsewa and the Tsang rulers and also founded medical schools. When the reputation of Tenzin Chökyi Gyalpo[658] began to spread, the schools were discontinued. However, later when they were covered by the religious and secular white umbrella of the Great Fifth, they were restarted. Later on his son Tseten Dorjé offered a word recitation of the Drathang *Four Tantras,* and the Great Fifth wrote a constitution for the school.[659] These factors were instrumental in raising the status of this tradition.

During the visit[660] to Drepung in the iron-monkey year (1680), I had the opportunity to engage Tseten Dorjé in conversation. He had followed his family tradition, and he gave at least the impression of being a lineage physician. However, despite his ability to pass the examination of reciting the words of the tantra and his possession of the family tradition, he did not have an in-depth understanding of medical science. Nevertheless, he was basically a very capable person who had initiated some far-sighted rules, and the schools still continue. However, he has since died. While memorization of the scriptures happens at the school, there is no one there to give teachings and so on. Moreover, various private activities go on that undermine even the focus on memorization, so that from the time of the rule of district governor Phukpa Tsangjin, all auspicious conditions for the school have been destroyed.

Other followers of the Gongmen tradition include the following: Gangpa Palgön Lhündrup who composed *Garland of Excellent Explanation: An Overview of the Science of Medicine* and *Method to Avoid Errors in Identifying the Four Times.* Drungtso Wangdenpa wrote *Hook of Wisdom: Messenger in Search of Excellent Explanation,* which answers questions on how eclipses of the sun and moon, the solstices and equinoxes, and so on affect the pulse. Chakdor Gönpo composed an outline of the Final Tantra and *Precious Garland Quintessence,* whose title he copied from Minyima's *Quintessence.* Depa Rongtso composed many works including *Mandala of Wisdom,* which answers questions on the identification of Sudarśana, the history of the lineage, and so on, and *Garland of Ambrosia Drops: Abridgement of Profound Instructions.* The Drukpa incarnation Pema Karpo composed *Treasure for the*

Benefit of Others: A Presentation of Four Tantras, and *Chapter on Treatment of Poisoning.* The Sixth Shamarpa Chökyi Wangchuk wrote *Death-Defying Ambrosia: Treatise on Medical Science.* Pawo Tsuklak Trengwa composed a history of medicine and a treatment for *kangbam.* Sokdokpa[661] composed *Essence of the Definitive: Four Tantras as Enlightened Speech.*

To summarize: the two most renowned medical traditions are the Upper and Lower traditions. The Upper tradition includes the Jang lineage, [224] by similarity the Gongmen lineage, the southern lineages, and so on. The Lower tradition includes the Surkhar uncle-to-nephew tradition and by similarity the Jarpo Panchen and Kyempa family traditions. These various lineages have preserved the tradition of medicine in this land of snow, and their literary output is beyond description.

18. The Great Fifth Dalai Lama and Desi Sangyé Gyatso

The contribution of the Great Fifth to the science of medicine

[225] THE THIRTY-SIXTH chapter of the *Mañjuśrī Root Tantra* says:

> When the doctrine of the Teacher on this earth
> has deteriorated in the extremity of time,
> he will without doubt appear
> in the form of a vow-holding king.[662]

The same text talks of his name:

> The letter *ma* and *youth,*
> loving the Dharma
> at the beginning and end.[663]

The *Book of Kadam: Father Teachings* predicts the sign of his birth year[664] and talks of his deeds:

> His birth at that time will be a birth from the seed of fire. Whatever Dharma he practices will be of great power. In particular, he will take great delight in and praise the meditation practices of the wrathful deities. He will be someone that the māras and their cohorts will not be able to withstand and he will defeat them utterly. Because of his great liking for the wrathful activities of mantra, again there will be much argument and much discussion. But he will not be defeated.[665]

Similarly the *Book of Kadam: Son Teachings:*

He will berate them, saying,
"The people of Tibet, of this land of snow,
like a heartless son despising his father,
now doubt me, the precious source of happiness."[666]

The *Chronicles of Ministers* says:

The body, speech, mind, qualities, and activities
of the great king Trisong Detsen,
the power of these five manifest
and unmistakably united as one;
two form bodies working for living beings;
a master of heaven and earth,
taming and cultivating the people of the north,
will come from the rains of Sahor.[667]

This verse predicts that the five manifestations—of the body, speech, mind, qualities, and activities—of the great ruler Tsangpa Lhayi Metok[668] will appear in order to guard the doctrines of sutra and tantra and that the power of all five will be united in one endowed being, who will care for his disciples comprising most of the people of the north, and who will be of Sahor ancestry.

Ratna Lingpa in his *Extensive General Transmissions* says:

A king with bodhi mind previously developed
will then appear in central Tibet as a manifestation of compassion,
his name meaning, "wise, powerful, and good."
With various means he guides living beings
and becomes a Dharma king with his own army.[669]

From the same work:

The center and Tsang[670] all gathered in his domain,
of great power and magical feats,
a master of the doctrine will appear.

These passages and others refer extensively to the basis of his emanation, the components of his name, the time of his coming, [226] his deeds, and so forth.

In Shikpo Lingpa's *Treasure Transmissions* it says:

> When the Tradruk stupa holding down the demoness[671]
> falls apart and becomes irreparable,
> the Sahor descendent from the Songtsen line
> brings the doctrine to the whole of Central Tibet and Tsang.[672]

Similarly, Dorjé Lingpa, Rikzin Sokdrup, Yölmo Trülku, Terdak Lingpa, Dawa Gyaltsen, and others produced predictions from the profound treasures. He was also clearly foretold by the predictions of Karmapa Mikyö Dorjé and others who were possessed of the visionary experiences of great beings.

My lama, great adherent to the tradition of the Bhagavān Buddha, is one whose nature is of love and affection for all beings of all worlds, even for those he has no cause to love. Long ago he arrived at the perfection of the great powers of the bodhisattva deeds, with the immeasurable qualities of the ten powers, the four confidences, and so on, and became the perfect buddha Rasmi Samudgata Śrīku Rāja, beautifully adorned with the marks and signs of enlightenment. In the impure worldly realms, in accord with the minds of disciples, he manifested as universally sovereign emperors, world monarchs, Indra, Brahmā, householders, monks, and so on. Like the single sphere of the moon effortlessly showing from its path in the sky its reflections in various and separate waters on this earth simultaneously, he appeared to the minds of the beings in this cool snowy land in the form of a monk king, with not a fraction of his auspicious birth and so forth distinct from that of a perfect buddha.

To illustrate his qualities by his name, he was the all-knowing mighty Ngawang Losang Gyatso Jikmé Gocha Thupten Langtso Dé. His great white-umbrella administration of religion and secular activities protected Tibet, China, and Mongolia, and having become a ruler of heaven and earth, he expanded and developed like the waxing moon the doctrine of the mighty Buddha, specifically sutra, tantra, and the other sciences.

In the field of medicine, he gave, not only as an enlightened being but in this present incarnation, too, all the transmissions of medical texts such as *Four Tantras,* [Dorbum Chökyi Drakpa's] *Vase of Ambrosia,* [Surkhar Nyamnyi Dorjé's] *Relic of Millions,* and the Gongmen texts of personal experience. [227] He practiced the instructions taught in the profound Yuthok *Heartdrop* and bestowed the *Illuminating Ambrosia Moonlight Initiation Rituals* comprising the *Stream of the Pure Initiations* from the *Vase of Ambrosia* treasure text, and so on. In doing so, he was the king of medicine, the combiner of lineages. However, to the minds of ordinary beings he memorized the three shorter tantras and studied their explanations, stone layout, practices, and recognition of medical plants only superficially, not displaying any in-depth knowledge or providing any such compositions of his own in his collected works.

Therefore, in response to the entreaties by Jang Ngö Nangso Dargyé, he urged Ācārya Döndrup Palwa and others to replicate the mother text of *Four Tantras: Essence of Ambrosia Secret Instruction Tantra on Eight Branches* located at Drathang Monastery. Publication of [the later Yuthok's] Eighteen Auxiliary Texts was requested by Darmo Menrampa Losang Chödrak and by others who offered him the mother text. Publication of Surkhar [Lodrö Gyalpo's] *Oral Transmission of Our Ancestors* commentary on the Root, Explanatory, and Final Tantra as far as the section on urine analysis was requested by Darmo Menrampa Losang Chödrak, and he [the Fifth] asked Namling Panchen to redact the text. In these undertakings my great lama did not make any in-depth revisions himself, providing only minimal input, thinking that at least it would be better than nothing. He gave without fuss all necessary prerequisites for the printing, and in so doing opened wide the door to an unending offering of Dharma in the form of published texts.

He ensured the continuity of two different medical institutes. One was the medical college Sorik Drophen Ling[673] to the west of Drepung Ganden Phodrang, whose first master was Drungchen Losang Gyatso of Nyithang and which was subsequently run by Jang Ngö Nangso Dargyé. The other was Drangsong Düpai Ling medical school in Shika Samdrup Tsé,[674] which was run by the Tsarong family. Consequently, it seems that the number of recitation examinations on *Four Tantras* increased at that time. He also established the medical schools in Lhawang Chok or Sharchen Chok run by Jang Ngö Nangso and subsequently by Darmo Menrampa. He also gave money and provisions to the students of Lhaksam and Nasa Lingwa.

In the tantra it says, "With gems there is nothing that cannot be dispelled."[675] They are the best remedy for the 404 kinds of illness, especially dual and complex disorders such as poisoning. They lengthen life and restore youth. Merely by wearing them on the body, you are protected from violent storms, hail, and weapons, and from the eight types of spirits. When made use of, they close the door to birth in the lower realms. Therefore, gem pills have great benefits. Many past nobles and high lamas, such as Gyantsé, [228] Yartöpa, Yargyap, Shamarnak, Drigung, and Tsechen, tried to make gem pills. However, they only used up to a maximum of eighty-three different medicines, they used the water in which rare gems had been soaked, and girls born in the tiger year were suddenly being killed, and so the process became tainted by crime.[676]

Therefore, because gem pills were not being manufactured correctly, the Great Fifth decided to perform a great act of giving in order to guard and protect the lives of living beings. He put a great deal of effort into collecting medicines from many other sources in search of those ingredients not found in his own storerooms. Moreover, when he visited the country of Tangkün people came to him like iron filings to a magnet to make offerings. Queen Dorjé Rapten Ma came from upper Mongolia, and Emperor Chung Wang also brought offerings. These offerings included many rare gems, holy relics of our Teacher and also of bodhisattvas, śrāvakas, and pratyekabuddhas, a handful of golden myrobalan, clockwise-coiled white conches, milk from a white lioness, whiskers taken from a live tigress, diamonds, beryl of various colors, amber, quartz, pearls, and other inconceivable vajra jewels of men, gods, and nāgas. All these he gave up without any sense of loss, as if they were stones on the ground, thereby seeding a wonderful and virtuous tradition that resulted in the large-scale production of many varieties of gem pills, such as the cold-ingredient precious compound, the hot-ingredient precious compound, the precious pill *tarima,* the poison-destroying bezoars as taught in the *Blazing Fire* speech tantra from the three body, speech, and mind Maheśvara tantras, together with their accompanying drinks. These were all blessed to become the immortality ambrosia of the gods, the death-defying ambrosia of the *asura,* and the happiness-creating ambrosia of humans.

He authorized and provided for the translations of texts in the great Potala palace by such translators as the great Lotsāwa Ngawang Phüntsok Lhündrup from Dar and the brahman Saṃnyāsin Godara Rañcara[677] from Mahora in western India. These texts were:

- *Essence of Āyurveda* [by Brahmaputra Hāsavajra]
- *The Remedies of Dānadāsa,* by the Indian Paha doctor Dānadāsa, with its seventy-two different remedial charm circles
- *Caraka Supplement to the Ocean-Like Brahmā Āyurveda* by the royal Āyurvedic practitioner Ragunātha from Mathurā
- *Miscellany of Beneficial Advice and Practices*
- *Meaningful to Behold: Opening the Eyes* by the Shājang doctor Manaho.[678]

With indigenous Tibetan material also, he arranged for many transmissions and oral instructions to be made available. These include the transmission of both the Mitrayogi and Tibetan traditions' treatments for recovering sight from Neluk, a specially invited Upper-tradition practitioner from Drachi; [229] works such as *Quintessence, Essential Compilation of Treatments, Golden Measuring Dish, Stream of Ambrosia,* and Jangpa Rikden Namgyal Draksang's *Extensive Commentary on the Explanatory Tantra* from Gelong Shenphen, holder of the tradition of Darma Gönpo from upper Tsang; and teachings on purifying mercury from the Druptop Orgyen tradition passed down to Namkha Lha from Nyanang. For the sake of living beings he encouraged the study of these works by local medical scholars, especially Darmo Menrampa and Lhaksam.

In keeping with the wishes of disciples he also encouraged medical compositions. In a commentary called *Loosening the Vajra Knots* Darmo Losang Chödrak and Namling Panchen together completed the unfinished section of *Oral Transmission of Our Ancestors,* beginning from the urine analysis chapter of the Final Tantra. Darmo Menrampa Losang Chödrak, Mermopa, and Larawa[679] composed *Golden Ornament of Excellent Explanation*[680] in the manner of a difficult-point commentary. This work left existing annotations in the text as they were but added annotations where there was no word commentary. In its commentary on the text, it followed previous commentaries where they existed but left untouched those parts for which there was no previous commentary. Larawa compiled from old manuscripts the biographies of the earlier and later Yuthok.[681] Also, in response to requests, the Great Fifth also wrote the colophons for the above works.

Quite a few authors of medical works appeared during the life of the Great Fifth. These include Nyithang Shapdrung Ngawang Shönu, who composed a commentary on the three shorter tantras; the learned Tibetan Mipham Gelek, who wrote *Anatomy of the Torso* and the *Explanation of the Tastes and Powers of Medicines;* and Lhünding Namgyal Dorjé, who wrote the *Great Adornment of the Stone Pillar.*

The contribution of Desi Sangyé Gyatso

As for myself, this person of brass masquerading as gold, when I was a child, I played by collecting various plants and pretending they were medicines, drawing diagrams in astronomy trays, and showing an instinct for teaching Dharma, taking part in religious processions, making tormas, and so on. I write of these only because those around me at that time have mentioned them. In my own mind, not only do I have no thoughts of being the incarnation of an ārya bodhisattva and the like, I do not even have any thoughts of being the incarnation of someone greatly trained in the sciences. [230]

Despite this, I was treated from an early age like a son by my master and father figure, the all-powerful, all-knowing Great Fifth, and from the age of eight onward, I had the great fortune of seeing him and hearing his words. He gave me the lay-practitioner vows that take hold of the three refuges. Then, in keeping with my age, he instructed me progressively, in an easygoing manner and to a level that I could assimilate, on all matters of religion and state. I remained in his service for many years afterward. Seeing a lump of earth as gold, he appointed me, and not in name only, as his representative in all affairs of religion and politics.

Then, as it says in *Chronicles of Kings:*

> At the end of time in the age of degeneration,
> after twelve different incarnations of the prince,
> there will appear in Tibet, this land of many snow peaks,
> a king of the noble class, a subduer of the poisonous hordes,
> possessed of the five auspicious signs of a king—
> deep thought, powerful speech, vast mind,
> ability to withstand, great power with discernment—
> and the military might and provisions of a king.[682]

Therefore, it is as if I am the thirteenth incarnation of Mutik Tsenpo, the son of Tsangpa Lhayi Metok.[683] Moreover, the Great Fifth would often talk of the subsequent births of Ngok Lekpai Sherap[684] from the *Book of Kadam.* The *King of Meditative Concentrations Sutra* states:

> Sun, moon, and stars may fall from the sky,
> the mountains, the earth, and its cities may be destroyed,
> space itself may change,
> yet you will never speak a word untrue.[685]

As we see here, it is the nature of a buddha never to claim that something is when it is not or that something is not when it is, thus it cannot be refuted. There are also quite clear predictions in the early and later treasures.

If I am the incarnation of that prince, consider the following from

Chronicles of Kings where, after saying that the births of Mutik Tsenpo included such great beings such as the ārya Asaṅga and the śrāvaka Aniruddha, it says:

> Concering the past, present, and future
> of Prince Jingyön Lekpai Lodrö,
> who I have named Mutik Tsenpo:
> eighty-four thousand eons in the past,
> in the presence of Sugata Nāgakula Pradīpa,
> while offering the *cittamaṇi* jewel...[686]

This refers to his developing the bodhi mind. The text continues:

> In the east of this billionfold world realm, [231]
> in a realm known as Viraja,
> he became a tathāgata, guide of living beings,
> teacher of gods and men, nourishing tens of millions
> with the name of Sugata Vimaladhvaja,
> a conqueror with all good qualities complete.

This passage explains that Mutik Tsenpo is also ultimately a buddha, with all faults vanquished and all good qualities perfected. How could I ever have such a hope?

Nevertheless, the Great Fifth taught me the *Wheel of Samantrabhadra*[687] section of Daṇḍin's work and gave me many teachings, both generally and specifically, on sutra and tantra. From Khewang Palden Phüntsok I learned the alphabet, the basis of being able to express oneself verbally. With Dar Lotsāwa I studied astronomy and, in the science of language, the Tibetan grammatical treatises *Thirty Verses* and *Use of Affixes* [by Thönmi Sambhota]. I continued my grammatical studies with Khewang Losal Phüntsok by learning the syllable tables of the grammatical treatises. I was only taught up to the half-curve astronomy diagrams and had no one to teach me more. However, the remaining diagrams, both explicit and implicit, as well as grammatical tables implied but not actually taught in the texts, and so on, became easy to understand by being a recipient of the great compassion of my kind lama. *Porthang* divination[688] and the contents of the three-section commentary to the *Arising Letters Tantra* were taught to me by the Lugo astrologer Ngakgi Wangpo.

Apart from these few studies I was not able to fill my mind to satisfaction with a full range of learning in the sciences. However, in the predictions of treasure revealer Drimé Künga it says:

> He with the name of Sangyé Lodrö Rinchen,
> born in the dragon or snake years,
> will compose texts in the horse or sheep year,
> and his own voice will emerge.[689]
> If he is able to overcome obstructions,
> he will complete his life and guide countless beings.[690]

This matches my name and my birth year.[691] Also it seemed that I had a few imprints for composition. Therefore, between the ages of about thirty and forty, using the more accessible scriptural traditions, I undertook various written compositions on the five sciences of grammar, logic, crafts, medicine, and the inner science of Buddhism amounting to twenty volumes. This I did incidental to supervision of the country.

Notwithstanding problems such as my speech defect,[692] I gave daylong explanations, which amounted to six monastic symposiums by today's standards, to congregations consisting of those from our own "Holders of the Yellow Hat" tradition from the three great monastic seats and so on during the consecration of the great reliquary; from the monastic community of Namgyal Phendé Lekshé Ling,[693] who were in service to the Great Fifth; [232] from those of Dorjé Drakpa Ewaṃ Chokgar and Mindröling monasteries[694] of the Nyingma school; to the Sakya monastic community from Yarlung Tashi Tsé Monastery on topics such as the sutra and tantra of their traditions, the three sets of the eight transmitted precepts of the early-translation school, and the Sakya Hevajra tradition.

For seven years at the Great Offering Ceremony,[695] I first gave the transmission and word commentary to the *Wondrous Eon* and, similarly, to the *Destruction of the Four Māras.* As illustrated by the teachings on an enlightened being not needing to purify wrong deeds and accumulate merit, I set about the immediate tasks of the organization and purpose of the offering ceremony itself. I gave teachings on how the master of our doctrine, the great Tsongkhapa, developed the bodhi mind but in reality was a buddha, on the deeds of the Buddha from the moment he first appeared in this world, a word commentary on the *Marvelous Eon* and so on. These became a important tradition for living beings and essential for fulfilling the aspirations that were the purpose of the Great Offering Ceremony itself.

Since the time of the arrival of the Great Sixth in Nyethang, I have given speeches, accessible to those of all walks of life, at important festivities in keeping with the needs of the occasion.

As is made clear in the Sumké constitutional document,[696] I had a great liking for the *pratimokṣa* vows, but apart from the lay-practitioner vows mentioned earlier and the eight daylong vows taken when opportune, they did not come my way.

The Great Fifth granted me outer and inner mandalas of secret mantra and [Guru Chökyi Wangchuk's] *Consummation of Secrets* to ripen my mind. I have completed meditation retreats to the required count on a number of deities and have even received direct signs concerning their progress. Without blame or condemnation from those around me, I spent a not inconsiderable amount of time in the practice of the generation and completion stages in the evenings and early mornings. I have maintained the bodhicitta dedication, keeping to my vow of not taking the life of a human except when powerless to do otherwise. Furthermore, in order to maintain the rule of law when governing the country, I have come close to harming the mind of compassion, but it is difficult to be of help in every case.

In the field of medicine, early on I memorized the three shorter tantras. I can remember Lingtö Chöjé Losang Gyatso distinctly. On the occasions when I saw Jang Ngö Nangso Dargyé up close—such as during the illnesses of my elderly mother, when Sakyong Trinlé Gyatso died, [233] and a few times when I was ill—I observed that he had the tantra quite firmly established in his mind but that he had little knowledge of any other oral instructions and was not someone who practiced clinical medicine. I also knew Mengom Drangyé, who apart from the remedies of the siddhas, for example, did not have an extensive knowledge of medical literature.

Lhaksam, or Sumga, I knew very well. He had only a rough knowledge of the text of the three shorter tantras. His practices were those of the *Vase of Ambrosia,* and he mainly followed the transmitted instructions Tsomé Khenchen, but his knowledge of medical literature was not extensive. Nevertheless, he had great compassion for his patients and worked hard. At times he could be gruff. Otherwise, he lived up to his name[697] and had a good mind toward everyone. As the tantra says, "With the mind of enlightenment holding the welfare of others as most important"; therefore, I think he fulfilled at least one of the six requirements.[698]

By way of the monastic community of Namgyal Phendé Lekshé Ling, by serving the Great Fifth and through the Great Fifth conferring upon him a few ripening practices of entering into mandalas, Darmo Menrampa had a strong and deep bond with the great protector and with me. He helped my great lama with his sight and provided me too with much support. His medical practice was mainly that of the transmitted instructions from the Upper tradition, and by undertaking it with great compassion, his merit in terms of medical practice was very great.

From the age of thirty onward, during those times when I came down with various ailments, and during the times I spent with them prior to that, I became very acquainted with Sumga and Darmo Menrampa. Therefore, incidentally, I saw that their precise identification of medicinal plants and the way they had gained their understanding of the tetxs was quite superficial.

There are other renowned physicians who are like Jetsün Mila's example of the snow mountains: they may be famous, but in matters of identification of plants, the layout of the medical tree, medical practices, and the ability to give extensive teachings on the medical texts, those who carry the responsibility of being elders trained in this medical tradition have very short tongues.

In the works of my great lama, the Supreme Fifth, crown jewel of samsara and nirvana, he says:

> However, with its tongue of erroneous and wayward teachings
> poking out of the hole of the behavior of these degenerate times,
> the poisonous snake that threatens the lives of beings,
> the lord of death disguised as a doctor...[699]

As his words indicate, these are very difficult times. [234] However, from Namgyal Dorjé of the Nya line as described earlier, I necessarily studied the identification of medical plants, the layout of the medical tree, anatomy, and so forth, and except for a few points, I was able to comprehend most of it. For those points I did not understand, I applied myself to a complete and detailed study of the translations of Indian commentaries found in the Tengyur, exemplified by Śūra's *Eight Branches* root text and commentary, as well as indigenous Tibetan commentaries. As a result, even those works I had not previously received word-by-word teachings on arose in my mind. Masters, especially Namgyal Dorjé, were able to clear up questions I had on the text of the Instruction Tantra and resolve doubts I had from other texts. Therefore, though I had initially memorized only the three shorter tantras and did not cultivate the actual words of the unmemorized Instruction Tantra—without which there can be no individual-word recitation examination—nevertheless, all the points of the tantra, especially the difficult points, were planted firmly in my mind.

In this hard-to-gain body of leisure and opportunities composed of six elements, this science pacifies all illness, and by providing the great elixir of physical, verbal, and mental happiness, it is the supreme wealth shared by all. In particular, the *Essence of Ambrosia Secret Instruction Tantra on Eight Branches* is, in the tradition of medical science, the undefiled word of our Teacher, the mighty Buddha, translated by the great lotsāwa Vairocana, and as explained previously, added to and redacted for the Tibetan context by Yuthok Yönten Gönpo, a king among physicians and a combiner of lineages; renowned as the glorious *Four Tantras,* it is the greatest of medical works, precious and prominent like the very peak of a banner of victory. However, with the exception of Jangpa Rikden Namgyal Draksang, Minyima Thongwa Dönden, and Surkhar Dharmaswami, those of the past spoiled this tantra like milk in the marketplace, and it lost its identity. Under the sponsorship of Yargyapa it was redacted by Surkhar Lodrö Gyalpo, who propagated the *Drathang Four Tantras,* as it became known, until its banner hoisted aloft upon the peak of samsara.

My lama the Great Fifth was in reality the omniscient one who ultimately saw all phenomena as many as there are, exactly as they are, as clearly as he would see a berry in the palm of his hand. However, in the eyes of the inferior and as his precious biography makes clear, in the discipline of medicine he memorized the Root, Explanatory, and Final Tantras, and apart from a seemingly superficial study of the outlines and the stone layout, he did not reveal any in-depth knowledge on the subject. [235] As I've already mentioned, I had met Jang Ngö Nangso Dargyé, and he was already advanced in age yet his understanding and ascertainment of the tantra was strong. However, he either did not comprehend the commentaries in great detail or, as the saying goes, "he prefers his father's cup," and so like other ordinary physicians, such as his disciples and entourage, he maintained that the Jang and Sur traditions held different assertions, for example, and made representations to the Great Fifth on the greatness of the Drathang edition of *Four Tantras*. Therefore, in keeping with this view, in the water-tiger year of the eleventh cycle (1662), the Great Fifth organized the woodblock carving of the Drathang edition and composed the print colophons.

However, in the iron-dog year of the same cycle (1670), while I was memorizing the three shorter tantras from the first printings of this new edition, a few thoughts arose in my mind. These were that the belief that the

Jang and Sur traditions held different positions, and so on, came to my great lama while he was busy reprimanding Künga Nyingpo [a.k.a. Tāranātha] of Jonang. Among the ranks of ordinary physicians, the differences in the identification of medical plants was attributable to geography; in terms of medical practices, the Upper and Lower traditions differed little. However, in terms of the primary topics of the literature, any later path depends upon an earlier path, and in that sense there were no differences.

Also the present Drathang tantra had a confusing layout, with many omissions and so forth, and I thought it no longer served as a trustworthy reference. Therefore I felt that the present publication colophon composed in verse and prose was a little excessive.[700] I reported all this in detail to the Great Fifth, and with delight he replied, "I merely accepted what Jang Ngö and others said. However, what you say is true. It would be excellent if you can look at it again, so do it." He therefore gave me permission.

While receiving the Yuthok *Heartdrop* initiation, he placed *Four Tantras* and [Yuthok's] Eighteen Auxiliary Texts upon my head as a blessing, and after he put them in my hands, the passage beginning, "From the minds of the five kinds of beings with their five poisons of ignorance" was recited up to:

> The four sections of this great tantra,
> with the final section making five,
> together with the Eighteen Auxiliary Texts,
> this initiation of every medical text and instruction:
> may it grant the power to understand exactly their meanings.[701]

This was followed by the granting of the mantra, and he beat a *ḍamaru* drum for a long time. At this time the meanings of those points of the text I had memorized earlier whose definitive comprehension had been so difficult, arose in my mind as my path. When the instruction to nourish the tradition of teaching was given, the thought to undertake this task immediately arose vividly in my mind. This was the blessing of great compassion entering my body, speech, and mind; all my deeds in the science of medicine I thought of as being solely the blessed speech of this great being. [236]

These were just thoughts, however, and I was unable to redact and reprint *Four Tantras* at that particular time. Later I concentrated my thoughts on this undertaking when beginning to write the *Blue Beryl* commentary. I had definitive reference works on tastes, powers, post-digestive tastes, natures, etymologies, and functions of medicines; I had been unable to memorize the Instruction Tantra, treat patients, and so on; and aside from the identification of plants, the channels, anatomy, and so on, restrictions on my time meant that I had not been able to devote much time to the great masters, and it was going to be difficult to undertaking this properly. Nevertheless, I diligently consulted the following important works:

- Various tantras, including the *Kālacakra, Vajraḍāka,* and *Ḍāka Ocean Tantra*
- Sutras, including *Sutra of Golden Light* and *Heap of Jewels Sutra*
- Vinaya texts, such as *Basic Vinaya* and *Short Vinaya*
- Works on Abhidharma, such as [Vasubandhu's] *Abhidharmakośa* and [Maudgalyāyana's] *Cause Terminology* and *Karma Terminology*
- Indian translations, such as [Pitṛceṭa's] *Treatise of Eight Branches,* its autocommentary, [Candranandana's] *Moonlight,* [Nāgārjuna's] *Hundred Medical Preparations,* [Ravigupta's] *Essential Medical Siddha,* [Nāgārjuna's] *Sutra of Life,* and [Bhalipa's] *Treatise on Mercury Preparation*
- Translations from Chinese, such as the *Somarāja*
- Shangshung translations exemplified by *Universal Emperor Compilation*
- Works from the early-translation Vajrayana lineages of Treasure and Transmission, such as the *Seven Ambrosia Fasicles,* the *Supreme Ambrosia Scriptures,* [Dorbum Chökyi Drakpa's] *Vase of Ambrosia,* and [Surkhar Lodrö Gyalpo's] *Clear Crystal Vase*
- Early Tibetan works, such as *Biji's Yellow Collection,*[702] *Illuminating Lamp of Thirty Instructions,* the great and lesser *Essence of Ambrosia,* the *Magic Key on the Difficult Fortress Path, Four Branches,* and the Eighteen Auxiliary Texts
- Many commentaries on the Root, Explanatory, and Final Tantras and other related works (nobody qualified to write a word-by-word commentary on the Instruction Tantra text has seriously appeared); Later Yuthok's *Golden Annotations* together with his *Copper Annotations* and *Explicit Annotations; Compositions for My Sons;* the "well-worn copy"[703] of the *Four Tantras;* the old Surkhar Gamnang edition of *Four Tantras; Fulfilling All Needs and Wishes*[704] by a great scholar of the Jang tradition; and others
- Other editions of *Four Tantras:* these include the Dzong Ga edition, a publication sponsored by Tri Sönam Dé—an incarnation of Mutri Tsenpo in Khung Dzong Karpo in the Gungthang district of Mangyül—that was undertaken by the monk Rinchen Palsang and

edited by himself along with the Awa monk Tashi, Chöjé Künga Gyen, and Rapjampa Chödé; the Gampo edition undertaken by Norbu Gyenpa (1589–1633) of [Daklha] Gampo, which was requested and edited by the physician Döndrup; the Takten edition undertaken by Jetsün Künga Nyingpo in Takten Monastery, [237] completed by his nephew Künga Gyaltsen, and edited by the master physician Tsojé Shönu Sö of Lhündrup Ding, also known as Dütsi Gyurmé, of the previously flourishing Nya family; and finally the Bodong edition
- Old handwritten manuscripts, copies of the chapters, and miscellaneous other works

In short, I studied assiduously, and with no shortcuts, almost every renowned medical text, both great and small, in this snow mountain land. In particular, I used the old Surkhar Gamnang edition of the tantra and the Chakdrekma copy as two fundamental reference works. In the Drathang *Four Tantras,* wherever there were missing words and so forth and this was replicated in the old texts, I used my own reasoning. For example, sometimes the number of divisions in the summary sections was incomplete; the remedies were omitted from the teachings on symptoms of illness; there was confusion in the outlines, and so forth; and there were incorrect and misspelled words. These I determined not with superficial inventions from my own mind but with sound scripture and reasoning. I also clarified archaic and difficult-to-understand terms. In this way, correcting and revising the tantra and publishing it opened the gateway to an unending offering of Dharma.

Composition of Blue Beryl and other works

Similarly, having turned onto the right path those who for a while had wandered off and those treading the wrong path, I began composing my commentary to *Four Tantras* called *Ornament to the Mind of Medicine Buddha: Blue Beryl Lamp Illuminating Four Tantras,* with about 1,200 pages.

Geshé Chakpa Chöphel had a greater ability to memorize than others, and so he was encouraged to memorize the tantra. Being continually distracted by affairs of state, I feared that I would lose what had been memorized, and so up to then any work had been in draft form like chalk on a writing board, and I had been unable to make any reliable redaction of the tantras. However, now I was able to supplement the words of the Root, Explanatory, and Final Tantras as well as the Instruction Tantra.

As a way for everyone from the scholar to the child to easily understand the entire meaning of the above as clearly as seeing a berry in the palm of one's hand, I commissioned a collection of medical paintings, something never before accomplished:[705] [238]

1. The first painting depicts the introduction to the first chapter of the Root Tantra. In the center of the manifested location of the medical forest and medical city, on the mountains endowed with the powers and the medicinal plants that act as effective remedies to hot, cold, simple, and complex disorders, is the celestial mansion of the external city of Sudarśana. Inside, endowed with the five perfections,[706] sits the teacher, Medicine Buddha, the king of beryl light. The five rishi brothers—whose natures are the mirror-like gnosis of purified ignorance, the emptiness gnosis of purified anger, the equality gnosis of purified pride, the analysis gnosis of purified desire, and the accomplishment gnosis of purified jealousy—teach the tantra to the assembled audience of Buddhists and non-Buddhists in the form of requestor and receiver. The painting is accompanied by a written description.
2. The second painting shows the emanation of Vidyājñāna and Manasija described in the second chapter of the Root Tantra. It also shows the third chapter's description of the two trunks of balanced and imbalanced humors arising from a single root—the condition of the body—as the basis of illness. From the first trunk arise the three branches of the humors, bodily constituents, and waste products. These branches together have twenty-five leaves. The second trunk has nine branches. These are: causes and circumstances, entrances, locations, pathways, times of arising, results, reaction imbalances,[707] and categories. These branches contain sixty-three leaves. In total the branches together have eighty-eight leaves. The flowers are those of good health and long life. They produce the fruits of Dharma, wealth and fortune, and happiness, represented by the depiction of the aggregates dissolving into the enlightened form.
3. The third painting shows the root of diagnosis producing the three trunks of observation, palpation, and questioning. The observation trunk has branches of the tongue and the urine, each branch having three leaves. The trunk of palpation has branches of wind, bile, and phlegm, each producing one leaf. The trunk of questioning also has

branches of wind, bile, and phlegm. On this trunk the wind branch has eleven leaves, the bile branch seven, and the phlegm branch eleven, making twenty-nine leaves in total. Therefore, there are three trunks, eight branches, and thirty-eight leaves.

4. The fourth shows the methods-of-treatment root with four trunks: diet, behavior, medication, and therapies. The *diet trunk* has six branches made up of food and drink corresponding to each of the three humors. The wind-food branch has ten leaves, the wind-drink branch four. The bile-food branch has seven leaves, the bile-drink branch five. The phlegm-food branch has six leaves, the phlegm-drink branch has three. This makes thirty-five leaves in total. The *behavior trunk* has three branches corresponding to the three humors, each branch having two leaves, six in total. The *medication trunk* has fifteen branches spread among those of taste, powers, pacification, and cleansing. [239] There are eighteen leaves of tastes and powers divided among the three humors, twenty-three leaves on the pacification branch, and nine leaves on the cleansing branch, making fifty leaves in all. The fourth or *therapies trunk* has three branches corresponding to the three humors and seven leaves. In total this root has four trunks, twenty-seven branches, and ninety-eight leaves. This painting also shows Vidyājñāna dissolving back into the heart of Medicine Buddha.

These are the four paintings depicting the Root or Mind Tantra.

5. The fifth painting depicts the emanation of Rishi Vidyājñāna described in the first chapter of the Explanatory Tantra and the formation of the body described in the second.
6. The circulatory system from the front as taught in the Explanatory Tantra and according to the tradition of Lhündrup Ding.
7. The posterior view of the same circulatory system.
8. Similes of the body as taught in the third chapter, and the quantities of bodily constituents in men and women up to the quantity of menstrual blood taught at the beginning of the fourth.
9. The ninth painting continues from the previous textual depiction and shows the description of the bone structure up to the three-and-a-half-cubit dimension of a poorly formed body.
10. The posterior view of the above.

11. The circulatory system of formation, existence, and connecting channels according to our own tradition.
12. The posterior view of the above.
13. The channels dividing up into 360 minor channels.
14. The anterior view of the network of a further division of minor channels throughout the body, the life channels,[708] and the bloodletting channels according to the Surkhar tradition.
15. The white water channels[709] running down from the brain and its connections to the outer channels.
16. An anterior view of the vulnerable points, from those of the flesh up to the textual description of the orifices.
17. Posterior view of the above.
18. A wonderful synopsis of the fifth chapter of the Explanatory Tantra, a classification by gender and by humor from the sixth chapter, and various signs from the seventh chapter, with supplementary material from Candranandana's *Moonlight.*
19. The seventh chapter's description of the omens seen by the doctor on his way to meet a patient, beginning from the auspicious sign of a full container of grain; supplemented by Candranandana's *Moonlight* on signs in dreams and descriptions of how dreams enter the mind.
20. Dreams auspicious for good health and long life, beginning with dreams of Brahmā up to the reversal of the signs of imminent death.
21. A wonderful synopsis of the eighth, ninth, tenth, eleventh, and twelfth chapters.
22. The thirteenth, fourteenth, and fifteenth chapters.
23. The wholesome diet taught in the sixteenth chapter, from rice up to light soup.
24. Wholesome diets starting from barley-beer stew in the section on prepared foods, up to the way food becomes poisonous explained in the seventeenth chapter on dietary rules, and including a synopsis of the eighteenth chapter.
25. A depiction of how medicines are formed from the five elements as taught in the nineteenth chapter and a depiction of medicines for the elimination of single-type disorders up to female stones from the twentieth chapter.
26. Single-type disorder medicines from golden sand up to the Indian bdellium tree.
27. Individual capability of medicines from pine resin up to gold spot. [240]

28. Individual capability of medicines from silver spot up to the *mṛdu* vine.
29. Individual capability of medicines from wickweed to angelica.
30. Individual capability of medicines from bull angelica to gecko lizard.
31. Supplementary material on the individual capability of medicines from banded agate to wild goosefoot.
32. Supplementary material on the individual capability of medicines from red goosefoot to black aconite.
33. Supplementary material on the individual capability of medicines starting from blue aconite and concluding with medicinal honey.
34. Standard cures for fevers from camphor to Sanchal salt, as taught in the twenty-first chapter.
35. The thirty-fifth painting continues the twenty-first chapter from onion and garlic up to Himalayan rhubarb, completing the chapter.
36. Medical instruments described in the twenty-second chapter.
37. The twenty-third chapter's teaching on good health, the twenty-fourth's on actual examination, the twenty-fifth's examination by guile, the twenty-sixth's examination of the criteria for accepting or rejecting a patient, the twenty-seventh's approaches to healing, and the twenty-eighth's specific medical tests.
38. Actual treatments as described in the twenty-ninth and thirtieth chapters.
39. The duties of the physician described in the thirty-first chapter, and Vidyājñāna dissolving into Medicine Buddha's crown.

Therefore, the Explanatory or Body Tantra is depicted by thirty-five paintings.

40. A depiction of the manner in which the Instruction Tantra was delivered, and an anterior view of the bloodletting, surgery, and cauterization points from the first to the ninety-second chapters.
41. Posterior view of the above.
42. Causes of wind disorders taught in the second chapter up to the causes of tumors described in the seventh.
43. Causes of anemic dropsy from the eighth chapter up to the causes of developed fever from the sixteenth.
44. The causes of empty fever from the seventeenth chapter up to causes of contagious fever from the twenty-third.

45. The causes of poxes from the twenty-fourth chapter up to the causes of male genital disorders from the forty-second.
46. The causes of female genital disorders from the forty-third chapter up to the causes of hemorrhoids from the sixty-fourth.
47. The causes of erysipelas from the sixty-fifth chapter up to the causes of demonic illnesses in children from the seventy-third chapter.
48. Causes of gynecological disorder from the seventy-fourth chapter up to causes of wounds from the eighty-second.
49. Anterior view of the channel-system grid for all relevant chapters of the Instruction Tantra and the cranial types described in the eighty-third chapter.
50. Posterior view of the above channel-system grid and head wounds described in the eighty-third chapter up to wounds on the limbs from the eighty-sixth.
51. From the eighty-fifth chapter, the anatomical grid of the trunk along with its vulnerable points.
52. Grid of the purulence locations within the trunk from the eighty-fifth chapter.
53. The compound poisons of the eighty-seventh chapter, and the food and natural poisons of the eighty-eighth and eighty-ninth chapters. [241]
54. The great elixir rejuvenation from the ninetieth chapter,
55. The lesser elixir rejuvenation from the ninetieth chapter and the causes and conditions for the topics of the ninety-first and ninety-second chapters.

Therefore, the Enlightened Qualities or Instruction Tantra is depicted by sixteen paintings.

56. The exposition of the Final Tantra, up to the movement of the spleen pulse in the late winter month in the seventh topic on pulse correspondence to the seasons and five elements.[710]
57. The movement chart of the seasons from the seventh topic of the pulse section up to pulse divination for victory over an enemy from the eighth topic.[711]
58. The quivering-liver pulse in the friend pulse description from the seven wonderful pulses of the eighth topic up to the causes of spirit affliction based upon the wood-element pulse.
59. Heart-pulse spirit affliction up to those of the spleen pulse of spring.

60. Spirit affliction in the lung pulse of spring up to examination of the pulses of mother and daughter in the substitution pulse diagnosis.[712]
61. Examination of the wife's pulse when the husband is sick in substitution pulse diagnosis from the eighth topic on the wonderful pulses up to the incomplete pulse of the natural pulse.
62. The elements of the months, days, and hours up to the tenth topic on the impossibility of hot and cold disorders occurring simultaneously in both the upper and lower body.
63. The death pulse in wind disorders from the eleventh topic of the pulse diagnosis chapter up to the section on provision for feast offerings and the practice of giving and offering as described in the twelfth topic on spirit pulses.
64. Examination of lifespan from the life-essence[713] pulse from the pulse diagnosis chapter up to the manner in which food and drink become urine as described in the second chapter of the Final Tantra.[714]
65. The section on the urine of a healthy person up to the *Somarāja* description of the colors of urine and the tantra's description of the way urine containing undigested butter suggests a cold disorder.
66. Indications of nondigestion described in the *Somarāja,* the three turtle diagrams for male and females in the urine indications of spirit possession section, and depictions of the harms of the nine types of spirit.
67. From the Urine Analysis chapter, identifying the nine harmful spirits, starting with the black-brown spirits, up to the *Somarāja* descriptions of urine divination.
68. Divination from urine vapor as taught in the *Somarāja,* and Jinamitra's and Yuthok's method of examination and ways to read unchanging urine.
69. Examination of the tongue from chapter 2 up to unsuitable conditions for medicinal oil therapy described in chapter 13.
70. Proper conditions for purgatives described in chapter 17 up to improper conditions for suppositories taught in chapter 17.
71. Improper conditions for enemas from the eighteenth chapter up to wind and blood-bile disorders as improper conditions for bloodletting in the twentieth.
72. The seventy-seven or seventy-nine bloodletting channels of chapter 20 together with the summary, and cauterization as taught in chapter 21. [242]

73. Anterior and posterior views of cauterization points taught in chapter 21 up to those of minor surgery explained in chapter 25.
74. Anterior view of cauterization points using supplementary material described in *Somarāja.*
75. Posterior view of the above.
76. Fomentation compress described in chapter 22 and minor surgery from chapter 25.
77. The concluding teachings from chapter 26 up to the "imputed" curable spirit ailments from chapter 27.
78. The "real" but curable illnesses up to "the vase of ambrosia resurrecting the dead."
79. Discussion of the secrecy or preciousness of the tantra in chapter 27 from the example of lion's milk,[715] and the depiction of the doctor becoming a buddha by dissolving into the enlightened body. Vidyājñāna absorbs into the secret place of the Buddha, Manasija absorbs into his tongue.

The Final or Enlightened Activities Tantra is depicted by twenty-four paintings. There are seventy-nine paintings in all.

I have gone to great lengths to acquire prime-quality medicines that are not produced by most doctors because of the rarity of good ingredients in this cold country. I have also newly created surgical instruments exactly as described in the texts without regard to the difficulties and shortage of necessary tools.

Because the Instruction Tantra reads very clearly, I had doubts about composing the supplement to it called *Camphor to Cool the Burning Torment of Pain: A Sword to Cut the Noose of Untimely Death.* However the Instruction Tantra has vital importance for medical practice and there were concerns about the one-to-one transmission of its core instruction being weakened, and I received clear omens that it would be beneficial to do so. When I was beginning this work, all that needed to be organized fell effortlessly into place. Among the omens, well-formed medical plants that had never previously grown in Tibet, such as the castor oil plant—which cured the illness of the middle-floor temple keeper of the Trülnang Lhasa temple[716]—were delivered to me. A few days before beginning, whether some medicine was being prepared the day before I cannot say, but the aroma of medicine pervaded the area, and illnesses such as *beké* subsided. Many such auspicious signs appeared.

The trained lineage physician Lhünding Namgyal Dorjé posted questions on the Rasa[717] stone pillar addressed to doctors in the area on the subject of the capacities of various medicines. He received no real answers to his questions, only those devoid of substance and resembling the ramblings of children. Therefore I composed *Answers to the Questions: The Arrow of Arjuna that Illuminates the True Flight.* [243]

I also composed many other short works on the science of medicine. These include one in response to queries on *Blue Beryl* expressed by Ngawang Palden, a maintainer of the medical tradition from Mindröling, and another to refute the errors in medicine and astronomy made by Tibetan Scholar Mipham Gelek,[718] who composed some reliable works on poetry, and who appeared to be someone who lived up to his title in the field of general knowledge, but who composed a few works only because he knew how to read, write, and string words together. [245]

Part 4

THE STUDY OF MEDICINE AND THE THREE SETS OF VOWS

19. The Reason to Practice Medicine

As a practice of purification and merit accumulation focused on the form of my kind root lama, the Great Fifth, I made one hundred thousand circumambulations of Jowo Śākyamuni from the Lhasa Barkor, the inner circumambulation path. After I had completed this practice I went to the Lingkor outer path in the manner of laying a stone at the Jorak shrine.[719] In the afternoon I went on a pilgrimage to Chakha Mountain.[720] I arrived at its summit—and although the early texts describe it as the exalted mountain of Vajrapāṇi, shaped like a lion leaping into the sky, to my mind, from its three and four sides,[721] I thought it looked just like the manifested city of Sudarśana—and some astonishing sights occurred. The Lhünding Ganden chief physician was sent to inspect the sides of the mountain and discovered they possessed hot and cold powers, corresponding perfectly with the sunny and shady sides, as well as many medicinal plants of these powers that no one knew were growing there.

This was one condition for the construction of the Chakri Medical College. Other reasons were to fulfill the hopes of my lama, the Great Fifth, who had instituted the Sorik Drophen Ling medical school to the west of Drepung but which fell into ruin and was no longer in operation. Also, as stated previously, the science of medicine has become the twin of the moon on the third day of the month.[722] Moreover, the five degenerations generally increase over time. The *Sutra of Going Forth* says:

> The lifespan of humans will decline. When it falls below five hundred, the five degenerations will predominate. These are the degenerations of lifespan, of mental afflictions, of living beings, of views, and of the times.[723]

Many other texts including the *Vinaya* speak similarly. In the medical literature also:

When the five hundred years of the end of time arrives,[724]
human behavior will degenerate under the control of desire,
practitioners of tantra will destroy the internal vajra bonds,
monastic communities bring about sectarian troubles,
heretics, Buddhists, and Bönpos will cast curses,
living beings will break their words, fight, and turn to butchery;[725]
at that time the *mātṛkā* and ḍākinīs will be disturbed,
and from the clouds of disease formed from their breath
will come Nepali illness, *gyuser, gaklhok,* and poxes.[726]

Therefore, sentient beings live in fear of the sufferings brought on by the many kinds of illness, and the science of medicine, as stated previously, is superior to other sciences in giving protection from these fears.

Furthermore, the *Sutra of Golden Light* says:

I have taught you how to cure disease.
If through this you heal living beings,
You will gain the greatest of fruits.[727]

In the sixth chapter of the Root Tantra it says:

Ripening into the fruits of Dharma, wealth, and happiness.[728]

In the thirty-first chapter of the Explanatory Tantra:

The fruits for the doctor are temporary and permanent.
The temporary is happiness in this life,
power, wealth, and joy.[729]

Also:

As for the permanent results:
having abandoned pretense and desire,
one engages in healing the sick
and walks the path to buddhahood.
This the king of physicians has said.[730] [246]

In the *Caraka* it says:

The fruits of such work
are temporary and ultimate.[731]

The great ācārya, the glorious Śūra, says in the later *Eight Branches:*

Abandoning pretense, devoid of desire,
those who engage the science of healing
will gain the fruit of becoming the supreme doctor.[732]

Yuthok Gönpo says in his *Quintessence:*

In this life: fortune and respect,
wealth and happiness in fame,
all accomplished without effort—
these are the results of practicing medicine.[733]

Therefore, one reason for practicing medicine is that it will accomplish your wishes in this and future lives. For accomplishing the welfare of others, in which living beings are held as supreme, it is able to relieve this human body of the sufferings of birth, old age, sickness, and death. For example, "Birth will come quickly and easily, without danger,"[734] and so on, thereby describing practices for relieving the sufferings of birth. Also:

The body with its signs of aging,
its sixteen kinds of decline,
(will develop the agility of the lion,
the strength of a bull,)[735] the sheen of a peacock,
and become sprightly like the best of horses,
with a lifespan to rival the sun and moon.[736]

This is from a section on rejuvenation procedures. Also:

In this way the ninety-eight techniques of healing,
if relied upon single-mindedly, with effort and respect,
will rescue you from the great swamp of disease.[737]

Further:

> A great warrior defeating the enemy of disease.[738]

These indicate the power of the science of medicine to pacify all illnesses, which are illustrated by the 404 types. Also:

> Protector of life, granter of fearlessness,
> vase of ambrosia, lifting one from death.[739]

This illustrates its ability to protect from the fear of untimely death.

Furthermore, Śūra in his *Eight Branches* says:

> Medicine is the hand lifting one from the swamp of disease.[740]

Caraka states:

> The eight branches of medicine, like a boat in the great sea,
> quickly rescues those from the great waves of unceasing illness.[741]

Nāgārjuna says:

> Targeted medical practices
> empty the ocean of disease.[742]

Therefore, through the practice of medicine, the bodhisattva will accomplish the welfare of others in accordance with his prayers. This is also a reason for practicing medicine. In *Engaging in the Practices of the Bodhisattva* it says:

> For all beings that are sick,
> may I, until they are all healed,
> be their medicine, doctor, and nurse.[743]

The scholar Kyegui Pal[744] also says: [247]

> In every realm of the ten directions
> may there be medicine, doctors, and nurses,
> suitable food, drink, and every provision.[745]

20. Devotion to a Master

THEREFORE, THE VALUE of the science of medicine is that it accomplishes the welfare of self and others. Therefore, whether they wish to become doctors and practice the science of healing or practitioners of the sacred Dharma of sutra and tantra, the essential inner science, students and practitioners of all sciences should seek out both a teacher and a master. The *Array of Trunks Sutra* says:

> Son of the lineage, in order to accumulate great virtue, do not be discouraged in seeking out the spiritual friend, never tire of seeing him, and never be sated in questioning him. Held by him you will not fall to the lower realms, turn away from the Mahayana, or run contrary to its practices. Therefore, put him in your mind and remain constantly in his presence.[746]

The *Bodhisattva Basket of Scripture* says:

> In short, acquiring and perfecting the activities of the bodhisattva, acquiring and perfecting the perfections, the levels, the forbearances, the meditative concentrations, clairvoyance, the *dhāraṇī* retentions, the types of confidence, the dedications, the prayers, and the phenomena of enlightenment all depend upon a guru. The guru is their root cause. From a guru they arise. From a guru they find their birth and their development. They are produced by a guru, increased by a guru. On a guru they rely. The guru is the cause.[747]

Gopadatta says:

> As the sick depend upon the doctor,
> so the wise rely upon a guru from the start.

> To cure their illness the patient earnestly attends
> to the doctor regarding the taking of medicine.
> Likewise, attend to the Dharma of the gurus.
> As the intelligent patient diligently follows
> the treatment exactly as explained,
> the wise by doing likewise will gain deathlessness,
> and by drinking of this ambrosia
> will attain the supreme.[748]

Therefore, the spiritual friend or guru and the fully qualified master of tantra are objects of great reverence. In particular, irrespective of which science you study, it is imperative you rely upon someone with experience and mastery of the subject. If this advice is not heeded, and you mix book study with your own made-up ideas, and so on, you will lack the continuum of the blessings of the Dharma, [248] and you will not be able to comprehend fully the meanings of those texts with profound, implicit, and deliberately veiled meanings. In his *Shoots of Wisdom* Nāgārjuna states:

> The study of great works of knowledge
> undertaken without the tutelage of teachers
> makes you repugnant in society,
> like a pregnant whore.[749]

The teachings of King Indrabodhi also say:

> Without the boatman you cannot cross the river.
> Without the guru, though you possess great qualities,
> there is no freedom from samsara.[750]

But what is the mark of a guru or master? The best gurus are the buddhas or bodhisattvas, who manifest in various forms for the benefit of disciples. The next best are those who have directly perceived the nature of reality. Otherwise, the minimum qualifications for an ordinary being is expressed in the *Kālacakra Root Tantra:*

> Stable, disciplined, and intelligent,
> patient, honest, and free from deception,
> knows mantra and the yogas of tantra,

is compassionate, wise in the treatises,
knows well the ten activities,
is wise in drawing mandalas,
a master skilled in explaining tantra,
of great faith with senses tamed.[751]

"Honest" is explained[752] to mean "abiding with an exceptionally kind and honest attitude toward living beings." The mind must be well trained by the discipline of bodhicitta. Without it one of the most important qualifications of a vajra master is missing.

"Knows mantra and the yogas of tantra" is rendered in the *Commentary on the Illusory Net Tantra* as "knows the yogas of the secret mantra tantras,"[753] and is explained by the author, Ānandagarbha, as referring to the ability to thwart hindrances by the yogas of mantra and medicine. In the *Commentary to the Vajraḍāka Tantra:*

> "Mantra" refers to the eight lines, and so forth. "Tantra" refers to medicine. "Yogas" refers to practices. "Knows" means skilled.[754]

Therefore, by using mantras and substances, he knows how to accomplish a host of actions by way of the four feats of pacifying, increasing, controlling, and wrath. However, if these are not mastered, he may have developed general insights on the path and be skilled in the preparation of rituals and so forth, but he still lacks the particular quality of a vajra master.

The *Vajrapañjara Tantra* explains "wise in the treatises" as "wise in all the sciences,"[755] [249] and therefore you have to know the inner science and with it the three baskets of scripture and so on. Therefore, holding yourself to be a vajra master yet not knowing any of the baskets of scripture is to be an ass posing as a lion.

The "ten activities" are explained in the last chapter of the *Ornament of Vajra Essence Tantra:*

The two rituals for repelling,
the secret and wisdom knowledge empowerments,
the ritual of separating, the ritual food,
vajra recitation, the ritual of wrathful expression,
consecration, and mandala meditation:
these are the ten secret activities.

Mandala, meditative concentration, mudrā,
standing posture, seated posture, recitation,
the fire ritual, offering, activity yoga, and concluding:
these are the ten outer activities.[756]

Therefore, ten inner and ten outer activities are taught. Vajra masters of the lower classes of tantra should know the ten outer activities. Vajra masters of the highest tantras should also know the ten inner activities. An explanation of these activities would be too much, and so their explanations should be sought elsewhere.

Also, in the eighth chapter of the *Vajrapañjara Tantra* it says:

Lo! Mantra taught by the qualified vajra master
will grow within the practitioner.
A guru who is stable, possessed of profound Dharmas,
who is wise in all the sciences,
knows the fire offerings, the mandalas, and the mantras,
has perfected the art of consecration and the ritual food,
possesses knowledge of the ten activities,
guards with the conduct of the śrāvakas
while revering the stages of the mantra vehicle,
whose form is a joy to behold,
who is skilled in the drawing of mandalas
and has completed the mantra repetitions
and vanquished all root downfalls,
who brings happiness and welfare to the world
through the great yogas of mantra and tantra:
when such a guru has materialized
let no one disparage him.[757]

In particular, the requirement that the guru not possess any of the root downfalls, as pointed out above and expressed also in the *Saṃvarodaya Tantra,*[758] is indispensable. The line "guarding with the conduct of the śrāvakas" illustrates the same point made in the *Vajra Garland Tantra,*[759] in the section on the qualifications of the vajra master, where it states that outwardly one holds the conduct of the *pratimokṣa* while inwardly delighting in the Guhyasamāja. Therefore, pure *pratimokṣa* conduct in keeping with the Vinaya is essential. [250] "Outwardly" refers to physical behavior while "inwardly" refers to the mind. These terms do not mean outside and inside one's dwelling.

"Completed the mantra repetitions" means having completed the required deity-yoga meditation commitment.[760] Moreover, it is taught that he who gives empowerments, performs consecration rituals, and so on without having completed the required deity-yoga meditation commitment harms himself. In the *Essentials of the Mandala Rite of the Four-Seat Tantra* it says:

> The vajra master of the supreme mandala
> has first completed the deity-yoga meditation
> and then, with mind completely trained,
> turns his attention to the mandala.
> If the deity has not been pleased, however,
> you will be rejected.[761]

Kṛṣṇacarya also said that if the deity has not been pleased by your deity-yoga meditation, you will be rejected.[762] The *Vajra Garland Mandala Rites* states:

> With a knowledge of the path to omniscience,
> first gather merit through deity-yoga meditation,
> weaken and destroy the hindrances.
> With no deity-yoga meditation there are no *siddhis*.
> Therefore, know well the two stages, live well in isolation,
> and meditate upon the deity assembly.
> When tired, repeat the deity's secret mantras.
> Repeat a hundred thousand of the principal deity,
> or a hundred thousand of one's own deity,
> and ten thousand of the mandala residents,
> This is prerequisite deity-yoga meditation.[763]

The *Vajra Garland Mandala Rites* also says:

> In this way, having comprehensively undertaken the prerequisite deity-yoga meditation, you will be able to instantaneously generate and withdraw the deity assembly of the mandala, complete in every aspect. Therefore, either because it has not been

> forbidden by the possessors of the mandala or because you have earned permission through your accumulation of merit, you can meditate on the mandala, perform consecration, gather disciples, and so on.[764]

On this point, the *Mañjuśrī Root Tantra,* [Jagaddarpaṇa's] *Kriyāsamuccaya,* the *Consecration Tantra, Ornament of Vajra Essence Tantra, Vajra Garland Tantra, Illusory Net Tantra,* and other tantras are mostly in agreement, although the wording is often different.

In early translation secret mantra, the Vajra Vehicle deity-yoga meditation is said to be of three kinds. These are the completion of "activity" deity yogas based on length of time and mantra count and, particularly, the requirement of a proper "close" deity yoga before undertaking any of the tantric activities.[765] Therefore, it can be understood that thorough familiarity with the yoga of the deity of the mandala [251] you are initiating disciples into—having at minimum completed a deity-yoga retreat with the required number of mantra repetitions—is an essential requirement for being a qualified vajra master.

From the point of view of the Sutra Vehicle, the glorious Nāgārjuna has said:

> Content, compassionate, moral,
> with the intelligence to dispel the afflictions—
> rely upon such beings;
> knowing this, honor and revere them.[766]

Candragomin says:

> Take them from a guru who abides in his vows,
> is wise, and has great ability.[767]

In *Engaging in the Practices of the Bodhisattva* it states:

> Never will I, though it may cost my life,
> give up the spiritual friend wise in the Mahayana
> and possessed of the supreme bodhisattva conduct.[768]

The *Commentary on Four Hundred Verses* says:

> The guru who knows the minds of disciples
> and is capable of caring for them
> should gather disciples;
> the ignorant should not collect disciples.[769]

Vinaya Light states:

> Those who are possessed of ethics,
> who know the rituals of Vinaya,
> who have compassion for the sick,
> whose entourage is without blemish,
> who are enthusiastic in benefiting
> with Dharma and with worldly goods,
> who teach at the right time,
> they are commended as gurus.[770]

The first chapter of *Ornament of Realization* says:

> With mind not discouraged and so forth,
> who teaches no nature and so on
> and dispels its opposing forces,
> is in all respects a guide and protector.[771]

There are many similar citations, but they can be summarized by the verse in the *Ornament of Mahayana Sutras:*

> Rely upon a spiritual friend who is disciplined,
> pacified, well pacified, of exceptional qualities,
> who has perseverance, is rich in scripture,
> has insight into reality, is wise in words, is of a compassionate nature,
> and who has put all discouragement behind him.[772]

Because he has ethics he is disciplined. Because he has meditative concentration he is pacified. Because he possesses wisdom he has well pacified the mental afflictions. Because his qualities are higher than others they are exceptional. Because he shows no laziness in working for others he has perseverance. Because of his great learning he is rich in scripture. He has gained insight into the nature of reality. He has great skill in speaking. He has a compassion that does not look to worldly gain. In teaching Dharma he is never discouraged. These are the ten qualities of a guru. Alternatively, he has the following five qualities:

> The bodhisattva has much learning,
> sees the truth, is wise in words,
> has compassion, is not discouraged;
> such a holy one is truly a great being.[773]

By his quality of knowing scripture he has much learning. By his quality of insight he sees the truth. [252] He is skilled in speaking. In his thoughts he has the compassion that does not turn to worldly gain. In thought and deed he is not lazy and so is never discouraged. Also:

> Vast, dispels doubt,
> worthy of regard, teaches two realities:
> this the perfect teacher of bodhisattvas.[774]

Being very learned he has vast learning. Because of his great wisdom he dispels the doubts of disciples. Because he is virtuous in word, deed, and thought, he is worthy of being regarded as a guru. He teaches the reality of the afflictions and the path of liberation.

These qualities are mostly found in ārya beings and so are difficult to find. However, there are three qualities that are essential: the wisdom of a scholar, an attitude of compassion, and activities endowed with patience. The first of these means being wise in the topic one is teaching and wise in the art of teaching itself. Wise in the topic means that its explanation possesses the support of scripture, reasoning, and oral tradition, by which one has the ability to remove the doubts of disciples. Being wise in the art of teaching means using clear and correct grammar and language; staying relevant to the topic at hand; teaching at a suitable depth and duration; and ensuring your words have relevance by evaluating them with the three criteria.[775] Moreover, the delivery should be elegant and inspiring, bringing joy to others.

Alternatively, the wisdom of a scholar here could mean being free from the eleven faults taught in the *Science of Explanation,*[776] or from the eight faults of teaching listed in *Ornament of Mahayana Sutras:*

> Lazy, unintelligible,
> not beginning the teaching at the correct point,

unsure, unable to dispel doubts,
unable to instill certainty[777]
though teaching without doubt,
becomes bored with teaching,
is miserly in teaching Dharma:
these are the faults of speech.[778]

This quality could also refer to being free from the eleven faults taught in the *Science of Explanation,* where it means being wise concerning the three types of behavior in yourself and the disciples, likened to the three types of containers.[779]

The second essential quality of a teacher is compassionate mind. In the *Mañjuśrī Manifestation Sutra:*

> To teach but with no compassion for the listeners is the work of Māra.[780]

The third quality, being endowed with patience, means not being discouraged by the hardships and fatigue experienced while teaching, and being patient with disciples' questions and the arguments of others. These three qualities are essential requirements.

Generally, the concept of the spiritual friend possessed of all excellent qualities found primarily in the inner, principal science of Buddhism can also apply to the other sciences. Daṇḍin talks of "being learned and without blemish,"[781] echoing the criteria discussed above. Here in medicine we talk of the six qualities needed to be a physician, as mentioned previously. Thumi Sambhota in his *Thirty Verses* says:

Listen to the texts from the lamas;
hold them as your masters.[782] [253]

Therefore, in whatever subject they are teaching, masters who teach should be regarded as spiritual friends.

21. The Pratimokṣa Vows

The three sets of vows

IN CONNECTION with such a person, the *Prophecy of Bhadra Māyākāra Sutra* from the twenty-first volume of the *Heap of Jewels* collection says:

> Bhadra, these four provide for the purity of bodhisattva practice. What are they? They are the purity of the three vows, the pure place, a pure wisdom, and a pure birth.[783]

On this topic Sakya Paṇḍita Künga Gyaltsen wrote:

> For the faithful who wish to practice
> in accord with the words of the Buddha,
> I will explain the three divisions of vows.[784]

All buddhas teach the Dharma in accordance with disciples' mental faculties and dispositions. For those disciples attracted to the lower paths, the lower-vehicle wheels of Dharma were turned by way of teachings on conduct free of desire. All these turnings teach the foundation practice of the exceptional training in ethics—encapsulated in the *pratimokṣa* vows of liberation, the very root of all good qualities—and the two practices that form the actual means to liberation. These are the exceptional training in concentration, encapsulated in the practices for developing *śamatha* quiescence, and the exceptional training in wisdom, encapsulated in the practices for developing *vipaśyanā* exceptional insight.

For those disciples disposed to the vast practices, the Perfection wheel of the Mahayana was turned. This turning taught the foundation practice of developing bodhicitta and the bodhicitta vows—the very root of Mahayana qualities—as well as the complete bodhisattva practices of training in the six perfections.

For those disciples inclined to the profound, the Dharma wheels of the four classes of tantra were turned by way of the application of desire. These teachings revealed the foundation practice of the vows and the common and exclusive pledges—the root of all tantric siddhis as well as provisional and definitive deity yogas and their supplementary practices as means to develop swiftly the two kinds of siddhis.

For these reasons, there is no doctrine of the Buddha not included within the three vows and the complete training in their commitments. Therefore, because it is recognized as being for the common good in general and because they are in particular indispensable endowments for spiritual friends, I will give a short presentation on these three. [254]

The pratimokṣa vows

In the explanatory *Vajraśekhara Tantra* it talks of the *pratimokṣa,* bodhicitta, and tantric vows:

> The vows of *pratimokṣa,* bodhicitta, and *vidyādhara* mantra.[785]

"*Prā* means complete" is the root,[786] to which can be added the affix *kti,* because "*kti* is suitable," (the *kṛt* affix *kti* can be added to roots to give the *bhāva* form). The particle *k* blocks the *guṇa* and so is elided. Because of the *nipāta* conjunction, the vowel *a* becomes shortened to leave *prati,* which can mean "first" and so on, but primarily it means "individual."

"*Mucḷ* means rescue or freedom." This is the root. "From *un, sa*" (untraced). Therefore, the affix *sa* and *vikaraṇa* affix *ap* are added. The vowel *ḷ* is an *anubandha* connecting particle and so is elided. The *ap vikaraṇa* causes the vowel *u* to become its *guṇa* letter *o.* The *c* becomes *k* because "*ku* for *cu*" (formations ending in the *ca* consonant group that are roots meeting consonants from *jha* to *sa,* or that are nominal stems meeting consonants from *ra* to *sa,* become their equivalents from the *ku* consonant group). "From *ku, i, la, sa* becomes *ṣa*" (when gender endings of the consonants in the *ka* group, the eight vowels beginning with *i,* and the five consonants *ha, ya, wa, ra,* and *la* take a following *sa,* it becomes *ṣa*). Therefore, the *sa* becomes *ṣa.* This leaves *pratimokṣa,* meaning "individual liberation."

To explain this term by its etymology, the word *prati* means "individual" or "separate," and when you receive the vows, the antidote to wrong activity is born, and so the mindstream rejects or separates from those traits to be abandoned. The term *mokṣa* means "liberation" or "to be freed." Directly you find liberation from wrong activity, and gradually you are freed from the lower realms and samsara. On this point *Buddha Vairocana's Teachings on Bodhisattva Practice* says:

> Keeping to the ethics of this *pratimokṣa* is like moving from the darkness into the light, like finding wealth when poor, like finding medicine when sick, like being plucked from a dark prison. This is the great preceptor of all and is not unlike the Buddha abiding in the world.[787]

The *Sutra of Pure Morality* says:

> Just as one without sight cannot see forms,
> one without ethics cannot see the Dharma.
> Just as one without legs cannot walk,
> one without ethics will not find freedom.[788]

In the *Sutra on What Is Precious to a Monk* it says:

> These *pratimokṣa* ethics are the greatest joy,
> these *pratimokṣa* ethics are the path to freedom,
> these *pratimokṣa* ethics are excellent qualities,
> these *pratimokṣa* ethics are the causes of buddhahood.[789] [255]

In the *Pratimokṣa Sutra:*

> The center and the very heart
> of the fathomless mountain lakes
> of the Vinaya of the Buddha
> is this *pratimokṣa.*[790]

Dharmaśreṣthin in his *Praise of Vinaya* says:

> Just as the roots of a tree
> are the foundation for its growth
> and for all it bears,
> so the roots and causes
> of all within the sacred Dharma
> is taught to be the Vinaya.[791]

In the same work:

> The teaching of the conquering Teacher
> is taught to be Sutra and Abhidharma.
> Vinaya is both teacher and teachings,
> therefore worthy of double reverence,
> like Buddha and Dharma as one.[792]

In this verse the scriptural baskets of Abhidharma and Sutra serve as the teachings but not as the teacher. The basket of Vinaya, however, functions as both teacher and teachings. It is therefore an exalted topic, and its subject matter can be ascertained under six major outlines:

1. Divisions
2. Abridgement
3. Definitions
4. Stages
5. Fixed number
6. Etymology

Divisions

The *Basic Vinaya* states:

> Ordination, purification ceremony,
> removal of prohibitions,
> summer retreat, animal hides, medicines,
> clothing, laying out the robes, Kauśāmbhi,
> formal acts, Pāṇḍulohita, persons, moving,
> removal from purification ceremony,
> dwelling places, arguments, and schism.[793]

These are the seventeen foundations of Vinaya.

Abridgements

These seventeen divisions can be condensed into three:

1. Ordination
2. Attaining clothing for the road and for dwelling, the seven reparation foundations, and repairing degeneration through formal acts
3. Guarding against degeneration by any of the remaining foundations

Alternatively, they can be condensed into five:

1. Purification of broken commitments
2. Supports for living
3. Supports for accomplishing all
4. Supports for reparation
5. Supports for all

Definitions

The definition of the subject matter that is taught is that from among the two ethical practices—adopting and discarding—it is primarily a practice of the first type. The definition of the actual teaching is the revealing of this subject matter

Stages

One attains what has not been attained, then protects what has been attained, and then repairs, if necessary, what has been weakened. This initial stage is taught by the ordination foundation [and purification ceremony];[794] [256] the next eight foundations constitute primarily the intermediate stages, and the remaining seven foundations constitute primarily a final stage. In this way the stages have a causal sequence.

Fixed number

For persons to attain the level of a high rebirth and the definitive happiness of nirvana, they must first enter into the doctrine as yet unentered. Having entered the doctrine, they have to guard their practices and when weakened repair them. Therefore, if there were less than seventeen foundations these stages would not be complete. With these seventeen the above requirements are met perfectly, and so more than seventeen is unnecessary.

Etymology

They are called *foundations* because they provide the foundations or supports for the perfect practice of the exceptional training in ethics. For a more extensive explanation of this topic, which here has been condensed into these six points, see the *Golden Victorious Myrobalan Vinaya Ceremonies* by my lama Ngawang Losang Gyatso, in reality the Buddha; the extensive and concise monastic advice of Mañjuśrī Tsongkhapa; and the works of Dülzin Drakpa Gyaltsen, the omniscient Gendün Drup, Panchen Sönam Drakpa, and others.

The essentials of this topic are summed up in Mañjuśrī Tsongkhapa's *Essence of the Ocean of Vinaya:*

> The eight daylong *upavāsa* vows, the male and female *upāsaka* lay vows, the male and female *śrāmaṇera* novice monastic vows, the vows of the trainee *śikṣamāṇā* nun, the vows of the fully ordained *bhikṣuṇī* nun and *bhikṣu* monk: these the eight types of *pratimokṣa.*[795]

This passage lists the eight types of *pratimokṣa,* which are those of the daylong *upavāsa,* the lay male *upāsaka,* the lay female *upāsikā,* the male *śrāmaṇera* novice monastic, the female *śrāmaṇerikā* novice monastic, the trainee *śikṣamāṇā* nun, the fully ordained *bhikṣuṇī* nun and the fully ordained *bhikṣu* monk. Alternatively, the master Atiśa and others list only seven kinds of *pratimokṣa,* omitting the daylong *upavāsa* vows because of their short duration.

If all of these vows are taken with a mind wholly renounced of samsara that works for the attainment of nirvana, then they become true *pratimokṣa* vows. Taken for the purposes of this life, such as for freeing from illnesses or from the punishments of authority, they are known as *ethics for protection from fear.* Taken solely in pursuit of the pleasure of the gods in future lives, they are known as *ethics aspiring to future benefit.* These last two are vows of lesser significance.

The fully ordained monk pledges restraint from the seven nonvirtuous physical and verbal acts[796] and other related nonvirtuous acts. These are known as the seven types of abandonment and their associates. Elsewhere these are described as the two hundred and fifty-three rules. The novice restrains from the three nonvirtuous physical acts and from the verbal act of telling lies, together with all associated acts. Alternatively, these are known as the forty coarse acts of abandonment.

Lay practitioners who vow to refrain from one nonvirtuous act, such as killing, are known as single-abandonment *upāsaka* practitioners. [257] Those who vow to refrain from two acts, such as killing and stealing, are known as partial *upāsaka* practitioners. Those who take vows against the three physical acts and the verbal act of telling lies are known as almost *upāsaka* practitioners. Those who add the vow of abstinence from alcohol are complete *upāsaka* practitioners. Those who take the vow of celibacy are known as celibate *upāsaka* practitioners.

The trainee nun adds six root restraints and six associated restraints to the vows of a female novice nun.

Apart from the proscription against accepting anything precious, the *upavāsa* vows correspond closely to those of the novice monastic.

Concerning the conditions necessary for the growth of these vows, the Sautrāntika school and others talk of instances of these vows even taking root in animals. However, regarding the accounts in the Vinaya and the sutras of the Bhagavān Buddha and his śrāvaka disciples bestowing lay *upāsaka* and one-day *upavāsa* commitments on male and female *yakṣa* demons, such as Hārini and Gopāla, and on nāga serpents, this was done merely to develop some minor virtue or to bind them to good behavior. The type of birth needed for a true production of these vows is that of a man or woman from the three continents and not of any other form. All the great monastic scholars of Vinaya are agreed on this.

According to the Buddhist Vaibhāṣika schools, the *upavāsa* vows must be taken from a fully ordained monk. However, a Vinaya passage talks of the householder Anāthapiṇḍada giving the vows,[797] and so the presence of an ordained monastic is not always necessary. The ceremony for taking the vows consists of going for refuge followed by taking the pledge three times. Then the commitments are recited. If you have decided to keep the commitments on every fifteenth, thirtieth, or eighth day of the month for a whole month or for a year, and so on, it is acceptable to undergo just one ceremony for that whole period. You can take the vows for a whole solar day or you can regard night and day as separate. The eight acts to be abandoned under the vows are the four root acts; drinking alcohol; singing, dancing, and wearing jewelry counted as one; sitting on high seats; and eating at the wrong time.

On becoming a lay *upāsaka*, the *Mahānāman Sutra* says:

> Mahānāman, it is like this: the householder who wears the white clothes, has the marks of a male, goes for refuge to the Buddha, Dharma, and Sangha, and utters the words, "Accept me as an *upāsaka*"—by this alone he becomes an *upāsaka*.[798]

In keeping with this passage, the Aparāntaka[799] Buddhist school and others assert that just by going for refuge one can become an *upāsaka* practitioner. For the Vaibhāṣika school, those who have not taken all five vows are not true *upāsakas*. The ceremony consists of going for refuge three times, [258] reciting the commitments three times, and saying, "Master, accept me as an *upāsaka* practitioner who will practice just this conduct." By this procedure the vows are generated. The coarse and subtle levels of the downfalls are similar to those of the *upavāsa.* The giving-up procedure is very similar to that of an ordained monastic.

There are four hindrances to the "attaining what is not attained" by way of the two stages of receiving ordination vows.[800] In the *hindrance to duration,* the recipient is in debt, is enslaved as a servant, does not have parental permission, or does not have permission from the king. In such cases, although the vows can be taken, they are soon lost. In the *hindrance to attractiveness,* the recipient is one born with white hair or with pale skin.[801] Here, the vows can be generated but the recipient's unattractive appearance could hinder the laity from developing faith in the teachings. In the *hindrance that is a specific obstacle to the development of qualities,* someone may take the vows but through ill health is unable to fulfill the commitments. *Hindrances to actually generating the vows* includes various types of unsuitable recipients, such as those who have committed heinous acts, hermaphrodites, eunuchs, spirits, and those living in the northern continent of Uttarakuru.

As well as being free from the above hindrances, you need the presence of five conducive conditions. These are place, continuity, signs, thought, and ceremony.

Place refers to places where the Buddha has appeared, where the Dharma has not disappeared. *Place* in the sense of "object" refers to a quorum of Sangha present to act as objects of request during the ceremony. The preceptor should fulfill the criterion of an elder by having been a fully ordained monk for more than ten years. The thirteen Sangha supplementary factors should be present, which include the monks present being fully ordained and learned in the Vinaya, not standing but sitting, not subject to actions such as punishment, and so on. At least one of the twenty-one sets of five criteria[802] should be fulfilled. The preceptor of the novice monk should be learned in giving the novice monk vows and explaining the commitments. The revealer of secrets preceptor is skilled in performing the ceremony of revealing hindrances to the ordination in a secret manner, and is ceremonially appointed by the Sangha after being verbally petitioned and then accepting the petition. There should be the ritual preceptor in the midst of the Sangha who knows by heart the words of the ordination ceremony and recites them without making the smallest mistake of even half a word. In a central land there should be a minimum of ten members of the Sangha present and in remote areas a minimum of five. [259]

Continuity means that the vows to be taken should not have degenerated in those present.

Signs means that the would-be novice monk should have all the signs of one to be ordained and be appropriately attired. The would-be fully ordained monk should have the three robes and the begging bowl blessed by the preceptor, and should be holding them correctly. He should also be washed and clean.

Thought means that the mind is at ease, with a heartfelt desire to take the vows; the recipient knows that the vows have been received; and the mind is taken with thoughts of definite renunciation.

With these conditions in place, there is a definite conferral of the vows of the earlier and later stages, the very root of the doctrine.[803]

Protecting the received vows from degenerating is done by five methods:

- Relying on a special spiritual friend
- Maintaining a pure mind
- Purifying the commitments
- Living in conducive circumstances
- Recognizing their opposing forces

The novice monk has entered the doctrine but not completely. Therefore, novice monk downfalls that contradict the commitments are not grouped under different headings but all fall into the single category of *faults (nyes byas, duṣkṛti).*[804] Of the thirty-six novice monk downfalls that transgress the vows taken, the four root downfalls are known as faults similar to the *defeats (pham pa, parājita)* of a fully ordained monk. These and the vow of holding on to robes and others that make up the seventeen and a half downfalls are non-downfalls for a novice monk. Apart from those, all novice monk transgressions of the commitments of fully ordained monks are known as *faults to be restrained.*

The downfalls that transgress the commitments of a fully ordained monk can all be put into five groups: defeats, punishable by excommunication, those that cause downfalls, those to be declared, and faults. The two hundred and fifty-three commitments and their associated faults, the boundaries for protection of the vows, and the causes for downfalls should be studied in greater detail.[805]

Concerning the restoration of generated vows: degeneration brought about by a defeat and intentionally concealed is like cutting the head off a palm tree and is described in the Vinaya as something that will not grow again. Therefore there is no procedure for restoring the vow in this situation.

Degeneration brought about by a defeat that is free of any intention to conceal it—and all manner of downfall below that—is capable of being restored, as explained in the ordination ceremony. [260]

The benefits of keeping just one commitment at particular times are immeasurable. The thirty-sixth chapter of *King of Meditative Concentrations Sutra* says:

> For as many millions of eons as there are grains of sand in the Ganges,
> with a pure and joyful mind, one may
> revere and honor billions of buddhas with food, drink,
> parasols, and banners, garlands of lights and lamps;
> but for one who at the disintegration of the Dharma,
> when the teachings of the Tathāgata are lost,
> holds to just one commitment for a day and night,
> the merit is by far the greater.[806]

Also:

> Praised and exalted by the buddhas of the past,
> those who hold to flawless ethics
> will draw many beings away from hell and sinful acts.
> Those holding to the flawless ethics praised by the buddhas
> are venerating every tathāgata past.[807]

The *Sutra Requested by Susthitamati Devaputra* from the twenty-second volume of the *Heap of Jewels* collection says:

> Buddhas who appeared in the past,
> those who have not yet appeared,
> and those who are presently appearing,
> do not gain the peace of enlightenment
> without abandoning many faults.
> Ordination has been praised by every tathāgata,
> and those who wish to please the buddhas
> should seize ordination in the Conqueror's teachings.[808]

There are many such passages.

22. The Bodhisattva Vows

Sakya Paṇḍita said:

> Generation of the mind is of two kinds:
> that of the śrāvaka and that of the Mahayana.[809]

Generation of the mind is found in both Great and Lesser Vehicles. The lower vehicle has a generation of the mind for an arhat, a pratyekabuddha, and a buddha, but this tradition did not spread to Tibet.

On the procedure for the ceremonial generation of the engaged bodhi mind of the Mahayana with its subsequent taking of the bodhisattva vows and their proper commitments, [261] many Tibetan scholars maintain that just as Maitreya and Ārya Asaṅga on the one hand and the glorious protector Nāgārjuna on the other, whose traditions are renowned as the two great chariots, professed the two different philosophies of Cittamātra and Madhyamaka, so on this topic also there are different assertions. Firstly, scholars maintain, there are differences in the type of person from whom you take the vows, because on this point the protector Maitreya begins, "Rely upon a spiritual friend who is disciplined, pacified, well pacified..."[810] and so on, whereas Nāgārjuna says, "Content, compassionate, moral..."[811] and so on. On the type of person who can take the vows, the Cittamātra position is summed up in the verse beginning, "The seven types of *pratimokṣa*" up to "these are fortunate, others are not,"[812] meaning that the one who takes the bodhisattva vows must hold one of the seven *pratimokṣa* disciplines. According to a Mādhyamika, the vows can take root in any of the six types of sentient being and in any person from a king to a butcher. They assert that this demonstrates a difference between these two traditions concerning the type of being who can take the vows. They also maintain there are differences in the way you guard the vows and restore them if they degenerate.

However, Khedrup Gelek Palsangpo, in his *Broom of the Buddha's Precious*

Doctrine: A Brief Presentation on the Three Sets of Vows, refutes any suggestion of differences between the two:

> Firstly, positing different types of person from whom one takes the vows is incorrect because the difference in those two passages is only in the wording. The definitions of the true spiritual friend they teach differ a little in terms of detail, but the meaning of each is the same.[813]

Also:

> Therefore, apart from differences in some secondary elements of the ceremony, the actual ceremony of taking the vows is essentially the same for the traditions of Ārya Nāgārjuna and Ārya Asaṅga. Ācārya Jetāri, whose assertions veered toward the Madhyamaka, also talked of the two stages of aspiring bodhicitta and taking the vows.[814]

Therefore, this topic is summarized by Maitreya and Asaṅga in the chapter on ethics from *Stages of the Bodhisattva* under nine categories, or outlines:

> Nature, the whole, difficulty, entrances,
> the special being, all aspects, loss and want,
> happiness here and elsewhere, and purification:
> with these nine points is ethics summarized.[815]

"Nature" refers to the general definition. "The whole" refers to all the divisions of the topic. As one is entering something difficult to accomplish, "difficulty" refers to the exclusivity of these ethics. "Entrances" describes the methods of entering this undertaking. "Special being" refers to the type of person undertaking these ethics. "Aspects" refers to all the aspects of ethics. [262] "Loss and want" refers to features of objects and actions. Future results of this practice of ethics is happiness both "here" and "elsewhere" in future lives, as well as "purification."

Of these nine categories in this topic of ethics, *general definitions* consists of the following:

- The object in front of which one takes the vows
- The form of the person who takes the vows

- The ethics to be guarded
- The way to protect bodhisattva ethics
- Causes for losing the vows
- Ways to restore degenerated vows

The object in front of which one takes the vows

This procedure can be undertaken in the presence of a master or without a master. In the first scenario, you take the vows from someone who themselves have generated the aspiring bodhicitta, who keeps the bodhicitta vows, who is wise in the Mahayana, who has memorized and can recite and enunciate the words of the ceremonial requests for the commitments and so on, and who is understandable. Ācārya Candragomin says in his *Twenty Verses on the Bodhisattva Vow:*

> The vows of the bodhisattva,
> a veritable treasure of every merit,
> are taken with the highest of minds
> from a guru dwelling in the vows
> who is wise and capable.[816]

Therefore, the vows are taken from a guru fully qualified to bestow them. If such a lama cannot be found, *Stages of the Bodhisattva* says:

> In front of an image of the Tathāgata, touch your head to the feet of the buddhas and bodhisattvas living and dwelling in the ten directions.[817]

Therefore, in front of an image such as that of Buddha Śākyamuni, you first perform the seven-branch practice and so on, and then ask the conquerors and their sons of the ten directions to hear your words; you pledge three times to train in the foundations of every practice of all bodhisattvas of the past, present, and future. In this way, you take the vows.

The form of the person who takes the vows

The Indian *siddha* Jetāri states: "A son or daughter of the family, with the perfect form and the perfect mind...."[818] Therefore,

> the forms of gods, nāgas, and so on, in which the mind striving for full enlightenment can be generated, are suitable simply for the generation of the aspiring bodhicitta. However, those forms of living beings grasped by the ceremony of aspiring bodhicitta, and who are fully qualified for the taking of the bodhicitta vows, will have, at the very least, states of mind in common with the paths of the lower and intermediate scopes, a mind well trained in the seven cause-and-effect transmitted instructions, [263] and so forth, by whose power some mind-affecting experience of bodhicitta has grown within their being.[819]

This is the position of Khedrup Jé. In *Light on the Path* by the master Atiśa it says:

> Those who possess without break
> vows of seven types of *pratimokṣa*
> have the good fortune for bodhisattva vows;
> others do not.[820]

On this verse Mañjuśrī Tsongkhapa, in conjunction with citations from [Atiśa's] *Autocommentary on Light on the Path to Enlightenment* and [Abhayākaragupta's] *Ornament to the Thought of the Buddha,* says in his *Highway to Enlightenment: An Exposition of Bodhisattva Ethics:*

> This has been stated. However, what it means is that if a beginner does not possess any of the seven *pratimokṣa* vows, he does not have the good fortune to develop any exceptional vow based upon ethics; and if he does not possess any natural abandonment[821] in common with the seven types of *pratimokṣa* vows, then he does not have the good fortune simply to develop the bodhisattva vows. It does not mean that if he is not a qualified holder of the seven *pratimokṣa* vows he cannot develop the bodhisattva vows.[822]

Also, if that were its meaning, you would have to accept that this statement means that bodhisattva vows could not develop in gods. However, on this point, both great chariot traditions are in agreement, and there are many accounts in the scriptures and canonical treatises of universal sovereigns generating the bodhisattva vows. Even though these beings may have already possessed various *pratimokṣa* disciplines, such as the lay *upāsaka* vows or the eight daylong restraints, these vows were seen as inferior to their receiving the bodhisattva vows. The *Sutra of the Good Eon* states:

> When the conqueror Hitaiṣin became a local governor
> and vowed in the presence of Tathāgata Ratnaśrī
> to restrain from killing for a day,
> he first generated the mind of enlightenment.[823]

Similarly, the *Sutra of Repaying the Kindness* recounts how when our Teacher was born as a brave being forced to drag a cart in the hell realms, he thought of the suffering of his companion and the mind of enlightenment was born within him.[824] Also when born as the merchant's son Abhinanda, as retold in the *Sutra of the Three Heaps;*[825] or as Mutoba in *Sutra of the Good Eon;* as King Prabhāvati and as the potter Vipulaprabhā in the Vinaya; as the beggar in the *Great Nirvana Sutra;* and as the brahman Samudrarajas, minister of King Aranemi, in the *White Lotus of Compassion Sutra:*[826] in all these accounts he developed the bodhi mind.

The same point can be illustrated using Avalokiteśvara. In the *Illusion-Like Samādhi Sutra* he was miraculously born as the son Ratnottama from the left and right lungs of king Śrītejas.[827] In the *Differentiating the Dharma and the Meaning Sutra* [264] he was miraculously born from the lap of Ratnaśrī, queen of Cakravartin Jayin, to become the son Ratnasambhava.[828] At these times too he developed the bodhi mind.

There have been many cases of there being no opportunity to take the *pratimokṣa* vows or instances where it has been impossible to keep them. Also, as long as you do not take them for competitive reasons and you have not been forced to take them against your will, it is not actually necessary for you to be endowed with the *pratimokṣa* vows in order to take the bodhisattva vows.

The ethics to be guarded

The bodhisattva Ārya Asaṅga has said:

> Bodhisattva ethics can be found in the householder and in one ordained. In brief, ethics are of three types: the ethics of having

> vows, the ethics of developing virtue, and the ethics of helping others.[829]

The work of the bodhisattva is twofold: ripening your own mind and ripening the minds of others; and the first of these is twofold: freeing yourself from wrong behavior and developing good behavior. This is the reason ethics has a threefold division. Moreover, the ethics of holding vows in keeping with those of the śrāvakas becomes the foundation for the other two, because as a sutra states, "Without freeing yourself, you cannot free others." Likewise, if you do not develop virtue in yourself first, you cannot truly fulfill the needs of others. The order of these three, therefore, is also appropriate.

Concerning the first of these, the ethics of holding vows found in the bodhisattva: if a bodhisattva holds *pratimokṣa* vows, this refers to those *pratimokṣa* vows firmly held by the Mahayana bodhi mind present in his mental continuum. If the bodhisattva does not actually possess *pratimokṣa* vows, it refers to an innate possession or deliberate development of the ethics of abandoning acts that are wrong by nature. This too is the ethics of having vows.[830]

Briefly, the ethics of developing virtue refers to the following. Having taken the bodhisattva vows properly, and with your whole continuum grasped by the Mahayana bodhi mind, you engage as appropriate in acts of gathering virtue by physical, verbal, and mental means through the practices of the six perfections, and so on. [265]

The ethics of helping others means the following. Having taken the bodhicitta vows and with your continuum grasped by the Mahayana bodhi mind, you work as appropriate for others in eleven ways. You help those in need of companionship, those confused in their way, those in need of help, those in danger, those tormented by grief, those bereft of possessions, those seeking a place to stay, those wishing for peace and harmony, those who have entered the correct paths, those who have gone astray, and finally you help by taming others with your supernatural powers.

The way to protect bodhisattva ethics

The bodhisattva Śāntideva in his *Compendium of Practice* says:

> The vows of the bodhisattva
> arise extensively within the Mahayana.[831]

Also:

> By never giving up the spiritual friend,
> by constant study of the sutras.[832]

These verses state that these are the methods for protecting ethics. Therefore, you should familiarize yourself with the points of practices and devote yourself completely to the spiritual friend who brings those practices to other disciples. These are the main methods for keeping your ethics. You should also apply yourself well to the study and contemplation of the precious Mahayana sutras and especially to *Stages of the Bodhisattva* and *Compendium of Practice.* If that is not possible, it is important to at least study thoroughly the ethics chapter of *Stages of the Bodhisattva* and to become learned and be able to eliminate misconceptions about all points of bodhisattva practice. Without doing that, you will remain confused on what is to be developed and what is to be discarded, which is the foundation of the practices of engaging and rejecting.

It might then be asked, to what extent should a novice bodhisattva engage in these practices taught in these sutras? The *Compendium of the Mahayana* says:

> There are limitless divisions of bodhisattva practices.[833]

Also, Ācārya Bodhibhadra in his *Commentary on the Twenty Verses on the Bodhisattva Vows:*

> The practices of the bodhisattva are immeasurable and without limit.[834]

Therefore, when divided extensively the practices or commitments of the bodhisattva are beyond number and measure. They can, however, be illustrated numerically. The *Medicine Buddha Sutra* mentions four hundred:

> The bodhisattva vows hold four hundred commitments.[835] [266]

Śāntarakṣita in his *Commentary on the Twenty Verses on the Bodhisattva Vows* says:

> There are many thousands of bodhisattva commitments.[836]

Blaze of Reasoning says:

> There are seven hundred points of bodhisattva practice.[837]

A sutra explaining the bodhisattva points of practice talks of ten defeats and forty-eight downfalls as the fifty-eight commitments of the bodhisattva. In *Precious Garland* it says:

> The four hundred practices of the bodhisattva.[838]

Buddha Vairocana's Teachings on Bodhisattva Practice also talks of ten defeats and forty-eight downfalls.[839] Therefore, in these and other passages, various numbers are mentioned commensurate with the capacity of disciples' minds.

However, the commitments of the bodhisattva can be summed up by the following verse from Ācārya Candragomin:

> Whatever to others and even to oneself
> is suffering but beneficial,
> is pleasurable and beneficial,
> these one should do.
> Whatever is pleasurable but not beneficial,
> one should not do.[840]

These days the most popular delineation of the commitments comes from the great Dharma king Mañjuśrī Tsongkhapa in his *Highway to Enlightenment,* where they are divided into defeats and faults. The defeats or root downfalls have been taken from the *Ākāśagarbha Sutra* by Śāntideva and put into verse in his *Compendium of Practice:*

1. Stealing possessions of the Three Jewels
   is asserted as a downfall by defeat.
2. The second, the mighty Buddha has proclaimed,
   is to abandon the sacred Dharma.
3. Toward monks—even those of fallen ethics—
   stealing their robes, beating them,

casting them into prison,
causing them to leave their ordination,
4. committing any of the five heinous acts,
5. holding to wrong views,
6. and destroying towns and suchlike
are said by the Buddha to be root downfalls.
7. Talking of emptiness to those with minds untrained,
8. turning away from full enlightenment
those dwelling in the way of the Buddha,
9. bringing others to the Mahayana
by causing them to leave the *pratimokṣa,*
10. maintaining that the śrāvaka vehicle
does not bring an end to desire and so forth,
and causing others to hold that view,
11. talking of your own qualities
for the sake of gain and reputation
while abusing others in verse and other writings,
12. falsely proclaiming that you realize the profound, [267]
13. punishing those intent on virtue
by taking that given to the Three Jewels,
14. and abandoning *śamatha,*
giving the possessions of those in meditation
to those reciting scripture:
These are the root downfalls,
causes for the great hells.[841]

On these the *Ākāśagarbha Sutra* it says, "Those of royal lineage empowered from the crown of their heads,"[842] and so on. This means that five root downfalls are labeled as *downfalls of the king,* five are *downfalls of the minister,* and eight are called *downfalls of beginners.* Lama Mañjuśrī Tsongkhapa's categorization of fourteen root downfalls or defeats and four branch downfalls is essentially the same.

Concerning the category of faults, *Stages of the Bodhisattva* lists forty-six faults to be abandoned. In brief, these are explained as being faults of miserliness and so forth—hindrances to the gathering of virtue as outlined by the practices of the six perfections—and faults that hinder working for the benefit of others.

Causes for losing the vows

Three causes for losing the vows have been taught: giving up the aspiring bodhicitta; following any action that is similar to a "cause for defeat" and that is accompanied by the complete binding factors;[843] and thirdly, returning the vows. Any of these constitutes a cause for losing the vows. If you are unable to keep the *pratimokṣa* vows and return them, you cut the merit of continuing in the vows, but the actual handing back of the vows is not in itself a great wrong. However, to hand back the bodhisattva vows is to transgress those vows you made by promising in the presence of all the buddhas and bodhisattvas to work for and to bring about the welfare and happiness of all living beings. It is a betrayal of both the buddhas and sentient beings, and consequently you will have to wander endlessly in the lower realms. *Engaging in the Practices of the Bodhisattva* states:

> If, when I have promised such,
> I do not accomplish it,
> I betray all those sentient beings;
> what kind of birth then shall I take?[844]

Ways to restore degenerated vows

Although striving not to be tainted by faults, if you should incur a fault by the four causes of downfall—ignorance, unawareness, a preponderance of mental affliction, and disrespect—you restore the vows in accord with the proper way. [268] As it says in the *Twenty Verses on Vows of the Bodhisattva:*

> For intermediate downfalls confess to three,
> for the remainder confess before one,
> for other afflictions and non-afflictions,
> confess just before your own mind.[845]

Therefore in the presence of a person suitable for confession, you confess from the depths of your heart and rise up from the fault.

A popular view these days is that the *pratimokṣa* and other vows do not possess form. Sakya Paṇḍita says:

> The vows of the bodhisattva,
> being born from mind, have no form.[846]

This is saying that they are not lost, even up to the attainment of enlightenment. If they did possess form, in the same way that the Vaibhāṣika school asserts the *pratimokṣa* to have form, and that meant that they remained until death destroyed them, this would render some uncertainty about the *upavāsa* vows found in their tradition that are taken for one day only. On the other hand, if vows had no form and this meant that they were not lost even after passing beyond death, then the Madhyamaka assertion that the *pratimokṣa* possess the nature of consciousness would mean that even after death they too would persist. Therefore, I am fairly sure that these divisions are created on the basis of time, in which you pledge to keep the vows until a certain event occurs or for a fixed length of time, and not on the basis of whether they are form.

To enter the secret mantra Vajrayana, these bodhisattva vows are also indispensable. The *Mañjuśrī Root Tantra,* in the first chapter on the collection of rituals, states:

> If three things are present, the practice of mantra will be complete. What are these three? Not to give up on all living beings, guarding the vows of the bodhisattva ethic, and never giving up one's mantra.[847]

The Guhyasamāja explanatory tantra, the *Vajraśekhara,* also says:

> In the order of their stages,
> train yourself in the six perfections;
> keeping in mind the welfare of living beings,
> engage in the practices of the bodhisattvas.[848]

The Hevajra explanatory tantra, the *Vajrapañjara,* states in the twelfth chapter:

> This I will do for the bodhi mind:
> to accomplish the wishes of myself and others,
> I generate the supreme bodhi mind.
> *Emaho!* Inviting all living beings as guests,
> I will emulate the great deeds of the enlightened
> and become a buddha for the benefit of living beings.[849]

On the benefits of following this great path of sutra and tantra combined, the *Gaṇḍavyūhasūtra* says:

> Son of the family, it is like this. Just one shaft of light may enter a house or a room and all darkness therein present for thousands of years is immediately dispelled and replaced by light. [269] Similarly, if just one generation of the bodhi mind enters the house of the mind of any sentient being, black with the dense darkness of ignorance, immediately the darkness and obstructions of karma and mental affliction accumulated over countless thousands of eons are dispelled, and the light of wisdom is born.[850]

Therefore, a genuine bodhicitta, just by being generated in the mind, can remove in an instant the mental obstructions accumulated over many eons. Also in the *Maitreya Prasthāna Sutra:*

> Son of the family, it is like this. The precious diamond, even when broken, still outshines all wonderful golden ornaments, does not lose the name "diamond," and will still dispel all poverty. Son of the family, similarly, the precious diamond of the mind generated toward omniscience, even when lax, still outshines all the ornaments of achievements of the śrāvakas and pratyekabuddhas, and without losing the name of bodhisattva will dispel all the poverty of samsara.[851]

Therefore, even when not engaged in the practices of the bodhisattva, if you have the aspiring bodhicitta, you are still a bodhisattva. The same sutra says:

> If the merit explained as the ripening
> of the bodhi mind were to have form:
> even if it filled up as many realms
> as there are grains of sand in the river Ganges,
> that would still be but a fraction.[852]

Śāntideva in his *Engaging in the Practices of the Bodhisattva* says:

> The moment the bodhi mind is born
> in those wretched beings bound in samsara's prison

> they become known as sons of the Tathāgata,
> to be revered by gods and men.[853]

Atiśa in his *Light on the Path:*

> The merit of the bodhi mind,
> were it to have form,
> would fill the realms of space
> and yet still be more.
>
> Someone may fill with precious jewels
> Buddha realms as many as sand grains in the Ganges
> and offer them to the lord of the world,
> yet he who puts his palms together
> and bows his mind toward enlightenment
> makes the greater offering.[854] [270]

Thus, the benefits of the bodhi mind are extensively described in the precious sutras and cannot be adequately reproduced here.

Also, in the *Sutra Requested by the Householder Ugra* found in the nineteenth volume of the *Heap of Jewels* collection:

> Householder, the bodhisattva householder living in a house should go for refuge to the Buddha, go for refuge to the Dharma, and go for refuge to the Sangha.[855]

And:

> Householder, furthermore, the bodhisattva householder holds completely the foundations of practice. It is like this: holding completely the five commitments of practice...[856]

Thus much is taught on the commitments of practice using the vows of a complete *upāsaka* practitioner as an illustration.

In the *Sutra Requested by Upāli,* from the twenty-fourth volume of the *Heap of Jewels* collection in the chapter "Determining the Vinaya," it states:

> Upāli, therefore, you should say that the practices of those of the śrāvaka vehicles are made pure by different actions and by

> different thoughts. Why is that? Upāli, the actions and the thoughts of those of the śrāvaka vehicles are one thing, and the actions and the thoughts of those bodhisattvas who have truly entered the Mahayana are another. Upāli, whatever is pure ethics for those of the Śrāvakayāna is impure ethics, improper ethics, for those bodhisattvas who have truly entered the Mahayana. Whatever is pure ethics for those bodhisattvas who have truly entered the Mahayana is impure ethics, improper ethics for those of the Śrāvakayāna. Why is that? Upāli, those of the Śrāvakayāna do not seek, even for an instant, to take rebirth in samsara. That is pure ethics for those of the Śrāvakayāna. That is impure ethics, improper ethics for those bodhisattvas who have truly entered the Mahayana.[857]

Also:

> Therefore, Upāli, you should say that the commitments of those bodhisattvas who have truly entered the Mahayana are to be guarded. You should say that the commitments of those of the Śrāvakayāna should not be guarded. [271] You should say that the commitments of those bodhisattvas who have truly entered the Mahayana are to be undertaken. You should say that the commitments of those of the Śrāvakayāna should not be undertaken.[858]

Also:

> Śāriputra, the first serious fault of the bodhisattva should be confessed in the presence of ten. The fault of taking a woman by the hand should be confessed in the presence of five. The fault of looking at her with a deluded mind should be confessed in the presence of one or two persons. The faults of the bodhisattva committing the five heinous acts, the faults concerning women, children, the hand, the shrine, the Sangha, and other serious faults should be confessed day and night solely in the presence of the thirty-five buddhas. The procedure of this confession is as follows: "I of such and such name go for refuge to the Buddha..."

The passage continues up to:

> To those who possess ocean-like achievements, exalted beyond number, I put my hands together and go for refuge.[859]

This confession is the *Sutra of the Three Heaps,* known these days as the Confession of Downfalls recitation. The text continues:

> Śāriputa, in this way the bodhisattva with his mind concentrated on the thirty-five buddhas and all the tathāgatas should purify all wrong acts.

These passages—on bodhisattva commitments, downfalls, confession procedures, and the differences between the *pratimokṣa* vows and the bodhisattva vows—which have not been elaborated on by commentators of the past, and on which there is little explanation, I have presented here only as an opener for further amplification. In the future, if any wise scholars wish to write extensively on the subject of bodhisattva vows, I would ask them to examine this sutra and flex their tongues. [272]

23. Vidyādhara Tantric Vows

Sakya Paṇḍita states:

> Having entered the Vajrayana path,
> if you wish to attain buddhahood soon,
> strive in the stages of ripening and liberation.

Also:

> For the ripening of the empowerment,
> seek out a guru with lineage undiminished,
> who does not confuse the procedures,
> who is wise in organizing inner and outer rituals,
> who is capable of planting seeds of the four bodies,[860]
> and who acts in accord with the words of the Buddha.
> From him take the four empowerments;
> through him one becomes a holder of the three vows.[861]

Therefore, the vajra master is one who is free from the faults of anger, pride, and so on, and who possesses the qualities of compassion and the achievements of the ten activities, as taught in [Aśvaghoṣa's] *Fifty Verses on the Guru.* He should possess the four oral transmissions: a lineage beginning from Samantabhadra or Vajradhara whose river not dried up, whose aroma of blessing has not vanished, whose stream[862] remains uncorrupted, and whose water satisfies the devoted mind. He should be one who is focused on the unerring traditional explanations of the practices of past gurus and on the correct rituals by way of a soundly referenced lineage of explicit teaching. He should be one who is able to introduce directly the bases for purification, the phenomena to be purified or removed, the purification processes, and the fruits of purification. Such a person is necessary for nourishing the disciple by bestowing the ripening empowerment and the liberating explanatory teachings and providing the support of transmission, in dependence on which you practice the generation and completion stages and so on.

The nature of an empowerment is that which has the power to actually create the special result of your future achievement. On the etymology of the term the *Hevajra Root Tantra* states:

> Meaning "to sprinkle" and "to pour,"
> it is therefore an "empowerment" *(abhiṣekha).*[863]

The root "*śīkṛ* means to wash or pour." To this root is added the particle *ta,* which is the middle-person plural of the *parasmaipād vartamāna* tense in the imperative *(loṭ)* mood in a benedictive sense. The *ṛ* is an *anubandha* indicatory letter and is omitted. The *vikaraṇa* in-between *ap* affix is added, causing *i* to become *e* by the *guṇa* process, and the resulting formulation is *śekta.* Because "letters change and weaken" and "the remainder can be known by worldly usage," the *śe* becomes *se* and the prefix *abhi* is added. "From *ku, i, la, sa* becomes *ṣa"* (when gender endings of the consonants in the *ka* group, the eight vowels beginning with *i,* and the five consonants *ha, ya, wa, ra,* and *la* take a following *sa,* it becomes *ṣa*), and also "for *sa, ṣa*" means that the *sa* becomes *ṣa.* This results in *abhiṣekta.* [273]

Alternatively, the root "*sic* means to sprinkle." To this is added *tip,* the first-person singular of the *parasmaipād vartamāna* present. The *vikaraṇa ap* affix is added because "For the agent, *ap"* (for expressing the agent from roots such as *bhū,* the in-between affix *ap* is added when followed by any of the eighteen affixes from *tip* to *mahe*). The *p* is elided as an *anubandha.* The *c* is brought to the vowel *a.* "From *muc,* etc., *mum*" (when roots such as *muc* meet *vikaraṇa* affixes such as *ap,* the *āgama mum* is added). Therefore, *mum* is added. "*Sa* and *tu* to *śa* and *cu*" (final consonants *sa* and those of the *ta* group brought to initial *śa* and those of the *ca* group become *śa* and those of the *ca* group). Therefore *na* becomes *ña.* The prefix *abhi* is added. As done previously the *si* becomes *ṣi* to form *abhiṣiñca.* (In the process, *tip* must also be elided, and the remainder of *mum,* being an *agama,* must also be elided.)

Therefore, in keeping with "sprinkling" and "pouring," as expressed in the first line of the verse above, just as water and fertilizer is added to a seed, the bodily sites of the empowerment—the crown, the tongue or throat, the heart, the navel, and the secret area—are progressively sprinkled and poured upon. Because of this the four empowerments will individually have the power to wash away the corresponding taints of these sites and develop the corresponding sprouts of the four bodies; hence the term "empowerment."

In keeping with the second line, receiving the four empowerments gives you power over the meditations on the four paths and power to attain the resultant four bodies, therefore it is called an "empowerment." Alternatively, the particle *ñca* means "to wash," and receiving the four empowerments will wash away the taints of not being aware that body, speech, and mind, together with mind and wind combined, dwell in the nature of the four bodies. Therefore it is an empowerment. Abhyākaragupta in his *Lesser Stalks of Oral Instruction* says:

> Because it cleans away the defilements
> of body, speech, and mind,
> it is an empowerment.[864]

The bases to be purified by the empowerment are the four primordial and naturally abiding vajras,[865] which form the goal of your practice. The phenomena to be purified or removed are the coarse and subtle temporal defilements that obscure these vajras. The purifying of these phenomena is by way of conferring an empowerment suitable to that disciple's capacity, thereby ripening the disciple to meditate on the corresponding path and gain the result. The effect of purification is the nourishing of the special seeds or potentials of the four bodies. This means that by conferring empowerment, which will bring about the transformation of the bases-of-purification four vajras into the fruit-of-purification four bodies, the suitable-vessel disciple has been planted with the seeds of the four bodies, which is secret mantra's way of activating the potential that is the naturally abiding lineage.[866] The *Mahāmudrā Drop Yoginī Tantra* states:

> When at the beginning the disciples
> are once conferred with empowerments,
> they become without doubt a suitable vessel
> for the explanation of the great secrets.
> No empowerment means no siddhi,
> as squeezing sand will produce no oil.
> Those who arrogantly give teachings on the tantras [274]
> without the conferral of empowerment,

> master and disciples, even if they have gained siddhi
> will land in hell as soon as they die.
> Therefore, with all your effort,
> seek empowerment from a guru.[867]

The *Vajra Garland Tantra* says:

> Empowerment is prime,
> all siddhis will forever be present.
> I will explain accordingly;
> therefore, first of all, listen well.
>
> Once the master confers perfect empowerment,
> the wise and intelligent disciple
> becomes a suitable vessel
> for the yogas of the completion stage.
>
> When perfect empowerment is absent,
> even though the practitioner knows tantra,
> disciple and master alike
> will fall to unending hell.[868]

If you enter the practices without receiving a proper empowerment, even though you know the tantra and through practice gain siddhi, the disciple will go to hell, as will the master. Receiving empowerment depends on entering the mandala and seeing the mandala. In the *Yoga Equal to All Buddhas Later Tantra:*

> Not having entered the mandala,
> disregarding all pledges,
> ignorant of the reality of the secret mantra:
> one may practice but to no avail.[869]

The *Little Saṃvara Tantra* says:

> The practitioner of mantra
> who has not seen the mandala
> and yet wishes to become a yogi

> is like one striking the air with his fist,
> like one drinking the water of a mirage.[870]

For the seven common empowerments there are the powder mandalas, and for the higher exalted mandalas:

> Body, secret organs, and the mind:
> these are always the three types of mandala.[871]

By seeing the appropriate mandala one has received empowerment. Then, as the great Dharma king Mañjuśrī Tsongkhapa says:

> Vajrayana, supreme among the Conqueror's teachings,
> brings joy to those of great intelligence.
> For those who enter it, the foundation of siddhi
> is the vows of the glorious Vajrasattva.[872]

Therefore, this leads to an explanation of the tantric vows or pledges:[873] [275]

1. The way to take the vows and pledges
2. Determining the downfalls that break the vows you have taken

The way to take the vows and pledges

This is under three headlines:

1. In order that the disciples know the vows to be taken, they are recited for a clear understanding. This is because at the time they are taken they must be held with a clear and unconfused concentration. Therefore, the vows are declared as taught in the *Vajraśekhara Tantra*.
2. Taking the vows
3. Conferring or not conferring empowerment on those taking or not taking vows

Declaring the vows

1. The individual vows of the five families
2. Pledges in common with all five families

The individual vows of the five families

> Go for refuge to the Three Jewels
> of the Buddha, Dharma, and Sangha;
> this is the firm pledge
> of the pure buddha family.[874]

Such an entreaty to go for refuge to the Three Jewels is the pledge of the Vairocana family. The lines, "this is the firm pledge of the pure buddha family" is as it appears in many texts. However, Mañjuśrī Tsongkhapa has "joyful buddha family."[875] "Firm" means that the pledges cannot easily be broken by destructive forces.

> You of great intelligence:
> hold the vajra, bell, and mudrā.
> Bodhicitta is taught to be the vajra,
> wisdom is taught to be the bell.
> Hold also the vajra master,
> for the guru is equal to all buddhas.
> These are taught as the pledges
> of the pure vajra family.[876]

This is urging that "you of great intelligence should hold the vajra, bell, and mudrā." How this is to be done is explained by the lines, "Bodhicitta is taught to be the vajra" and so on. Moreover, the vajra master also should be held with reverence. These are the pledges of Akṣobhya.

> For the supreme jewel family,
> three times in the day and at night,
> practice constantly four kinds of giving:
> wealth, fearlessness, Dharma, and love.[877]

"Jewel" refers to the family of Ratnasambhava. The verse is saying that three times in the day and three times in the night you should practice without fail the four kinds of giving: those of material wealth, gifts of fearlessness, Dharma, and love. These are the pledges of Ratnasambhava.

> You should hold the sacred Dharma
> of the outer, inner, and secret vehicles.[878]
> These are the pledges and vows
> of the pure lotus family.[879]

Holding the whole Dharma without discarding any of the three vehicles and so on is the pledge of Amitābha. [276]

> For the supreme-activity family,
> hold well all vows taken
> and perform offerings as best you can.[880]

Keeping all the vows you have taken and making offerings as best you can are the pledges of Amoghasiddhi.

These have been the specific pledges of the deities belonging to the tathāgata, vajra, jewel, lotus, and activity families.

Pledges held in common by all five families:

1. Root pledges
2. Secondary pledges
3. Conclusion

Root pledges

> Fourteen, other than these,
> are explained as other-inflicted defeats.
> Don't abandon and discard them;
> they are explained as root downfalls.
> Three times in the day and at night,
> day after day, recite them.
> When they degenerate, the yogi
> has committed a gross fault.[881]

There are common pledges other than the individual pledges of the families, and these too are not to be abandoned in the mind or discarded by verbal and physical acts. What are these pledges? First the root pledges are taught. These are proscriptive rules for the fourteen acts described in the tantras as *other-inflicted defeats,* whose alternative name is *root downfalls*. These actions break the vows and inflict defeat upon their disciplining powers. They are called *other-inflicted defeats (phas pham pa, pārājika)* because a destructive power from "over there" comes to inflict defeat "over here."

Concerning the identity of these fourteen, some say they refer to transgressing the pledges concerning the Three Jewels in the first buddha family; the vajra, bell, and vajra master in the second; the four types of giving in the third; the three Dharma pledges of the fourth; and just the offering pledge of the fifth family. These total fourteen. Others say they refer to the fourteen acts beginning with five contraventions, from non-killing of living creatures to abstaining from alcohol.[882] However, they should be understood as the fourteen root downfalls taught by the great Mañjuśrī Tsongkhapa and which will be listed below.

Secondary pledges

1. Pledges of abandonment
2. Pledges of reliance
3. Other pledges of reliance

Pledges of abandonment

> Do not kill living creatures,
> do not take what is not given,
> do not engage in perverse desire,
> do not tell lies,
> and do not take alcohol, the root of all ruin.
> Leave behind all improper activity
> not included in the taming of others.[883]

The four acts of abandonment from not killing to not telling lies [277] plus the abandoning of alcohol are the five practice foundations that act as foundations for the attainment of siddhi. Also, you should leave behind all improper activity of body, speech, and mind. However, for some sons of the Conqueror who properly guard their tantric vows, there are occasions when the seven physical and verbal activities, such as killing, are permitted when performed for the sake of taming others, and at those times such actions are not included in the above.

Pledges of reliance

> Devote yourself to the holy beings,
> give respect and service to the yogis.
> The three activities of the body,
> the four of speech, and the three of mind—
> develop them as much as you can.[884]

Devote yourself to the spiritual friend from which comes the development of mantra wisdom. Show respect to the yogis by not belittling them, and dedicate yourself to the ten white activities as much as possible.

Other pledges of reliance

> Have no desire for the lesser vehicles,
> don't turn your back on working for others,
> do not leave samsara behind,
> never develop a fondness for nirvana.[885]

The lesser vehicles have a smaller intention of working for others and aim for a lesser enlightenment. These are the paths of the śrāvakas and pratyekabuddhas, and you should have no desire to travel down them. Do not turn your back on others by being lazy in your task of working for countless living beings and so on. For as long as samsara exists, wear the armor of working for others. Abandon desire for the nirvana that is the mere freedom from the bondage of existence. Abandon these causes of turning away from the Mahayana.

> Do not despise gods, demigods, and *guhyaka;*
> do not walk upon mudrā, mounts,
> weapons, and implements.[886]

"Gods" are both mundane and supramundane. The *guhyaka* are a type of *yakṣa* spirit. "Mudrā" refers to drawings of deities. "Mounts" are the representative forms of deity mounts and the modes of transport of the guru. "Weapons" are deity weapons such as swords and spears. "Implements" are deity implements such as wheels and vajras. Toward all of them, do not commit the faults of despising them or walking on them.

Conclusion

The conclusion of the common pledges of the five families:

> These have been explained as pledges;
> guard them always.[887] [278]

This applies to all the pledges previously announced. The text continues:

> Extensive teachings on related vows
> are to be found in the secret tantras.[888]

Extensive teachings on vows or commitments of practice related to those already explained can be found in all the tantras. This has been said in order to dismiss any thought that the above explanations were exhaustive.

Taking the vows

1. The request
2. Taking hold of the vows

The request

In the *Vajraśekhara Tantra:*

> Master, grant me the vows.
> Sun of the Sage, every buddha,
> please hear this request.[889]

To this request by the disciple the guru says:

> Great being, do you wish
> to hold fully the secrets
> of the pure *mahāguhya* family?[890]

The guru asks if the disciple wants to take the vows. If he does not want them from his heart, they will not grow and are therefore forfeited. If the disciple is truly seeking the vows, he requests the vajra master, "Master, please listen to me,"[891] and proceeds to.takes the vows.

Taking hold of the vows

The *Vajraśekhara* states, "Master, as you have repeated, so I will do." This promise is dealt with under three headings:

1. Generating bodhicitta
2. Actually taking hold of the vows
3. Concluding promises

Generating bodhicitta

> Just as the guardian buddhas
> of the past, present, and future
> have single-pointedly developed
> their minds for enlightenment,
> I too generate this peerless and supreme mind.[892]

This is the aspiring bodhicitta, thinking, "When I become Vajrasattva I will lead all beings also to this enlightened state," as well as the engaged bodhicitta whose nature is the practices—giving and so forth—of this bodhicitta path. These two will produce the peerless result, and they are therefore "peerless and supreme."

Actually taking hold of the vows

> The practice of ethics,
> the ethics of gathering virtue,
> and the ethics of working for living beings:
> this vow of the buddha family yoga
> I will hold firmly.
>
> The Buddha, Dharma, and Sangha,
> the peerless Three Jewels:
> from now on I will firmly hold. [279]

This is the Vairocana vow.

> For the supreme vajra family,
> the vajra, bell, and mudrā

I will firmly hold.
The master too I will hold.

This is the Akṣobhya vow.

For the beautiful pledge
of the supreme jewel family,
six times a day
I will perform the four acts of giving.

This is the Ratnasambhava vow.

For the great lotus family
arising from the great enlightenment,
I will hold the highest Dharma
of the outer, inner, and secret vehicles.[893]

This is the Amitābha vow.

For the supreme activity family
I will hold well all vows taken,
and perform offerings as best I can.[894]

This is the Amoghasiddhi vow. These verses are for the taking of the individual vows.

Concluding promises

Having generated the bodhi mind,
peerless and supreme,
for the sake of all living beings,
I will keep well all vows.
Those not free I will free,
those not delivered I will deliver,
and those in torment I will comfort;
I will bring living beings to nirvana.[895]

The first two lines illustrate the aspiring and engaged bodhicitta. The next two lines encapsulate the five sets of vows. "Those not free" refers to Brahmā and others who are bound by the chains of the two obscurations—ignorance and so on. "Those not delivered" are the śrāvakas and pratyekabuddhas who are not delivered from the obscurations to omniscience. "Those in torment" refers to hell beings and the like. "I will bring living beings to nirvana" refers to bringing all living beings to the nonabiding nirvana.[896]

Conferring or not conferring empowerment on those taking or not taking vows

[Ānangagarbha's] *Sarvavajrodaya Vajradhātu Mandala Ritual* says:

> To those not taking the vows, do not say, "Now, today you..." and so forth. As master, do not confer permissions or empowerments.[897]

This is a section on empowerment not being conferred on those who are not taking the vows, and a second section on refuting objections on this point and taking the vows through empowerment.[898]

The *Vajrā Garland of Mandala Rituals* says:

> The six empowerments of garland, water, and so on grant power to activate the antidote to ignorance and are therefore called *wisdom empowerments*. Disciples who are conferred with these empowerments are empowered to hear, teach, and perform the mantra practice of the action and performance tantras.[899]

Abhayākara is saying that, apart from the two higher classes of tantra, when conferring empowerments such as the *Bhūtadamaka* and other mandalas taught in his *Vajra Garland of Mandala Rituals,* [280] it is acceptable to set aside the vows of the five families and to just confer the common vows. This is because they are just disciple empowerments for listening to, teaching, and practicing action and performance tantra, and that if the master empowerment is not conferred, the vajra-master vows are not given. This is the third section under this heading, dealing with which vows are conferred in action and performance tantra.

Pledges can be compiled under the headings of the four common root downfalls, the twelve *pāramitā* root downfalls, the thirty root downfalls of action tantra, the fourteen root downfalls of performance tantra, and so on.

Determining the downfalls that break the vows you have taken

Here there are three headings:

1. Identifying the person in whose mindstream the downfalls occur
2. Types of prescribed downfalls in that person
3. Explanations of each type

Identifying the person in whose mindstream the downfalls occur

This person must possess two features. He must have received exclusive secret mantra vows and not given them up, and he must be in a normal state of mind. If you have no vows, you might commit natural faults but you would not incur a prescribed downfall. Secondly, if you go insane, for example, and your memory becomes deranged, it is said you cannot incur a downfall.

Types of prescribed downfalls in that person

These are of two types. The *Vajrāvalī of Mandala Rituals* states:

> The downfalls of one who possesses the Vajrasattva vows are of two kinds: root *(mūlā)* downfalls and gross *(sthūlā)* downfalls.[900]

Explanations of each type

1. How not to be tainted with a root downfall
2. Restoring degenerated vows

How not to be tainted with a root downfall

1. Identifying the downfalls
2. Generating desire to guard the vows and not be tainted by downfalls
3. How to guard them

Identifying the downfalls

> For this reason Vajradhara has said
> that siddhis follow from the master;
> to disparage him is the first root downfall.[901]

For this reason of bringing all sentient beings to the attainment of the four bodies, which is the perfection of abandonment and insight, the all-pervading master and conqueror **Vajradhara has said that** [281] the accomplishments of the two types of **siddhis**—the mundane and supramundane—taught in the precious tantras come from or **follow from the** practices of proper devotion to the guru, or **master**. Therefore, **to disparage him** with contempt and to disrespect the body, speech, mind, and deeds of any masters, from those who have conferred on us all four empowerments down to those who taught us just one verse, **is the first** heavy **downfall** and is the **root** of even the fourteen primary downfalls that I, Śūra,[902] have compiled from the many coarse and subtle faults in mantra that are explained in the great texts.

> Transgressing the words of the Sugata
> is said to be the second downfall.[903]

Treatise of Valid Cognition says, "By his achievement of a threefold elimination of causes he is the **Sugata**."[904] In other words, because there is no creation of a basis for the sufferings of samsara, he has "gone beautifully." Because all seeds of the view of self have gone, he has "gone without return." Because all phenomena to be eliminated have disappeared, he has "gone entirely." Therefore, he dwells in the path of happiness, a buddha who has gone *(gata)* beautifully to happiness *(su)*. To **transgress** any of the three sets of vows he has taught within the mighty ocean of his **words**, especially the prescriptions of the tantric vows, accompanied by the deliberate intention to ignore them, **is said to be the second** of the fourteen root **downfalls**.

> Anger toward a vajra brother or sister
> is spoken of as the third fault.[905]

Those who have taken pledges from the same vajra master, the same mandala, or the same male or female consorts are *special* **vajra brothers and sisters.** Those who take pledges from different masters and so on are *individual* vajra brothers and sisters. All those who have entered the Mahayana are *close* brothers and sisters. To become angry from the depths of your heart at another brother or sister who has received all four empowerments within the same mandala of this vehicle of the vajra *(rdo rje)*—whose etymology is that, being the lord *(rje)* of all stones *(rdo)*, so hard and solid, it cannot be broken or split by anything—or even with someone with whom one has received a single verse of tantra teaching, **is spoken of as the third fault.**

> Abandoning love for sentient beings
> the Conqueror has declared the fourth.[906]

The six types of beings do not remain as one particular type but repeatedly circle and migrate in samsara [282] and are therefore called "migrators." Alternatively, by possessing a body that acts as the basis for consciousness, they are "embodied beings" who possess the nonmaterial sentience or mind that knows pleasure and pain, and so on. To wish that even one of these **sentient beings** has no happiness at all, thereby **abandoning love** in the sense of casting it far from your mind, the **Conqueror,** meaning he who has won the battle over millions of Māra hordes, **has declared** to be **the fourth** root downfall.

> Bodhicitta is the root of Dharma,
> to abandon it is the fifth.[907]

The 112th chapter of the *Avataṃsaka Sutra* says:

> Son of the family, the bodhi mind is like the seed of all the Dharmas of the Buddha.[908]

As this sutra says, the essence or the root of the Dharmas of the Buddha is exclusively the generation of the mind that thinks, "I will attain the enlightenment, the ultimate achievement of insight and abandonment, and bring all beings to the nonabiding nirvana." Therefore, to think "I cannot attain that state of enlightenment for the sake of limitless sentient beings," and thereby **abandon** the aspiring **bodhicitta is the fifth** root downfall.

> Deriding the doctrines of one's own
> or others' tenets is the sixth.[909]

Although the commentary asserts one's own tenets as referring to the secret mantra Vajrayana and the tenets of others as being the Perfection Vehicle, Nagpopa says that one's own doctrine refers to Buddhism while "others" refers to non-Buddhist tīrthikas, and I wonder if this is not correct. A tantra says:

> Deriding the non-Buddhists
> will send Vairocana far away.[910]

Also, something similar can be found in the commitments of taking refuge, which is indispensable to all vehicles. Therefore, whether it refers to Buddhist and non-Buddhist, or to the four great tenets of the noble land of India, to sutra and tantra, and to the more well-known traditions these days in the snowy land of Tibet—the Sakya, Geluk, the Karma, Drukpa, Dakpo, and Shang traditions of the Kagyü, the Shijé tradition, and so on—if you initially belong to any such grouping, leave it for another, and then deride your own former tradition, or alternatively if you deride and wholeheartedly reject the traditions and tenets of others more generally, this is the sixth root downfall.

> Proclaiming the secrets to beings
> completely unripe is the seventh.[911]

Beings are unripe in five ways. Those said to have base desires are those with wrong views [283] in whom the criteria necessary for secret mantra are incomplete and so are unripe in the sense of not being suitable vessels. Those who have not received the vase empowerment, even though they may be free of wrong views, have not been ripened by ritual. Those who have not received the knowledge-gnosis empowerment have not been ripened completely. Those who have not restored a broken root downfall are unripe by their degeneration. The fifth are those unripe because of their fear of the profound. Carelessly proclaiming to any of these types of beings the realities of the secrets of mantra, such as the two stages, is the seventh of the root downfalls.

> Aggregates are entities of the five buddhas;
> to despise them is the eighth.[912]

The five aggregates of form, feelings, discrimination, formations, and consciousness have the entities or nature of the five naturally pure buddhas or tathāgatas—Vairocana, Ratnasambhava, Amitābha, Amoghasiddhi, and Akṣobhya, respectively. They are to be given offerings with the inner fire-offering ritual and should be treated well and made to feel at ease. The eighth root downfall is to deliberately despise or torment the body, and to foolishly pursue behavior such as self-denial, casting yourself into pits, demeaning acts, improper feats of endurance, self-mutilation, and fasting—with a mind not grasped by the Mahayana and seeing these practices as causes for liberation.[913]

> The ninth is to doubt
> the natural purity of phenomena.[914]

This refers to entertaining doubts of validity or uncertainty over phenomena's lack of nature, the purity of emptiness free of fabrication, and also, as mentioned previously, toward the pure and nonsectarian Dharmas of one's own and other traditions, and particularly to the profound and authentic Dharmas practiced by my guru, the Great Fifth.[915] Such doubts constitute the ninth downfall.

> Constantly showing love to the wicked
> is asserted as being the tenth.[916]

Even toward wicked sentient beings that possess the ten criteria for being an enemy of the doctrine, such as disparaging the Three Jewels and the guru, destroying the teachings, and so forth, you should of course maintain a level of consciousness that cares for them with great compassion. However, while it is acceptable to behave in this compassionate manner for a while, to nurture love for these beings constantly over a long period of time without being able to remove[917] them with a compassionate mind, is, [284] as I Bhavila[918] assert, to commit the tenth root downfall.

> To give concept toward phenomena
> that are devoid of names and so on
> is the eleventh.[919]

The eleventh root downfall is using the philosophical analysis of tenet study to conceptualize with terminology and so forth marked by a grasping at true existence of those profound phenomena that ultimately are free of fabrication by name, words, verbalization, and the like. Alternatively, having found the perfect view of the no-self of phenomena, you then have to maintain it continuously; if instead you turn away from it, this is also the eleventh.

> Turning the minds of beings with faith
> is said to be the twelfth.[920]

"Beings" refers to any living being possessed of a great devotion of faith and disposition for the path of the supreme secret mantra of Vajrayana. With the wish to reverse their faith in that vehicle, you use derision and disparagement to uproot their aspiration again and again or even just once. This is the twelfth root downfall.

> Not using the pledges as they are found,
> this is the thirteenth.[921]

This means that at properly conducted ceremonial feasts or hero and heroine festivities, not purifying though the power of thought the five meats, five nectars, and other pledge substances, and consequently not partaking of them as they are. It also means not using pledges in the sense of not wanting to partake of pledge substances in the form of evening meals and so forth. This constitutes the thirteenth root downfall.

> Disparaging women, nature of wisdom,
> is the fourteenth.[922]

With "wisdom" referring to the great-bliss gnosis, and "nature" meaning "arising here," the agent that produces this wisdom in the yogi is woman, whose etymology is as follows. During the first eon close to the time of the development of male and female reproductive organs, a goiter-like protuberance appeared on the bodies of beings. In some beings it grew and became the sign of a male. Therefore, such a being was known as man (*skyes pa,* "growth"). In others it developed an opening and did not protrude. This was the sign of a female, and so she became known as woman (*bud med,* "with no protuberance"). "Woman" here can refer to those of supramundane qualities or any being that fulfills the criteria of being a woman. To disparage those women because of your stubborn attachment to the desire-free path of the *pratimokṣa,* or being motivated by a desire to find fault in them, is the fourteenth root downfall of those who follow highest yoga tantra.

These downfalls have been summarized by Ācārya Śūra or Bhavila, crown jewel of Indian scholars. Similarly, they are found in father tantras such as the twelfth chapter of the *Vajra Essence Ornament Tantra,* [285] the explanatory tantra *Vajraśekhara,* the seventeenth section of the *Black Yamāri Tantra,* the eighteenth chapter of the *Red Yamāri Tantra,* where apart from few differences in internal divisions and in translation, they number fourteen. In the fifteenth chapter of the mother tantra *Vajrapañjara,* ten downfalls are listed,[923] but they contain nothing that is not included in the fourteen explained above.

Summary

The teachings on these downfalls are prescriptive rules for the prevention of serious faults. The principal objects through which these faults can occur are those who teach us the Dharma, our practitioner friends, and the Dharma to be practiced.

Faults arising from focusing on the first of these are prevented by the prescription for the first downfall. Friends are of two kinds: true friends and false friends. The prescription of the third and twelfth vow stops us from acting wrongly to the first type of friend. The tenth prevents us from acquainting with the second type of friend. Dharma is of two types: scripture and practice. Practicing with disregard to the scriptures, slandering teachings by denying that they are the words of the Buddha, and teaching the unsuitable are prevented by the second, sixth, and seventh prescription.

Dharma in terms of practice refers to the basis of the path, the nature of the path, and branches of the path. The *basis* of the path refers to the bodhi mind developed for sentient beings, and the fourth and fifth vows prevent us from acting wrongly to those sentient beings and from giving up the very nature of that mind.

The *nature* of the path consists of the generation stage and completion stage. The eighth prescription prevents us from mistreating the aggregates, which are the bases of the deities we meditate on. The ninth and the eleventh vows prevent us from abandoning emptiness from the very outset of the completion stage and, even though it has been perceived, giving up mental engagement in it.

There are two *branches* of the path: the pledges as the foundation of the path and women companions. The thirteenth and fourteenth prevent not partaking of the pledges and the disparagement of women.

Generating the desire to guard the vows and not be tainted by downfalls

1. Reflecting on the advantages of guarding the vows
2. Reflecting on the faults of not guarding the vows

Reflecting on the advantages of guarding the vows

If mantra practitioners avoid these,
they will without doubt gain siddhi.[924]

The *Treasury of Secrets* says:

If given pure empowerment,
they will be empowered life after life, [286]
and in seven lives even without meditation
will gain siddhi.[925]

In *Five Pledges* it says:

If there are no downfalls,
siddhi in sixteen lives.[926]

Vibhūticandra says likewise.[927] Therefore, if you have not been tainted by the root and secondary faults—and even if you have been tainted, if you have properly restored them—thereby guarding the vows and pledges well, you will achieve siddhi within sixteen lives. Furthermore, until that time you will be happily protected by the conquerors, the bodhisattvas, and the great male and female warriors. Qualities will continue to grow, and the māras will find no opportunity to attack. These and many other bounteous benefits will follow. Therefore, develop great enthusiasm and inspiration in guarding the vows.

Reflecting on the faults of not guarding the vows

Or, if they degenerate their pledges,
such degenerates are seized by Māra.
They will experience great suffering
and, facing downward, go to hell.[928]

Saraha says:

> Conversely, if their pledges degenerate,
> forget the gaining of siddhi,
> even human birth will be difficult.[929]

Many texts make the same point. In short, if you transgress the pledges and prescriptions and they degenerate, then in this life you will be seized by Māra and other wayward spirits and experience all manner of misfortune, thereby bringing much suffering to body and mind. In the next life you will be turned upside down and fall to hell.

Therefore, the benefits and the corresponding disadvantages are huge, and consequently you should be very clear about what is to be developed and what is to be abandoned.

How to guard the vows

> Therefore, destroy your pride,
> do not deceive yourself,
> and be knowledgeable.[930]

The benefits of guarding the vows are immense; the drawbacks of not guarding are likewise huge. Therefore, if you are not knowledgeable about the threshold between downfall and no downfall, then that lack of knowledge becomes a cause for downfall. Therefore, its remedy is to thoroughly know the root and branch downfalls.

Even if you are knowledgeable, if you have no respect, even for practitioner friends and for the prescribed rules, then such disrespect becomes a cause for downfall. Therefore, destroy your pride and develop respect.

Even with respect, if you do not cultivate mindfulness, awareness, and conscientiousness, such a lack of conscientiousness becomes a cause for downfall. Therefore, do not deceive yourself and arm yourself with conscientiousness and so on in all you do.

Though you may behave conscientiously and with great respect, if you are troubled by much mental affliction, such a predominance of affliction will become a cause for downfall. [287] Therefore, as illustrated above with pride, whatever other affliction predominates, apply yourself to its antidote and reduce it.

The *Vajraśekhara* says:

If you degenerate the pledges,
you will not gain these fruits.
This will become your water of hell.
Break your pledges and you will burn.[931]

Restoring degenerated vows

In meditation make offerings to the guru
of whatever you have.
Then beginning with refuge in the Three Jewels,
if you want to benefit yourselves
with the vows of bodhicitta and so on,
you mantra practitioners should
take them with great determination.[932]

If you guard the vows as described above but still incur a root downfall, such as disparaging the guru through a lack of conscientiousness, straight away make preliminary offerings to the guru by sitting with the single-pointed mind of meditation and offering whatever you have—meaning according to your ability—to the visualized assembly. Then confess the transgressions. If you want to benefit yourself now and in the long term, retake the vows.

Mañjuśrī Tsongkhapa says:

The pioneering *Kālacakra Tantra*
has a different tradition of explanation
from other sutras and tantras.[933]

In Kālacakra literature, which my guru the Great Fifth calls a nondual tantra, there are many slight variations on the topics explained above. For example, on the taking of the vows, it says in the *Initiation* chapter, "For the desire Vajra family, the vajra, bell, mudrā, and guru are venerated on the crown"[934] and so on. Also, on the lines teaching the fourteen root downfalls: "Disturbing the mind of the glorious guru is the first root downfall for the son,"[935] and so on. These indicate a difference in content.

Vows in the early translation schools

In India this tradition was so secret that it existed as a one-to-one oral tradition. In Tibet, as designated by the time of its translations, it became known as the "early translation" tradition. Generally, in this tradition this topic can be dealt with under eight headings:

1. Nature of the pledges
2. Etymology
3. Divisions
4. Bases of the pledges
5. Benefits of keeping the pledges
6. Disadvantages of breaking pledges
7. Repairing broken pledges
8. Guarding the pledges [288]

Nature of the pledges

The power that is the mindstream bound by the tantric vows prevents the breaking of one's oaths. The *Supreme Pledges Tantra:*

> "Pledge" means bind:
> a vajra hard to break,
> a permanent guard.[936]

Etymology

The *Supreme Pledges Tantra:*

> In general, "pledge" *(dam tshig)* means
> divorced of all pretense
> in a mind with no anger *(tshig pa)*.[937]

Divisions

Generally, the tantra tradition talks of root and secondary pledges. The root pledges are divided into enlightened body, speech, and mind pledges. There are twenty-five secondary pledges—five headings each containing five: those to be known, those to be accepted, those not to be abandoned, those to be practiced, and those to be accomplished.

Specifically, in this tradition, there are seven divisions: those of view, practice, accomplishment, common pledges, specific pledges of enlightened body, speech, and mind, secondary pledges, and essential pledges. In the *Tantra of the Self-Appearing Mind* it says:

> A summary of the pledges taught
> in the great collections;
> hold them in your mind:
> pledges of the view bringing insight,
> pledges of continual practice,
> general pledges of accomplishment,
> the general common pledges,
> pledges of body, speech, and mind,
> pledges counted as secondary,
> and the essential definite pledges.
> These and other pledges
> are taught in brief and extensively.[938]

Bases of the pledges

This refers to the master and to the disciple brothers and sisters. The *Tantra of the Self-Appearing Mind* says:

> The pledges inconceivable to the mind
> are taught in brief as being two—
> those of the master and those of the disciple—
> and are known as foundations for the guarding of pledges.
> The cause for guarding pledges is the master,
> the guardian of pledges is the disciple.[939]

Vajra brothers and sisters are determined as being of four types. The same text says:

> Vajra brothers are explained by four characteristics:
> common, close, joined, and joined by the mandala vase.[940]

All those who have entered the teachings, and especially those who have entered tantra, are *common* vajra siblings. Those who follow the same Dharma are *close* siblings. Those brought together by the same guru are *joined* siblings. Those conferred empowerment at the same ceremony in the same mandala by the same lamp, the same vase, are all *closely joined* vajra siblings.

You should know that all these are objects whose risk factor is multiplied seven times.

Masters are also of four types. A commonly recognized master is one universally conferred with that title. [289] A guiding master is he who brings one to Dharma. The empowering master confers pledges and vows. The scriptural master passes on oral instructions. The *Tantra of the Self-Appearing Mind* says:

> Master too are of four kinds:
> masters in general, guiding masters,
> the pledge empowerment master,
> the scriptural instruction master.[941]

On the etymology of the terms master *(lopön)* and disciple *(lopma),* the text continues:

> The etymology is as follows:
> Liberating from ignorance into knowledge,
> he is the teacher *(slob).*
> Bringing one to the great perfection,
> he is the powerful one *(dpon).*
> The etymology of disciple:
> Listening without distraction
> he is the student *(slob).*
> Becoming a vessel for instructions,
> he is the mother *(ma).*[942]
> In this way, such a master and disciple
> dwell equally in this perfect state.
> With the pledges it is thus.[943]

Benefits of keeping the pledges

The *Tantra of the Self-Appearing Mind* says:

> For those dwelling in the pledges,
> correctly bound to the pledges,
> all hopes will be fulfilled.[944]

The *Māyā Tantra* says:

Those dwelling in the supreme pledges
will be blessed and regarded as sons and brothers
by the supremely great and the great.[945]

Disadvantages of breaking pledges

The *Tantra of the Self-Appearing Mind* says:

If broken, both guru and disciple will burn.
If the body pledges are broken,
they will boil in the vajra hell
and be born in a place of great wailing.

If the speech pledges are broken,
all light will disappear
as you are born in a place of great darkness.
Even when freed from there,
you will be born dumb.

If the mind pledges are broken,
you are born in places of mental turmoil,
of constant quarrel, endless strife,
fighting, and great suffering.
Alternatively, you lose your mind,
struck down with the illness of madness,
to be born finally in the hell of wailing.[946]

Also, further on:

Signs of broken pledges are:
experiencing various misfortunes,
plagues, and other infectious diseases,
being murdered by demons and spirits and sent to hell,
going blind, becoming deaf,
never succeeding in whatever is attempted,
your skin erupts in sores and leprosy,
being punished by the king and robbed by bandits,
getting infectious illnesses not caught by others,
and seeing your wife and children die. [290]

Everyone becomes an enemy;
all efforts are for naught.[947]

Repairing broken pledges

This is under three outlines. On repairing broken pledges of the enlightened body, the *Tantra of the Self-Appearing Mind* says:

Recitation of the vast scriptures,
extensive *gaṇacakra* offering ceremonies,
and meditation on the three-circle purity.[948]

For repairing broken pledges of the enlightened speech:

Perform the ceremony of the hundred lamps,
recite the *Hundred Abandonment Reparations*
and undertake various confession practices
and you will see the achievement of purification.[949]

Abandonment Reparations[950] refers to the *naraka* confession ritual.[951]

For repairing broken pledges of the enlightened mind:

Make offerings to please the guru,
exalted offerings of whatever you have.
If you perform confessions in this way,
all thoughts will be realized,
all wishes will be fulfilled,
and all works will be accomplished.[952]

Guarding the pledges

Seeing the advantages and disadvantages, bind the mind with mindfulness and pure awareness. The *Tantra of the Self-Appearing Mind* says:

Dwelling perfectly in the pledges,
not forsaking them even at the eon's destruction,
is the way to guard the great pledges.[953]

The master possesses knowledge of the tantra and the levels of the pledges and guards those pledges by the tenfold knowledge. The disciple does not possess this knowledge and guards the pledges by following the instructions of the master. These ten are: knowledge of the meanings of text, knowing how to answer questions, knowing the right time and occasion for empowerment and instruction, knowledge of the wide view, knowledge of the great desire of meditation, knowledge of profound reality, knowledge of being unmixed with samsara, knowledge of dwelling at a supramundane level, and knowledge of the defining characteristics of general and specific phenomena and the features of phenomena. The *Tantra of the Self-Appearing Mind* says:

> As a method of protecting the pledges,
> the ten features within a single consciousness is exalted.
> In one with fewer than that,
> conduct yourself according to the master of pledges.[954]

There is much explanation to be given on the specific pledges of the enlightened body, speech, and mind and on the supremacy of the peerless pledges, but this will suffice. [291]

The eight gross downfalls

These are taught in the works of the glorious guide, Ācārya Nāgārjuna.[955]

1. "Taking wisdom by force" is to take by force a consort not fully trained.
2. "Taking her ambrosia by force" is to take the ambrosia of the above by force.
3. "Not keeping the secrets from unsuitable vessels" is to show paintings, statues, texts, the six types of tantric ornaments, and so on to unsuitable vessels, such as those who have not received the empowerment and those who have no faith.
4. "Fighting during the ceremonial feast" is to quarrel or fight during the *gaṇacakra* feast or festivities of heroes and heroines.
5. "Showing another Dharma to those with faith" means, for example, teaching conventional truths to those who ask about the meaning of the ultimate truth.
6. "Staying seven days with a śrāvaka" means staying for seven days or more in the house of a śrāvaka who rejects and has contempt for secret mantra.

7. "Falsely having the pride of being a yogi" means to have and to teach with great conceit knowledge of reality merely by relying on a deity sādhana.
8. "Teaching Dharma to those with no faith" means giving empowerment to those who are not ripened by empowerment and lack faith in mantra, or to teach the secrets of mantra to those attracted to non-Buddhist Dharma.

These are the eight serious downfalls. "If they degenerate, undertake confession."[956] Therefore, if these vows are broken through ignorance and so on, undertake the confession practices according to the procedures.

Dwelling purely in the vows and pledges means that at best you will become a buddha in this life; if not, then in the intermediate state; and at the very least within seven lives or sixteen lives.

The Vajrayana has been extensively praised. Mañjuśrī Tsongkhapa says, for example:

> So hard to find, this peerless path;
> to discard it, how extraordinary!
> Therefore, enter this profound path,
> the Conqueror's supreme vehicle,
> the Vajrayana, rarer than the Buddha himself,
> a treasure source of the two siddhis,
> and practice with determination for a long time.[957]

Also:

> Ultimate teaching of the mighty[958] Buddha,
> the glorious highest yoga tantra.

The manner in which the resultant mantra vehicle is superior to the causal vehicle is taught in several precious tantras and propounded by many Indian scholar practitioners, and has been extensively dealt with elsewhere. [292] Nevertheless, as the saying goes, where there is great profit there is great danger, and of the three vows, those of mantra are the hardest to guard and keep. The great being [Atiśa] Dīpaṃkara said in the miscellaneous section of the *Book of Kadam: Father Teachings:*

> I am never tainted by faults in my *pratimokṣa* vows. However, I have been tainted by one or two small faults in my bodhisattva commitments. In my tantric vows, faults occur constantly, but these faults have never accompanied me for more than a day.[959]

Therefore, as can be clearly understood, we should be very careful.

24. Changes in Vow Status and the Preceptor Question

Changes in the status of the three vows

THERE ARE MANY scriptural references on whether the three vows change their individual status[960] in the mindstream of vajra-holding tantric practitioner who possesses all three vows. These can be rendered into common and exclusive assertions. On the first Sasang Mati Paṇchen says:

> The *Abhidharmakośa* says, "Separate, they are not mutually exclusive." Therefore, even when they exist in the mindstream of a single person, these three vows are quite separate. Were it otherwise, when the vows of a fully ordained monk are given up, all three would be given up. However, it is taught that when the vows of a fully ordained monk are given up, one reverts to being a novice monk, and when these are given up, one possesses the vows of a lay *upāsaka*. Because they are not mutually exclusive, their nonrevelatory[961] aspects can exist individually in the mindstream of a fully ordained monk who has entered the doctrine in successive stages.[962]

The great scholar Butön Rinpoché says:

> However, when a person takes the vows in successive stages, he increases his renunciation by adding, for example, the five remaining vows of a novice monk to the five lay *upāsaka* vows to make ten. Are they all separate? Like stacking coins on top of each other, they are substantially different and distinct from each other—the three vows of renouncing killing up to the three vows of renouncing alcohol are produced with distinct characteristics, and it is the same with renouncing singing and dancing and so on. So what are these differences? Differences exist because the

> bases are different. The wish to take on many different bases of commitment involves turning away from many different areas of pride and negligence. [293] Also the basis of, say, killing is different from the basis of, say, eating at the wrong times. There are also differences in the way you engage in the various foundations of restraint.[963]

[Chim Jampaiyang's] *Ornament to Commentary on Abhidharmakośa* says:

> The vows of the *upāsaka* and so forth all remain separate. The former do not transform into the latter, nor do they all become one.[964]

In his *Broom of the Buddha's Precious Doctrine: A Brief Presentation on the Three Sets of Vows,* Khedrup Rinpoché Gelek Palsangpo, having refuted the views of others, says:

> The correct view is as follows. The development of the three vows in the mindstream of one person requires three separate processes, constituting the initial collections of causes in the form of three distinct ceremonies. Because of this, the causes for giving up these sets of vows must also be individual. However, in between these times, guarding a lower vow becomes a causal condition for the higher vows to be held by a special motivating force, and for as long as that condition is present, the lower vows are a branch of the higher vows. However, this is not a case of these two being substantially the same or of sharing a mutual type or mutual continuum, in which one would disappear if the other were taken away. For example, if a jewel such as an emerald were placed in clear water in a clear and clean receptacle, the color of the water becomes part of the color of the jewel, but removal of either the jewel or the water would not remove the other.[965]

This means that, without the two lower vows, the higher vows suffer the fault of not having all parts complete. There are also statements that seem to say that the two lower sets of vows are necessarily taken within the ceremony creating the higher vows. These statements are made on the basis of a special intention of the author. Furthermore, there are assertions that state, for example, that the true bodhisattva vows are only made complete on the basis of already being a fully ordained *pratimokṣa* monk. Many scriptural sources also state that the qualification of a true vajra master is incomplete within a spiritual friend without the *pratimokṣa* of a fully ordained monk. For example, the *Kālacakra Root Tantra* states:

> Except for those on ārya levels,
> householders should not be gurus of kings.
> Of those whose learning is complete,
> who possess the signs...[966] [294]

However, my guru the Great Fifth, in reality the omniscient one, states in his *Golden Victorious Myrobalan Vinaya Ceremonies:*

> For those of lesser minds, the boundaries of the tenets of the great scholars are hard to ascertain. Nevertheless, like Milarepa knowing his own cave in Nyanang, in keeping with the merit of beginner disciples who take *pratimokṣa* according to the śrāvaka tradition, Paṇchen Śākyaśrī and Vibhūticandra, who are learned in this tradition and belong to the lineage of the great alms-seekers of Kashmir, maintain that the three vows are separate in terms of substance.[967] Vibhūticandra says:
>
> > From the ocean of the Paṇchen's mind,
> > with its vast wisdom and compassion,
> > I have taken this garland of jewels on the three vows.[968]
>
> Therefore, Vibhūticandra composed *Garland of Light on the Three Vows,* in which the three vows are taught as being separate in substance, in accordance with the thinking of Paṇchen. In it he says:
>
> > Therefore, to say the union of all three
> > exists in the vidyādhara vows alone is not correct.
> > If it were, the lower two would be produced
> > without need of the ceremony.
> >
> > A common ceremony for all three vows
> > the mighty Buddha did not teach.
> > The thought behind the praise

> that by vidyādhara vows alone,
> one comes to possesses all three,
> is not from the resultant point of view.
> If it were, omniscience would be
> of supreme and inferior types.[969]

The three vows in the mindstream of an ordinary being are substantially different from each other. The creation of the higher vows requires the previously created foundation of the lower vows, and therefore the three vows have different times of creation. The *pratimokṣa* vows dissolve at death while the other two are not lost, therefore they possess different causes for their dissolution. If you steal the possessions of the Three Jewels and your action is accompanied by the complete binding factors, your bodhisattva vows are destroyed, but that is not true of your *pratimokṣa* vows. Despising women out of great affliction breaks a tantric vow, but it does not incur a defeat in *pratimokṣa.* Feeling repulsion for and refusing pledge substances such as meat, alcohol, and the five nectars is to incur the thirteenth root downfall of the tantric vows, but such acts are to be abandoned in *pratimokṣa*. Therefore, the three vows are different in terms of substance.

When the sun, moon, and stars are all present in the sky, the latter two are outshone by the sun and remain unseen, even though they are not nonexistent. In a similar way the *pratimokṣa* and bodhisattva vows are outshone by the tantric vows. From this it can be inferred that the three parts of the *pratimokṣa* existing in one person are separate [295] but that the full monastic vows predominate with the other two remaining not evident. They are not nonexistent, just as when water, alcohol, and milk are poured one after the other into a single bowl; the smell of the alcohol and the color of the milk predominate, but this does not prove the absence of water. Similarly, the *Garland of Light on the Three Vows* says:

> When one endowed with the *pratimokṣa*
> takes those of the bodhisattva,[970]
> the first remains unseen in the foundation consciousness.
> Having taken the vows of the vidyādhara,
> the lower two remain unseen.
> For example when the stars appear in the sky
> they shine with a little light,
> but when the face of the moon rises,
> the world is lit and the stars' light fades.

> In turn, when the seven horses of the blazing sun appear,
> the world is bright and the moon's light dims.[971]

Therefore, the lower the vow the fainter it becomes. The higher the vow the stronger it is. This is also the position of my great guru.

In the *Essence of Secrets Tantra* the early translation school also says:

> The ethics of the might of the Vinaya
> and its inconceivable vows
> are all complete and pure
> in the pledges of the supreme and peerless.[972]

Therefore, in the mindstream of a three-vow vajra-holding tantric practitioner the three vows are complete and yet have changed their status. This is because the *pratimokṣa* and bodhisattva vows have transformed into tantric vows. They way they change is as follows. The clinging to appearances aspect of the *pratimokṣa* and bodhisattva vows, which is not held in the approach of the great equalizing wisdom, is completely given up. The *pratimokṣa,* with its aspect of relinquishing harming others, and the aspect of engaging in the welfare of others found in the bodhisattva vows are both complete and intact within the skillful means of effortlessly accomplishing the welfare of others that arises from the sphere of the great equalizing wisdom of the tantric vows. Moreover, it is explained that by becoming higher in terms of substance, these two vows have changed their status to become the substance of the tantric vows.

Who can give the pratimokṣa and bodhisattva vows?

It cannot be said with any certainty that there is only one kind of preceptor who necessarily bestows the *pratimokṣa* vows, because in the Vinaya there is reference to the householder Anāthapiṇḍada bestowing full monastic vows. [296] Also in the third fascicle[973] of the *Sutra Requested by the Householder Ugra* from the *Heap of Jewels* collection:

> Then the Bhagavān Buddha said to bodhisattva Maitreya and bodhisattva Viśuddha, "You great beings, ordain these householders with the full monastic vows." With the permission of the Bhagavān Buddha, the bodhisattva Maitreya and the bodhisattva

> Viśuddha performed the ordination. The bodhisattva Maitreya ordained nine thousand householders, and the bodhisattva Viśuddha ordained seven thousand householders.[974]

Therefore, although these bodhisattvas were in the form of householders, they clearly acted as preceptors for ordination.

Also the term "monk" cannot be applied solely to those with shaven heads, bare feet, and wearing the three robes. In the *Ten Cakra Kṣitigarbha Sutra* it says:

> Son of the family, furthermore, there are four kinds of monk. What are they? They are the ultimate monk, the conventional monk, the monk like a stupid sheep, and the shameless and immodest monk.
>
> Who is the ultimate monk? The Bhagavān Buddha, the great bodhisattva monk possessed of great achievements, with control over all phenomena, or those of pratyekabuddha enlightenment, the arhat, the nonreturner, the once-returner, and the stream enterer: these seven types of being make up the category of ultimate monk. Also, those beings who live in houses, do not shave their heads and their beards, do not wear the three robes, have not taken all the monastic *pratimokṣa* ethics, do not take part in requesting, ceremonies, purification rituals, and monastic activities: if they possess the dharmas of the āryas and they possess the fruits of those dharmas, they are also known as ultimate monks. This is the meaning of being an ultimate monk.
>
> What is a conventional monk? He who shaves his head and beard, dons the orange robes, and goes forth to become endowed with the *pratimokṣa* ethics is a conventional monk.
>
> Who is the monk like a stupid sheep? He is ignorant of whether he has weakened his root vows or not. [297] He is ignorant of whether the fault is heavy or light. Although he incurs various small breaches, he shows no remorse and does not declare them. He does not think about the faults he commits and pays no heed and has no qualms over minor faults. He does not devote himself to wise beings. He does not, from time to time, honor or serve the learned and those of great wisdom. He does not approach them respectfully and ask them questions. He does not ask, "What is

good? What is bad? What is not bad? Why is this good? Why is this wrong?" Such a person is a monk like a stupid sheep.

Who is the shameless and immodest monk? He approaches and is ordained into my doctrine merely for a livelihood, is without shame, breaks all the ethics of the *pratimokṣa,* and pays no heed to and has no fear of the suffering coming in the next life. Full of filth and decay, he is like the *kāla* worm.[975] He behaves like a dog at the sound of the conch. He constantly lies and does not know words of truth. He is in the grip of miserliness, jealousy, and ignorance, and is far from the three supreme activities. Attracted to gain, honor, and reputation, he delights in the six objects of the senses. Distracted by desire he is drawn to objects of form, sound, smell, taste, and touch. Such a person is shameless and immodest and is included among those who ridicule and slander the holy Dharma. This is the shameless and immodest monk.[976]

Therefore, those we assert these days to be pure monks are conventional monks, while ultimate monks are taught to be those endowed with the Dharmas of the āryas and the fruits of those Dharmas. Because of this, Saraha, preceptor for the full ordination of the glorious guide Ārya Nāgārjuna and one who had already crossed the vast ocean of Vinaya, said:

Taking the arrow maker's daughter as consort,
until yesterday I was not a monk;
from today onward I am a monk.[977]

Similar statements can be found in many biographies of Indian pandit practitioners. Here in Tibet, too, Ra Lotsāwa Dorjé Drakpa (1016–1198) said:

Partaking of meat and alcohol is the ceremonial feast, [298]
killing those who break their vows is a tantric pledge,
relying upon women is *karmamudrā:*
when I came to understand this,
it did not conflict with being a Vinaya-holding monk.[978]

Similarly, there were many other great beings, such as the Shangdro abbot Yudrakpa,[979] Bodong Paṇchen Jikdral,[980] and the Takten incarnation Künga Nyingpo,[981] who externally were adorned with the red robes, but internally their minds were integrated with the gnosis of the mahāmudrā, and they were able to make use of meat, alcohol, and women while at the same time acting as ordination preceptors in order to develop and take care of their disciples. These beings, for whom there was no contradiction between meditation and post-meditation, I think also demonstrate the point of the above citations.

However, don't confuse fish and turnips by including here people such as Salmo Drakpa, the Gyalwa Karmapa attendant Gyedra Rapjampa Küntu Sangpo, the Jamgön incarnation, and many others who shamelessly indulge themselves in drinking alcohol and sleeping with women while at the same time acting as ordination preceptors, ācāryas, and so on. They do not have even a billionth of the knowledge or realization of these great beings and are merely like the jackal who tries to follow where the tiger jumps.

To illustrate this point in the context of the object from which you take the bodhisattva vows, the Perfection Vehicle spiritual friend or master is illustrated in the *Avataṃsaka Sutra* in the Flower Ornament chapter.[982] Sudhana, the son of a merchant in the southern Indian town of Sukhākara received a prophecy from Mañjuśrī and devoted himself to a hundred and ten spiritual friends, beginning with the monk Meghaśrī and ending with bodhisattva Maitreya, in a great building adorned with the ornaments of Vairocana. They include rishis such as Bhayāgrasvara from the region of Sucinala; brahmans such as Uṣmanāyatana from Parīṣṭi; girls such as Maitrī, daughter of Siṃhaśrī, the king of the city Siṃhavijṛmbhita; youths such as Īṣvara from Sumukha; goddesses such as Mahāmāyā; householders such as Sucandra; and Nāvikaśūra from the town of Kūṭāgāra on the coast. From these beings he took the vows without the need for any formal basis *(rten)*.

In the first fascicle of *Encouraging the Exceptional Thought* it says: [299]

> Bhagavān, from now on, when we see someone of the bodhisattva vehicle enjoying the five sense pleasures, be they a householder or a monk, if we show disrespect or dishonor to them, or refuse to recognize them as teachers, then we are failing the Tathāgata.[983]

In the single-fascicle *Prophecy of Aśokadatta Sutra* it states:

> Subhūti said, "Girl, it is extraordinary that while dwelling in a house you dwell in such Dharma and give such a pure teaching!"
>
> The girl replied, "Venerable Subhūti, do not think of the

> mahāsattva bodhisattvas in terms of laymen or monks. Why? They are to be distinguished by their minds, by their wisdom, by their gnosis."[984]

In the third fascicle of *Teaching the Five Perfections Sutra:*

> If a bodhisattva dwells in a house and goes for refuge to the Three Jewels, dedicating all for the attainment of the omniscient mind, even though he enjoys the five sense pleasures, by doing just this much he dwells in the ethics of the bodhisattva and is endowed with the ethics of the bodhisattva. The bodhisattva who dwells in the ethics of the bodhisattva is not divorced from the perfection of ethics.[985]

Therefore, as long as you are not without the bodhi mind, your attire and behavior is of no regard. In particular, the ninety-fifth fascicle of the *Buddha Avataṃsaka Sutra,* in accordance with the prophecy of his spiritual friend Gandhaka Samantadarśin:

> Sudhana went to the land of Tāladhvaja to search for King Agni. On his arrival he asked the people for the whereabouts of King Agni. "Son of the family," they replied, "King Agni is sitting on the lion throne performing the activities of a king. He is protecting the kingdom. Those who deserve to be punished, he is punishing. Those who deserve to be rewarded, he is rewarding. Those who are deceitful he is questioning. On those with disputes, he passes judgment."[986]

And so on. The text continues:

> Sudhana, the merchant's son, went to where the king was sitting. There he saw him, in the prime of youth, [300] of handsome and attractive form, adorned with special marks, dwelling in regal splendor and might, immune from the harm of the forces of others in this world, sitting there with the might and power that fears no enemy, with an entourage of ten thousand ministers all working to fulfill the king's needs.
>
> In front of the king were those in charge of carrying out

punishments. They were men resembling the guardians of hell or the attendants of the lord of death. They were covered in fearful armor, wrathful, unbearable and terrifying to look at, with red eyes, fangs, the three lines on their brows knit to form a dreadful grimace. They carried weapons and instruments such as swords, axes, daggers, arrows, clubs, and spears. Their bodies and faces were ugly and frightening. Standing there like black clouds, angrily emitting fearsome snarls, their presence was unbearably frightening. He gazed upon these figures who would tear the hearts out of a hundred thousand creatures, as they strove to punish those beings that had been deemed worthy of punishment.

Among the offenders were those who had committed all manner of crimes: thieves who had stolen the wealth of others, those who had misused the possessions of others, bandits who had ambushed and robbed on the roads, those who had burned down villages, cities, towns, and farmsteads, those who had burgled and attacked villages. There were committers of atrocities, poisoners, slanderers, killers, and adulterers—perverse, malicious, and lustful committers of countless evils. He watched as many thousands of them, each tightly bound by five chains, were brought in front of the king and were handed down the appropriate sentence. Then, commanded by the king, some had their hands and feet cut off, some their ears and nose, some had their eyes plucked out, some had parts of their body cut off, some were burned alive, some had boiling nitrous water poured over their bodies until their skin blistered. He watched as they endured these dreadful and unbearable barbaric punishments and killings. [301]

On the killing ground he saw the hands, feet, ears, eyes, noses, heads, and other body parts of those who had been killed piled up like a mountain. He watched as the ocean of blood rose to a depth of three leagues and many leagues wide. He watched as the place became filled with jackals, foxes, dogs, vultures, eagles, and *kurara* hawks,[987] picking apart and devouring the thousands of bones, arms, legs, and headless torsos. Some of the corpses became discolored and turned blue. Some began to decay, some became putrid, and some were infested with maggots. He watched this terrifying and chilling scene unfold before him.

While being executed, so many dreadful atrocities were done

to them that they cried out in terror, begging for mercy. When Sudhana heard these anguished cries, he trembled with fear and was filled with revulsion. They were sounds like the sounds of the great Mountain Crushing Hell.

Having witnessed this furious and frightening slaughter, Sudhana thought to himself, "In order to help and bring happiness to all living creatures, I have entered the path of the unsurpassed and perfect enlightenment. I have sought out and made efforts in the practices of the bodhisattvas. I have asked spiritual friends what virtuous deeds are to be cultivated, what nonvirtuous deeds are to be left behind. But this King Agni has no virtue; he engages in great wrongs; his thoughts are those of violence; he engages in the killing of other living beings; he works to bring torment to other beings; he pays no heed to future lives; and he is standing on the edge of the great cliffs of hell. What bodhisattva practice is there to be gained from him?"

With these thoughts he stood there in doubt and hesitancy. Suddenly, celestial beings from the realms above called out to this greatly compassionate being; "Son of the family, do you not remember the instructions given to you by your spiritual friend Rishi Jinoṣman?"

He looked up to the sky and replied, "I remember." [302]

The gods continued, "Son of the family, do not have such doubts about your teacher's instructions. Son of the family, the spiritual friends teach truly and flawlessly and do not mislead. Son of the family, the bodhisattvas' knowledge of skillful activities is beyond comprehension. Their knowledge of ways to gather sentient beings is beyond comprehension. Their knowledge of ways to help sentient beings is beyond comprehension. Their knowledge of how to destroy sentient beings is beyond comprehension. Their knowledge of ways to exalt sentient beings is beyond comprehension. Their knowledge of ways to purify sentient beings is beyond comprehension. Their knowledge of ways to protect sentient beings is beyond comprehension. Their knowledge of ways to bring in sentient beings is beyond comprehension. Their knowledge of ways to ripen sentient beings is beyond comprehension. Their knowledge of ways to tame sentient beings is beyond comprehension. Therefore, son of the family, go ask him about the practices of the bodhisattva."[988]

This passage teaches that because this was a bodhisattva of the high levels who had shown himself in the form of a king performing evil acts for the sake of living beings, Sudhana should regard him as a spiritual teacher and devote himself without entertaining wrong views and doubts.

Also, the fifty-third branch of the *Wish-Fulfilling Tree of the Bodhisattva's Lives* by King Kṣemendra tells of the time our Teacher, while still on the path, was Subhāṣitagaveṣa, king of Vārāṇasī, and of how he went in search of wise counsel:[989]

> His chief minister Sumati said,
> "In the remote forest roams a hunter
> who is known as Lubdhakrūraka.[990]
> From him you will gain counsel,
> new and precious and consistently wise."[991]

With this prediction the king, adorned with a priceless string of jewels, set off and traveled alone through the forest:

> Searching with great resolve,
> he found the hunter on a mountainside,
> busy in his fervent love of hunting,
> enemy to the contentment of elephants,
> skilled in spearing and clubbing animals.
> In his left hand and like his own mind
> was a crooked and fearsome bow,
> the adversary of all those in the forest;
> accomplished solely in the art of killing, [303]
> his right hand held the arrows that bring
> the elephants to liberation.[992]

To this hunter, this lover of killing, holding in his hands a bow and arrow, the king offered the priceless string of jewels and made a request for wise counsel. The hunter replied:

> By the pledge of virtue
> I will give you wise counsel.
> As soon as you receive the counsel,
> you must throw your body from this mountain.[993]

The hunter said he would give the king wise counsel if he immediately jumped off the cliff upon hearing it. The king pledged that he would. The hunter recited one verse, which in essence said, "Do not touch wrong deeds and mental affliction that torment your path to happiness."[994] Having received this verse he jumped off the mountainside without hesitation.

Also in the hundred and seventh branch of this *Wish-Fulfilling Tree of the Bodhisattva's Lives,* the householder Śuddhodana offered a huge pile of jewels for just the smallest of wise counsels from the daughter of King Brahmadatta. The text says, "With the jewel of wise counsel firm in their hearts, they are bound by excellent qualities,"[995] and so on. These accounts talk of teachings being received without recourse to an object[996] of wise counsel.

In the third[997] fascicle of the *Boxed Arrangement* it says:

> "Son of the family, in the great town of Vārāṇasī there is a Dharma teacher who holds in his mind the great six-syllable mantra, who recites it and contemplates it correctly. Son of the family, when you see this Dharma teacher, do not have doubts, for if you do, son of the family, you may fall from the bodhisattva levels and be reborn in the lower realms. That Dharma teacher will have degenerate ethics and degenerate behavior and will be surrounded by wives, sons, and daughters. He will even cover the orange robes with excrement and urine, and his behavior will be unrestrained."
>
> Then Viṣkambhī said to the Bhagavān, "I will do as the Bhagavān has instructed." He went to Vārāṇasī, bowed his head at the feet of that Dharma teacher, and listened to the six-syllable mantra.[998]

This point is taught extensively in this sutra.

Also Aśokadatta, the daughter of King Ajātaśatru, pleased the Teacher by not rising from her seat in the presence of the śrāvakas.[999] [304] She surpassed Śāriputra, Maudgalyāyana, Mahākāśyapa, Subhūti, Rāhula, and others with her Dharma oratory, and the Teacher prophesized that at the end of seven countless eons she would become enlightened in the world known as Vimalaprabhā.

Even the beer seller Vinasa taught the Dharma and brought others to the path of ripening and liberation.

Natasthāpana was a servant of Queen Śyāmāvatī, who in some accounts is the queen of King Paurastya but most say was the queen of King Ajātaśatru. Natasthāpana taught the Dharma from behind closed doors. Because of this the queens did not realize the truth. They asked the Bhagavān why this was, and he replied that through reverence it could be realized. So Natasthāpana was placed on a high seat where she taught Dharma, and soon the queens realized the truth. This is an account where no formal object is relied upon but where an object of reverence is of importance.

Furthermore, the householder Surata, the householder Ugra, Sūbahu, Sumati, the girl Vimaladatta, the girl Vimalaśraddhā, the merchant Bhadrapāla, Licchavi Vimala, the goddess Śrīmālā, and others have all taught fully ordained monks and others without possessing the *pratimokṣa* as a basis.

In the Vajrayana Buddha Śākyamuni himself taught the highest yoga yantras such as the nondual Kālacakra, the father tantra Guhyasamāja, the mother tantra Cakrasaṃvara, and so on, with teacher and audience all manifested solely in the form of desire. Later in the land of Oḍḍiyāna as King Indrabodhi, he taught the father tantra Guhyasamāja and also many tantras of the early translation school. These works are the fundamental texts of tantra.

Similarly, there were many lay Indian pandits such as Candragomin, and here in Tibet the Dharma king Songtsen Gampo gave the Mahākaruṇa teachings at Pabongkha, and many hundreds of "long-haired" *(ral pa can)* practitioners were brought to the path of ripening and liberation. The great master Atiśa, founder of the Kadam tradition, had a body of disciples, including monks, as vast as the ocean, but he entrusted the complete tradition to his main disciple Dromtön Gyalwai Jungné in his form of an *upāsaka* lay practitioner:

> My teachings I entrust to you;
> yet no matter how many qualities you may possess,
> no one person could take them all on.
> They will be divided, therefore,
> among eighty others of fortunate merit,
> and by this they will prosper.[1000]

Those who built the foundations of the Sakya tradition, such as the three white-robed practitioners[1001] [305] and Drokmi Lotsāwa; those at the root of the Kagyü tradition such as Marpa, Tsurpa, Mila, and Shangpa Nigu; also Rongpa Galo, Tanak Gö Lotsāwa, the Kashmiri Somanātha, and many other spiritual friends, without relying on any ordained basis, brought beings to ripening and liberation in the form of lay practitioners. Therefore, there is nothing decisive about the need for an ordained basis.

My guru, the Great Fifth, says in his *Silken Robe Biography,* in the *ka* volume, page 129b:

> It is said dismissively, "Oracles who reveal deities, painters of deities, young monks, and so on mistake the non-ordained for gurus." If this refers to lay people, then you should know that not only in the Nyingma but also in the new translation schools there are many lay gurus, including Drokmi, Mal Lotsāwa, Marpa, Mardo Lotsāwa, Gö Lotsāwa, Sachen Künga Nyingpo, Ra Bumseng, Khubön, and Ga Lotsāwa Namgyal Dorjé. If you say, "They are different because they are practitioners of tantra," then you should know that in India there were those such as King Kṣemendra and in Tibet, King Songtsen Gampo and Rikden Namgyal Drakpa.[1002]

However, in terms of their nature, they should possess all the necessary qualities mentioned previously, and it is especially important, as emphasized by the story of the servant Natasthāpana, that they are objects of reverence.

25. Benefits

The benefits of their teachings

As for the benefits of the teachings given by those worthy of teaching Dharma, the *Lion's Roar of Maitreya,* from twenty-third volume of the *Heap of Jewels* collection, says:

> Giving away as much gold as would fill
> the great thousand-world realm
> would not match the benefit gained
> from teaching just one four-line verse.
>
> For those wishing to benefit others,
> of far greater benefit than bestowing on a single being
> every happiness of every living being in the three realms
> is to teach that person one verse of the Buddha's doctrine,
> for it will deliver that being from suffering.[1003]

Also:

> Were one person to fill with precious jewels
> world realms as many as the grains of sand in the Ganges
> and with a joyful mind offer them to the king,
> while another gave just a single verse to a single sentient being,
> that great gift of jewels would not amount to a fraction of—
> would not even compare to—the gift of the verse offered in
> compassion.
> If that is so, how could we possibly conceive the merit
> of giving the same to two or three beings?[1004] [306]

The *Sutra Teaching the Benefits of Giving* states:

> Giving the gift of Dharma results in the ripening of remembering past lives.[1005]

In the *Ten Thousand Perfection of Wisdom Sutra:*

> Subhūti, it is like that. Just as you have said, it is like that. Should a son of the family or a daughter of the family, on the eighth, the fourteenth, or the fifteenth day of the month recite or teach this Perfection of Wisdom, the accumulation of merit created is immeasurable, uncountable, limitless, inconceivable, and inestimable. Should such a person recite or teach this Perfection of Wisdom, they will come to dwell among the retinue of gods.[1006]

In *Encouraging the Exceptional Thought:*

> Maitreya, should a bodhisattva, working hard as my attendant, fill this great billionfold world realm with shrines made from the seven precious gems, that would not please me, it would pay me no reverence, it would not venerate me. But Maitreya, should a bodhisattva take at the very least a four-line verse of the Perfection of Wisdom and commit it to memory, keep it in his mind, read it, understand it, or teach it, that is paying me reverence, seeing me as guru, venerating me, pleasing me. Why is that? Maitreya, the enlightenment of the tathāgatas arises from learning. It does not arise from the possession of material things.[1007]

In the *Seven Dharmas Requested by Avalokiteśvara:*

> Were one person to fill to overflowing with precious jewels
> world realms as many as the grains of sand in the Ganges
> and with a joyful mind offer them to the king,
> while another gave a single verse to a single person,
> that vast gift of precious jewels
> would not be fraction of—would come nowhere near—
> the gift of a verse offered with compassion.
> If this is so, how could we possibly conceive
> the merit of doing it two or three times?[1008]

These passages speak of the merit of giving the minimum of just a single verse. *Differentiating the Middle Way and the Extremes* from the works of Maitreya states:

> Writing, making offerings, giving,
> listening, reading, memorizing,
> preaching, recitating, contemplating, and meditating:
> the merit of these ten activities is incalculable.[1009] [307]

Preaching a text, or reading a text, has been described as one of the four verbal Dharma activities,[1010] and is one of the ten causes producing an incalculable amount of merit. The commentary to *Differentiating the Middle Way and the Extremes* states:

> Preaching the meanings or the words means to teach Dharma with great enthusiasm to those who are suitable.[1011]

Therefore, the benefits of teaching are inconceivable.

The benefits of listening

In the fourth chapter of the *Sutra Requested by Pūrṇa:*

> Ānanda, do not think that scents, aromatic powders, perfumed lotions, incense, victory standards, banners, beautiful clothes, the sweet sounds of cymbals, and songs of praise to the tathāgatas are the best offerings. Ānanda, do not hold these to be the best type of offerings. Listening to these profound sutras, taking them to your mind, remembering them, reading, reciting, receiving transmissions, and practicing them exactly as they are taught are the best offerings. Such activities, therefore, are offerings to the tathāgatas, are acts of service, of veneration, of respecting them as gurus, and are words of praise to them.[1012]

Therefore, listening to Dharma and receiving transmissions are far superior to making material offerings.

The twenty-seventh chapter of the *Meeting of Father and Son Sutra* says:

> Śāriputra, say a son of the family or a daughter of the family who has entered the bodhisattva vehicle practices for ten eons the first five perfections divorced from the perfection of wisdom. Śāriputra, one dwelling solely in the single-minded concentration of the bodhisattva who hears just this teaching accumulates far greater merit.[1013]

Merely listening to the profound Dharma is of greater benefit than the five perfections—giving, guarding one's ethics, developing patience, increasing effort, and abiding in meditative absorption.

In the *Qualities of the Buddha Realm of Mañjuśrī* from the fifteenth volume of the *Heap of Jewels* collection:

> Son of the family, someone may fill with the seven types of precious gems as many buddha realms as can be seen by the unobstructed sight of the tathāgatas [308] in the ten directions and offer them to each tathāgata. Another will listen to this particular Dharma, take it to their mind, hold it, read it, understand it, or practice it. The merit of the former does not approach a hundredth of the latter, a thousandth of the latter.[1014]

In the third chapter of *Sutra Requested by the Householder Ugra:*

> Ānanda, someone who listens to and comprehends this particular Dharma, who teaches it extensively and perfectly to others in order to preserve the sacred Dharma and to ensure that the family of the Buddha does not die out, and who dwells in the practices is one who is making offerings and performing devoted service to the bhagavān buddhas of the past, present, and future.[1015]

In the *Sutra of the Gradual Arising of Enlightenment:*

> Ānanda, those who wish to see the Tathāgata, and who wish to perform the deeds of the Buddha for sentient beings, should listen to this particular Dharma, take it into their minds, keep it there, read it, and teach it to others.[1016]

From the second chapter of the *Lion's Roar of Maitreya:*

> Kāśyapa, someone may fill this billionfold world realm with oil whose height reaches from the oceans to the world of Brahmā, plant a lamp wick the size of Meru, and light it as an act of offering to the Tathāgata. Yet another who sits in front of their preceptor or master with a perfect mind and intention and receives one four-line verse, recites it, and then takes seven steps earns by far the greater merit.[1017]

In the second chapter of *Encouraging the Exceptional Thought:*

> Because I yearned for enlightenment,
> I gave away my limbs thousands of times.
> If I am never sated by listening to Dharma,
> why do they become bored with listening?
>
> For the sake of a single four-line verse,
> I turned from my wife and child.
> If I renounced my kingdom and possessions,
> how can the scholars not listen to Dharma?[1018] [309]

In the one-fasicle text called *Sutra Requested by the Girl Sumati:*

> Therefore, Mañjuśrī, the bodhisattva mahāsattvas should with all effort strive to write these precious sutras, to transmit them, to hold them in their minds, to read them, and to teach them to others, for this will be the legacy of my doctrine.[1019]

In the *Prophecy of Aśokadatta Sutra:*

> Ānanda, someone may fill this billionfold world realm with various jewels and give them away. Another may simply listen to this particular Dharma. If this latter action creates so much more merit than the former, what need to speak of the merit of working hard to take this Dharma to mind, to comprehend it, to not forget it, to read it, and to transmit it in the appropriate language?[1020]

In the second chapter of *Sutra Requested by Vimaladatta:*

> Receiving, reciting, and remembering the teachings,
> addressing others with words pleasing and attractive,
> tirelessly teaching the Dharma,
> and cultivating the signs of meditative concentration:
> devoting yourself to these four practices
> develops power and the memory of previous lives,
> the memory of thousands of eons gone by,
> and the attainments of the supreme guide.[1021]

In the *Sutra Requested by Kāśyapa* from the *Heap of Jewels* collection:

> Kāśyapa, a son of the family or a daughter of the family may fill as many world realms as there are grains of sand in the Ganges with the seven kinds of gems and give them as offerings to the tathāgata arhat fully enlightened and perfect buddhas. For as many bhagavān buddhas as there are grains of sand in the Ganges, they may build temples of each tathāgata constructed from the seven types of precious gems and numbering as many as the grains of sand in the Ganges. For as many bhagavān buddhas as there are grains of sand in the Ganges, they may serve and honor with every form of pleasure and comfort for as many eons as there are grains of sand in the Ganges the immeasurable number of communities of śrāvaka monks of each tathāgata. They may build shrines to all those tathāgatas who have passed into nirvana. [310] But a son of the family or a daughter of the family filled with faith who takes a transmission of one verse from the Mahayana *Heap of Jewels* collection, and having taken it does not forsake it, generates merit far, far greater.[1022]

In the *Eight Thousand Perfection of Wisdom,* in the Types of Merit chapter:

> "Kauśika, more than that, a son of the family or a daughter of the family, in order to venerate the tathāgata arhat fully enlightened and perfect buddha who has passed into nirvana, may undertake the building of many millions of shrines built of the seven gems and containing tathāgata holy relics at its core. And once the shrines are constructed, that son or daughter of the family for the rest of his or her life may make many celestial offerings to those

shrines consisting of celestial flowers, celestial incense, celestial perfumes, celestial garlands, celestial lotions, celestial silks, celestial parasols, celestial victory standards, celestial bells, and celestial banners, and ring the whole shrine with garlands of lamps. With such a host of celestial offerings, he or she may revere it, venerate it as a teacher, prostrate to it, make offerings to it, honor it, and worship it. Kauśika, what do you think? From this practice would that son of the family or a daughter of the family create much merit?"

Indra replied, "Much merit, Bhagavān. Much merit, Sugata."

The Bhagavān continued, "Kauśika, this son of the family or daughter of the family will create merit much more than the previous. Yet he or she with great faith in this perfection of wisdom who thinks on it, who has great liking for it, who with joyful mind generates the bodhicitta and with an exceptional state of mind listens to it, takes it into their mind, keeps it in their mind, studies it, comprehends it, reads it, teaches it, teaches it well, transmits it, recites it, teaches it extensively to others, explains its meanings, contemplates it, and examines it with his or her development of wisdom; who works for the sacred Dharma to be preserved for a long time, praying, 'May the way of the Buddha never cease; [311] may the sacred Dharma not disappear'; who turns it, if small, into a bound volume of text and keeps it and preserves it so that it may prove beneficial for the bodhisattva mahāsattvas, because it possesses the way of the Buddha; who offers all kinds of offerings to this perfection of wisdom such as flowers, incense, perfumes, garlands, lotions, powders, silks, parasols, victory standards, bells, and banners, and encircles it with garlands of lamps; who reveres it, venerates it as a teacher, prostrates to it, makes offerings to it, honors it, and worships it; Kauśika, that son of the family or daughter of the family will create merit immeasurably greater."[1023]

Pandit Candranandana says:

Through transmission of the teaching, understanding of the text is gained.[1024]

Ācārya Sthiramati in his *Commentary to Differentiating the Middle Way and the Extremes* says:

> When listening to others reading, listening with respect.[1025]

Therefore, many precious sutras talk of the limitless benefits gained from studying, listening, or receiving transmissions of the sacred Dharma. [313]

26. Qualities of a Master of Medicine

On the characteristics of a master of medicine, or physician, the thirty-first[1026] chapter of the Explanatory Tantra from *Four Tantras* says:

> The healer who heals,
> the doctor who practices:
> this section has the headings of
> causes, nature, etymology,
> types, function, and results.[1027]

Therefore, there are six sections: the causes of a doctor, the nature, etymology, types, function, and results.

Causes

> The causes are intellect, a virtuous mind,
> keeping the pledges, well skilled,
> endeavor, wise in traditions of the world.[1028]

The main causes for becoming a wise doctor are possessing an intelligent mind capable of discriminative analysis; possessing a supremely virtuous and exceptional state of mind that wishes to be of benefit to all living creatures; holding the pledges, which will be listed later; being manually, verbally, and mentally well skilled; endeavoring in the proper activities at the proper time; and being wise in the ways and customs of the world.

Now the extensive explanation:

> Possessed of great intellect, stable, and careful,
> he comprehends all healing practices, extensive and brief;
> in all procedures he fears no hindrance,

and with his wisdom a subtle clairvoyant discernment arises.
This is the most important of the causes.[1029]

The first of the six causes is intelligence. Generally the term "intellect" *(blo)* refers to a wisdom capable of great discernment and analysis, though the term "intelligence" *(blo gros)* is more widely used. Therefore, a doctor has a great intellect capable of comprehending all the scriptures. It is not distracted by extraneous circumstances and is therefore a stable intellect. It is careful because it proceeds in all matters by way of prior examination. With genuine possession of these three qualities, a doctor comprehends the meanings of all the short and extensive texts that primarily explain practices for healing. With this learning he does not have the fear and apprehension of being hindered or obstructed by a lack of knowledge, and he undertakes with ease every medical practice the occasion calls for. [314] Even with those practices not taught in the scriptures, because of his untainted wisdom, he has a subtle clairvoyance-like discernment that arises appropriately for the occasion. Of all the six causes, this intelligence is the most important.

A virtuous mind means possessing bodhicitta—
its preparatory, actual, and subsequent practices.
The first is seeing the suffering, wanting to help, developing faith,
having firm equanimity toward the good and bad, the loved and the hated,
with compassion, love, joy, and equanimity,
and generating the yearning bodhicitta.
To engage in actual practice is to practice without limits.
Subsequent practice is to hold in esteem without resentment,
which makes your curing easier,
allowing you to become a support to the lives of many.[1030]

The second cause is to be endowed with the bodhicitta that recognizes all living beings as your parents. As a topic it is divided into preparatory, actual, and subsequent practices. The preparatory practices of attitude are seeing these three realms as nothing but suffering, developing a sustained state of mind that wishes to help all living creatures—none of which have not been your parents—having a faith in the Three Jewels as the unfailing refuges, and from the depths of your being having a mind of equanimity toward the good and the bad such as gold and clods of earth, toward the loved and the hated such as friends and enemies, and so on. From this attitude you abide in the compassion that cannot bear the suffering of the lower realms, the love that regards living beings as a mother would regard her only child, the joy of seeing any being freed from suffering, and the equanimity of being divorced from all attachment and aversion. These four are known as dwelling in the four realms of Brahmā. Then comes the generation of the mind of supreme enlightenment that yearns to attain the state of a buddha for the sake of all sentient beings.

The actual practice is to work solely for the benefit of others and, in terms of time and number, to practice without limits and without partiality. Subsequently, if you hold the practice of medicine in high esteem and treat the sick with an exceptional state of mind that carries no resentment for any patient whatsoever, your patients become easier to cure, and you become a support for many lives.

Keeping the pledges

> Of the pledges, six to keep in the mind,
> two to hold, and three to know. [315]
> In the first are those of the master,
> speech, medical literature,
> your brothers, patients, and pus and blood.
> These are like the Buddha, the rishis' speech,
> the transmission of enlightened speech,
> friends and brothers, children, and dogs and pigs,
> these six pledges of the mind to be guarded.
>
> For the second, the medicine vidyādharas and their instruments,
> hold them as oath-bearing protectors and their implements.
> Medicines like gems, ambrosia, and offering substances—
> these are the three recognitions;
> they are gems fulfilling needs and desires,
> ambrosia curing all disease,
> and the ritual food offerings for the vidyādhara.[1031]

"Keeping the pledges" refers to six to be kept in the mind, two to be held, and three to be known. Concerning the first of these three sets, the six refer to your master, his words, medical literature, your brother-like companions, patients, and the blood and pus of patients. These six are to be kept in the mind and guarded as being, respectively, the actual Buddha, the speech of the rishis, the actual tantra as the speech of the Conqueror, your vajra brothers, children, and as objects that engender the behavior of dogs and pigs.[1032]

The two pledges to be held concern the vidyādhara medicine rishis and their instruments—the bloodletting funnel, and so on. These should be regarded as pledged protectors of medical science and their implements, respectively.

The third set of pledges is that all medicines should be recognized as gems, ambrosia, and offering substances. Indirectly, relying on medicine fulfills all your needs and desires, therefore, medicines should be regarded as wish-fulfilling jewels. Because they quickly and easily cure patients of their illnesses, they should be regarded as ambrosia. Medicines in the form of ritual food offerings[1033] please the vidyādhara rishis and are to be regarded as offering substances. The extensive explanation of this topic involving deity meditation, eulogies, prayers for auspiciousness, and mantra recitation has been dealt with elsewhere.

Well skilled

> "Well skilled" means manually, verbally, and mentally skilled.
> Skilled with his hands, he is wise in medical techniques;
> with sweet words he is capable of bringing joy to the sick;
> of bright intellect, his mind is clear and unconfused.
> Knowing these, he becomes a master among craftsman.[1034]

"Well skilled" from the six causes means he is manually skillful, verbally skillful, and mentally skillful. Skilled with his hands, [316] he knows techniques of medical preparation and medical practice, such as using the enema medicine pipe, bloodletting lancets, and splints. Being verbally skilled in using pleasant and reassuring words, he is able to bring joy to patients. Being of a bright intellect, he remains clear and unconfused in the recognition of symptoms, medicines, medical techniques, and so on. Knowing these he becomes a master or supreme among craftsmen.

Endeavoring in activities

> Effort in activities concerns yourself and others.
> For yourself this means training in the causes,

devoting yourself to causal conditions,
making effort with regard to your companions,
and endeavoring to complete your development.[1035]

Exerting yourself in work as a cause for becoming a doctor therefore involves:

1. Endeavor for yourself
2. Endeavor for others

Endeavor for yourself

1. Training yourself in the basic causes
2. Devoting yourself to acquiring the necessary conditions
3. Endeavor with regard to your companions
4. Completing your development

These four are presented in the verse in outline.

Training yourself in the basic causes

The basic cause for all achievements in the field of knowledge is a good comprehension of writing and reading. Therefore, from the beginning you must complete and master these skills. Why? Because the line between having and not having great qualities, and being skilled and not skilled in teaching, composition, and debate, is determined primarily by ability in reading and writing. The *Thirty Verses* says:

The foundations of all training,
the cause of the wise orator,
the foundation for the expression of words,
is explained as the construction of letters.[1036]

Also:

With this order of study,
even those of little effort
will soon find wisdom;
therefore begin your studies here.[1037]

My own guru the Great Fifth also said:

> Grammar, logic, crafts, medicine, Buddhism, poetry,
> lexicography, metrical composition, drama, astronomy—
> nothing is not worth studying.
> So without ever being satiated
> cut wrong notions about learning.[1038]

It is important to sever all mistaken notions about the five major and five secondary fields of knowledge. For scholars these are the main gateways, or subjects of study and contemplation. The *Sutra of Repaying the Kindness of the Skillful Buddha* says: [317]

> Why should bodhisattvas study the great treatises on grammar? They will be adorned with accurate language, whereas with inaccurate language they will not be able to explain the meanings. Moreover, they will come to know and comprehend all topics. For these and other reasons they should study the treatises on grammar.[1039]

Therefore, study of the science of grammar primarily brings knowledge and comprehension of all topics. It eradicates all errors of language and meaning that oneself and others fall into. If you do not know this science, you will similarly not understand the grammatical formations, etymologies, and so on found in medical literature, and you will be incomplete as a scholar.

The *Sutra of Repaying the Kindness of the Skillful Buddha* says:

> Because one will come to know of all errors, and because one will be able to distinguish the words of the Tathāgata from the words of the worldly, the bodhisattva should study the treatises on reasoning.[1040]

The great Mañjuśrī Tsongkhapa said:

> If you do not wash the eyes of your mind
> again and again with the ambrosia waters of reasoning
> flowing from the great Dignāga, defeater of false orators,
> let alone not seeing the supremely profound,

your misconceptions are likely to proliferate
even when examining the meaning of lesser texts.
Though you find conviction merely through correct affirmation,
you will not be able to eliminate doubts
through the power of valid perception that establishes and refutes.[1041]
You become like a stake driven into mud—
unable to secure any stable and valid imprints.[1042]

If you do not become learned in the science of reasoning or valid perception, defeater of all those dwelling in errors of meaning and destroyer of all wrong views, then let alone not understanding the profound meanings of the teachings of the Buddha and the treatises, you will not even be able to develop any stable and valid imprints concerning the meanings of coarser scriptures, and meanwhile your misunderstandings will increase.

The Great Fifth said:

This great wheel of the compounding of medicine,
with its spokes of heat and cold finely balanced,
glorious magical blades of a thousandfold knowledge,
cutting through the nets of disease
for the health of all living creatures—
how amazing![1043]

This death-destroying, ambrosia-like science that grants longevity without old age, and is the antidote to all 404 types of disease, is the main topic and practice of this work. Therefore, there is no need to dwell on it here. [318] Also:

Supreme jewel wealth of the science of crafts:
great ocean that knows no end,
the arts and crafts of body, speech, and mind,
the measure of the distance to its farther shore
gained by the three signs that training is complete.[1044]

There is no art and no science that cannot be included in physical, verbal, or mental skills. Therefore, the science of crafts and skills is the most important and is indispensable knowledge for a physician, as taught above in the section on being well skilled.

> The inner science, revealing the supreme path
> of great renunciation, bodhi mind, and liberation.[1045]

The inner science of the 84,000 Dharma collections or the twelve branches of scripture are gathered into the three baskets of scripture and the four classes of tantra and contain a subject matter of sutra and the new and old-school secret mantra; he who has correctly entered their paths will accomplish great waves of benefit for himself and others. Its need and importance, therefore, is unimaginable.

In medicine also, the inner science is of great significance, such as in the practices for consecrating medicine. Therefore, you should have mastered the stages of generation and completion and the invocation of enlightened activity, having completed at the very least the stipulated deity-yoga meditations of Dorjé Trapring[1046] or other meditation deities. Furthermore, knowledge of this science is necessary on occasions, because if you cannot even explain the divisions of the sutras, old and new tantra, the four classes of tantra, the great and the two lesser vehicles, and so on, then any attempts at teaching, composing, and debating will be like arrows fired in the dark. This science then is the most important area to persevere in.

Also:

> A king proud of his youth but unadorned
> is a target of gossip.
> Similarly a work shorn of poetics
> is not ranked as a work of the wise.[1047]

You may be proud of the excellence of a composition, but if it lacks the devices of poetics, then like a man in the prime of youth wandering around unclothed, it is not a thing of beauty. Therefore, with their beautifying verbal adornments of a thousand moods and expressions,[1048] you should pursue a study of the treatises on the art of poetry.

> The lexicographer with his brush of communication
> paints a variety of beautiful word pictures
> on the broad new silks of the mind;
> arranged in series, a show of lexicography.[1049]

The treatises on lexicography[1050] are not only essential for teaching and composing, but in the medical sutras and treatises also, much depends on lexicography. [319] Therefore, you should study *Treasury of Immortality,*[1051] *Various Clarifications,*[1052] and other works.

> The beautifully woven brocade of *vṛtta* and *jāti* meters
> adorned with the patterns of light and heavy sounds,
> well made into the clothing of well-constructed Sanskrit,
> is worn by many a scholar in the land of snow.[1053]

To learn how to construct a line of verse, study thoroughly the treatises on metrical composition, such as *Jewel Source Treatise of Metrics* by Ratnākara.

> In the Sindhuvari grove of worldly knowledge,
> their slender bodies blend prose and poetry,
> their smiles skillfully welcome the guests of well-told tales;
> the saffron heads of drama sway to and fro.[1054]

There are many special reasons for studying the art of drama, such as to curb ignorance of different languages and dialects.

Of particular importance:

> A never-before-seen mirror
> of elemental and astrological calculation,
> the *Victory in Battle Tantra* clearly revealing images
> of phenomena subtle and hard to perceive—
> does it steal the pride of the omniscient mind?[1055]

The *Victory in Battle Tantra,* or *Arising Letters (Svarodaya Tantra)* contains many practices essential for the science of medicine, such as divination diagrams for medical practices, the auspicious ambrosia times, lunar remainders[1056] calculation, and so on through which the doctor is able to ascertain when medicine and medical practice becomes ambrosia-like in its benefits; the outer, inner, and secret inauspicious *kulika* times, which if not known can mean the medicine becoming poison and so forth; fortune and life divinations for life-and-death prognoses—not always used for medical purposes; and so on.

Astrology,[1057] so called because it primarily teaches the examination of constellations, calculates planetary and stellar combinations,[1058] and so on. Using it one calculates the times, directions, and dates when the collecting, preparation, and taking of medicines becomes effective and auspicious. There is a great difference between these benefits and the disastrous consequences that come from not knowing this astrology.

Black [or, elemental] calculation is so called because it spread from the country of black clothes.[1059] It describes pulse evaluation—calculating mother, son, enemy, and friend pulses—and urine analysis in conjunction with turtle diagrams and so on, topics that are of prime interest for medical literature. It also covers subjects such as karma calculation, which can predict lifespans and foretell whether one will survive an illness without medical intervention. It deals with the examination of the year, month, day, and hour to divine whether various therapies are appropriate and to calculate the auspicious and inauspicious times for compounding medicines, for performing various medical practices, and so on. It also covers the consulting of land guardians[1060] to divine auspicious and inauspicious directions. [320] In particular, using only illness divination and time divination, you can make prognoses and learn which demon is causing the illness and what rituals are to be performed, all without resorting to guesswork or relying on other forms of divination, oracles, and the like. In this way elemental calculation has a very strong connection with medical science.

Astrology, elemental calculation, and *Arising Letters* divination generally can be applied to all phenomena, and together with the location of the life force[1061] and so on, they are in all respects indispensable tools.

Devoting yourself to acquiring the necessary conditions

The necessary condition is devotion to the master,
dealt with under three headings:
definition, manner of devotion, and reason.
The definition of a master is one extensively learned,
in possession of the oral tradition, patient,
of little guile, compassionate, and worthy of reverence.

Devotion should be one of trusting without doubt,
of carrying out tasks without duplicity,
of behaving always in harmony with his thoughts,
and of making effort in constant thought of his kindness.

The reason for such devotion is that
you learn quickly and become wise.[1062]

Therefore, having trained yourself in all forms of knowledge, as illustrated by the previous topic of reading and writing, you devote yourself to the causal condition for becoming learned in medicine. This is the master, and this topic is under the three headings of definition of a master, the way to devote oneself, and the reason for such devotion. The definition of a master is someone who has extensively examined his own and others' medical traditions and become wise and learned in their words and meanings. He possesses not just one but as many oral traditions as possible, and he is not miserly with them. He is calm and patient. "Of little falsehood" means with little guile and deceit.[1063] He has compassion for the sick and for his students, and is deemed worthy of reverence by those of noble status. The student should devote himself to such a person.

Having found a master with such qualities, the way of devotion is with single-minded trust devoid of the doubt that asks, "Through him will I master my studies? Should I study with him or not?" You follow his instructions exactly, whether in his presence or not. All your behaviour should be in harmony with his thoughts. Even if you have made only meager development, think of it as being the result of his kindness, and steadily persevere.

The reason for such devotion is that it allows you to quickly master the medical texts and become learned.

Endeavor with regard to your companions

Endeavor with regard to your companions
is to ask and make enquiries of them,
and to memorize and contemplate without laziness.
Why? Laziness is a hindering enemy.[1064]

Not only should you rely upon the master, but toward your companions you should do as follows. [321] To some ask, "What does this mean here in this text?" To others ask, "What is such and such?" Do not be lazy in retaining texts and the words of the master and others, or in contemplating their meanings. Why? Because laziness is an enemy that hinders such contemplation. Therefore always generate perseverance.

Completing your development

> Completing your development means
> practicing what is seen and heard,
> taking, becoming familiar, and eliminating all doubt.[1065]

Having learned how to read and write, devoted yourself to a master, and shown willing endeavor to your companions, you will complete that scholarship or development by ensuring that whenever you see or hear that someone, whether high or low, has even a morsel of a good teaching, you endeavor to request it and to put it into practice. In this way you take all teachings into your mind and become familiar with them, thereby eliminating the taint of doubt.

Endeavor for others

> Endeavor for the activities of others
> is effort for the sake of the patient,
> where without the interruption of delays—
> like someone under threat of death
> carrying melted butter on a wall—
> you endeavor with concentration,
> administering treatment at the right time.[1066]

Here "activities of others" refers to the patient, for whose sake you must concentrate single-pointedly, uninterrupted by delays or by other activities, not just once but until it is certain that the patient will either live or die. Concentrate like someone walking on top of a high and narrow wall carrying a bowl full of melted butter who is threatened with certain death if he spills a drop, and endeavor to administer—at the right time and without delay—the treatment indicated by your examination of the symptoms.

Wise in traditions of the world

> To be wise in the traditions of the world
> refers to worldly ethics, the spiritual, and both.
> For the first, become learned,
> care for others with gentleness,

and subdue others with toughness;
with these three desires are met.

With wisdom in spiritual matters
comes a disciplined mind, affability, and contentment,
bringing benefits to self and others.

With both comes concern and compassion for the deprived,
and those on high will fulfill your needs.
Endowed with these six collections,
results will undoubtedly arrive.[1067]

The last of the six causes is to become wise in world traditions. It is dealt with under three headings: to follow the traditions of the human world, [322] to follow spiritual or celestial traditions, and to train yourself in both.

For the first of these, you train to become learned in the behavior that conforms to the traditions of the world. Toward those you aim to benefit, use appropriate methods. For some show concern, reassuring them with gentle speech and movements. For others use tougher means to subdue them. With these three your wishes will be met.

Similarly, on the spiritual path, if you have a disciplined mind, are easy to get on with, and have contentment concerning desires, you will benefit yourself and everybody else.

Being learned in both worldly and spiritual ethics gives you a special compassion for those made wretched by disease and deprived by poverty, and you care for them with a pure intent. When this happens those on high, such as lamas and dignitaries, will remark, "This is truly a bodhisattva physician!" and they will ensure that all your needs are met.

Therefore, endowed with this collection of six causes needed to become a learned physician—being of an intelligent mind and so on—you will gain without doubt the temporary benefits of this life, such as celebrity and wealth, as well the ultimate fruits.

The nature of a physician

To understand as appropriate the characteristics
of humors, the vulnerable, and remedies
is asserted as being the nature.[1068]

The nature of a physician is asserted as being a knowledge that has understood by way of sharp or middling faculties as appropriate all the characteristics of the three humors, the ten vulnerable bodily phenomena,[1069] and all salutary medical practices.

Etymology

As for the etymology of *physician:*
"medicine" by curing illness, aiding the body;
"hero" by applying surgery to the disease;
"physician" by protecting all beings like a father;
regarded as lords by kings.[1070]

This is the etymology of the term *physician (sman pa/dpa').*[1071] Because he alleviates the pain of illness and brings relief to the body, he is "medicine" *(sman).* When he uses surgical instruments such as surgical spoons and cutters for serious illnesses, he is brave and fearless *(pa/dpa').* Therefore he is a "hero of medicine" *(sman pa/dpa').* Alternatively, he is a "physician" because he protects all living beings like a father.[1072] Also, kings are as gods of the world, and even they revere physicians as lords. Therefore, they are known as *lhajé,* or "lords of the gods." [323]

Types of physicians

Types are the unsurpassed, the special, and the ordinary:
unsurpassed in eliminating the three poisons, their causes, and their effects.
clearly know the minds of others and are loving, upright, and true;
those of conferred lineage, their trained followers, and those familiar with practice—
these are the friends of living beings;
those with desire who suddenly appear in the guise of physicians—
these are the butchers of lives.
However, they are identified as the best and the worst.[1073]

Concerning the types of physician, there is the unsurpassed physician, the special physician, and the ordinary physician. The physician who eliminates desire, aversion, and confusion, the ignorance that causes these three poisons, together with the wind, bile, and phlegm disorders that result from the three poisons is the blessed Buddha. He is the physician surpassed by no one. In the *Mañjuśrī Illusory Net* it says:

> The best and lord of physicians,
> unsurpassed reliever of pain.[1074]

The special physician possesses clairvoyance that knows the minds of others as well as immeasurable love and compassion. Therefore those made wretched with suffering he brings to happiness, while his own mind is upright and true.[1075] *Caraka* says:

> All these great rishis
> possess the fivefold clairvoyance
> and know the eighteen supreme fields of knowledge.[1076]

The ordinary physician is of two types, the first of which is of three kinds. There are those who have been conferred as chief physicians of genuine Dharma kings, manifestations of the three buddha families, a distinction that is passed down through their lineage. There are those who are not of the lineage of chief physicians of kings but who have followed after them and have trained well in their medical studies. Still others do not possess the qualities of being highly trained in medical studies but through observation of their master's practice have become familiar with the work of a physician. These three are allies of the lives of living beings.

Those who know nothing but, out of desire for food and clothing, suddenly appear in the guise of a physician are the butchers of life. However, among the divisions of ordinary physicians, those of conferred lineage, trained followers, and those familiar with practice are identified as the best physicians, while the second type are identified as the lowest of physicians. This division into "best" and "worst" is made primarily on the basis of worldly standards. On this point the *Small Collection Illuminating Lamp*[1077] commentary on the Explanatory Tantra says:

> Physicians of "conferred lineage" refer to those conferred as physicians of kings and who then possess a physician lineage. [324] "Trained followers" are those physicians who follow the great scholars and train accordingly. Those "familiar with practice" are

those who do not know the medical scriptures but have relied on the oral traditions and have become familiar with practice by watching the master at work and developing their own practice. Physicians who train hastily through desire have no mastery or familiarization but, driven by desire, merely assume the guise of a physician.

The last are of four types: the physician familiar with the patients' means, the physician limited by scrolls, the physician who has picked up a few manuscripts, and the physician who is little more than a salesman. The first is a physician who treats others having calculated the benefit the patient will be to him. The second is a physician whose practice is based on having seen a few scrolls of the profound oral tradition. The third is a physician whose practice is based on hearsay, something someone has written down, or some mediocre medicine and writings stolen by thieves. The fourth is a physician whose practice is based on knowing a little and who sells general medicines that treat all parts of the body saying, "This medicine is good for this." These physicians are butchers of lives.[1078]

Concerning the "best physician":

> Of a venerable race, intelligent, dwelling in pledges,
> wise in scripture, penetrating to the essence of oral traditions,
> complete mastery, working primarily for Dharma,
> desire left behind, disciplined, skilled,
> a great mind of love for others, undistracted,
> considering the welfare of others as his own,
> clear and informed in all medical practices,
> the best physician, sole protector of the sick,
> a son in the lineage of the vidyādhara rishis:
> thus has spoken this manifestation of the life-granting
> medicine king.[1079]

The best physician is born of a venerable race such as that of the royal, noble, or brahman classes. He has the intelligence to distinguish between what is correct and incorrect and constantly dwells within the pledges. He is wise in the meanings of both small and extensive scriptural traditions and penetrates with certainty the precise essence of the profound oral traditions. He has gained complete mastery in all medical practices, and by mainly striving solely for the Dharma, he leaves behind desires motivated by the eight worldly attitudes. He is disciplined physically, verbally, and mentally and likewise skilled physically, verbally, and mentally, and he has exceptional love and compassion for others. Without being distracted for an instant, he considers the welfare of others to be more precious than his own. [325] He is clear and informed on all the meanings of scriptures of all medical practices of all traditions. Such a one with such qualities is the best physician of all those who claim to be physicians. He is the sole protector of those beings brought down by sickness, a son holding the lineage of the vidyādhara medicine rishis. I, Vidyājñāna, manifestation of the life-granting medicine king, the beryl king, have spoken this.

Also, as it says in the twenty-sixth chapter:

> The physician ascends to the dais of the scholar,
> knows the scriptures, observes the work, and is pure.[1080]

A physician ascends to the heights of intelligence, training, fame, and veneration—likened to the dais of a scholar—where he is elevated by his knowledge of the five sciences, especially the science of medicine. Through the tantras, treatises, transmissions, and oral traditions, he knows the meanings of all the scriptures. He has observed the work of his master in areas of examination, medicines, therapies or surgery, rules of diet, and behavior and integrated them accordingly. He is pure and clean because he is without the faults of being of poor or mixed ancestry, he does not possess a mind that covets the wealth of his patients, he is not partisan in his compassion, and he is not someone who messily spills blood in simple medical procedures. A physician must possess these sixteen attributes.

In the Entrustment Chapter of the Enlightened Activities, or Final Tantra, of *Four Tantras:*

> A suitable vessel for the entrustment of this tantra
> is possessed of the pledges and raises the guru to his crown.
> Able and willing to give up wealth or life,
> he has no sense of loss for either.
> Of great intelligence he discerns
> contradictions and connections in the text.

Of great bodhi mind primarily concerned for the welfare of others,
he has a mind entrusted to Dharma, with no guile and pretense.
To the fortunate ones possessed of these six causes
will this tantra of the great rishis be entrusted.[1081]

Endowed with the pledges he will properly venerate the gurus and masters. In order to develop excellent qualities, he is willing and able to sacrifice his life and any kind of wealth without a sense of loss. Endowed with great intelligence he is able to discern all contradictions and connections in the texts and oral traditions. With a great bodhi mind he primarily works solely for the sake of others. [326] With his mind entrusted solely to the Dharma, he is divorced of the guile and pretense that seeks to deceive others. Surkhar[1082] asserts these six causes taught in the Final Tantra to be the same as the six taught in the Explanatory Tantra in the chapter on physicians, but these two have different meanings.

Also *Caraka:*

The doctor who is intelligent and wise,
whose qualities are perfected,
his mind moist with compassion,
is the crown jewel of all physicians.[1083]

In the introduction to the *Treatise of Eight Branches:*

The physician on the dais of the scholar,
knowing scripture, observing the work, and pure.[1084]

In *Illuminating Lamp:*

The healer is pure and wise,
strives for understanding,
has senses calm and disciplined,
and is well learned and good-natured,
compassionate to others,
knowledgeable, and skilled;
on the dais of the scholar,
knows the scriptures.[1085]

In *Essence of Eight Branches:*

> A physician well learned in the texts
> is a good scholar wise in the transmissions;
> familiar with the practices and virtuous
> is the good physician, the exalted physician.[1086]

Therefore, a physician must have these excellent qualities. However, as *In Devotion to the Ultimate Truth* says:

> Because of these *kaliyuga* times of trouble,
> qualities and faults are mixed within gurus;
> none are completely without fault.
> Disciples will come to rely on those,
> discovered after careful examination,
> to have a predominance of good qualities.[1087]

Therefore, in these *kaliyuga* times it is rare to find masters with all these good qualities present. Rely on those whose good qualities outweigh their bad.

27. Examining Disciples and Studying with the Master

Examination of disciples

ON THE TANTRA POSITION in general, the *Fifty Verses on Guru Devotion* states:

> Guru and disciple suffer equally
> any degeneration of pledges.
> Therefore the brave one examines
> the relationship between guru and disciple.[1088]

In the *Vajra Garland Tantra:*

> Just as a jewel is tested by rubbing
> and gold by heating and cutting,
> the disciple is examined for up to twelve years. [327]
> In this way, mutual examination should proceed.
> If this is not done, obstacles will arise,
> destroying siddhis and bringing suffering.[1089]

Also:

> Just as one should not pour
> the milk of a lioness into an earthen pot,
> so the Mahāyoga tantras should not be given
> to those vessels who are unsuitable.
> The disciple meets death in that moment,
> ruined in this and future lives.
> If instruction is taught to unsuitable vessels,
> the master suffers degeneration of siddhi.[1090]

Thus, this point is forcefully made. The twelve years referred to means that if after examination you cannot come quickly to a decision, continue for a maximum of twelve years. If you are able to decide quickly, twelve years are not necessary.

If it is not possible to find one with all the necessary characteristics complete, as taught in the tantras, then rely on one who has eliminated most faults and, with the most important branch qualities complete, possesses a predominance of good qualities. The action tantra called *Tantra Requested by Subāhu* states:

> One with such qualities complete
> is very rare in this *kaliyuga,*
> so rely upon a mantra friend
> with half, quarter, an eighth of these qualities.[1091]

Therefore, examine for worthy and unworthy vessels. On the actual faults of disciples, the *Vajraḍāka Tantra* states:

> Those angry, too intellectual, too old,
> those who are actual monks,
> those bound by attachment and desire:
> jewels without worth, do not teach them.[1092]

The *General Rituals Secret Tantra* states:

> Leave behind those of coarse speech,
> of little enthusiasm, those who kill,
> those who steal, and false friends.[1093]

Also:

> Duplicitous, false ethics, little faith,
> little effort, a poor mind, uncertain, distracted,
> little respect for the master and his vajra brothers:
> such a one is not suitable for empowerment.[1094]

There are many similar passages. So what are the qualities of a true disciple? The *Vajraḍāka Tantra* states:

Without pride, pretense,
with no clinging to self,
entrusting self to the Dharma:
to these impart the instructions;
to others, a downfall occurs.[1095]

Also:

Of faith and great striving,
never tired of listening or learning,
respectful toward guru and brothers:
such a one is fit for empowerment.[1096]

The *Illusory Net Tantra* says:

Taking joy in meditation,
always respectful toward the guru, [328]
constantly making offering to the gurus:
one with such qualities is a disciple.[1097]

The *Great Illusion* says:

Of intelligent mind, great enthusiasm,
Of gratitude, from a good family,
devoid of pride, good-looking,
in the prime of life, of healthy complexion.[1098]

From the *Essence of Secrets Tantra:*

If possessed of faith, effort, conduct, insight,
give the benefiting initiation,
the power initiation, in order.[1099]

From the *Vajraśekhara Tantra:*

Belief in the Three Jewels,
fear of committing wrong deeds,
good discipline, faith, and pure joy:
to such a one give the pledges.[1100]

From *Four Hundred Verses:*

> An unprejudiced, hard-working, and intelligent
> listener is a suitable vessel;
> other qualities will not be projected onto the speaker
> nor upon the listener.[1101]

Therefore, the mind of a true disciple is unprejudiced, capable, brave, and stable. With great endeavor he cracks the whip of perseverance in order to remember the teachings, contemplate the meanings, resolve all contradictions and errors, ask questions about them, and so on. He possesses the eye of intelligence, meaning he has an intellect that comprehends the words of the teaching profoundly, clearly, quickly, and without difficulty. He is someone with the intelligence to understand, the aspiration to work hard, and a respectful attitude devoid of pride.

As for the qualities of the medical disciple the *Caraka* says:

> Intelligent, happy to give, of gratitude,
> kindhearted, without desire, striving in discipline.[1102]

In *Eight Branches* by Śūra:

> Possessed of generosity, ethics, and compassion,
> of pure conduct,[1103] appreciative, and kindhearted,
> relying upon the elixirs, life and merit will increase.[1104]

One with these qualities fulfills the definition of a disciple. One with opposite qualities is an unsuitable vessel and not to be accepted. In *Caraka:*

> A bad person, of corrupt intelligence,
> a mere reflection of a physician
> should not even be spoken to,
> let alone taught.[1105]

Aśvaghoṣa says:

> Placed in a rotten vessel
> it immediately becomes poison.[1106]

Also:

> Not knowing with any certainty the treatises,
> absorbed merely into the words,
> holding in his hands the noose of Yama:
> cast far away this wicked physician.[1107] [329]

Also, in the Final Tantra, in the section on entrusting the compiled teaching for safekeeping:

> Keeping the master secret while promoting himself,
> stealing by stealth, making gains by flattery,
> deceitfully preying on the wealth of others,
> seized by pride and conceit, devoid of compassion.[1108]

In the Explanatory Tantra, from the above section on the activities of the doctor:

> Not endowed with such qualities,
> possessing the faults of this lowest type,
> this doctor without a lineage,
> like a jackal that has seized a kingdom,
> is revered by no one.
>
> This doctor ignorant of scripture,
> like a blind person being shown various things,
> cannot discern various disorders and treatments.
>
> This doctor without the familiarity
> that comes through observation,
> like one walking on an unfamiliar path,
> wonders about symptoms and surgical technique.
>
> This doctor who cannot diagnose,
> like someone wandering friendless in a foreign land,
> does not recognize a single disorder.
>
> This doctor ignorant of pulse and urine,

like a messenger unable to carry a message,
cannot articulate disorders as hot or cold.

This doctor ignorant of prognosis,
like a leader who cannot talk,
is struck with embarrassment and a poor reputation.

This doctor ignorant of treatment techniques,
like someone shooting at a target in the dark,
his remedies never strike the disorder.

This doctor ignorant of behavior and diet
is like a king whose kingdom has become his enemy:
the disorder grows in strength,
the bodily constituents grow weak.

This doctor ignorant of pacification compounds,
like a farmer ignorant of farming,
compounds wrongly, too little or too much,
and the disorder merely increases.

This doctor ignorant of purging techniques,
like pouring water on a hill of sand:
causing illness and harming the bodily constituents.

This doctor without surgical instruments,
like a warrior without armor and weapons,
cannot overcome the enemy of disease and its army.

This doctor ignorant of moxabustion and bloodletting,
like a burglar without inside information,
is confused about the disorder and the therapy.

Therefore, such bad physicians
with invariably erroneous ideas,
their remedies are likewise erroneous;
demons in the guise of physicians,

holding the noose of the lord of death—
they are the levers that topple the fortress of life.
Therefore, have no connection with them,
lest your circle of dependents be ruined.[1109]

Also, from the Final Tantra:

To such a unmeritorious and an unworthy vessel—
like a jewel in the throat of a sea monster,
never emerging from its mouth though shaken for an age—
it should remain secret.[1110] [330]

How the disciple studies with the master

With the above faults eliminated and the right qualities acquired, the way in which the disciple listens is described under two headings:

1. Eliminating the three faults using the analogy of pots
2. Developing the six recognitions

Eliminating the three faults using the analogy of pots

If one pot is upside down, another the right way up but unwashed, and another clean but leaky, even rain from the gods would not fall in to the first. If it fell into the second pot, it would become polluted and unfit for drinking, and so forth. It would remain clean in the third but would soon leak away. Similarly, the student may be present where the Dharma is being taught but not paying attention. He may be paying attention but understands it wrongly, his motivation is wrong, and so on. He may have been free of those two faults, but the words and the understanding gained at the time of listening were not embedded firmly in his mind, and he forgets them. If these and other similar failings occur, the great purpose of listening to Dharma will not be realized. Therefore, you should be without these faults.

As a remedy for these three faults a sutra says, "Listen well, and take it to your mind."[1111] In the *Stages of the Bodhisattva* it says:

> Listen with the desire to know everything, with a single-pointed mind, with attention on the teaching, with a mind of respect, and with the whole of the mind.[1112]

Developing the six recognitions

In the Flower Ornament chapter from section 110 of the *Avataṃsaka Sutra:*

> Son of the family, develop the recognition of yourself as a sick person, of the spiritual friend as the doctor, of the teachings as medicine, and of conscientious practice as the cure for your illness.[1113]

This teaches four recognitions. Recognizing yourself as a sick person is taught in *Engaging in the Practices of the Bodhisattva:*

> If we must follow the advice of a physician
> even when afflicted with an ordinary illness,
> what need to mention when we are constantly afflicted
> with the manifold illnesses of desire and so forth.[1114]

We need to develop this recognition because we are constantly plagued with mental afflictions such as desire that create dreadful and long-lasting sufferings difficult to cure.

Recognizing the Dharma teacher as the doctor is accomplished as follows. If we are seriously suffering from a wind disorder, a bile disorder, or some other ailment, and we set out in search of an experienced doctor. [331] When we meet him we feel joy. We listen to what he says and respectfully minister to his needs. It is the same with the Dharma teacher. We seek him, and when we find him we do what he says and serve him respectfully, "wearing it as an ornament not as a burden." In *Bhagavān Jewel Qualities* it says:

> Therefore, by seeking the highest enlightenment,
> destroy the pride that comes from being learned with arrogance,
> and like the sick who depend on the doctor to be cured,
> devote yourself without distraction to the spiritual friend.[1115]

Recognizing his teachings as medicine means that just as a sick person would cherish the medicine prepared for him by the doctor, you should recognize the teachings and advice given by the Dharma teacher as being of great importance, and go out of your way to cherish them and not let them go to waste by just forgetting them, and so on.

Recognizing conscientious practice as the cure of the illness means that just as the patient understands that if he does not take the medicine prepared by the doctor, the illness will not be cured, you should understand that without putting into practice the teachings given by the Dharma teacher, you cannot eliminate desire and so on. Therefore, engage in conscientious practice and do no pursue mere words, devoid of practice, just to build up a large collection of terminology.

In this way, seeing yourself as a sick person is very important. With that recognition the others follow. If this first recognition is nothing but words, you will not attempt to follow or put into practice the advice in order to eliminate the afflictions, and you will remain instead a mere listener. You will be like a sick person who searches out a doctor but does not take the medicine, for he only seeks the preparation of medicine; in doing so he does not recover from his illness. The *King of Meditative Concentrations Sutra* states:

> A person is sick and his body is in pain;
> for many years he know no relief.
> Tormented for so long by his illness,
> he seeks out a doctor in search of a cure.
>
> Again and again he searches, and finally
> he finds a wise and learned physician,
> who takes great pity on him, saying,
> "Take this medicine," and hands it to him.
>
> If he takes such excellent and beneficial medicine,
> he will be cured, but should he not take it,
> the doctor is not at fault, nor is the medicine;
> the fault lies with the patient himself.
>
> Likewise, having been ordained into this doctrine, [332]
> having learned about all the powers, concentrations, forces,
> putting no actual effort, no proper effort
> into the practice of meditation,
> how will nirvana be attained?[1116]

Also:

> I teach this excellent Dharma but if you,

having heard it, do not apply it well,
you are like the sick person
holding a bag of medicine
unable to cure his illness.[1117]

In *Engaging in the Practices of the Bodhisattva:*

I will put these into practice,
for what is achieved by mere words?
Is merely reading the medical texts
of any use to the sick person?[1118]

The term "conscientious"[1119] in the line "Recognition of...conscientious practice as the cure of your illness" applies to putting into practice that to be cultivated and that to be discarded as taught by your spiritual friend. To do that you have to know these practices. To know them you have to learn them. Therefore, this term also applies to the necessity of learning and of gaining understanding from that learning. Therefore, adopting a practice that accords with your learning capacity is an important principle.

Vasubandhu in his *Science of Explanation* says:

Arrogant, lacking faith and aspiration,
distracted, withdrawn, and bored—
these are the contaminants of listening.[1120]

The true disciple has abandoned these faults.

With the aims of protecting living beings from the sufferings of sickness in the short run and of bringing them ultimately to peerless enlightenment, the medical student holds the virtuous thought of wanting to study, contemplate, and teach the great texts of the medical tradition, and sits upright on a low seat in the presence of the master. There, with joy and a disciplined mind, he should listen with great respect for the teacher and the teachings. In the *Ten Cakra Kṣitigarbha Sutra* it says:

With undistracted faith and respect listen to the Dharma;
do not belittle or disparage it.
Make offerings to the Dharma teacher;
see him as being like a buddha.[1121]

In the *Garland of Past Lives:*

> Sit on a very low seat,
> generate the serenity of a disciplined mind,
> gazing with eyes of happiness,
> drinking in the nectar of words.
>
> Have respect and with concentration
> and a mind pure and joyful—
> like a patient listening to a doctor—
> show reverence and listen.[1122]

Also:

> Come together at the right time without interruption, [333]
> sit still with firmness of purpose,
> and with great devotion welcome the teachings to your ears.[1123]

Every word should be heard, comprehended, and contemplated—and even repeated aloud—with concentration:

> With clear mind ascertain the words and understand meanings
> and contemplate them constantly without laziness;[1124]
> until familiarized, repeat and concentrate.
> These are the factors for remembering teachings;
> abandon those which are their opposites.[1125]

Also:

> However, mind wandering off elsewhere, forgetfulness,
> vagueness on what are virtuous, nonvirtuous, and neutral minds—
> these do not receive the blessings of Dharma
> and render all as meaningless:
> Vajrasattva and other tathāgatas
> do not bless a forgetful mind.[1126]

In *Engaging in the Practices of the Bodhisattva:*

> That done by a wandering mind becomes meaningless,
> the knower of reality has said.[1127]

It is very important to have great enthusiasm for the words and meanings of the Dharma devoid of any mental wandering. Listening to Dharma is a very rare occurrence and arises from eons of merit accumulation. The *Sutra of Inconceivable Secrets* says:

> Alas! Faith and the listening to Dharma such as this
> will not be found in a hundred eons.[1128]

In the *Sutra of Great Play:*

> It is possible to encounter no Dharma
> for a hundred thousand million eons,
> and yet you have found it today;
> dispel all inattentiveness.[1129]

Therefore, it is very important to embrace the conduct of listening to Dharma conscientiously with body, speech, and mind.

As for the benefits of listening in such a way, the *Bodhisattva Basket of Scripture* states:

> Virtuous and nonvirtuous dharmas—
> without listening you will not know them.
> Through listening you know all dharmas;
> listening you do not engage in wrong,
> listening you eradicate harmful acts,
> listening you pass into nirvana;
> wanting to listen, your listening increases,
> and listening increases your wisdom.[1130]

Also:

> Listening one comes to know Dharmas,
> listening one turns from the nonvirtuous,
> listening one eradicates the meaningless, [334]
> listening one gains liberation.[1131]

Also:

> One with sight and a lamp sees forms.
> Similarly, through listening,
> one knows virtue and nonvirtue.[1132]

Detailed Vinaya Presentations states:

> Much listening has five great benefits: you will be learned in the aggregates, learned in the sensory realms, learned in the sensory sources, learned in dependent origination, and for giving teaching and advice on these, you will not have to rely on others.[1133]

From the *Garland of Past Lives:*

> Dispelling the darkness of ignorance, listening is a lantern;
> never stolen by thieves and robbers, it is the greatest wealth;
> destroying the foes of confusion, it is a great weapon;
> showing ways and giving advice, it is the greatest friend,
> the greatest glory, the greatest fame, and the greatest treasure;
> when meeting those of high status, it is the greatest gift;
> in the midst of others, it pleases the learned;
> shining on opponents, it is like the light of the sun.[1134]

Also:

> You become disciplined and grow clarity of confidence;
> fame and reputation quickly arrive.
> It is the cause of a very special ease and skill in speech.
> With the confidence and fearlessness of listening,
> you clearly understand the meanings.
> Endowed with listening you dwell
> without contradiction on the path of the three circles.
> It bequeaths essence to practice,
> and you attain liberation without hardship
> from the fortress of birth.[1135]

From the *Uttaratantra*:

> Should one person, striving for the highest enlightenment,
> offer constantly to the great Dharma king
> golden realms adorned with jewels,
> as many as atoms in a Buddha realm,
> and should another hear words from this treatise,
> and on hearing them take great liking to their meaning,
> the latter would bring much more merit
> than the virtue produced by the giving.
>
> Should persons of intelligence, wishing for enlightenment,
> protect effortlessly through their body, speech, and mind,
> and without the slightest taint, their ethics for many an eon,
> and should another hear words from this treatise,
> and on hearing them take great liking to their meaning,
> the latter would bring much more merit
> than the virtue produced by this guarding of ethics.
>
> Should a person with the meditative absorption meditation
> that smothers the fires of afflictions of the three realms
> gain the realms of the gods and of Brahmā
> as a method to attain enlightenment without the process of death,
> and should another hear a few words from this treatise,
> and on hearing them take great liking to their meaning, [335]
> the latter would bring much more merit
> than the virtue produced by this meditative absorption.
>
> Why is this? Giving produces wealth, ethics gains high birth,
> and meditation suppresses the afflictions,
> but because wisdom eliminates all afflictions
> and all obstructions to omniscience,
> it is supreme, and its cause is listening to this.[1136]

From the *King of Meditative Concentrations Sutra:*

> The knower of reality as it is, the Tathāgatha Buddha, has taught that there are ten good qualities of much listening and learning. What are these ten? One will not engage the mental afflictions, one will not develop a harmful state of mind, one will separate

> from doubt, one's views will become pure, one will abandon wrong paths, one stays on the path, one stands at the door of no death, one becomes closer to enlightenment, one shines among all living beings, and one is no longer frightened by the lower realms.[1137]

There are many similar passages. There are great benefits of listening in accordance with the stages of the various vehicles, and finally if you listen to the definitive teachings and are not afraid, the benefits are even greater. The *Sutra of the Good Eon* says:

> Greater than bringing to enlightenment
> all the beings of these world realms
> is the special merit of one who hears
> the teaching on no aggregates and is not afraid.[1138]

In the *Abridged Perfection of Wisdom in Verse:*

> The supreme perfection of wisdom is not seen,
> the bodhisattva and the bodhicitta are not seen;
> those who hear this and are not confused, not afraid,
> are engaging in the wisdom of the Sugata.[1139] [337]

28. Chakri Medical College and the Author's Own Practice of Medicine

ALTHOUGH IT WAS difficult to nourish the development of such a teaching environment and methodical approach as described above, I nevertheless began the Chakri Vaidūrya Drophen Tana Ngotsar Rikjé Ling (Vaidūrya Sustenance to Living Beings, the Wondrous to Behold Center of Knowledge),[1140] a college for the major and minor sciences, with an education based on the works I have composed. The numbers in the beginning, including some senior monks appointed as memorization teachers, came to about thirty, whereas these days it has grown to about seventy monks. Examinations on the tantra and its supplements are held, and during the great offering and prayer festivals, many are conferred as Menrampa medical scholars.

Those medicinal plants found in one-to-one lineages that lack any special stipulations of time, stellar, and planetary position, and so on, are collected according to each lineage's own stipulations. Generally, however, the Final Tantra says:

> Roots, branches, and stems—all classified under stems—
> cure diseases of the bones, channels, and flesh.
> When the sap[1141] has dried in the autumn
> is the recommended time for collecting.
>
> Leaves, milk, and shoots—all classified under leaves—
> cure diseases of the hollow organs, marrow, and spirits.
> When leaves and petals are fullest in the rainy season
> is the recommended time for collecting.
>
> Flowers, fruits, and tips—all classified under fruits—
> cure diseases of the eyes, solid organs, and head.
> During autumn winds, the time of ripening,
> is the recommended time for collecting.

Bark, inner bark, and resins—all classified under bark—
cure diseases of the skin, fibers, and limbs.
When buds appear in the spring
is the recommended time for collecting.

Gather purgatives when sap dries up and the force of the
plant fades,
and emetics when buds are drawn upward.
Ideally, during the auspiciousness of the waxing moon,
these should be gathered by a pure child, washed and adorned,
while reciting mantra and auspicious words.[1142]

Therefore, medicinal plants are to be collected according to various stipulations of time. Supported by traditional accounts stating that the majority of plants are ready during the time of the face of rishis,[1143] the usual collecting times for most ordinary medicines are not hugely contradictory. Therefore, each year students were sent out to gather as well as to identify medical plants from neighboring areas such as Drak Yerpa and Nyangdok. When I had the time, during the time of the rishis I gave, as appropriate, transmissions of the tantra and other works, and introductions to their meanings.

All this has resulted in a significant contribution to the continuing growth of medical science. For example, the number of medical plants identified is more than twice the number previously identified by local and outlying doctors of the past. [338]

However, as the first chapter of the *Sutra Requested by Rāṣṭrapāla* says:

Lacking modesty, consideration, and care,
shameless like crows, coarse and uncultured,
spiteful with jealousy, pride, and arrogance:
monks like these will enter my doctrine.[1144]

At a time even more degenerate than the age of degeneration, people dressed in the garb of fully ordained monks will have minds and behavior displaying a lack of shame and modesty even worse than lay men and women. The passage continues:

They will increase in number like the laity,
with accumulated possessions, servants, and entourages.[1145]

These people of sordid conduct, with their wealth and possessions gained from others and their many servants and helpers, will entice the people to have faith and a great liking for them. However:

> Those with pure ethics and endowed with good qualities,
> who hold to the Dharma and work for the good of others
> and who are disciplined and abide on the perfect path,
> will in later times be abused by sentient beings.[1146]

By the power of spirits who delight in evil, those who conscientously pursue the Dharma will no longer be attractive in the minds of others and, far from being objects of faith and aspiration, will simply become objects of abuse. Such an illustration has parallels in general to the practice of Dharma these days.

For the great Lhajé physicians also, with the six causes of a physician complete, capable of vast accomplishments for the welfare of others, possessed of the innate or developed skills of wisdom, the *King's Chronicle Extracted from a Pillar* says:

> At that time evil forces will spread
> and change the minds of people,
> who will engage in nonvirtuous behavior.[1147]

In the *Teachings on the Self Arising Self Appearing* from the northern Treasure tradition:

> In the decrepit times when the lifespan is fifty years, there will come to Tibet māras and all kinds of wrong practices endorsed by the great spirit Pehar.[1148]

My guru the Great Fifth also said:

> Alongside the never-ending demons of the past,
> the new hostile spirits of these times
> rise up like a lake in summer.[1149]

Everywhere, demons such as pledge-breaking spirits and troublesome spirits are changing things, and people are turning away from this Āyurveda science of life even more than from the study of knowledge in general. They pursue their various other studies by merely nodding toward achievements and studying them as they would taste food to check saltiness.[1150] [339] Even those who do engage in this field of study and conduct themselves properly suffer much harm and abuse and do not get the things they wish for. The *Sutra Requested by Candragarbha* says:

> Those who unerringly walk the way of the sacred Dharma are slandered and disparaged. They have little wealth and few possessions and suffer much harm and illness.[1151]

Sakya Paṇḍita says:

> Fools hold the monkey entertainer
> in higher regard than the scholar.
> The monkey owner is showered with food and money;
> the scholar goes on his way empty-handed.[1152]

The glorious protector Nāgārjuna:

> Of the joker and the scholar,
> the foolish hold the joker in higher regard.
> The joker is bestowed with wealth,
> the scholar goes without.[1153]

The omniscient Butön also:

> Alas, I have so very little merit,
> born in this snowy realm, this land of Tibet,
> where Dharma declines and wrong teachings increase,
> where those engaged in Dharma are abused,
> where fools are revered and scholars cast aside like grass.[1154]

Not differentiating the fool from the true scholar has led to a lessening of beneficial activity for sentient beings. There are many who are deceivers at heart without an iota of the qualities that come from knowledge or learning, who have not the slightest idea of the practices involved in collecting and compounding their own medicines, but procure oral-tradition medicines from others and hand them out as if they were "one medicine to cure a hundred diseases." These people may open the door of beneficial activity when they come into contact with minor illnesses that do not actually require treatment.[1155] However, as it is said:

> Fools may accomplish good works,
> but it is by luck and not by design.[1156]

To summarize, the *Sutra Requested by Candragarbha* says:

> During the period when my doctrine is drawing to a close, the protectors of the Dharma will also not be happy, and non-Dharma practices will increase in strength and power.[1157]

Also:

> During those times the gods and nāgas that delight in the Dharma will leave the land. Māras and other hinderers of the Dharma will take their place, and the power and force of non-Dharma will increase.[1158]

In *Tales of the Kaliyuga* by Maticitra:

> In the world in these Kaliyuga times,
> weapons of pretense and deceit are strong.
> The goodness of the soil is consumed by the earth, [340]
> all natural materials lose their power,
> and the gods do not send the rain.
> Fierce winds blow, harvests do not ripen,
> and crops fail, while those that grow are struck by hail.
> Under the weight of the Kaliyuga
> the earth produces no fruit.[1159]

Also:

> Those with great qualities are not revered,
> whereas to the wealthy, unworthy of offering,
> confused beings make offerings.

Yama is undoubtedly leading the world to suffering.
How will he be stopped?

Those possessed of the force of immorality
threaten and wipe out those of pure ethics.
The deceitful, with the power of their love of evil,
will destroy the sacred Dharma.[1160]

Also:

All good works smeared by corruption,
the meritorious disappear, their time passes.
Everywhere the force of goodness is weak;
māras descend upon it and destroy it.[1161]

There is much more of the same in this work.

In the *Chronicles of Ministers:*

By the perverted pride of the deities,
trust is placed in those with false teachings.
The light changes into darkness.

And so on until:

Troublesome spirits enter the hearts of men,
demonesses enter the hearts of women,
and air spirits[1162] enter the hearts of children.[1163]

From *Sutra Requested by Sāgaramati:*

Though there be thousands of companions on the dark side,
this is my sole friend on the bright side.[1164]

Ārya Nāgārjuna states:

Devoting themselves to evil beings
who seek the destruction of virtue.[1165]

Therefore, during the period of the degeneration in the final five hundred years of the doctrine, and specifically when powerful malicious spirits arise who delight in the dark side and push living beings into the ways of error, where they will only follow wrong paths and diminish their store of virtue, there is great doubt that in the future the help and assistance needed for living beings and the preservation of the doctrine will transpire as wished.

From my own side, I engaged in the extensive provision of medicine by compounding not-insignificant quantities of medical powders, pills, decoctions, and so forth for smallpox sufferers, who had increased in number over time, and for the supervisors and craftsmen, including laborers, who were involved in the construction of the central and ancillary structures of the Ornament of the World reliquary for the Great Fifth.[1166]

Every year, for the treasury of death-destroying ambrosia medicine, I performed detailed calculations concerning the sun and moon, planets and constellations, their elemental combinations, land guardians, and so on. In particular the nāga and *kulika* and the two ambrosia periods are given prime importance.[1167] [341]

In accordance with actual instructions found in the tantra and its oral-tradition supplements, and aided by instructions received indirectly from various one-to-one lineages and so on, I measured, weighed, and compounded with great precision and great care various medical substances. I performed the consecration rituals according to the authoritative source for each of these compounds and repeated the individual mantras to develop their powers.

Of those who came to me begging for medicine because of my position, there were those who for some reason claimed to be chronically ill or feigned illness. As *Wise Counsel* says:

> When taxes are levied, they count their wealth,
> when they have to go, they don't feel well,
> when they see food and drink, they rush in,
> when they see hardship, they skillfully avoid it.[1168]

Others who came begging were actually chronically ill, and some had received treatment from various physicians, but it had not worked and they were abandoned. They were not beggars from the beginning. No matter who they were, I examined them using only the question-and-answer technique, because I was unable to conduct visual or physical examinations through urine and pulse.[1169] Therefore, I looked at their condition and examined what other doctors had said, and satisfied my mind that their hot and cold elements did not seem seriously out of balance.[1170] For those who had been abandoned by their doctors because they had exhausted all treatments, and for the poor who had no one to examine them, I sent via messengers medicine that I thought would help them, even though they had not made contact with me first.

I helped Lampa Lama Ngawang Tenzin from Mongolia. He had seen many doctors—Darmo Menrampa, Kyipewa, Epa Lhündrup, and others—who had examined him and made contradictory prognoses and then abandoned him, placing him almost in the mouth of the lord of death. I was able to help Gungsep Norlha, who was suffering with a particular menstrual illness that had gone unrecognized and was treated unsuccessfully by many physicians. These and other helpful treatments I have given.

During the offering and prayer ceremonies, I gave compounded medicines and the compounding ingredients to the medical college students and doctors. Also I gave to all those who requested a variety of precious medicines, such as the six excellent medicines,[1171] which are of definite benefit to the sick.

I have developed, like the autumn full moon, an exalted state of mind that works on behalf of the medical tradition and of living beings. As it has been said in this literature:

> Able and willing to give up wealth or life,
> with no sense of loss for either.[1172]

This passage is from the section on the six causes of a doctor. Also, in the ninth chapter of the action tantra *Requested by Subāhu:*

> Always place your mind in love for those living beings tormented by illness.[1173] [342]

In the *Jewel Lamp Dhāraṇī:*

> There will be kings, ministers, envoys,
> and fearless physicians, wise in text and practice,
> and they will be great trees in the wilderness,

an endless supply of medicine and jewels,
wish-fulfilling jewels, wish-granting trees,
showing the way to those who lose the path.[1174]

The *Liccavi Vimalakīrti Sutra* says:

In the intermediate eon of illness,
he becomes the supreme ambrosia,
liberating sentient beings,
restoring health, and bringing happiness.[1175]

And in the *Pāramitā Synthesis* by the great scholar Śūra:

Bringing no aging and no death in this world,
supplying countless stores of the best of medicines.[1176]

In this way I think I have followed the great waves of bodhisattva conduct.

Conclusion

29. Dedication

Bhagavān, supreme physician,
arising as the enemy of disease born of ignorance:
from your kindness exalted wisdom arises as the ambrosia of life
to produce the phenomenon of health, free of disease,
the foundation for a life extended to its fullest,
for Dharma, for wealth, and for all happiness;
the peak of all sciences—causes for knowing all things,
that cares for sentient beings, the supreme science
for the healing of body and mind!

Having fully understood its supremely virtuous doctrine,
exceptionally virtuous minds work to preserve it without decline,
their fingers of pure and courageous wisdom
skillfully pulling out the fierce and angry teeth of the evil deeds
that drink bodies and minds, causing the pain endemic to living beings.
Those peerless beings—Kumāra[1177] and others,
especially the ranks of lineage and trained follower physicians—
why would the intelligent not have faith in them? [343]

Their wisdom of comprehending the tantra exists like stars in the daytime,
yet at the mere sound of the thunder of fame, reputation, and wealth,
they are conceived in the womb of "physician in name alone."[1178]
On whether patients will live or die they are uncertain,
riddled with doubt, merely guessing, these brothers of Yama:
for such doctors, not even in dreams does the saliva of faith arise.

Not determining the meanings of texts
free of the fearful prejudice of attachment and aversion,
nor weighing the goods to be discarded or cultivated

with the scales of scripture and valid perception:
you writers of history, each preferring the cups
used by their old father of blind partisanship,
you can rest easy now.

Friends, here the crooked speech of prejudice is left far behind,
with the navigator of investigative intelligence
aboard a boat of great learning
upon the ocean of Buddha word and commentary
on the traditions of the outsider, Buddhist, Deva, and Rishi,
greatly famed in the lands of India and Tibet,
a vast resource plumbing the depths of medical science,
not to be refuted by scripture and reason,
the wound of error inflicted by the knife of the rishi curse
piercing the body of the science of life,
transformed immediately by incisive writing into a pure eye,
this **well-explained history** of the **glorious science of medicine**,
a vast and pure realm, deep as a Himalayan mountain lake,
a great **mirror of beryl** reflecting a form never before seen,
its humors in balance, its activities of body, speech, and mind pure,
pleasing even the **rishis** who from the corners of their eyes are attracted—
like Brahmā to his daughter born from his own imagination.

By the merit of composing this **festival of joy,**
I pray that the cataracts in the eyes of all beings,
brought on by the demon of prejudice
are erased forever, and that by examining and investigating
with nonpartisan intelligence, they come to see clearly,
and that those of clear minds with all causes of a doctor complete
will enter this jeweled house of the path of the sciences,
built on its foundation of desire for happiness and freedom,
with the wish to benefit others. [344]

By its power may many beings be free—
as the egg given by Rishi Tārakākṣa gradually matured,
and Damayantī was freed from the lowly state of servitude
when her mother died an untimely death—
and may they live their lives to completion,

and the bright white light of the winter moon,
with its glorious camphor stream of pacifying coolness
of Dharma, wealth, and happiness, wax forever.

For my forebears, too, this virtue is dedicated.
The false images drawn with the inks of ordinary provisional meanings
in the form of wicked deeds, the faults and downfalls
of my supreme root guru, the Great Fifth,
buddha in the guise of a bodhisattva,
master in bringing the jewel rains of siddhis of samsara and nirvana:
may they be erased, and may his pure wish
solely to benefit the Dharma and living beings be fulfilled.

As the intention of this great protector
was to blossom the sweet-smelling utpala lotus of benefit
to doctrine and living beings when the time is apt,
may the sun of the Great Sixth shine
from the great sky realm of *Akaniṣṭha*
as a light in this world forever.

With the shade offered by its golden wheel,
heaven-ordained and arcing across the sky,
may the parasol of the rule of the Palace of Completion of Joy[1179]
adorned with jewel of sovereign authority
never fall and remain for all existence.
By its power may this land ringed by snow mountains
be free of civil strife arising as chariots of evil,
of disturbance, wars, epidemics, and famines,
and may all come to dwell in an era of completion.

May the creator of this, endowed with the power of a specially
virtuous mind,
by the instincts planted, by teaching and composing, even by the
flow of speech,
be victorious in the battle over the hindering enemy hordes
of those humans and nonhumans of poison minds.
Having perfected the indestructible life force,
whose vajra of longevity sunders the mountain of the lord of death,

may the vast amulet within the container of my thoughts
be forever full with the jewels of my wishes fulfilled. [345]

In the future, too, after the sun of this life has set,
may I be cared for without separation in every birth
by the mighty guide, the fifth great emperor,
as promised with his vajra words spoken
with an unchanging white-toothed smile.

Finally, having become a fully enlightened buddha
with the supreme gem of the four bodies,
a result of being cleansed a hundred times
in the mighty river of a bodhisattva's deeds,
may I become a great guide for all beings.

The monastic community practicing, studying, and memorizing this science,
on **Chakri** hill symbolizing the creation of the nectar of immortality,
from which flows the Āyurveda ambrosia stream
of the king of medicine shining with **beryl** light,
of **sustenance to all living beings,**
the mountainsides and the environment inseparable
from the **beautiful-to-behold** town of Sudarśana;
by its practice of the **wondrous** science of medicine,
even though all dharmas have no self,
may the wheels of this **place of knowledge—**
with a hub of teaching and practice
and vast rim of study and contemplation—
grind to dust the armies of the ferocious three poisons' diseases;
and with its spontaneous enlightened activities for self and others
swelling like the cascade of summer rivers,
may all beings gain victory over untimely death.

30. Previous Histories of Medicine

EARLIER HISTORIES of medicine include:

- *Great Garuḍa History of Medicine*[1180] found in the Eighteen Auxiliary Texts composed by earlier Tibetans, with sections on: the greatness of *Four Tantras;* deeds of our Teacher the fully enlightened Buddha, such as the turning of the wheels of Dharma; explanations of the major sciences; and the establishment of the science of medicine as the word of the Buddha.
- *Beautiful Rainbow Overview,*[1181] also found in the Eighteen Auxiliary Texts, has an opening section similar to the above and a main body of text on the outlines of the Explanatory Tantra chapter.
- *History of Medicine: Illumination of Knowledge* by Drangti Palden Tsojé deals generally with the way great beings cared for living beings, and specifically on the coming of the buddhas of the good eon, with special reference to the appearance of our Teacher the Buddha; presentations of the doctrines of Buddha, bringer of happiness, [346] and the three trainings; and the way the sciences and especially the science of medicine developed in India and Tibet. In his assertions that *Four Tantras* was taught by Medicine Buddha, compiled by the rishis, translated into Tibetan by Vairocana, presented to the Dharma king Trisong, who then concealed it as a treasure that was discovered by Drapa Ngönshé and disseminated by Yuthok, he is more or less in agreement with my guru the Great Fifth.
- *Stream of Beryl: A History of Four Tantras* by Tsoknyi Gyatso of Phenyül Drosawa. Generally, this work is in keeping with most of the early-translation medical canon. It asserts *Four Tantras* to be the word of the Buddha taught in the land of Oḍḍiyāna during the middle turning of the wheel of Dharma, that it belongs to the Vinaya basket of the three scriptural divisions, but that it is not a revealed treasure.

- *Wish-Granting Tree: Verses on the Ascertainment of Four Tantras as Word of the Buddha,* by Jangpa Lhatsün Tashi Palsang. He asserts that *Four Tantras* was taught in Bodhgāya.
- *Sunlight that Opens the Lotus Grove of the Science of Medicine*[1182] by the Jang physician Sönam Yeshé Gyaltsen, son of the above. This work has a general presentation on the doctrines of the Buddha and a commonly accepted history of medicine, but with the unique assertions that *Four Tantras* was taught by our Teacher Vajradhara in the land of Oḍḍiyāna, that it is found in both Treasure and Transmission traditions, and that the two streams combined within the Jang tradition.
- The biographies of the main physicians of the Jang tradition up to and including Minyima Thongwa Dönden, his son, and Sönam Yeshé Gyaltsen.
- *Jeweled Lamp History of Medicine,* composed by a Jang physician who came after Minyima Thongwa Dönden and his son, whose style of composition is similar to Drangti's *Illumination of Knowledge.* He asserts that *Four Tantras* was taught in Oḍḍiyāna by Vajradhara.
- *Mirror of White Silver: A Well-Composed History of Medicine* in verse by Tsomé Khenchen Kawa Śākya Wangchuk. Its general message is in keeping with Drangti's *Illumination of Knowledge* and Jangpa Tashi Palsang's *Ascertainment of Four Tantras.* This work contains the particular assertions that *Four Tantras* was taught by our Teacher in Oḍḍiyāna and entrusted to Rishi Manasija, and that later our Teacher manifested miraculously in the Himalaya Mountains and emitted light from his mouth from which Manasija appeared. *Four Tantras* was then again taught to Kumāra Jivaka. Jinarṣabha or Rājānaka Vajra Mārajit, the son of Vaiśravaṇa, was appointed guardian of *Four Tantras,* and so on. [347]
- *Golden Sheaves: A Well-Composed History of Medicine,* by Jarpo Panchen Dorjé Palam. This work has five major sections: a general description of the five sciences; early and later medical traditions; translations; dissemination; and the deeds of the great physicians. Asserting that *Four Tantras* was taught in Oḍḍiyāna by our Teacher manifested as Medicine Buddha, he refutes mistaken notions by resolving doubts concerning such things as porcelain bowls and elemental divination not existing in India. He also explains how Yuthok supplemented the tantra and clarified obscure and confusing sections, and how the Eighteen Auxiliary Texts were composed.

- *A Treasure for the Benefit of Others* is an explanation of *Four Tantras* by Drukpa Pema Karpo, who asserts that our Teacher took Kumāra Jivaka to Gandhamārdana Mountain to break his pride, after which he taught him the glorious *Four Tantras* by having him repeat it back.
- *History of Medicine: Endowed with the Five Ambrosia Perfections,* by Lhajé Mipham Sangpo, a contemporary of the Jangdak Dharma king Wangpo Dé.[1183] He asserts that our Teacher taught *Four Tantras* in Bodhgāya in India, and that it is to be included in the *Enlightened Qualities Ambrosia Tantras* from the early-translation tradition.
- A very similar but more extensive work was written by the Dechen Chökhor physician Ratna Mingchen.[1184]
- *Ornament to the Thoughts of the Rishis: A History of Medicine* by the foremost Kyishö physician Rinchen Ding Bodhisattva Losang Gyatso. This is a history covering the Dharma in general and the five sciences, with particular reference to the origins of medical science. On the Dharma he covers listening and teaching. He asserts that *Four Tantras* was taught by our Teacher manifest as Medicine Buddha in the land of Oḍḍiyāna, that it is to be classified as action tantra, that it was translated into Tibetan by Vairocana and revealed by Drapa Ngönshé, and so on. In this he is very much in accord with the assertions of my master, the Great Fifth.
- *Treasury of Jewels: A General Explanation of the Science of Medicine* by a disciple of the Dakpo physician Karma Künphen.[1185] His establishment of *Four Tantras* being the word of Buddha and a revealed treasure follow generally accepted assertions. His particular assertions are that *Four Tantras* was taught by our Teacher, compiled by the rishis, entrusted to Śrīmālā, chief of the ḍākinīs, from whom it was requested by Yuthok, who checked and settled various points of the text. He investigates the possibility that Śākyamuni Buddha and Medicine Buddha are not the same being, citing passages from Songtsen Gampo's work on the lives of the Buddha. In this he differs a little from previous commentators.
- *Granting Wishes: Well-Explained Overview of Medicine* by Lata or Kyempa Tsewang. In it he divides the tantra into outer, inner, and secret tantras.
- *General Knowledge History: The Wide-Open Door to the Unending Ceremonial Offering,* also known as *Dance Delighting the Rishis* by Surkhar Lodrö Gyalpo or Lekshé Tsöl, who lived around the time of Jarpo Paṇchen. [348] Its first chapter called "External Causes of Harm"

together with related material deals with the external world. The second is on the internal world. The third is a general presentation of the doctrine, beginning with our Teacher's development of bodhicitta up to the disappearance of his teachings. The fourth details how the science of medicine developed in the celestial and human worlds. The fifth explains how medicine appeared in the noble land of India. The sixth describes how it spread to Tibet. The seventh is a presentation and refutation of other traditions. The eighth is on the science of medicine itself and includes a biography of Yuthok and the beginnings of a biography of his disciple Sumtön Yeshé Sung. From then he should have continued with biographies up to his own time, but for some reason he did not, and the biography of Sumtön was left unfinished. The last chapter is on practice and was planned under three outlines, but contains only a very brief explanation of the five sciences plus a presentation on the alphabet. This whole work on the world, its inhabitants, the deeds of the Buddha, and so on is a very extensive collection of words presented in an affected and ostentatious manner by someone writing about medicine and history as he sees it. The unfinished sections were completed by Drukpa Sangyé Dorjé (1569–1645), who in a work on Madhyamaka refutes Jetsün Tsongkhapa.

- A work known as *Quick Path for the Fortunate: A Religious History* by someone called Tsarong Ayu.[1186] The first four or five pages on the praises and so forth are copied from Surkhar Lodrö Gyalpo's *Dance Delighting the Rishis*. This is followed by connected and disconnected passages that have simply been copied from the above. From the biography of Sumtön onward, it seems like his own work.
- *Well-Explained Ocean-Like Overview: A Dance to Delight the Rishis* by Ruddha Ānanda, a Sukhar disciple. It is arranged under two main headings: a history in the form of an overview and a commentary in the form of textual explanation. The first section deals with the external world, the inner world of sentient beings, the buddhas of the fortunate eon, in particular the twelve deeds of our Teacher, the councils, sutra and tantra from the Kangyur and Tengyur, how Maitreya will appear in the world, the origins of the science of medicine, a presentation on what is Kangyur and what is Tengyur, [349] how medicine spread in Tibet, a materia medica, biographies of physicians from Jivaka to Yuthok, and so on. It is an extensive text that essentially follows Lodrö Gyalpo.

Similarly, there are many compositions in the Sur tradition following on from the above—such as the Root Tantra commentary, *Garland of Core Instructions*—that assert the tantra was the work of Yuthok, but like the misfit of an upper jaw of a lion and a lower jaw of a camel, assert that the place where the tantra was taught was the eastern land of Beryl Light, and so on.

Other histories that assert our Teacher to be the author of *Four Tantras* and so on—though whether they have other scribal or substantive errors is not determined—include the early work, *Heap of Jewels; Illuminating Beacon* by Chejé Shangtön Shikpo; *Sunlight Clarity of Meaning* by Phaktön Śākya Gönpo; *Great Overview* by Mentön Shönu Rinchen; *Lamp Illuminating the Four Points* by Nyemo Chökyi Wangchuk; *Histories* by Nyemo Künga Döndrup; and *Short Work on Sources* by Pal Khachö Wangpo. These and other early works I have not seen.

Histories on the theme of *Eight Branches* include:

- *Compendium of Knowledge Blazing from Atop a Victory Banner,* by Chejé Shangtön Shikpo, presents the development of the bodhi mind by our Teacher, his accumulation of merit, the twelve deeds, the teaching of the *Clearly Seeing Knowledge Tantra* during the second turning, the greatness of the rishis, a biography of Śūra identifying and refuting all wrong assertions about his birthplace, the composition of *Essence of Eight Branches,* its translation into Tibetan, a classification of word of Buddha and treatise, the seven medical traditions, the four medical literature collections, and the two translation periods.
- A synthesis of the above, called *Shorter Blazing from Atop a Victory Banner,* by Lhatsün Tashi Palsang.
- A medical history by Yuthok Gyatso beginning with a general presentation of the five sciences, an outline of our Teacher's development of the bodhi mind and deeds, followed by an alternative biography of Śūra and the generally accepted biographies of Āryadeva and others, together with an account of how *Essence of Eight Branches* was composed.

Stream of Ambrosia by Thazhi Śīlasaṃgha, a medical history by Minyak Mikyö Dorjé,[1187] *Garland of Narrative, Overview, Thirty Instructions History,*[1188] and *Essence of Ambrosia History* are also examples of histories, but I have not seen these. [350] There are later works, such as *Knowledge of All Sciences* by Taktsang Lotsāwa Sherap Rinchen, that are all like filling a water pot from here, there, and everywhere.[1189]

Despite the existence of all these histories, I had not seen one that covered the whole body of the science of medicine, and thus the aspiration to write a medical history began when I was about thirty. However, distractions and an increase in the number of other compositions meant that it was not taken up and remained as an idea. The work was actually begun in the male water-horse year of the twelfth sixty-year cycle, in the *aṣaḍha* month on the fifteenth day, which is the day commemorating the Conqueror's entry into the womb, and was also a Monday coinciding with an auspicious stellar combination of the *śrāvana* constellation.[1190]

Most of the previous medical histories mainly include topics such as the formation of the world, the deeds of our Teacher beginning from his development of the bodhi mind, and explanations of the five sciences, all presented according to the authors' experience. However, these days such topics have been fully explained elsewhere.

31. Colophon

THEREFORE, WITH A DISCUSSION of the complete literary corpus of the science of medicine, as well as a presentation on masters and students in terms of the study of this science, a section on the vajra-holding master possessing all three vows as an offshoot of the previous topic, and a section on the characteristics a teacher of the Dharma, this has been *Mirror of Beryl: A Well-Explained History of the Glorious Science of Medicine, A Feast to Delight the Rishis.*

A manuscript says:

> Driphak, Gyama, Yasang,
> Tsalpa, Jayül, and Lhadruk:
> these the six regions of Ü;
> Ngari, Latö, Lhojang,
> Chumik, Shalu, and Jangdrok:
> these the six regions of Tsang;
> and Yardrok, in neither Ü nor Tsang.
> These are the thirteen regions.[1191]

In the Tsalpa region of these thirteen, containing the feudal district of Uru Shöchen[1192] divided into upper and lower regions, and of these two, in the lower region, where the sky hosts the Dharma wheel of eight spokes, the earth is laid with the eight petals of the lotus, and on all sides are paraded the eight auspicious symbols; it is a place where all ten virtues are complete. There under the protection of the nearby backdrop of wonderful mountains, whose interior contains the actual palace of Śrī Cakrasaṃvara and whose exterior hosts a parasol covering the three realms, an auspicious clockwise white conch, and a banner of victory in all directions—all three self-arising phenomena as clear as the moon's reflection in water—in Nyang Dren Drongmé—meaning the area of those who were serfs *(dren)* to Nyang

Tingsin, in the lower *(drongmé)* of the two upper and lower communities—I was born into a family that made its living by collecting taxes and was descended, it is said, from Tsurtön Wangi Gyalpo.[1193] [351] From the moment of my birth, I was lovingly cared for as a parent would a child by my father-like lord and master, the all-knowing, mighty king of kings, the Great Fifth. Externally, he conferred or granted me religious and secular rule in its entirety; internally, he recognized me from the Oral and Treasure traditions and secret documents as an incarnation of an earlier, celestially descended king; secretly, he conferred on me completely numerous four-empowerment initiations into highly secret mandalas of suchness and enthroned me as a vajra master, thereby caring for me in these and other ways with a kindness that went beyond mere words. I, who am known as Buddha Apti[1194] in the well-constructed language of Sanskrit and as Sangyé Gyatso in the language of this land of snow, was awarded the Explainer of All title for competence in the Vyākaraṇa[1195] texts with the names One with the Intelligence Pleasing Sarasvatī and One with the Newfound Youth of Proud Ṣaṇmukha. In my fiftieth year plus one, 2,663 years after the Conqueror Siddhārtha, accomplisher of all, manifested his birth in the town of Kapilavastu, 2,583 years after he withdrew his physical form in Kuśinagarī, in the era of the practice of ethics, 105 years after the Kālacakra *kaliyuga* era of troubles began, 721 years before the *caturyuga* era of completion that dawns after Rudracakrin has destroyed the barbarians; in the year known as *bhānu* in the celestial language of Sanskrit or "sun" *(sūrya)* according to the *Cakrasaṃvara Commentary,*[1196] as *gei wei* in the language of Greater China, in this land as the female sheep year[1197] of the water element in harmony with the *wangthang* power element—a year possessed of four elements, a moon-element year with the sun occupying the mansion of Gemini—in the Jyeṣṭha month and the middle summer month according to Kālacakra coarse astrology, in the early autumn month and greater iron-monkey month according to Chinese Porthang divination, on the third Victory lunar day[1198] of the bright side or waxing phase whose *Kālacakra Tantra* vowel is *ṛ,* consonant *ga,* element fire, and sensory pleasure taste; whose *Arising Letters Tantra* vowel is *u,* consonant *kha,* element fire, and sensory pleasure is form; whose development, in common with both traditions, is that of the youth; whose day of the seven-planet week is the powerful Son of the Moon (Wednesday) joined in nuptial joy with the activity lunar-mansion goddess Anurādhā[1199] to form the yoga of ambrosia joy; whose correspondence is *kumara,* whose element combination is that of the youth, whose lesser correspondence is Increase of the Day, whose astrological yoga is *sādhya,* whose *karaṇa* sector is *taitila,* whose link from the twelve links of dependent origination is "craving" according to the *Kālacakra Tantra* and "compositional factors" according to *Arising Letters Tantra,* whose sun is the fire tiger,[1200] whose date *parkha* trigram is *li,* and whose date *mewa* is four and green: on this day when planets, date, and constellations are in auspicious combination, [352] and when the lord of the seven horses is moving through the houses of the *gola* firmament on his southern passage, at the earth-rabbit hour of the second half of dawn, when the time *parkha* is *kun,* the time *mewa* is five and yellow, when the *tatkāla* ascendant is Cancer, the semigod star of coarse calculation is *sthāvara,* at the Jupiter ambrosia period, when the true moon remainder is "excellence," at this virtuous hour, I have completed this work.[1201]

Up until the age of fifty, all my compositions, even the most modest of letters, were written in my own hand partially because dictation meant that my speech defect caused scribes to hear incorrectly, leading to mistakes. However, since the age of fifty my ability to write by hand has declined, and in the mornings and evenings poor sight has made it difficult to see clearly. Therefore, the task of writing has been undertaken by the scribe Pema Sönam of Chakar.

May there be fortune and prosperity at all times and in all places.

Notes

1 See, for example, Dr. Barry Clark, *The Quintessence Tantras of Tibetan Medicine* (Ithaca NY: Snow Lion Publications, 1995); Vaidya Bhagwan Dash, *Encyclopedia of Tibetan Medicine* (Delhi: Sri Satguru Publications, 1994); Desi Sangyé Gyatso, *Tibetan Medical Paintings* (New York: Harry N. Abrams, 1992).

2 Desi Sangyé Gyatso borrowed heavily from previous histories, which he lists as an appendix, and he often quotes verbatim from these for a few pages without criticism. This sometimes makes for a few internal contradictions in the book as a whole, such as the same title attributed to different authors.

3 Kachuwa Chölothar, *Bod kyi gso dpyad rig pa thog ma'i 'byung khung la rob tsam dpyad pa gzur gnas dgyes pa'i gtam* (Dharamsala, India: Tibetan Medical Institute, 2000).

4 *Four Tanṭras* is to be regarded as a single work, each "tantra" corresponding to a chapter. Its full title is *Essence of Ambrosia Secret Instruction Tantra on Eight Branches* (see bibliography).

5 See p. 148. Unless otherwise indicated, most of the following account of the orgins of Tibetan medicine is taken from the text itself.

6 "In the sources translated above, 'Galenos' is said to be 'from Tazig or Rome' and 'from Rome in Tazig,' a confusion also found in the Chinese *Hsin T'ang Shu,* where it is stated that Rome was under Arab sovereignty. Because of the consistent use of the name Rome (written in Tibetan either *Phrom* or *Khrom*) in close connection with Tazig, there is no doubt but that, as proved long ago by Schaeder, the Greek 'Eastern Roman' or Byzantine Empire is meant." Christopher I. Beckwith, "The Introduction of Greek Medicine into Tibet in the Seventh and Eighth Centuries," *Journal of American Oriental Society* 99.2 (1979), p. 300.

7 Jampa Trinlé, *Gangs ldzong gso rig bstan pa'i nyin byed rim byon gyi rnam thar phyogs bsgrigs zhes bya ba* (Dharamsala, India: Tibetan Medical Institute, 1991), p. 26.

8 Pawo Tsukla Trengwa, *Feast for the Wise: An Historical Record [Chos 'byung mkhas pa'i dga' ston]* (Sarnath, India: Vajra Vidya Institute, 2003), p. 1412.

9 Christopher I. Beckwith, "Tibetan Treacle: A Note on Theriac in Tibet," *Bulletin* (Bloomington, Indiana: The Tibet Society, 1980), pp. 49–51.

10 "Since the title *biji* (variously written *bidzi, bibyi, bitsi, biche)* is specifically said to be a foreign word meaning 'physician,' possible Indo-Iranian origins come first to mind." Beckwith, "The Introduction of Greek Medicine into Tibet," p. 303.

11 Tsering Thakchoe Drungtso, *Tibetan Medicine: The Healing Science of Tibet* (Dharamsala, India: Drungtso Publications, 2004), p. 318.

12 *Four Tantras,* Final Tantra, 26.660.6.
13 Orgyen Lingpa, *Lotus Chronicles,* 85.503.3.
14 Or *Grugu.* Identified as present-day Yugu in northwestern Tibet, "north of Ngari and south of Khoten" (*Great Tibetan-Chinese Dictionary,* p. 1332).
15 *Dol po;* in north-central Nepal, west of Mustang.
16 *Khro ru tshe rnam gyi gsung rtsom thor bu phyogs bsgrigs* (Lhasa: Bod ljongs mi dmangs dpe skrun khang [Tibetan People's Printing Press], 2003), pp. 38–41.
17 See p. 454.
18 *Wish-Fulfilling Tree: List of Practices from the Yuthok Heartdrop,* Collected Works, *nga,* 1.2.
19 Desi Sangyé Gyatso, *Tibetan Medical Paintings.*
20 These and following details of Desi Sangyé Gyatso's life have been taken from Prof. Losang Tenzin's introduction to the new critical edition of *Mirror of Beryl* published by the Institute of Tibetan Classics. Dr. Losang Tenzin Rakdho is dean of the faculty of medicine in the Tibetan Medical Department Central Institute of Higher Tibetan Studies, Sarnath, India.
21 See, for example, Glenn H. Mullin, *The Fourteen Dalai Lamas* (Santa Fe, NM: Clear Light Publishers, 2001), pp. 239–72.
22 This version of events is as described by Prof. Losang Tenzin.
23 At the time of writing, Dr. Khenrab Gyatso is chief lecturer at the Tibetan Medical Institute, Dharamsala, India. His hitherto untranslated composition is a work in progress and deals with the history, theory, and practice of Tibetan medicine.
24 Drungtso, *Tibetan Medicine,* p. 302.
25 This phrase and the following description of unworthy physicians are taken from the text on p. 460.
26 Jampa Trinlé, *Gangs ldzong gso rig bstan pa'i nyin byed rim byon gyi rnam thar phyogs bsgrigs zhes bya ba* (Dharamsala, India: Tibetan Medical Institute, 1991); Troru Tsenam, *Khro ru tshe rnam gyi gsung rtsom thor bu phyogs bsgrigs* (Lhasa: Bod ljongs mi dmangs dpe skrun khang [Tibetan People's Printing Press], 2003).
27 The five major sciences are linguistics, logic, medicine, arts and technology, and "inner meaning," or Buddhism.
28 For a more recent appraisal of the state of Tibetan medicine in Tibet see Tibet Information Network (compiler), *Tibetan Medicine in Contemporary Tibet, Volume 2: Health and Health Care* (London: Tibet Information Network, 2004).
29 *Vaidūrya.* It would appear that *vaidūrya* is the gem family beryl. Desi Sangyé Gyatso composed works called *White Beryl, Yellow Beryl,* and *Blue Beryl* as well as this *Beryl Mirror,* and the gem beryl, likewise, appears in various colors, such as the blue-green aquamarine, golden-yellow helidor, pink or peach beryl, dark blue beryl, emerald, light green, pink morganite, red beryl, and the colorless goshenite. When used to describe the color of Medicine Buddha, it refers to the color aquamarine. See "Vaidurya," by Marianne Winder, *Bulletin of Tibetology,* November 1990.
30 The first object of veneration in these verses is the Fifth Dalai Lama, mentor and father figure to the author. This is followed by homage to Śākyamuni Buddha in his aspect of Medicine Buddha. The other figures are the five rishis, in particular Vidyājñāna and Manasija, speaker and requestor of the tantra, respectively; the Buddhist and non-Buddhist audience of the original teaching of *Four Tantras;* Jivaka, the famous physician at the time of the Buddha; Nāgārjuna, as a writer of

medical texts; the Indian master Śūra, identified as the author of the renowned *Treatise of the Eight Branches;* his grandson Candranandana; Padmasambhava, the tantric adept who visited Tibet; Tsongkhapa, the great scholar practitioner; Vairocana the translator; his contemporary King Trisong Detsen; and Muné Tsenpo, the king's son. For identifications of the remaining figures, see corresponding notes.

31 Words in bold are the name of the Great Fifth immortalized as the buddha Rasmi Samudgata Śrīku Rāja *('Od zer kun nas 'phag pa dpal brtsegs kyi rgyal po).*

32 *Lta na sdug.* Sudarśana or Dṛśākāṅkṣya.

33 The five rishis are seen as manifestations of the five wisdoms of an enlightened being. See p. 86.

34 Epithet of Brahmā.

35 The eight, or seven, rishis are well known in ancient Indian literature, where they are held to be the originators of the brahman caste. Their names vary according to tradition. See p. 103.

36 *Videha (lus 'phags)* literally means "superior body."

37 Literally, "raised by Kumāra"; Kumāra here refers to King Bimbisāra's other son, Kumāra Abhaya, who raised his younger stepbrother, Jivaka, who is the object of homage here. The story is told later in the section on the life of this famous physician.

38 *Yang tsha.* But see later section on Candranandana, where he is said to be Śūra's grandson.

39 The verse is homage to the physician Candranandana, whose name and most-renowned work is woven into the lines. *Moon* is "Candra," and *Abhirati,* which possibly refers to Akṣobhya's western buddha realm, can also be written as "Nandana." His work is *Moonlight: A Commentary on the Essence of Eight Branches.*

40 "Flower of the god Brahmā" is an epithet of King Trisong Detsen, who is said to be an earlier incarnation of the Great Fifth Dalai Lama, who in turn is said to be a manifestation of the buddha Rasmi Samudgata Śrīku Rāja.

41 Ninth-century son of King Trisong Detsen. Purgyal, the "the kingdom of Pu," is an ancient name for Tibet.

42 Treasure revealer who unearthed *Four Tantras;* his biography appears later in the text.

43 This homage to Sumtön Yeshé Sung, a disciple of Yuthok, includes a play on his name: Sumtön ("revealing three," although Sum [*sum*] is a place name rather than the number three [*gsum*], and this phrase technically translates as "teacher from Sum") Yeshé ("gnosis") Sung ("meditative retention").

44 Refers to minister Drangti Gyalnyé Kharpuk, reputed to be royal physician and minister to Dharma king Tridé Tsukten Mé Aktsom, seventh-century father of Songtsen Gampo.

45 The Tangut tribe; see note 583 about him below.

46 Jangdak Namgyal Drakpa Sangpo (1395–1475) is the founder of the Tibetan Jang medical tradition.

47 Minyima Thongwa Dönden, a disciple of Jangdak Namgyal Drakpa Sangpo. Minyima *(mi'i nyi ma)* means "the sun of humanity."

48 This is homage to the Nya family lineage. Nya *(gnya')* here means "shoulder," hence the play on words. The first in the Nya family medical line was Nyapa Chösang,

one of the nine wise physicians of Tibet, who are briefly identified later in the text. According to Trinlé (p. 68), the family name Nya was given to Chösang's father by locals who said that because of his great love for others, he should be carried on the shoulders of all. The Dorjé is Lhünding Namgyal Dorjé, a seventeenth-century contemporary of the author.

49 Surkhar Nyamnyi ("equal") Dorjé ("vajra") (1439–75) is the founder of the Sur medical tradition. Terdak Lingpa Gyurmé Dorjé (1646–1714) was a teacher and student of the Fifth Dalai Lama. A Nyingma treasure revealer, he founded Mindröling Monastery in 1670.

50 Rājānaka Vajra Mārajit is a wrathful *yakṣa*-like protector, whose tantric practice was discovered by treasure revealer Drapa Ngönshé in Samyé where he discovered the *Four Tantras*. The four activities usually refer to those of pacification, increase, subjugation, and wrath.

51 These are clearly three wrathful protectors. I cannot find much about them. However, see p. 164.

52 The Tibetan translation of *Āyurveda* here is *tshe yi rig byed,* literally "science of life," which is often used as a synonym of *gso ba'i rig pa* or *sman dpyad rig pa,* meaning the science of healing or medicine.

53 Here the title of the work is woven into the verses. This work belongs to a genre called *khog 'bubs* or *khog 'bugs,* which usually refers to the history of the development of medicine. Literally, it means "to erect a structure" or "create an enclosure" in the sense of erecting a tent, building the exterior of a house, or even opening an umbrella. Here the author has incorporated the two syllables of this term into the verse. *Khog* means "structure," "interior," "something hollow," "the mind," "stomach," etc.; *'bubs* means "to erect" or "to cover."

54 *Mirror of Poetics (Kāvyādarśa),* Toh 4301 Tengyur, sgra mdo, *se,* 318b7.

55 *Uttaratantra,* 5:16, Toh 4024 Tengyur, sems tsam, *phi,* 72b3.

56 Toh 353 Kangyur, mdo sde, *ah,* 190a1. Translated from the Chinese.

57 *Mahāyānasūtrālaṃkāra* 12:60, Toh 4020 Tengyur, sems tsam, *phi,* 15b4.

58 *Yogacaryābhūmi,* Toh 4035 Tengyur, sems tsam, *tshi,* 161a2.

59 These are listed on p. 228.

60 *Bodhisattvabhūmi,* Toh 4037 Tengyur, sems tsam, *wi,* 51b7.

61 Ibid., 56a4.

62 Ibid., 57a2.

63 According to the commentary to this text by Sāgaramegha (Toh 4047), wisdom that "engages" *('jug pa)* is the wisdom of a bodhisattva who "practices by faith" and has not attained the first ārya level. The second, which is "engaged" *(zhugs pa),* is that of the ārya bodhisattva.

64 *Bodhisattvabhūmi,* Toh 4037 Tengyur, sems tsam, *wi,* 113a6.

65 Ibid., 114b4.

66 Ibid., 133b6.

67 Sakya Paṇḍita Kunga Gyaltsen, *Various Compositions: A Bouquet of Flowers,* Collected Works, *tha,* 32b4.

68 *Well-Composed and Illuminating Commentary on the Kālapasūtra Grammar Work,* Sa skya pa'i bka' 'bum [Sakya Canon] (Tokyo: The Toyo Bunko, 1968), vol. 8, 2a3.

69 Citation untraced.

70 Ngawang Losang Gyatso, *Stream of the Ganges: An Account of Teachings Received,* Collected Works, *ka,* 4a6.

71 Grammar, poetic theory, prosody, drama, and lexicography.

72 *Mi dge ba.* This probably refers to the fact that disease is a karmic fruit of nonvirtue, but the term also means "bad" or "unfortunate" and may just be referring to the general adversity of ill health.

73 Chap. 4, Toh 343 Kangyur, mdo sde, *ah,* 189b4. Translated from the Chinese.

74 *Yogacaryābhūmi,* Toh 4035 Tengyur, sems tsam, *tshi,* 187a5.

75 *Bodhisattvabhūmi,* Toh 4037 Tengyur, sems tsam, *wi,* 50b1.

76 *Four Tantras,* Root Tantra, 2.4.7.

77 *Four Tantras,* Explanatory Tantra, 1.15.12.

78 *'Du ba.* One of the names for the body's three humors of wind, bile, and phlegm, whose excess, deficiency, and disturbance provoke illness.

79 *Four Tantras,* Final Tantra, 27.665.4. Generosity is often classified into three types: generosity with material things, generosity with Dharma, and generosity that grants freedom from fear.

80 *Essence of Eight Branches (Aṣṭāṅgahṛdayasaṃhita),* chap. 1, Toh 4310 Tengyur, gso rig, *he,* 44b3. For more on the figure of Pitṛceṭa, see below, pp. 128–43.

81 Untraced.

82 Untraced. As it says in the text below, Āyurveda emerged from the face of the god Brahmā.

83 Untraced in Taktsang Lotsāwa's works, but cited in volume 2 of the Collected Works of the Great Fifth, *tsa,* 179b3.

84 Again, *'du ba,* here referring to the three humors of wind, bile, and phlegm with the addition of blood.

85 The six branches *(rig byed kyi yan lag, vedāṅga)* are articulation *(bslab pa, śikṣā),* grammar *(vyākaraṇa, brda sprod),* metrics *(chandas, sdeb sbyor),* etymology *(nirukta, thos pa),* astronomy *(jyotiṣa skar rtsi),* and rites and ceremonies *(kalpa, rtog pa).* The two subsidiary treatises are those on love *(dran pa, smara)* and Dharma *(chos).*

86 Such citations from the Vedas are well known in Tibetan literature, but as the original texts were not translated into Tibetan, the citation cannot be sourced. However, this citation and the following two are quoted in Surkhar Lodrö Gyalpo's *General Compendium of Knowledge Indispensable to Physicians,* pp. 159–60.

87 Ibid.

88 Ibid.

89 Śūra is an alias of Pitṛceṭa, *Aṣṭāṅgahṛdayasaṃhita,* chap. 1, Toh 4310 Tengyur, gso rig, *he,* 44b3.

90 *Viśeṣastavaṭīkā,* Toh 1110 Tengyur, bstod tshogs, *ka,* 10a1.

91 Ibid., 13a6.

92 Making the final *a* in *sura* ("god") long turns it into *surā,* or alcohol. The prefix *a* is a negating particle.

93 *Devātiśayastotraṭīkā,* Toh 1113 Tengyur, bstod tshogs, *ka,* 57a5.

94 This is the name as transliterated in the text. Degé has Praca. Elsewhere the father of Dadhici is Atharvan.

95 In most versions of this popular legend, the sun god's wife is referred to as Saṃjñā or Saṃjañā.

96 *Devātiśayastotraṭīkā,* Toh 1113 Tengyur, bstod tshogs, *ka,* 46a6.

97 Śālihotra, *Śālihotrīyāśvāyurvedasaṃhitā,* Toh 4345 Tengyur, lugs kyi bstan bcos, *ngo,* 161b4.

98 *Sor mo la spyod,* but other editions have *ser me la spyod.* Either way, it remains unidentified.

99 Śālihotra, *Śālihotrīyāśvāyurvedasaṃhitā,* Toh 4345 Tengyur, lugs kyi bstan bcos, *ngo,* 162b4.

100 *Amarakoṣaṭīkākamadhenu,* Toh 4300 Tengyur, sgra mdo, *se,* 242a6.

101 *Vibhāvanālaṃkāra (srid pa can gyi rgyan),* literally, "causing to appear." According to Monier-Williams this device of Sanskrit poetics is "the description of effects, the causes of which are left to be conjectured." According to the *Great Tibetan-Chinese Dictionary* it is a device used to show effects from obscure causes and is one of the thirty-five *embellishments of meaning (arthālaṃkāra, don gyi rgyan).*

102 *Bodhisattvāvadānakalpalatā,* chap. 1, Toh 4155 Tengyur, skye rabs, *ke,* 4a1.

103 *Four Tantras,* Instruction Tantra, 89.544.6.

104 Pitṛceṭa, *Aṣṭāṅgahṛdayasaṃhita,* chap. 34, Toh 4310 Tengyur, gso rig, *he,* 313b6.

105 In the verse the horse is identified merely as *thor thos* (untraced as a Tibetan word) and the *apsaras* goddess as "goddess" *(lha mo).* The identifications as translated come from Puṇḍarīka's *Vimalaprabhā* commentary on the *Kālacakra Tantra* in the Peking Tengyur. According to Monier-Williams, the *apsaras* goddess who appeared at the churning was was Rambhā.

106 Cited in Puṇḍarīka, *Stainless Light (Vimalaprabhā),* Toh 845 Kangyur, rgyud, *śrī,* 430a7.

107 *Pramāṇavārttika,* 1:343, Toh 4210 Tengyur, tshad ma, *ce,* 107b2.

108 This refers to the four ages of the Buddha's doctrine: the age of perfection *(rdzogs ldan, caturyuga),* the age of three *(gsum ldan, treatyuga),* the age of two *(gnyis ldan, dvāparayuga),* and the age of troubles *(rtsod ldan, kaliyuga).*

109 *Mañjuśrīmūlakalpa,* Toh 543 Kangyur, rgyud, *na,* 194b1.

110 Ibid., 194b3.

111 Ibid., 194b4.

112 *Sa zhag.* Glistening film or skin left after rainwater has dried up.

113 Better known as Taktsang Lotsāwa (b. 1405).

114 Author of *Commentary on Praise of the Exalted,* quoted previously.

115 Pitṛceṭa, *Aṣṭāṅgahṛdayasaṃhita,* chap. 39, Toh 4310 Tengyur, gso rig, *he,* 328b6.

116 *Arura: Terminalia chebula Retz;* renowned as the king of medicinal plants. See glossary, chebulic myrobalan.

117 Possibly *atha,* meaning "then." In the Degé edition of the quote below it says, "The syllable *oṃ* and the word 'then' *(de nas).*"

118 Candranandana, *Candrikāprabhāsa,* Toh 4312 Tengyur, gso rig, *ko,* 3a4.

119 Anubhūti, *Sarasvatīvyākaraṇsūtra,* 1:1–9, Toh 4297 Tengyur, sgra mdo, *se.*

120 *Vajraśekharatantra,* chap. 2, Toh 480 Kangyur, rgyud, *nya,* 156a2.

121 Citation untraced. Probably to be found in *Vinayavastuṭīkā.* Toh 4113 Tengyur, dul ba, *tsu.* "Measure" *(tshad, mātrā)* probably refers to the intonation length of the syllable. This is one meaning of *mātrā,* a term cognate with "meter."

122 On this difficult verse, both this edition and the Degé edition quote "activity" *(las)*, but according to Prof. Losang Tenzin, "body" *(lus)* is more probable.
123 Bhāvaviveka, *Tarkajvālā*, Toh 3856 Tengyur, dbu ma, *dza*, 297b6. *Sattva, rajas,* and *tamas* are the three qualities *(guṇa)* or constituents of all existence, according to much ancient Indic literature.
124 Ibid., 298a3.
125 Cited in Puṇḍarīka, *Vimalaprabhā*, chap. 3, Toh 845 Kangyur, rgyud, *śrī*, 228a5.
126 *Hevajratantra*, chap. 5, Toh 417 Kangyur, rgyud, *nga*, 6a7.
127 Toh 1190 Tengyur, rgyud 'grel, *nga*, 1b2.
128 Cited in Puṇḍarīka, *Vimalaprabhā*, chap. 3, Toh 845 Kangyur, rgyud, *śrī*, 228a5.
129 Candrakīrti, *Pradīpodyotana*, chap. 14, Toh 1785 Tengyur, rgyud 'grel, *ha*, 118a5.
130 Śrīdharasena, *Abhidhanaśāstraviśvalocana*, Toh 4453 Tengyur, sna tshogs, *po*, 90b1.
131 *Candrasūtra*, Toh 42 Kangyur, sher phyin sna tshogs, *ka*, 283a3.
132 These are five classes of texts teaching mantra recitation for achieving various feats.
133 *Mahāmantrānudhārisūtra*, Toh 563 Kangyur, rgyud, *pha*, 154b4.
134 *Klu 'bum khra bo*, by Tönpa Shenrap, published in Delhi, 1977, by Khedrup Gyatso.
135 The thirtieth or last day of the lunar month, when the sky is "empty" of the moon.
136 *Gola* is a Sanskrit term that refers to the dome-shaped canopy of the sky through which the sun, moon, stars, and planets travel.
137 Desi Sangyé Gyatso, *Phug lugs rtsis kyi legs bshad baidūrya dkar po*, 57.17.
138 *Shed bu*; *mānava* or *manu*, from which the English word "man" comes.
139 Possibly *vimalagotra* or *vimalamutra*.
140 *Vinayavastu*, Toh 1 Kangyur, 'dul ba, *ka*, 179b5.
141 Ibid., 277b6. This is a summarizing verse that comes at the beginning of a section and as such is little more than a listing of topics. The first topic is general medicines permitted for the monastic community. Other topics are medicines or foods that have come to be permitted due to a specific incident. Permitted fats allowed are of five types: fish, frog, crocodile, bear, and pig. This came about when a monk was told to eat fat because no other medicine would cure him. Another was prescribed astringents for scabrous skin. Another monk went insane and had to be force fed raw meat. Pilinda, or the son of Pilinda, was constantly ill, and as a result monks were allowed to carry medicine pouches. Revati was a monk who doubted everything and was called Doubting Revati; his doubts led to certain food being allowed. Acidic juice refers to Indian gooseberry *(amla)* juice with salt.
142 Seven-day medicines must be consumed within seven days. Life-long medicine can be taken for the duration of life.
143 *Vinayavastu*, Toh 1 Kangyur, 'dul ba, *ka*, 278b1.
144 Some of the seven bodily constituents are not listed here as they usually are elsewhere (see glossary). Maybe this is because the text was translated from the Chinese. "Fatty tissue" *(klad rgyas)* would normally read "fat" *(tshil)*. Prof. Losang Tenzin said this could be rendered as "brain." "Essence" *(ro)* is normally "plasma" *(dangs ma)*, and "element" *(khams)* is usually "semen" *(khu ba)*.

145 This list differs from the eight branches detailed in *Four Tantras,* which are: internal illnesses, children's illnesses, women's illnesses, demonic influence, wounds and surgery, poisons, illnesses affecting the elderly, and aphrodisiacs.

146 Of the six types of chebulic myrobalan, King or Conqueror *(vijaya, rnam rgyal)* is supreme and is usually found only in the celestial realms. The verse plays with its name: "form" *(rnam),* "king" *(rgyal).*

147 Chebulic, emblic, and baleric myrobalan, black pepper, long pepper, and ginger.

148 *Sutra of Golden Light: King of the Supremely Victorious Sutras,* chap. 24, Toh 555 Kangyur, rgyud, *pa,* 130a2.

149 There are three versions of *Sutra of Golden Light* in the Degé Kangyur: *Sutra of Golden Light: King of the Supremely Victorious Sutras* (Toh 555); and two versions under the name *Sutra of Golden Light: Mighty King of Sutras* (Toh 556 and 557). The sutra quoted at length above is Toh 555, the version translated by Chödrup from a Chinese text. The version of the sutra translated from the Sanskrit into English by R. E. Emmerick is Toh 557 (Oxford: Pali Text Society, 1979).

150 Dza Yeshé Sung, twelfth-century medical scholar.

151 Orgyen, or Urgyen, in Tibetan. The Indian spelling has several variants as well, e.g., Uḍḍiyāna, Oḍiyān. Oḍḍiyāna was the seat of the early development of Buddhist tantra. Its exact location is a subject of some debate.

152 A.k.a. Tsenpashilaha. See the account of his life later in the text.

153 Cited in *Oral Transmission of Our Ancestors* by Surkhar Lodrö Gyalpo, 19a6.

154 These are the four mountains, mentioned in *Four Tantras,* that surround Sudarśana. The Dakchenpa referred to here is presumably an early master from the Sakya tradition, but I am unable to identify him.

155 These assertions are all cited in Surkhar Lodrö Gyalpo, *Oral Transmission of Our Ancestors,* 21b4. The identities have been inserted as annotations in between the text, but here the author has included them as main text.

156 In Tibetan medical literature there is much discussion on whether *Four Tantras* is the word of the Buddha or composed at a later date. The author investigates this matter later.

157 Famous Indian doctor at the time of the Buddha to whom a whole chapter is dedicated below.

158 One of the four mountains surrounding Sudarśana.

159 *Treasure for the Benefit of Others: A Presentation of Four Tantras,* Collected Works, *ka,* 3b2.

160 *Oral Transmission of Our Ancestors,* 22a2.

161 Collected Works, *ya,* 78a6. The author is saying that Surkhar Lodrö Gyalpo rests his assertion on the line in bold.

162 An edition of the Kangyur, or collected words of the Buddha, deposited in the fifteenth century in Palkhor Chöde Monastery in Gyantsé. See Paul Harrison in Cabezón and Jackson, eds., *Tibetan Literature: A Study in Genre,* p. 80.

163 Toh 505 Kangyur, rgyud, *da,* 284a2.

164 *Yum chen mo,* but "Prajñāpāramitā" in the actual tantra.

165 The guardians of the four directions in the Cāturmahārājika heaven: Vaiśravaṇa (= Kubera), Dhṛtarāṣṭra, Virūḍhaka, and Virūpākṣa.

166 *Lalitavistara Sutra,* Toh 95 Kangyur, mdo sde, *kha,* 54a7.

167 The whole story is found in *Vinaya Kṣudrakavastu,* Toh 6 Kangyur, 'dul ba, over volumes *tha* and *da,* 310–33.

168 *Abhiniṣkramaṇa Sutra,* Toh 301 Kangyur, mdo sde, *sa,* 15a4.
169 *Yojana,* a distance reckoned to be around either four or nine miles.
170 Here "five hundred" is a term of quantity meaning "a considerable number."
171 Orgyen Lingpa, *Five Chronicles,* 24.499.1.
172 *Oral Transmission of Our Ancestors,* 19a4.
173 Untraced.
174 *Khams, dhātu.* This term can be used for the four elements of earth, water, fire, and air that make up the body or it can refer to the seven bodily constituents or tissues (see glossary).
175 In the *Great Garuḍa History of Medicine* (p. 10) from Eighteen Auxiliary Texts, one of the reference history books used by the author, it states that *Four Tantras* was taught at the time of this sutra.
176 Although the tantra clearly talks of four distinct mountains, according to Prof. Losang Tenzin, Desi Sangyé Gyatso asserts these mountains should be seen as possessing one side each. Otherwise, each mountain would have sides facing all four directions, which would contradict the descriptions in the tantra detailing the different types of medical plants growing on these mountains depending on the particular direction they faced. Surkhar Lodrö Gyalpo in his *Oral Transmission of Our Ancestors* also says that this is one mountain with four sides and that the names of actual mountains given to these sides—Gandhamārdana, Himavat, Vindhya, and Malaya or Malabar—are not to be taken literally.
177 Possibly the large vases that stand on the roofs of palaces.
178 Cited in *Oral Transmission of Our Ancestors,* 23b6.
179 Here in his description of the setting for the teaching of *Four Tantras* the author is interspersing his text with actual text from the introduction to *Four Tantras.*
180 Found in *Medicine Buddha Sutra (Bhaiṣajyaguru-vaidūryaprabhāsyapūrva-praṇidhānaviśeṣavistāra-sūtra),* Toh 504 Kangyur, rgyud, *da,* 174b2.
181 *Ratnākarasūtra,* vol. 7, Toh 124 Kangyur, mdo sde, *tha,* 289b4.
182 *Śūraṅgamasamādhi Sutra,* Toh 132 Kangyur, mdo sde, *da,* 296a3.
183 Ibid., 309a1.
184 This may be the *Vajraśekhara Explanatory Tantra,* Toh 480 Kangyur, rgyud 'bum, *nya.*
185 Candrakīrti, *Bright Lamp (Pradīpoddyotana),* Toh 1785 Tengyur, rgyud 'grel, *ha,* 9b1.
186 The largest area of world realms in Buddhist cosmology.
187 *Mahāsahasrapramardana,* Toh 558 Kangyur, rgyud 'bum, *pha,* 80b5.
188 *Māyopamāsamādhisūtra,* Toh 130 Kangyur, mdo sde, *da,* 219a2.
189 *Saṃghāṭasūtradharmaparyāya,* Toh 102 Kangyur, mdo sde, *nga,* 247a6.
190 *Mañjuśrīparipṛrcchā,* Toh 172 Kangyur, mdo sde, *ma,* 4a7.
191 *Abhisamayālaṃkāra,* 8:9, Toh 3786 Kangyur, shes phyin, *ka,* 11b5.
192 *Sarvabuddhasamayogatantra,* Toh 366 Kangyur, rgyud, *ka,* 155b4.
193 *Yang dag sgrub pa, saṃsiddhi.*
194 *Sarvabuddhasamayogatantra,* chap. 5, Toh 366 Kangyur, rgyud, *ka,* 155b3.
195 *Abhidhana-uttaratantra,* chap. 35, Toh 369 Kangyur, rgyud, *ka,* 323b5.
196 *Ekavīrākhyāśrīcaṇḍamahāroṣaṇa-tantrarāja,* Toh 431 Kangyur, rgyud, *nga,* 320a3.
197 These days a region of western Nepal.
198 *Four Tantras,* Final Tantra, 26.660.6.

199 *Yid las skyes,* Manasija. As there is no extant Sanskrit original, the rendering of Tibetan names in Sanskrit presents some problems, mainly those of choice. Here and elsewhere I have mainly followed Lokesh Chandra and Vaidya Bhagwan Dash.

200 "Treasure" *(gter ma)* refers to the unearthing of texts previously hidden; "transmission" *(dka' ma)* refers to the unbroken transmission of a text from early Indian times without any intervening hidden period.

201 *Gzhan 'phrul dbang byed;* usually described in Buddhist texts as a class of gods "able to enjoy the pleasures of others," but also described as being the abode of Māra. So here presumably it is the name of the kind of māras that live there.

202 According to the *Eighteen Accessory Texts,* the *Crystal Mirror Medicine Tantra* was taught to Ānanda during the second turning of the wheel of Dharma.

203 Some of the following three citations from this sutra I have translated according to the edition translated from the Sanskrit (Toh 120, mdo sde, *tha*); it seems to make the greater sense. The two editions broadly agree but there are differences in detail.

204 This is according to the translation from the Sanskrit. The other, from the Chinese, has "testing" *(bgam).*

205 The text has *btsa',* "to be born." I have gone with Degé, *'tsho,* "to live."

206 *Mahāparinirvāṇasūtra,* Toh 119 Kangyur, mdo sde, *nya,* 35b7.

207 *Mahāparinirvāṇasūtra,* Toh 120 Kangyur, mdo sde, *tha,* 34a1.

208 Ibid., 110a1.

209 *Vajraḍākatantra,* chap. 49, Toh 370 Kangyur, rgyud, *kha,* 111b3. This cryptic verse is best explained by the commentary to this tantra (Toh 1415 Tengyur, rgyud 'grel, *tsha*), which says that Vajrasattva manifested as Mahādeva and consort, producing great light and fire, thereby terrifying the gods, demigods, siddhas, etc. This fire was the fire of a passion that melted the two into drops, and the buddhas saw that these drops were to be scattered around the world by the māras. Through the medium of song they beseeched Vajrasattva to awake from his passion and prevent this from happening. This is the origin of mercury, or quicksilver.

210 In Tibetan medicine myrobalan is usually described as being of five types. These seven types broadly correspond with the seven types mentioned in Indian Āyurveda. (Dash, *Encyclopedia of Tibetan Medicine,* p. 8.)

211 *Vajraḍākatantra,* chap. 49, Toh 370 Kangyur, rgyud, *kha,* 112a5.

212 Ibid., 114a5.

213 *Glang shu.* See glossary.

214 *Vajraḍākatantra,* chap. 49, Toh 370 Kangyur, rgyud, *kha,* 116b5.

215 *Ḍākārṇavatantra,* Toh 372 Kangyur, rgyud, *kha,* 215a1.

216 *Cakrasaṃvara/Saṃvarodaya Tantra,* Toh 373 Kangyur, rgyud, *kha,* 266a7.

217 Ibid., 288a4.

218 Ibid., 289a2.

219 *'Chi ba blu ba.*

220 *Cakrasaṃvara/Saṃvarodaya Tantra,* Toh 373 Kangyur rgyud, *kha,* 298a1.

221 The following verses from the *Condensed Kālacakra Tantra* are very difficult to interpret, and the translation has been made according to the *Vimalprabhā,* Butön Rinpoché's *Annotations to the Inner Chapter of the Vimalaprabhā,* and Khedrup

Jé's *Illuminating Reality: An Extensive Explanation of the Stainless Light, the Great Commentary on the Glorious Kālacakra.*

222 *Kālacakratantra,* 2:3, Toh 362 Kangyur, rgyud, *ka,* 40a7.

223 *Kālacakratantra,* 2:107, Toh 362 Kangyur, rgyud, *ka,* 51a1.

224 *Kālacakratantra,* 2:109, Toh 362 Kangyur, rgyud, *ka,* 51a4.

225 *Kālacakratantra,* 2:110, Toh 362 Kangyur, rgyud, *ka,* 51a6. The yogas described here are those of *prāṇāyāma* and vase yoga in the Kālacakra system. Their full application can be found in Khedrup Norsang Gyatso, *Ornament of Stainless Light,* p. 475.

226 *Kālacakratantra,* 2:111, Toh 362 Kangyur, rgyud, *ka,* 51a7.

227 *Kālacakratantra,* 2:112–13, Toh 362 Kangyur, rgyud, *ka,* 51b3.

228 *Stainless Light (Vimalaprabhā),* the commentary to the *Condensed Kālacakra Tantra,* states that "a few days" means three years and three fortnights.

229 *Kālacakratantra,* 2:115, Toh 362 Kangyur, rgyud, *ka,* 51b6.

230 Here urine is referred to as "Akṣobhya."

231 Black pepper, long pepper, and ginger are the three hot foods.

232 *'Byung po, bhūta,* but referred to in the *Vimalaprabhā* as *preta,* or ghost.

233 *Kālacakratantra,* 2:118, Toh 362 Kangyur, rgyud, *ka,* 52a4.

234 See following note.

235 *Kālacakratantra,* 2:119, Toh 362 Kangyur, rgyud, *ka,* 52a5. On this verse the *Stainless Light* commentary quotes the famous maxim, "As without, so within the body" to explain the substances mentioned here, all of which have external and internal counterparts. For the yogi the external and internal counterparts are undifferentiated. "Meditative absorption" *(bsam gtan, dhyāna)* refers to winds being drawn into the central channel. Externally "flower" refers to the juice of the *bhṛṅgarāja* flower, which according to Khedrup Jé is the *vaśaka* flower and grows in Nepal; internally it refers to menstrual blood. According to Khedrup Jé (p. 285), ingesting is inhalation through the nose. The five lamps are the five meats, which are the flesh of dog, ox, horse, human, and elephant. Bee vomit is honey or mead.

236 *Kālacakratantra,* 2:120, Toh 362 Kangyur, rgyud, *ka,* 52a6.

237 *Kālacakratantra,* 2:121, Toh 362 Kangyur, rgyud, *ka,* 52b1.

238 *Kālacakratantra,* 2:122, Toh 362 Kangyur, rgyud, *ka,* 52b2.

239 The mantra, according to *Stainless Light,* is *oṃ phreṃ viśvamātaḥ vajra kāṇḍakāna nāśaya nāśaya māma kuru kuru svāhā,* where *phreṃ* is made of letters of water, fire, and air, and *vajra kāṇḍakāna* refers to smallpox.

240 *Kālacakratantra,* 2:123, Toh 362 Kangyur, rgyud, *ka,* 52b4.

241 *Kālacakratantra,* 2:124, Toh 362 Kangyur, rgyud, *ka,* 52b5. The seven constituents are the seven bodily constituents mentioned above.

242 *Stainless Light* says these ingredients with ground pyrites, or marcasite *(mākṣika),* are placed in an open-top melting pot and the fire is blown vigorously until only the gold is left.

243 *Srang, pala;* a measure of weight, especially of gold, estimated by Monier-Williams to be about 120 grains troy (around 8 grams), but many other estimates exist. Here, it might just be referring to proportionate weights.

244 This verse contains instructions for producing gold to sustain the practitioner. Khedrup Jé speculates that "semigold" may refer to this substance being half silver, half gold.

245 *Kālacakratantra,* 2:125–28, Toh 362 Kangyur, rgyud, *ka,* 52b6.
246 Where necessary, the aromatic substances in this passage have been translated or listed according to Sanskrit synonyms listed in the *Stainless Light* commentary on this text.
247 *Kālacakratantra,* 2:129, Toh 362 Kangyur, rgyud, *ka,* 53a5.
248 This is a magic-square yantra in which any line of four numbers, as listed in the text, adds up to thirty-four. The sixteen numbers are represented by Kālacakra word numerals. In order they are 7, 12, 1, 14, 2, 13, 8, 11, 16, 3, 10, 5, 9, 6, 15, 4.
249 *Kālacakratantra,* 2:140, Toh 362 Kangyur, rgyud, *ka,* 54a6.
250 This means to be consecrated by the mantra *oṃ āḥ hūṃ amukāya (such a person) garbha (womb) śūlaṃ (pain) hara hara (destroy) svā hā.*
251 *Kālacakratantra,* 2:143, Toh 362 Kangyur, rgyud, *ka,* 54b3.
252 Cited in Surkhar Lodrö Gyalpo's *General Compendium,* 175.13.
253 Surkhar Lodrö Gyalpo, *General Compendium,* 175.16.
254 Usually the seven rishis *(saptarṣi)* include Pulaha and not Kaiṭabhajit, who is seen as an incarnation of Viṣṇu.
255 The author is making reference to a verse from the Root Tantra of *Four Tantras,* which describes the rishi entourage of the Tantra.
256 This is a possible rendering of *rkos gdab,* as found in the *Eighteen Accessory Texts.* The text here has *dkos ston,* which makes little sense.
257 *Par/bar bkab;* but the Eighteen Auxiliary Texts has *spar khab,* "covering with the hand." Surkhar Lodrö Gyalpo, in his *General Compendium* 250.18, has "gold" instead of "sun and moon."
258 *Mahāmayūrīvidyārājñī,* Toh 559 Kangyur, rgyud, *pha,* 112a5.
259 As written.
260 *Four Tantras,* Final Tantra, 26.660.6. See previous citation, page 86.
261 Viśākhadeva, *Vinayakārikā,* Toh 4123 Tengyur, 'dul ba, *shu,* 61b5.
262 *Bud me rin po che, strīratna;* one of the seven treasures of a king.
263 According to Mukhopadhyaya (p. 6560) this is the Buddhist monk Ātreya and not the ancient rishi.
264 *Pad ma snying po;* possibly "Puṣkarasārin."
265 Jivaka means "physician," and this is the name he is usually known by.
266 Usually refers to an army or force consisting of cavalry, elephant, chariot, and infantry divisions.
267 A coin commonly used in ancient India; "the weight of one *kārṣā*" (Mon).
268 *Dmu chu.* Usually translated as third stage edema or dropsy. However, in its etymology, *dmu* is a disease-causing spirit, and *chu* is the water or lymph accumulation in the body brought on by the spirit. The etymology is obviously closer to the meaning in this story.
269 *Vinayavastu,* Toh 6 Kangyur, 'dul ba, *tha,* 265a6 and 273a3.
270 Probably because dried cow dung is known to stupefy scorpions.
271 This passage suffers from considerable cropping of the original story. In the Degé Tengyur Kāka suffers from leprosy, and the medicine Jivaka surreptitiously administers cures him. He is left on the side of the mountain with the two elephants. These are the "three cherished by the king." His words are to the local people.
272 This may be a mischievous insertion.

273 *Bzod pa;* usually referring to a level of attainment where realizations are not immediately overcome by fear, doubt, and so on, but gain a foothold in the mind.

274 Vedalī was in the south of India, in what is now Andhra Pradesh. The Tibetan *vai dha (be ṭa* or *be ta)* also sometimes refers to Vidarbha, in what is now Maharashtra.

275 *Laṅkāvatārasūtra,* Toh 107 Kangyur, mdo sde, *ca,* 165b4. The Joyous level is the first of the ten bodhisattva *bhūmis.*

276 *Rma bya chen mo;* Great Peacock; one of the five great *dhāraṇī* or spells.

277 *Mañjuśrīmūlakalpa,* Toh 543 Kangyur, rgyud, *na,* 308b6.

278 *Mahāmeghasūtra,* Toh 232 Kangyur, mdo sde, *wa,* 187b7.

279 *Kālacakratantrottaratantra,* Toh 363 Kangyur, rgyud, *ka,* 132b3.

280 *Tārākurulullekalpa,* Toh 437 Kangyur, rgyud, *ca.*

281 Written as Senda; Buddhist sect opposed to the Mahayana.

282 Nāgas are (1) born in the ocean, which here is likened to the dharmadhātu, or realm of ultimate truth; (2) live between the animal and spirit realm but not in either; (3) famed for their jealous guardianship of treasures; and (4) have fiery eyes and breathe fire from their mouths.

283 *Fundamental Stanzas on the Middle Way (Mūlamadhyamakakārikā), Sixty Verses of Reasoning (Yuktiṣaṣṭhikā), Seventy Verses on Emptiness (Śūnyatāsaptati), Finely Woven Scripture (Vaidalyasūtra), Refutation of Arguments (Vigrahavyāvartanī),* and *Precious Garland (Ratnāvalī).*

284 *Rgyud kun la btus pa.* Butön also mentions this work, but it is not listed in either the Degé or Peking Tengyur.

285 *Yogaśataka,* Toh 4306 Tengyur, gso ba rig pa, *he,* 1a2.

286 *Jīvasūtra,* Toh 4307 Tengyur, gso ba rig pa, *he,* 8b5.

287 Only the first of these is listed in the Tengyur (Toh 4308, gso rig, *he*). In *Tibetan Medicine* (p. 66) Dash lists nine other Sanskrit medical works attributed to Nāgārjuna. One of these nine—the *Rasaratnākara*—appears to be the fourth in this list.

288 In tantra *bodhicitta* can mean blood or semen, but this use would be unusual here. Other sources say the blood turned to milk as it flowed.

289 Literally, a *krośa,* which is an eighth of a league (*yojana,* about four miles). In other words, the temples went from more than fifteen miles apart to being a half mile apart.

290 *Pha khol.* Pitṛceṭa is the literal translation. As author of *Essence of Eight Branches (Aśṭāṅgahṛdaya),* he is often referred to as Vāgbhaṭa by Sanskrit scholars. However, he is known by many names, as the author points out below. Even the following citation refers to him as Mātṛceṭa.

291 *Mañjuśrīmūlakalpa,* Toh 543 Kangyur, rgyud, *na,* 308b1.

292 Pema Karpo, *Chos 'byung bstan pa'i padma rgyas pa'i nyin byed,* Collected Works, *kha,* 36b2.

293 Referring to Tāranātha's *Dam pa'i chos rin po che 'phag yul du ji ltar dar ba'i tshul gsal bar ston pa dgos 'dod kun 'byung,* 64b5. Translated by Lama Chimpa and Alaka Chattopadhyaya as *History of Buddhism in India* (Delhi: Motilal Banarsidass, 1997).

294 *Cleaning the Dirt from Vaidūrya to Reveal Its True Face [Bai dūrya g.ya' sel don gyi bzhin ras ston byed],* Collected Works of Desi Sangyé Gyatso, vol. 4, section 2, 176b4.

295 Epithet of the god Śiva.

296 Cited in Surkhar Lodrö Gyalpo's *General Compendium,* 210.9.

297 Surkhar Lodrö Gyalpo, *General Compendium,* 210.17.

298 *Pha khol ma khol.* This seems to be a play on the Tibetan word *ma,* which means both "mother" and "not." As indicated previously this term was used to indicate his obedience to his parents—"obedient to father, obedient to mother"—and here to mean almost the opposite—"obedient and disobedient to father." However, this cannot work with the Sanskrit term *pitṛceṭa-mātṛceṭa,* which does not carry the sense of disobedient.

299 *Yod;* although other versions have *yong* (come).

300 For this narrative and the verses see Butön's *Bde bar gshegs pa'i gsal byed chos kyi 'byung gnas gsung rab rin po che'i mdzod,* Collected Works, *ya,* 101b4.

301 Only the third and fourth of these are found in the Tengyur. See bibliography under Pitṛceṭa.

302 Cited in Surkhar Lodrö Gyalpo's *General Compendium,* 215.17.

303 In all Sanskrit sources the authorship of this work is attributed to Vāgbhaṭa. According to Mukhopadhyaya (p. 791) the *Aṣṭāṅgasaṃgraha* and the *Aṣṭāṅgahṛdayasaṃhitā* were composed by two distinct authors, both named Vāgbhaṭa.

304 *Khrag mkhris, raktapittam;* forms of hemorrhage.

305 Cited in Tāranātha's Collected Works, *ma,* 143b3.

306 *Ngo bo gnyis med pa.* But possibly Asvabhāva *(ngo bo nyid med pa).*

307 Toh 4309 Tengyur, gso rig, *he,* 13b2.

308 Written here and in Degé as *dpal chen dga' ba* (Saubhāgyānandana), but cited previously in the list of names of Aśvaghoṣa—and below, as well as in Surkhar Lodrö Gyalpo's *General Compendium*—as *dpal chen dge ba* (Saubhāgyaśubha).

309 *Rgyud shes,* but the Degé edition has *rgyun shes,* which would render it "with the wisdom of Ātreya."

310 *Padārthacandrikāprabhāsanāma-aṣṭāṅgahṛdayavivṛti,* Toh 4312 Tengyur, gso rig, *go,* 304a5.

311 Ibid., 304a3.

312 *Aṣṭāṅgahṛdayasaṃhita,* Toh 4310 Tengyur, gso rig, *he,* 334a6.

313 Rendered below as Śrī Ānanda. See Martin, p. 11, where his name is also rendered Pra-a-nan-ta.

314 *Klo.* These days the region of the Lhopa *(lho pa)* people in the south of the country.

315 Also called Lhathori Nyentsen (Lha mtho ri gnyan brtsan). Tibet's twenty-fifth king; 348–468 C.E. (Rechung). Twenty-eighth king, 254–74 C.E. (Dungkar). A contemporary of Vasubhandu according to Tāranātha.

316 *Gnyan po gsang ba.* During the reign of King Lha Thothori, a box fell from the sky containing three texts and a golden shrine. At first no one knew what they were, and the king called them the Secret Signs and placed them in a box in his palace.

317 *A zha.* According to the *White Annals,* quoted in Dungkar, p. 1834, this area is now part of Mongolia. Others say it is in the region of Kansu and the Blue Lake (Tso Ngön) in the north, but Dungkar rejects this, saying that it refers to an area on the far eastern reaches of Tibet. According to Kachuwa Chölothar, p. 8, it is in Domé Tsongka. Trinlé, p. 16, quotes the Fifth Dalai Lama as saying it is near Blue Lake. Others place it in Ngari.

318 For more on this locale, see in the introduction on p. 2–4.

319 Cited in Surkhar Lodrö Gyalpo's *General Compendium,* 288.10.
320 *'Tsho byed sman pa. Tsho byed* is also another term for a doctor or healer and is the Tibetan rendering of *Jivaka,* the name given to the renowned doctor who lived during the time of the Buddha. *Sman pa* means physician.
321 According to some accounts, this prince died before the marriage took place.
322 Thirty-seventh king of Tibet usually known as Tridé Tsukten (b. 704) (Dungkar, p. 396).
323 Orgyen Lingpa, *Five Chronicles,* 24.499.4.
324 Trinlé (p. 48) says that the name is in the language of Trom. Elsewhere in the text he is called Tsenpashilaha, but it appears to be of Sanskrit origin, possibly Campaśīla. See Martin (p. 15) and Beckwith ("The Introduction of Greek Medicine into Tibet," p. 303).
325 *Lhung bzed* (begging bowl), but Surkhar Lodrö Gyalpo has *lhu med* (whole, complete).
326 Trinlé (p. 47) points out that these works are rare indeed these days, although a copy of the *Works of Biji* exists in the Jong Medical Institute in Tibet.
327 *Dmag* (army), but Surkhar Lodrö Gyalpo has *dmangs* (ordinary people).
328 Dates for this figure vary: 742–97 (Dungkar); born 754 (Rechung); 755–94 (Beckwith).
329 Trinlé states that this is evidently the same Tsenpashilaha or Tsampashilaha described previously.
330 For *thor* read *thur* (Prof. Losang Tenzin). *Thor* is often an abbreviation of *thor bu* "miscellaneous" and *thur* an abbreviation of *thur ma,* "surgical instrument." More than once these two terms have been confused leading to doubt as to whether the correct reading is "miscellaneous treatments" or "surgical treatments."
331 Lodrö Gyalpo reading *mi tra* preferred. He also has *caṇḍa.*
332 *Gshal;* this is Lodrö Gyalpo's reading.
333 *Che tsho;* amended as per Lodrö Gyalpo from *che tshe.*
334 *Book of Kadam: Son Teachings,* 143.20.
335 Ibid., 203.1.
336 Ibid., 203.4.
337 Padmasambhava.
338 A district on the Tsangpo river to the west of Lhasa; these days called Nyemo Dzongsang Richü (Dungkar, p. 1399).
339 Orgyen Lingpa, *Lotus Chronicles,* 68.405.6.
340 Milk, butter, and yogurt are the three white foods; sugar, molasses, and honey the three sweet foods.
341 Dorjé Lingpa (1346–1405), *Great Mask: A Biography of the Translator Vairocana.*
342 Orgyen Linpga, *Lotus Chronicles,* 70.410.4.
343 *Dngul chas.* I have gone with Trinlé's reading here rather than *lus chas,* as written.
344 Here rendered as *rdo rje gdan, vajrāsana:* "vajra seat."
345 This is the first instance in this account of Ganjak being called by his well-known name of Vairocana.
346 Dorjé Lingpa (1346–1405), *Great Mask: A Biography of the Translator Vairocana,* p. 156. Parts of the letter and the description of the horses below have been translated in accordance with this edition.
347 Orgyen Lingpa, *Lotus Chronicles,* 85.503.3.

348 Ka Lotsāwa Paltsek and Chok Lotsāwa Lui Gyaltsen were two famous early translators of the Nyingma school. Rinchen Sangpo (958–1055), mentioned in the next line, has a section devoted to him in the text below.
349 Untraced. Ngok Lotsāwa Loden Sherap (1059–1109), a nephew and disciple of Ngok Lekpai Sherap (1018–1115), was a lineage holder of the Kadam school, holding the Sangphu lineage of Atiśa's stages of the path *(lam rim)* teachings.
350 Untraced.
351 In other words, *Four Tantras.*
352 Biji or Tsenpashilaha.
353 Orgyan Lingpa, *Lotus Chronicles,* 85.501.5.
354 Untraced.
355 Referred to in the homage as Apsé.
356 *Gru gu* or *Dru gu.* Identified as present-day Yugu in northwest Tibet, "north of Ngari and south of Khoten" (*Great Tibetan-Chinese Dictionary,* p. 1332).
357 In some versions "he" is replace by "I."
358 Text here and elsewhere has *'khug* or *khyug.* Amended to *mkhyud* on the advice of Prof. Losang Tenzin.
359 *Be du ra;* also found as Verura. Surkhar Lodrö Gyalpo has Vaidūrya.
360 *Ba che;* variously spelled *bir che, be che,* and *bi byi.* The last is also the name of Tsenpashilaha mentioned earlier and also of a doctor who came to Tibet from India during the reign of Thothori Nyentsen. See introduction, p. 4.
361 In Gongkar region west of Lhasa.
362 Of the nine previously mentioned Tibetan doctors, it would seem that Yuthok Gönpo is not included here.
363 Previously listed as *One Thousand and Ninety-One Treatments.*
364 Previously listed as being by the Nepalese master Anara.
365 Also Urpaya. See Martin, p. 14.
366 According to Martin (p. 12), could refer to an Uighur place name.
367 Ordained Ngari king of the tenth century responsible for inviting Atiśa to Tibet.
368 *Aṣṭaṅgahṛdayanāmavaidūryakabhāṣya;* Vāgbhaṭa's own commentary to *Essence of Eight Branches.*
369 Written as Nārotava.
370 Also known as Lu Kargyal, a Tibetan shepherd possessed by a demon who, aided by various magical powers, preached a heretical doctrine in Tibet.
371 As written.
372 As mentioned before, nowhere does the author refer to the composer of this text with a name that translates as Vāgbhaṭa.
373 Possibly Huitsung (1333–70), last of the Yuan emperors.
374 In this section "scripture" refers mainly to *Eight Branches.*
375 See note 349 above.
376 Written *na lendra.*
377 As written. Surkhar Lodrö Gyalpo has Candrali.
378 Citation untraced.
379 *La stod btsan yul mtshon la so nam byed.* This is the reading according to Orgyen Lingpa in the *Lotus Chronicles,* p. 561. The present text, however, has *bon* instead of *mtshon* and *gso* instead of *so.* Prof. Losang Tenzin suggests that *mtshon* refers to *mtshon cha,* weapons.

380 Orgyen Lingpa, *Lotus Chronicles,* 42.561.2.

381 Ibid., 42.561.7.

382 *Dud kha'i snye ma.*

383 Orgyen Lingpa, *Lotus Chronicles,* 42.564.4.

384 *Thems* or *them;* precise meaning here is unclear. The term usually refers to the threshold of a door.

385 Cited in Jamgön Kongtrül Lodrö Thayé, *Store of Precious Treasure,* vol. *ha,* dkar chag, 122.

386 *Gyad;* literally, "strong man."

387 The following seven sections deal with seven serious conditions or diseases *(gnyan nad).* A serious condition is described as being caused by the coming together of harmful external organisms and innate internal blood organisms. There are eighteen serious conditions (Dungkar, p. 974). The seven here are described in the glossary.

388 Treasure texts often use enigmatic language. The actual text of *Great Vase of Ambrosia* as found in *Store of Precious Treasures* talks of illnesses and disease riding the horses of the four elements; hence the following imagery of roads, regions, and households to describe bodily entrances and locations for diseases. The "three black forces" refers to a pandemic when harmful external and internal organisms combine, and infectious disease, fever, and wind disorder arise simultaneously (*Great Tibetan-Chinese Dictionary,* p. 1499).

389 *Las mtha' bsgyur;* described in the *Ambrosia Vase* itself as "designating specific powers to the particular medicine."

390 *G.ya'i bdud rtsi ma lha mo'i khrag.* Identified as a synonym for *daryakan* (Dungkar, p. 2616). *G.ya'i ma* is also identified as Chrysoplenium carnosum Hook (Pas, p. 234) and as Pyrola incarnate (Clarke, p. 157) Although there are twenty-five types of *daryakan,* this is not among them. *G.ya'* usually means dust, rust, or any type of accretion that gradually appears on a surface, In some accounts of the origin of this panacea, it refers to the mossy growth on rocks.

391 Described in the actual *Ambrosia Vase* text (p. 548) as "the rider of a fierce infectious disease on the fire stallion of bile driven by the spurs of the wind humor, surrounded by the army of phlegm."

392 *Kśaya;* "end" or "destruction." Refers to the incurable stage of a bile disease.

393 The *Ambrosia Vase* itself states that the text was hidden in the heart of "Eclipsing the Arrogant," identified previously as Hayagrīva, from whom the treasure was recovered. There is an annotation to the *Ambrosia Vase* noting that "Eclipsing the Arrogant" refers to the *upāsaka* general *Yangleber (yang le ber).* He is a convert to the Buddhist pantheon, previously existing as a Tibetan mountain deity. He is foremost in the retinue of Vaiśravaṇa, one of the four guardian kings. Red in color, he rides a wild horse.

394 *Mkhar chen bza',* also known as Yeshé Tsokgyal, the consort of Padmasambhava.

395 *Mde'u;* can also mean "pebble" or "slingshot." These days the term means "bullet," so presumably the medicine acted like a bullet to penetrate to the cause of the illness.

396 *Rgya nad;* the term *rgya* can be an abbreviation of *rgya gar* (India) or *rgya nag* (China).

397 *Bdag mo;* presumably the female personification of the illness or "owner" of the illness.
398 *Chung gsum bskyed;* the *Ambrosia Vase* describes these as three medicinal substances and mantras given to newborn infants before their first food.
399 The last two of the six are missing in the text, and have been added from the *Ambrosia Vase* itself.
400 This chapter is omitted in the text and has been added from *Ambrosia Vase* itself.
401 The meaning of these is difficult to decipher as Desi is either picking out lines from the text or copying someone else who has done just that. This and so much of this section is really a list of verbatim notes. The source text, being an enigmatic treasure, is often not revealing either.
402 Only eleven are listed. The author is copying because the *Ambrosia Vase* also speaks of thirteen scrolls but lists them at the end, and it might be that the dedication and summary make up the last two scrolls.
403 *Spyang ki;* can mean wolf also, but presumably refers to medicines, behavior, and food that "cleans up." The text itself seems to bear this out.
404 The *Ambrosia Vase* recounts the origin of this substance. The beautiful sons of Brahmā and Prajpāti were playing by a lake in the Himalayas when they were spotted by some maidens from the eight castes of nāgas. Overcome by desire they joined with each other on a rock. The red and white seeds were spilt; the white seed fell on the rock, the red fell between the rock. A resinous substance formed on the rock. It was known as *chongshi* ambrosia (calcite) or resinous *daryakan.* It is a panacea that has the power to cure all 404 diseases.
405 *Sdig ru can.* In *Lives of the Treasure Finders* from Jamgön Kongtrül's *Great Store of Treasures* (vol. *ka,* p. 42), this famous place for the recovering of treasures is said to resemble an entanglement of scorpions *(sdig ru 'dzings).*
406 In Lhodrak.
407 By Ngawang Losang Gyatso, the Fifth Dalai Lama.
408 Text has *tshan* (division) but should be read as *mtshan* (name) according to Prof. Losang Tenzin.
409 Although *dri chen* can mean excrement as well as referring to the medicinal plant asafoetida *(shing kun),* Prof. Losang Tenzin says that here it means excrement.
410 This appears to be the name of a single person from Kashmir who practiced the Bön religion but could possibly refer to a whole community.
411 Demons who take the form of birds and threaten the lives of children.
412 Possibly Tai Tsu (927–76), Chinese emperor, military leader, and founder of the Sung dynasty. However, this rendering of the line is taken from the *Lotus Chronicles,* where it reads, *ta'i tus brtsigs pa'i rtsigs pa stugs pa o'ng.* This is vastly different from the rendering produced in this text: *skabs su gcig las gcig nyid sdug pa yod.* Prof. Losang Tenzin suggested the former reading was more probable.
413 Probably short for Jing Gir Han (Genghis Khan), although he is usually credited as being born in the twelfth century while Drapa Ngönshé is said to be born in the eleventh.
414 Orgyen Lingpa, *Lotus Chronicles,* 92.562.15.
415 This is the seven-story clay reliquary on the northeast side of the monastery.
416 The author comments on the identity of this figure below.
417 Khutön Tsöndrü Yungdrung (1011–75) was one of Atiśa's three main disciples

from central Tibet along with Ngok Lepai Sherap and Dromtön Rinpoché Gyalwai Jungné. He had a reputation for vanity.

418 Although *ngönshé* was explained earlier as meaning "knowing the Abhidharma," it can also mean "clairvoyance," with *ngön* meaning "clear" *(abhi)* and *shé* meaning "to know."

419 Citation untraced.

420 Written *drug dmar* but according to Dungkar (p. 1875) should be *gru dmar,* "red corners."

421 *Khal.* A measure of about thirty pounds (14 kg).

422 Untraced citation. To emanate and withdraw mandalas is the practice of emanating and withdrawing the deities and mandala assemblies from oneself, as found in the generation-stage practices of highest yoga tantra.

423 This refers to the life story of Yuthok, in which these stories are told in full: Darmo Menrampa, *Brilliant Jewel Treasury: The Sealed Manuscript Biography of the Earlier Noble Yuthok Yönten Gönpo. Rje btsun g.yu thog yon tan mgon po rnying ma'i rnam par thar pa bka' rgya ma gzi brjid rin po che'i gter mdzod* (Beijing: Mi rigs dpe skrun khang, 1982). Translated as part of *Tibetan Medicine* by Rechung Rinpoché (Delhi: Sri Satguru Publications, 2001).

424 Darmo Menrampa, *Brilliant Jewel Treasury,* p. 45.

425 Ibid., p. 47.

426 Ibid., p. 52.

427 Ibid., p. 74.

428 The present account is of the eighth-century Yuthok Yönten Gönpo. The later Yuthok, or Yuthok the younger, was born in the twelfth century, and a short biography of him follows in the next section.

429 This person's name is very close to that of Dharmaśīla, mentioned earlier as one of the nine royal physicians and also from Nepal.

430 Referred to as Candradeva in Trinlé and in Darmo Menrampa.

431 A text with the same was mentioned above as belonging to Tsenpashilaha.

432 In other words, Darmo Menrampa's *Brilliant Jewel Treasury* biography.

433 Darmo Menrampa, *Brilliant Jewel Treasury,* p. 168.

434 He did this in order to escape, because they wanted to suck his blood and chop him to pieces.

435 Jowo Śākyamuni is the main statue of Buddha in the Jokhang temple in the heart of Lhasa. It was bridal gift to King Songtsen Gampo from his Chinese bride, Wen Cheng, in the seventh century. The fivefold self-arisen statue is a statue of eleven-faced Avalokiteśvara in a chapel of the Jokhang. It contains within a self-arisen sandalwood statue of the same deity. King Songtsen Gampo and his two brides also dissolved into the main statue, hence its name.

436 Ārya Vati Sangpo, in Mangyül near Tibet's border with Nepal, is a pilgrimage site for viewing one of four statues of Avalokiteśvara constructed in Nepal from a single sandalwood tree.

437 These days the "month of miracles" refers to the first Tibetan month.

438 Darmo Menrampa, *Brilliant Jewel Treasury,* p. 256.

439 Consort of Padmasambhava.

440 Darmo Menrampa, *Biography of the Younger Yuthok Yönten Gönpo,* p. 325.

441 There are multiple instances of a text of this name. Whether they all refer to the same work I cannot say. For sure, they do not refer to the *Ratnakūṭa Sutra.*
442 Present-day Sri Lanka (Dungkar, p. 2040).
443 Sometimes identified as Sumatra.
444 Darmo Menrampa, *Biography of the Younger Yuthok Yönten Gönpo,* p. 332.
445 Ibid., p. 330.
446 *Zad par zil gyid gnon pa'i skye mched.* A group of *samādhis,* or meditative concentrations, focused on the elements, shapes, colors, and so on, in which the appearance of the object appears however one wishes and totally eclipses all other appearances.
447 Text has *zong,* but Prof. Losang Tenzin says it should be read as *zangs.*
448 *Vajrahṛdayālaṃkaratantra,* chap. 9, Toh 451 Kangyur, rgyud, *cha,* 50a7.
449 *Aparimitāyurjñāna,* Toh 675 Kangyur, rgyud, *ba,* 218b1.
450 Puṇḍarīka, *Vimalaprabhā,* Toh 845 Kangyur, rgyud, *śrī,* 16a5.
451 *Yogānuttaratantārthāvatārasaṃgraha,* Toh 3713 Tengyur, rgyud 'grel, *tsu,* 104b5.
452 Ibid., 105a7.
453 *Gshon pa.* As a verb this is the past and future of *zhon pa,* "to ride," and as a noun it refers to that which is to be ridden—say a horse or a mule.
454 *Yogānuttaratantārthāvatārasaṃgraha,* Toh 3713 Tengyur, rgyud 'grel, *tsu,* 106a4.
455 Orgyen Lingpa, *Lotus Chronicles,* 27.179.6.
456 Collected Tantras of the Nyingma, vol. 10, no. 153. Unable to locate citation within this text.
457 Longchenpa, *Treasury of the Supreme Vehicle,* 38b5.
458 *Gegs,* although other editions have *gags. The Nyingma School of Tibetan Buddhism,* p. 333, has *'gags,* translated as "conclusion."
459 Untraced.
460 *Mañjuśīnāmasaṃgīṭīkāvimalaprabhā,* Toh 1398 Tengyur, rgyud 'grel, *pha,* 225b3.
461 Collected Works, *ba,* 2b5.
462 *Subahuparipṛcchā,* chap. 1, Toh 805 Kangyur, rgyud, *wa,* 118b2.
463 Collected Works, *ga,* 12b2.
464 Collected Works, *kha,* 8a2.
465 Khedrup Jé, Collected Works, *nya,* 13b4
466 Bodong Choklé Namgyal (1326/76–1451).
467 Untraced in the works of Bodong Choklé Namgyal.
468 *Ratnolkānāmadhāraṇī,* Toh 145 Kangyur, gzungs 'dus, *pa,* 60b3.
469 Collected Works, vol. 1, 785.13.
470 Untraced in the text.
471 Untraced.
472 *Vajrajñānasamuccaya,* Toh 447 Kangyur, rgyud, *ca,* 284b7.
473 *Vajravārahī Tantra,* chap. 7, Toh 378 Kangyur, *ga,* 65b6.
474 *Grog mo mgo rdum;* a saying that none of the Tibetan scholars I consulted have been able to recognize.
475 Ngawang Losang Gyatso, Collected Works, *nga,* 195a2.
476 Jñānaśrī, *Eliminating the Two Extremes in Vajrayana, Vajrayānāntadvayāpoha,* Toh 3714 Tengyur, rgyud 'grel, *tsu,* 115b2.
477 *Sekoddeśaṭīkā,* Toh 1351 Tengyur, rgyud 'grel, *na,* 222a7.
478 *Mañjuśrīnāmasaṃgītivṛtti,* chap. 1, Toh 1396 Tengyur, rgyud 'grel, *pha,* 96b3.

479 According to some the Kālacakra was taught in the Buddha's last year and therefore all tantras were also.

480 Toh 372 Kangyur, rgyud, *kha,* 264a4.

481 Cited in Lodrö Gyalpo's *General Compendium,* 117.16.

482 Toh 373 Kangyur, rgyud, *kha,* 291a3.

483 *Buddhakapālatantra,* chap. 1, Toh 424 Kangyur, rgyud, *nga,* 143a6.

484 *Vajrahṛdayālaṃkaratantra,* chap. 11, Toh 451 Kangyur, rgyud, *cha,* 51b1.

485 Ibid., 51a6.

486 These verses teach the lineages and tantras of action tantra. The line-break divisions between the verses indicate the sections on the three main lineages—tathāgata, vajra, and lotus—and the two worldly lineages, as explained in the three Indian commentaries on this tantra. There are various readings across the different editions of the tantra and its commentaries. The lineages and tantras are set out in more detail in Khedrup Jé's *General Presentation of the Tantras* and in Tsongkhapa's *Stages of Mantra,* the latter translated by Jeffrey Hopkins in *Deity Yoga* (Ithaca, NY: Snow Lion Publications, 1981).

487 According to *Notes Explaining the Text of the Questions of Subāhu Tantra* (Toh 2672), these numbers refer to the verse count.

488 *Gsang ba pa.* The "secret ones." This is the reading of the Degé Kangyur and the three Indian commentaries to the *Questions of Subāhu Tantra* in the Tengyur. The second Indian commentary *(Notes Explaining the Text of the Questions of Subāhu Tantra)* explains this as "taming the *yakṣa* and others." However, the Dharamsala and Lhasa editions of *Beryl Mirror* have *gsung ba po* ("speakers").

489 *Phyag drug pa.* This is the reading from Degé Kangyur. The Lhasa and Dharamsala editions have *bcu drug pa* (sixteen). This line is omitted from the commentaries.

490 Identified in *Notes Explaining the Text of the Questions of Subāhu Tantra* as Hari, wife of Pañcaka.

491 *Notes Explaining the Text of the Questions of Subāhu Tantra* identifies Pūrṇa as Vaiśravaṇa.

492 *Bstan bcos, śāstra.*

493 Vasubandhu, *Abhidharmakośa,* 1:25–26, Toh 4089 Tengyur, mngon pa, *ku,* 3a1.

494 Although this phrase is not reproduced in the text, I have included it here as it is found in the commentary to show that the commentary is quoting from another work entitled *Entering Gnosis.*

495 *Lhan cig,* "together." The quote as cited in Gendün Drup's commentary to the *Abhidharmakośa (Dam pa'i chos mngon pa'i mdzod kyi rnam par bshad pa thar lam gsal byed)* has *lhag cig,* meaning "more than," and is a source for asserting the existence of more than eighty thousand collections.

496 Degé has "this collection of Dharma" *(chos kyi phung po 'di),* but I have gone with the reading from the text *(chos kyi phung po'i mdo 'di).* According to Abhidharma tradition, this sutra was compiled by Śāriputra.

497 Yaśomitra, *Abhidharmakośaṭīkā,* chap. 1, Toh 4092 Tengyur, mngon pa, *gu,* 47b5.

498 The Sanskrit *cakra* ("wheel") has many meanings, one of which is "gathering," or "assembly."

499 *Abhisamayālaṃkārаṭīkāprasphuṭapadā,* Toh 3796 Tengyur, sher phyin, *nya,* 19a7.

500 Toh 353 Kangyur, mdo sde, *ah,* 167a6.
501 *Mahāmeghasūtra,* Toh 232 Kangyur, mdo sde, *wa,* 172a3.
502 *Śūraṅgamasamādhisūtra,* Toh 132 Kangyur, mdo sde, *da,* 300a3.
503 The *Avataṃsaka* has its own system of numbering, and "an indescribable-beyond-indescribable number" is an actual number somewhere near ten to the power of 136. However, see Cleary, vol. 2, p. 201.
504 *Avataṃsakasūtra,* chap. 4, Toh 44 Kangyur, phel chen, *ga,* 32b3.
505 Untraced.
506 *Grog ga, kṛtti.*
507 The citations giving the meanings of the verbal roots are from the *Sutra of Roots (Dhātusūtra)* by Pūrṇacandra. The grammatical rules, or *sūtras,* are from the *Sarasvati Grammar Sutra* by Anubhūti. I have added explanations of the rules in parentheses. They are from the commentary on this sutra by Troru Tsenam.
508 This refers to *bka'* (words) or to *chos* (Dharma), both in their sense of being the words of the Buddha.
509 *Yogacaryābhūmiviniścayasaṃgraha,* Toh 4038 Tengyur, sems tsam, 187a2.
510 Ibid., 187a4.
511 *Vyākhyāyukti,* Toh 4062 Tengyur, sems tsam, *shi,* 36a4.
512 Vasubandhu mentions entourages of queens and young friends.
513 It is not clear what four dharmas Vasubandhu is referring to here. There is no further glossing of this term within Vasubandhu's text, although he does refer to them as "the four dharmas of the monks." He also quotes another explanation of *certainty:* "Monks, killing is not Dharma; restraining from killing is Dharma." (36b)
514 Untraced.
515 Vasubandhu, *Abhidharmakośa,* 8:39, Toh 4089, Tengyur, mngon pa, *ku,* 25a3.
516 Maitreya, *Mahāyānasūtralaṃkāra,* 12:1, Toh 4020, Tengyur, sems tsam, *phi,* 13a5.
517 *Vajrayānāntadvayāpoha,* Toh 3714 Tengyur, rgyud 'grel, *tsu,* 115b2. The question part of this citation does not appear in the Degé edition.
518 Normally one would expect the reverse—nonabiding ascertained by ultimate perception and that taught as valid ascertained by conventional perception—but a case can also be made for this pairing.
519 Nāgārjuna, *Fundamental Stanzas on the Middle Way (Mūlamadhyamakakārikā),* 24:8, Toh 3824 Tengyur, dbu ma, *tsa,* 14b7. This citation was so well known in monastic Tibet that the title and author did not need to be mentioned.
520 *Aṣṭasāhasrikāprajñāpāramitāpañjikāsārottamā,* Toh 3803 Tengyur, sher phyin, *tha,* 2a2. These have been translated according to Śāntipa's own explanation in the same work.
521 *Bdag rkyen.* Refers to a cause that determines the nature of the effect even though it may not actually be its substantial cause. The eye is said to be the determining cause of visual consciousness even though it is form and not in the nature of consciousness. Likewise there are instances of Buddha's speech, such as blessed speech, in which the teachings are not delivered directly from the person of the Buddha but are determined by him.
522 *Uttaratantra,* Toh 4024 Tengyur, sems rtsam, *phi,* 19b5.
523 A meter of four lines and eleven syllables per line.

524 *Kṛt* suffixes are primary suffixes added to roots to form nouns or nominal stems *(ming, nāman)*. "*Ti, si,* and so forth" refers to conjugational and case endings added to roots and nouns to create "word forms" *(tshig, pada)*. As the *Sarasvatī Sutra* says, "With no case ending, a noun; with case ending, a word form."

525 Quotes that describe the meaning of the root or stem are from the *Root Sutra*. All other citations of rules are from the *Sarasvatī Sutra*.

526 This paragraph has been inserted by author as a gloss on the previous paragraph.

527 Vasubandhu, *Science of Explanation (Vyākhyāyukti)*, Toh 4061 Tengyur, sems tsam, *shi*, 123a2.

528 *Mi ldan pa'i 'du byed.*

529 *Pañcaskandhavivaraṇa*, Toh 4067 Tengyur, sems tsam, *si*, 2b1.

530 *Yogacaryābhūmiviniścayasaṃgraha*, Toh 4038 Tengyur, sems tsam, *zhi*, 196b4.

531 The eight investigations are those on: oceans, water, and land; jewels and precious stones; clothing; mountains and trees; men; women; horses; and elephants (Dungkar, p. 1018).

532 The discipline or Vinaya teachings of the Buddha are in four categories: *Basic Vinaya (Vinayavastu, 'Dul ba gzhi), Detailed Vinaya (Vinayavibhaṅga, 'Dul ba rnam par 'byed pa), Later Works (Vinayauttaragrantha, 'Dul ba gzhung bla ma),* and *Short Vinaya (Vinayakṣudrakavastu, 'Dul ba phran tshegs)*. Together they comprise the first seven volumes of the Kangyur.

533 The eight topics and chapters of *Ornament of Realization*.

534 *Commentary to the Collected Verses on Precious Qualities of the Bhagavān* by Haribhadra and *Commentary on the Collected Verses* by Buddhaśrījñāna.

535 Probably a synthesis of the *Abridged Perfection of Wisdom in Verse (Prajñāpāramitāsañcayagāthā)*.

536 *Susaṃskṛta (legs par sbyar ba):* well joined, well connected; a sacred composition.

537 *Tshad ma;* often rendered as "valid cognition" but refers generally to a state of validity.

538 *Yogacaryābhūmiviniścayasaṃgraha*, Toh 4038 Tengyur, sems tsam, *zhi*, 197b2.

539 Ibid., 197b4.

540 *Mirror of Poetics*, chap. 1, Toh 4301 Tengyur, sgra mdo, *se*, 322a1.

541 *Padārtha-candrikā-prabhāsa-nāma-aṣṭāṅga-hṛdaya-vivṛti*, Toh 4312 Tengyur, gso ba rig pa, *ko*, 1a4. Degé has some differences in the wording.

542 Ibid., 1a3. Degé has some differences in the wording.

543 As noted in the introduction, one of the pieces of evidence put forward by those who maintain *Four Tantras* is not the word of Buddha is the mention of white china or porcelain tea bowls, which they say were not found in India during the time of the Buddha.

544 Untraced.

545 Untraced.

546 One of Yuthok's main disciples.

547 Ngawang Losang Gyatso, *Wish-Fulfilling Tree: List of Practices from the Yuthok Heartdrop*, Collected Works, *nga*, 1a2.

548 Traced to the two-page table of contents at the beginning of Sumtön Yeshé Sung's *Sunlight of Compassion Clearing the Darkness of Suffering*, 2a4.

549 The following paragraphs, beginning with this line, describe the main sections of Yuthok's renowned *Heartdrop Collection*.

550 One *dré (bre)* is one twentieth of a *khel (khal)* or load; one *phül (phul)* is one sixth of a *dré*.
551 Probably Gampopa Sönam Rinchen (1079–1153), the well-known early master of the Kagyü school.
552 Darmo Menrampa, *Biography of the Younger Yuthok Yönten Gönpo,* p. 329.
553 Ibid.
554 Ibid. (1982 ed.), p. 344.
555 Probably referring to seven royal manifestations of Avalokiteśvara. The Fifth Dalai Lama was said to be an incarnation of King Trisong Detsen, who was held to be a manifestation of Avalokiteśvara.
556 Found in *History of the Heartdrop: Hook of Virtue,* 4b2.
557 Jñānadhara is the Sanskrit rendering of Yeshé Sung.
558 Twelve years, the time it takes to complete the cycle of twelve animals in the calendar.
559 The twenty-eighth year of a sixty-year cycle; possibly 1174.
560 As mentioned in the introduction, the sages Vidyājñāna and Manasija were emanations of Medicine Buddha that acted as teacher and requestor of *Four Tantras.*
561 Untraced.
562 Here he is playing with names. Tsojé Shönu was Kumāra Jivaka, the celebrated physician at the time of the Buddha and next in the *Four Tantras* lineage after Manasija.
563 Untraced.
564 According to Trinlé (p. 116) the dates of this ruler in the line of the kings of the past are not known but he was said to have established a great Dharma celebration in Ngari in 1076. This would have put him prior to Yönten Gönpo.
565 Kampoché: possibly Kampuchea. According to Gö Lotsāwa's *Blue Annals* (p. 390), Avadhūtipa lived in East Bengal, Atiśa's native region, though Atiśa is well known for having traveled widely.
566 *'Gro lding;* said to be another name for Oḍḍiyāna.
567 *Dbyug bcos:* medical investigation using a small stick to tap the site of illness, pioneered by Phadampa Sangyé and others.
568 Other editions have Drangti Drakpa Bum, Drangti Jotsün.
569 Karma Pakshi (1204–83) was the Second Karmapa.
570 *Rgya tsho;* smallest unit of administration in Tibet; a subdivision of a *dzong.*
571 Son of Yuthok Jampal (Trinlé, p. 168).
572 According to Trinlé (p. 168), this refers to the Sakya family lineage.
573 Possibly Chejé Śākya Pal and Minyak Dorjé Bum, who appear to be contemporary physicians.
574 *Four Tantras* in the later versions is categorized into four compilations *(mdo),* eleven main sections *(gnas),* and fifteen divisions *(skabs).*
575 According to Trinlé (p. 171) and to the *Sa skya sman grong pa'i man ngag dngul bre ma,* the Drangti lineage eventually became the *khu dbon bla sman* tradition, popularly known as the Sakya Mendrong medical tradition.
576 The works commencing from *Revealing Mirror Commentary* by Mara Gomchen is listed in Surkhar Lodrö Gyalpo's *General Compendium* and are grouped there under those works that rely mainly on *Eight Branches* as opposed to *Four Tantras.*

577 Above this work was stated as being translated by Jñānamitra, as the colophon of the Degé edition confirms.

578 Text with identical name attributed to Biji Leklo above.

579 *Me chu go ldog,* literally "Fire and water reverse," in which the pulse of a close relative of the patient is taken when the patient himself is inaccessible.

580 The list is only 55 lines, compared to the declared 56 traditions, but one line may include two traditions. The source text is untraced.

581 *Pur rgyal* or *spur rgyal,* "the kingdom of Pur," the old name for Tibet.

582 The physicians listed in the previous chapter span up to the thirteenth century. This section deals with the end of the fourteenth century onward.

583 Tibetan and Western sources agree that this dynasty was founded in 1038 by the Tangut (Tib. *tang zhang chang*) tribe and took the Chinese dynastic name Hsi Hsia. This was corrupted in Tibetan to *shis zha,* and then to *si hu* and *se'u.* (*Great Tibetan-Chinese Dictionary,* p. 2069). Minyak is now in Kansu province, in the Yellow River northern loop, and was previously known as Ning-hsia (Tib. *nying zha*). According to Fairbank and Reischauer, the Tanguts were actually Tibetans (p. 124).

584 The Sechen emperor was the Mongolian Kublai Khan, the grandson of Genghis Khan (1215–94). Western and Tibetan sources are in general agreement on his dates: he came to the throne in 1260, moved his empire from Karakorum to Beijing in 1264, and became the first ruler of the Mongolian Yuan dynasty in 1271.

585 The wood-pig year of the seventh cycle is 1395, and Dungkar explicitly states this year. However, if Jangpa were born in 1395, he would have been born a hundred years after his father's benefactor, Kublai Khan, died in 1294. Trinlé says that Jangpa was born in 1295, which would fit but does not correspond to the wood-pig year of the seventh cycle.

586 *Yongs 'dzin,* one who "protects completely" from the extremes of samsara and nirvana.

587 Vanaratna is said to be the last of the great Indian pandits to visit Tibet—in 1426. See *Tibet Chronology,* compiled by Dan Martin at www.thdl.org.

588 The "high-lineage Dharma king" is Jangpa, who chronologically could have received these awards from a Ming emperor because the Ming dynasty did not begin until 1368, and Jangpa was born in 1395. Kunga Tashi Gyaltsen Palsang was born in 1349 and visited the emperor in 1413. By calling him a high-lineage *(kalkī)* Dharma king, the author is indicating that Jangpa is an incarnation of King Sucandra.

589 King Sucandra was the king of Shambhala who first received the Kālacakra tantra from the Buddha in India.

590 1475.

591 Thus emulating the passing of King Sucandra of Shambhala, of whom he was an emanation.

592 Untraced.

593 These are kings Songtsen Gampo, Trisong Detsen, and Tritsuk Detsen, or Ralpachen.

594 *Mtha' drug tshul bzhi.* These are modes of interpretation of enigmatic tantras. One interpretation of these concepts is found in Dudjom Rinpoche's *Nyingma School of Tibetan Buddhism,* pp. 290–92.

595 *Bu ram shing,* "sugar cane." *Ikṣvāku,* one belonging to the sugar-cane lineage—the ancestral race of the Buddha.

596 Tib., *kun da.* Here probably refers to the white lotus flower that blossoms at night; sometimes refers to the *kumuda* flower.

597 *Sgrib shing.* Literally, "hindrance stick," the wearer of which cannot be harmed by spirits.

598 *Drang srong* in Tibetan; has the etymology of being upright—without pretension *(drang)* and honest *(srong).*

599 *Dge gnyen;* literally, "moving closer to virtue." Lay practitioner who has the basis of the five basic vows of liberation.

600 *Rigs ldan,* "holder of the lineage." Some say that, strictly speaking, the first seven rulers of Shambhala, of which Sucandra was the first, are not referred to as *kalkī* but as Dharma kings. The *kalkī* lineage actually begins with Mañjuśrī Yaśas, who began the vajra lineage by initiating the non-Buddhist rishis.

601 *Byang rong.* Either two districts or two families. May refer to the clashes between the Latö Jang rulers in southern Tsang and the Rinpungpas in central Tibet.

602 *Ta (ta'i) dben* (Ch. *da yuan*), general name given to the Mongol or Yuan dynasty that began in the thirteenth century. Tibetan masters who served as spiritual preceptors to Mongolian rulers were known as *ta'i dben ti shri.*

603 Künga Tashi Gyaltsen Palsang, who was born in 1349 and visited the Chinese emperor in 1413.

604 Probably a form of Padmasambhava.

605 According to Trinlé (p. 267) this was in 1453.

606 *Thang stong rgyal po.* This famous yogi lived for 125 years. According to Dungkar his dates are 1361–1485. According to the *Great Tibetan-Chinese Dictionary,* 1385–1509. Others give the dates 1385–1464. For more on this figure, see Cyrus Stearns' *King of the Empty Plain: The Tibetan Iron-Bridge Builder Tangtong Gyalpo* (Ithaca, NY: Snow Lion Publications, 2006).

607 *G.yas ru byang pa/bdag.* Literally, the "northern lord of Yeru."

608 A technique of reading the pulse as a means of divination. See Drungtso, p. 264.

609 Better known as Tāranātha (1575–1634).

610 This line has been translated according to Trinlé (p. 271).

611 Sakya Paṇḍita, Collected Works, *tha,* 1b6.

612 A cuckoo does not naturally kill, but one reared in a hawk's nest will copy the behavior of the hawk.

613 Text has "not passed," but that makes little sense because none of the other lineages came through Biji.

614 In the section on the Drangti lineage it states that the father of Drangti Jampal Sangpo was Drangti Sönam Büm and that the latter only met Yuthok Jampal later as a teacher. Therefore, the term "son lineage" means only that it began with the sons of Yuthok and not that each successive transmission has to be passed down from father to son.

615 *Lus 'dar,* "body shakes." Some editions have *lus 'dir,* "in this body," which also makes sense.

616 Orgyen Lingpa, *Lotus Chronicles,* 24.167.1.

617 The *Crystal Rock Lotus Chronicles,* another name for the *Lotus Chronicles,* is an account of the life of Padmasambhava, and this particular verse tells of Padma-

sambhava's acquisition of medical knowledge. Desi's comment here is a reference to the Treasure lineage listed above, which explicitly states that Padmasambhava received the transmission from Kumāra Jivaka himself and not his son. The sixth grammatical case corresponds approximately to the genitive.

618 Untraced.

619 The dates of Surkhar Nyamnyi Dorjé are commonly agreed to be 1439–75.

620 *Guṇa* (Tib. *yon tan*), the Sanskrit rendering of Yuthok's name.

621 Untraced.

622 *E rong*, a Nyingma hermitage seventy-five miles southeast of Lhasa.

623 Found in *Yuthok Heartdrop*, but a work of a similar name was composed by Yeshé Sung.

624 Translation of the following list has been assisted by Prof. Losang Tenzin and by comparison with the *Relic of Millions* edition found in the Smanrstis shesrig spendzod collection, vol. 58 (Leh: Tashigangpa, 1974), which varies considerably from the edition used by the author. There are many corruptions and variations in spelling. More research needs to be done on verification.

625 These are seven types of medicinal plants. See glossary.

626 *Byang wa*. Other editions have *bde ba*.

627 This idiom indicates a medicine so expensive, a pill the size of a louse would cost the price of a horse, a pill the size of a louse egg would cost the price of a sheep.

628 The substance that carries the medicine in the body.

629 Trinlé (p. 210) identifies these six places as being in present-day Lhokha, in southern Tibet.

630 Kyempa Tsewang is elsewhere in the text called Lata Tsewang. According to Trinlé (p. 212), he was born in 1479.

631 *Mdun na 'don*. A phrase that in earlier translations referred to brahman priests *(purohita)* who recited scriptures to the king (Dungkar, p. 1136).

632 According to Dungkar (p. 1485) Jarpo Panchen's dates are 1447–1506.

633 *Sman sgom*, "physician and meditator," indicating that he, like so many doctors of those times, was also a great practitioner.

634 The Seventh Karmapa (1454–1506).

635 This center is said by Trinlé (p. 216) to be the Lekshé Ling Dharma center in Tsurphu Monastery.

636 "Jarpo" because he was from the region of Ja, and "Panchen" *(paṇḍita)* because of his great learning (Trinlé, p. 217).

637 *Zhwa dmar ba;* presumably the Fourth Shamarpa, Chödrak Yeshé (1453–1524).

638 Son of Minyima of the Jang lineage.

639 This must refer to the basis of medical science, the practices, and the beneficial results of treatment.

640 As the author makes clear below, this refers to Rinpung Jikten Drakpa *('Jig rten grags pa)*, which must be a variant spelling of Rinpung Ngawang Jikmé Drakpa *(Rin spungs Ngag dbang 'jigs med grags pa)* born 1482 or 1542, the son of Rinpung ruler Ngawang Namgyal.

641 *Dra thang*. Also known as Dranang *(dra nang)*, Drathang Monastery is in Lhoka (Trinlé, p. 220).

642 *Yar rgyab*. An official, but I am unable to say more.

643 I cannot place the crow reference.

644 A disciple of Dharmaswami Surkhar Nyamnyi Dorjé.

645 *Treasury of Wise Sayings,* Collected Works, *tha,* 9a2, Collected Works of the Sakya, vol. 5, 108a2.

646 A helmet that should protect the wearer from outside dangers has itself been broken from the inside, because Lodrö Gyalpo has himself gone against his own tradition. This criticism is of the previously listed text and probably a work by Lodrö Gyalpo called *Lamp Dispelling Darkness: Presentation of Four Tantras Being the Word of the Buddha and Treatise,* in which Lodrö Gyalpo presents these three views of *Four Tantras.* His own position is somewhat ambiguous. In his work on the history of medicine, *General Compendium* (p. 312), after listing the many positions of others, he says he cannot say whether *Four Tantras* is the word of Buddha or a later treatise, and that declaring the word of Buddha as not being so is just as bad as declaring something not the word of the Buddha to be so. He also says that spending so much time arguing over this matter is pointless, and that we should be able to infer its origins in the same way we infer fire from smoke and the presence of water from ducks. Kachuwa Chölotar (p. 26) states that although Lodrö Gyalpo presents all three positions, we can clearly infer that he believes *Four Tantras* to be the work of Yuthok Yönten Gönpo. This whole section is actually a continuation of listing the works of Lodrö Gyalpo begun previously. However, Sangyé Gyatso does not even mention *Lamp Dispelling Darkness* by name but is possibly referring to it as "that one" in the next paragraph.

647 *Four Tantras,* Final Tantra, 27.665.17.

648 This is the text cited as *General Compendium* in earlier notes.

649 Very loud and impressive but essentially empty because no one has ever seen a dragon (Prof. Losang Tenzin).

650 This is Lodrö Gyalpo's own verse, which he used to mock the Rinpung ruler who refused to sponsor his publication of *Four Tantras.*

651 The Fourth Dalai Lama (1589–1616).

652 Of the four tantras in *Four Tantras,* the Root, Explanatory, and Final Tantras are the three shorter tantras. The Instruction Tantra is the longest.

653 Ngawang Losang Gyatso, *Stream of the Ganges.*

654 According to Trinlé (p. 285) this medical school, also known as Sharchen Chok, was situated in the Potala.

655 *Bi ma la,* although other editions have *rje mi la* (Lord Milarepa).

656 In this paragraph, there is no pronoun "I" at all and no unambiguous indication that the agent was Desi Sangyé Gyatso. Even Prof. Losang Tenzin had doubts about this.

657 *Gong sman,* literally, "doctor of high position."

658 Title given to the Mongolian chieftain Gusri Khan by the Fifth Dalai Lama.

659 The school was Drangsong Düpai Ling ("Place of the Assembled Rishis") in Shigatsé (Trinlé, p. 257).

660 There is no explicit subject to this verb, and it is not clear if it refers to Tseten Dorjé because it is in high honorific *(chibs bsgyur).* It is tempting, therefore, to think that the subject is the Fifth Dalai Lama.

661 Sodokpa Lodrö Gyaltsen (1552–1624).

662 *Mañjuśrīmūlakalpa,* Toh 543 Kangyur, rgyud, *na,* 325a7.

663 Ibid. There are many such cryptic predictions in the *Mañjuśrī Root Tantra.* Ac-

cording to Prof. Losang Tenzin, "the letter *ma*" refers to *mati (blo)* meaning "mind," part of the Great Fifth's name, Losang. He "loved the Dharma," meaning he devoted himself to Buddhist practice at the beginning and end of his life, whereas in between he ruled the country.

664 The Great Fifth was born on the twenty-third day of the ninth month of the fire-snake year, or 1617 (Trinlé, p. 290).

665 From the Prophecy chapter of the *Book of Kadam,* one of three supplementary chapters to the Father Teachings that may be a later addition. Not included in the Institute of Tibetan Classics edition.

666 *Book of Kadam: Son Teachings,* 167.19.

667 Orgyen Lingpa, *Five Chronicles,* untraced.

668 Another name for King Trisong Detsen.

669 Untraced.

670 Tsang can be said to be southwestern Tibet, in the vicinity of Shigatsé, and the "center" in this line is the area around Lhasa.

671 A famous temple in the Yarlung valley built by King Songtsen Gampo as one of four temples built at certain Tibetan locales that correspond to the shoulders and hips of a demoness.

672 Untraced.

673 Founded in 1643 (Trinlé, p. 296).

674 More commonly known as Shigatsé.

675 *Four Tantras,* Final Tantra, 11.621.13.

676 According to Prof. Losang Tenzin, rather than procure rare gems for use in medicine they instead used the water in which these gems had been soaked. In order to obtain some medicinal part of the body, such as bile, one or more young girls born in the tiger year were killed.

677 "Godara Rañcara" is as transliterated.

678 Of these five works, all but the fourth are in the Degé Tengyur as written. The third however is attributed to Sarvahitāmṛta Datta, and the fourth may well be Toh 4442, *Advice from the Royal Āyurvedic Practitioner Ragunātha from Mathurā,* which has become confused with the third.

679 Mermo Lodrö Chöpel and Larawa Losang Dönden were disciples of Darmo Menrampa.

680 According to Trinlé this work is on the Instruction Tantra of *Four Tantras.*

681 Darmo Menrampa, *Biography of Yuthok the Elder and the Younger.* According to Trinlé (p. 294), Mermopa was also involved in this work, and according to the colophon of the Yuthok biography, it was compiled by their teacher Darmo Menrampa, with these disciples as scribes.

682 Orgyen Lingpa, *Five Chronicles,* chapter on "Predictions at the End of Time," 213.13.

683 Tsangpa Lhayi Metok was King Trisong Detsen, of whom the Great Fifth was an incarnation. His third or fourth son was Mutik Tsenpo.

684 Ngok Lotsāwa Lekpai Sherap (1018–1115), the renowned disciple of Atiśa. His Ngok ancestry is traced to a minister of King Trisong Detsen, which provides the connection to the passage above. Desi Sangyé Gyatso describes Ngok Lotsāwa as an incarnation of Prince Mutik Tsenpo in his *Yellow Beryl* as well.

685 *Samādhirājasūtra,* chap. 14, Toh 127 Kangyur, mdo sde, *da,* 47a2.

686 Orgyen Lingpa, *Five Chronicles*, 209.23.

687 *Kun bzang 'khor lo.* According to TBRC (code T1418) this is "a poetic adornment described in the third chapter of the *Kāvyādarśa* of Daṇḍin comprising wheels of words in which the syllables read in any direction have a meaning."

688 *Spor thang.* A system of divination originating in China based on applying six elements to the sixty-year cycle to give 360 possibilities.

689 This idiom is explained by Desi Sangyé Gyatso himself in his *Yellow Beryl* as "having the capability of founding a new tradition," and he says in the same text that his name "Sangyé" (buddha) will become an actuality.

690 Untraced.

691 Sangyé Gyatso was born in the water-snake year of 1653.

692 According to Prof. Losang Tenzin, Desi Sangyé Gyatso apparently suffered from a serious stammer.

693 Monastery generally said to be founded by the Great Fifth in 1651 primarily for rituals to protect the state. According to Dungkar (p. 1231), however, it dates back to the time of the Third Dalai Lama and was founded when he was invited to Mongolia in 1579.

694 Dorjé Drakpa Ewaṃ Chokgar was founded in 1632, and Mindroling was founded by Terdak Lingpa, teacher of the Great Fifth, in 1676. Together, they were the two main Nyingma monasteries in Central Tibet.

695 Great Offering Ceremony was set up by Desi in 1694 (Dungkar, p. 1716), twelve years after the Fifth Dalai Lama passed away and when details of his death were no longer secret. The teachings mentioned all emphasize the point that a being may be an enlightened being but in the eyes of the world still has to undergo the trials and tribulations of ordinary life. This is a reference to the fact that although the Fifth Dalai Lama is already an enlightened being, he nevertheless passed away, and offerings, such as this great ceremony, are needed to ensure that he returns. Therefore, the "aspirations" refer to the wishes of the Fifth to return, but he can only do so if the merit of his people is ripe. The titles are untraced but according to Prof. Losang Tenzin may have been written by Desi himself.

696 According to Prof. Losang Tenzin, these days this document is to be found in the Potala.

697 "Lhaksam" *(lhag bsam)* connotes an uncommonly caring attitude toward others.

698 The requirements for becoming a doctor; these are explained below.

699 Untraced.

700 Each of the four tantras in the Drathang edition had a colophon composed by the Fifth Dalai Lama that praised the work fulsomely.

701 Untraced.

702 See under Tsenpashilaha.

703 *Phyag dreg ma,* literally, "hand-stained." In other words, the handwritten copy of *Four Tantras* was stained by so much thumbing of the pages.

704 Probably *Practices of the Science of Medicine: Fulfilling All Needs and Wishes (Gso dpyad kyi lag len dgos 'dod kun 'byung)* by Dütsi Gyurmé.

705 Seventy-seven of the seventy-nine paintings are in included as color plates in *Tibetan Medical Paintings* (London: Serindia Publications, 1992). That volume does not include paintings 6 and 7 below.

706 The five perfections: perfect teacher, Dharma, entourage, time, and place.

707 *Ldog rgyu;* I have gone with Clark in the translation of this term, although "side effects" is a possibility.

708 Described in the painting notes from *Blue Beryl* as being "like the life force" *(bla).*

709 "Water" or "white" channels are usually nerves and tendons. Red channels are blood vessels.

710 The first chapter of the Final Tantra is on pulse diagnosis and has thirteen topics. The five elements here are earth, fire, water, wood, and metal.

711 The eighth topic from this chapter of the Final Tantra deals with the "seven wonderful pulses" that are taken from healthy people and used as a form of divination.

712 Literally, *me chu go ldog,* "fire and water inversion." In the substitution pulse diagnosis, the pulse of someone close to the patient (mother, father, and so on) is examined when the doctor cannot access the patient.

713 *Bla rtsa.*

714 The Urine Analysis chapter has the following headings: (1) Prerequisites, (2) Time of examination, (3) Container, (4) How food and drink become urine, (5) Urine of a healthy person, (6) Urine of a sick person, (7) Urine indicating death, and (8) Urine indicating spirit possession.

715 The analogy rests on the idea that the milk of a lioness would crack an ordinary clay pot and be lost and must therefore be kept in a precious container. Similarly, unsuitable disciples are not able to retain the elixir of this teaching.

716 Better known as the Jokhang.

717 Old name for Lhasa.

718 Mipham Gelek Namgyal, 1618–85. The prefix Tibetan Scholar *(bod mkhas pa)* was affixed to his name like a title, a fact to which the author refers in the same sentence.

719 Jowo Rakkha: a mound of stones, originally erected as a dam, standing on an embankment of Lhasa's Kyichu River. It was an annual tradition to bring stones to this mound. What exactly is being referred to here I cannot say.

720 Also known as Chakpori or Chakri, this is the hill on which Desi Sangyé Gyatso founded the famous Chakri Medical College.

721 The Chaka mountain is actually three sided, but Sudarśana, as it appeared in Desi's vision, is four-sided (Prof. Losang Tenzin).

722 This is an expression meaning "fragile," as the moon on the third lunar day is barely visible.

723 *Abhiniṣkramaṇasūtra,* Toh 301 Kangyur, mdo sde, *sa,* 4b3. The degeneration of lifespan means that on average lifespan will shrink to about fifty years. The degeneration of mental afflictions means that anger, desire, ignorance, and so on will become more prevalent. The degeneration of living beings means that behavior, attitudes, and wealth will decline. The degeneration of views means that the number of nonbelievers in the Three Jewels, cause and effect, and past and future lives will increase. The degeneration of the times means that epidemics, famines, wars, and poor harvests will become widespread.

724 The last five hundred years of the five thousand years that the Buddha's doctrine will last.

725 *Mna' thab shan dmar byed.* Here *thab* means "fire" or "fireplace," and Surkhar Lodrö Gyalpo's *Transmission of Our Ancestors* (p. 328) renders it accordingly, but I

have gone with the Dharamsala edition of *Four Tantras,* which has *'thab,* meaning "fight."

726 *Four Tantras,* Instruction Tantra, 23.243.5.
727 *Suvarṇaprabhāsottamasūtra,* chap. 24, Toh 555 Kangyur, rgyud, *pa,* 132a4.
728 *Four Tantras,* Root Tantra, 6.14.7.
729 *Four Tantras,* Explanatory Tantra, 31.101.4.
730 Ibid., 31.101.11.
731 Untraced.
732 Pitṛceṭa, *Aṣṭāṅgahṛdayasaṃhitanāma.* Untraced.
733 Yuthok Yönten Gönpo (Later), *Yang snying bsdus pa.* Untraced.
734 Untraced.
735 These parenthetical lines are found in the Dharamsala *Four Tantras.*
736 *Four Tantras,* Instruction Tantra, 90.549.15.
737 *Four Tantras,* Root Tantra, 5.13.9.
738 *Four Tantras,* Final Tantra, 27.665.5.
739 Ibid., 27.665.8.
740 Pitṛceṭa, *Aṣṭāṅgahṛdayasaṃhitanāma,* chap. 14, Toh 4310, Tengyur, gso rig, *he,* 334a5.
741 Untraced.
742 Untraced.
743 Śāntideva, *Bodhicaryāvatāra,* 3:7, Toh 3871, Tengyur, dbu ma, *la,* 6b7.
744 Possibly Kyegu Künga Tsowa Sangpo (fifteenth century).
745 Untraced.
746 *Gaṇḍavyūhasūtra,* Toh 44 Kangyur, phal chen, *a,* 283b4.
747 *Bodhisattvapiṭaka,* Toh 56 Kangyur, dkon brtsegs, *ga,* citation untraced.
748 *Teachings of Respect for the Teacher of Dharma and for Listening to Dharma,* Toh 4172 Tengyur, spring yig, *nge,* 4a1.
749 *Nītiśāstraprajñādaṇḍa,* Toh 4329 Tengyur, lugs kyi bstan bcos, *ngo,* 112a4.
750 Indrabodhi, *Gnosis Accomplishment Sādhana (Jñānasiddhināmasādhana),* chap. 14, Toh 2219 Tengyur, rgyud 'grel, *wi,* 51a2.
751 Found in Puṇḍarīka, *Vimalaprabhā,* chap. 4, Toh 845 Kangyur, rgyud, *śrī,* 262a7. This passage is also found in Aśvaghoṣa's *Fifty Verses on the Guru (Gurupañcāśikā),* Toh 3721 Tengyur, rgyud 'grel, *tshu.*
752 Here and in the following explanations on these verses, the author is citing Jé Tsongkhpa's commentary on *Fifty Verses on the Guru,* his *Fulfilling All Hopes of the Disciples.*
753 *Māyājālamahātantrarājaṭīkā,* Toh 2513 Tengyur, rgyud 'grel, *i,* 196b7.
754 Bhavabhadra, *Vajraḍākatantravivṛtti,* Toh 1415 Tengyur, rgyud 'grel, *tsha,* 204b3.
755 *Vajrapañjaratantra,* chap. 8, Toh 419 Kangyur, rgyud, *nga,* 48b6.
756 *Vajrahṛdayālaṃkāratantra,* Toh 451, Kangyur, rgyud, *cha,* 57b7.
757 *Vajrapañjaratantra,* chap. 8, Toh 419 Kangyur, rgyud, *nga,* 48b5.
758 Also called the *Cakrasaṃvara Tantra.*
759 *Vajramālābhidhānatantra,* chap. 65, Toh 445 Kangyur, rgyud, *ca,* 271b2.
760 *Bsnyen pa.*
761 Āryadeva, *Catuḥpīṭhatantra-maṇḍalavidhisārasamuccaya,* Toh 1613, Tengyur, rgyud 'grel *ya,* 114b3.
762 Kṛṣṇacarya, *Cakrasaṃvarasādhana,* Toh 1446 Tengyur, rgyud 'grel, *wa,* 277a4.

763 Abhyākaragupta, *Vajrāvalī,* Toh 3140 Tengyur, rgyud 'grel, *phu,* 6a6.
764 Ibid., 6b3.
765 Presumably "activity" refers to the duration of the meditation retreat determined by the activity of performing a required number of mantras or remaining for a requisite length of time. "Close" may mean remaining in the retreat until signs of becoming close to the deity have appeared. According to Je Tsongkhapa in his *Stages of Mantra,* the third of these deity-yoga meditations is based upon "signs." "Tantric activities" refers to activities of pacification, control, increase, and wrathful expression.
766 *Precious Garland of Advice for the King (Ratnāvalī),* 5:92–93, Toh 4158 Tengyur, skyes rabs, *ge,* 125b4. The last two lines of this verse are a little different in Gyaltsap Jé's commentary.
767 *Twenty Verses on the Bodhisattva Vow (Bodhisattvasaṃvaraviṃśaka),* Toh 4081 Tengyur, sems tsam, *hi,* 166b2.
768 Śāntideva, *Bodhicaryāvatāra,* 5:102, Toh 3871 Tengyur, dbu ma, *la,* 14a5.
769 Candrakīrti, *Catuḥśatakavṛtti,* chap. 6, Toh 3867 Tengyur, dbu ma, *ya,* 110a6. Wording here differs slightly from the Tengyur.
770 Śākyaprabha, *Śrāmaṇeraprabhāvati,* Toh 4125 Tengyur, 'dul ba, *shu,* 155b6.
771 Maitreya, *Abhisamayālaṃkāra,* 1:37, Toh 3786 Tengyur, sher phyin, *ka,* 3a7.
772 Maitreya, *Mahāyānasūtralaṃkāra,* 18:10, Toh 4020 Tengyur, sems tsam, *phi,* 25b2.
773 Maitreya, *Mahāyānasūtralaṃkāra,* 14:8, Toh 4020 Tengyur, sems tsam, *phi,* 18a1.
774 Maitreya, *Mahāyānasūtralaṃkāra,* 13:5, Toh 4020 Tengyur, sems tsam, *phi,* 16b6.
775 Inference, experience, and convention.
776 Vasubandhu, *Vyākhyāyukti,* Toh 4061 Tengyur, sems tsam, *shi,* 63b6.
777 In this line the word for certainty *(brtan pa)* is taken from Gyaltsap Jé's commentary (p. 144). The Degé Tengyur and the root text as reproduced in Gyaltsap Jé's commentary has *brten* (reliance), while both citations as quoted in our text have *bstan* (teach).
778 Maitreya, *Mahāyānasūtralaṃkāra,* 13:12, Toh 4020 Tengyur, sems tsam, *phi,* 17a3.
779 A dirty container, a leaky container, and an inverted container. See also the discussion of the three "pots" below on p. 471.
780 *Mañjuśrīvikurvāṇaparivarta,* Toh 97 Kangyur, mdo sde, *kha,* 251b6.
781 Daṇḍin, *Mirror of Poetics (Kāvyādarśa),* chap. 1, Toh 4301 Tengyur, sgra mdo, 322a1.
782 *Vyākaraṇaliṅgāvataraṇa,* Toh 4348 Tengyur, sna tshogs, *co,* 161b2.
783 *Bhadramāyākāravyākaraṇa,* chap. 21, Toh 65 Kangyur, dkon brtsegs, *ca,* 28a1.
784 *Treatise on the Classification of the Three Vows.* Collected Works of the Sakya, vol. 5, 1b3.
785 Toh 480 Kangyur, rgyud, *nga,* 199b5.
786 As in previous glossing of Sanskrit terms, the rules quoted are from Anubhūti's *Sarasvatī Grammar Sutra* and their explanations in parentheses from the commentary by Troru Tsenam.
787 Toh 256 Kangyur, mdo sde, *za,* 74a6. This text entered the Kangyur from the Chinese.
788 *Śīlasaṃyuktasūtra,* Toh 303 Kangyur, mdo sde, *sa,* 127b2.
789 *Bhikṣupriyasūtra,* Toh 302 Kangyur, mdo sde, *sa,* 126b6.
790 *Pratimokṣasūtra,* Toh 2 Kangyur, 'dul ba, *ca,* 1a4.

791 *Vinayastotra,* Toh 4136 Tengyur, 'dul ba, *su,* 133a4.
792 Ibid., 133b2. Last line read *chos* (Dharma) instead of *khyod* (you) as in Degé.
793 *Vinayavastu,* vol. 1, Toh 1 Kangyur, 'dul ba, *ka,* 1a5.
794 As the Great Fifth, Ngawang Losang Gyatso, points out in his *Golden Victorious Myrobalan Vinaya Ceremonies* commentary (6b6), this stage also includes the purification ceremony. In this way the count of the stages comes to seventeen.
795 Collected Works, *kha,* miscellaneous, 61a5.
796 There are the three physical acts—mentioned several times below—of killing, stealing, and sexual misconduct, and the four verbal acts of lying, gossip, slander, and harsh language.
797 *Basic Vinaya (Vinayavastu),* Toh 1 Kangyur, 'dul ba, *ka,* 304b2.
798 Sutra untraced.
799 Avantaka, *nyi 'og pa;* usually asserted to be a western division of the Vaibhāṣika school.
800 The first of these refers to taking the *upāsaka* vows and the intermediate ordination of leaving the life of a householder. The second stage is the taking of the main vows.
801 Usually explained as referring to albinos.
802 These refer to sets of criteria necessarily fulfilled by the preceptors.
803 It is not clear if this sentence refers to *ceremony,* the last of the five conducive conditions. Normally, *ceremony* refers to the whole procedure consisting of preparation, actual ceremony, and conclusion. The earlier stages refer to the presence of the *upāsaka* and probationary vows.
804 The downfalls of fully ordained monks, in contrast, are grouped under five headings.
805 Although it is deemed inappropriate to make details of the vows and downfalls accessible to the general public, they can be found in the Pali translation of the *Pātimokkha Sutta* in *Sacred Books of the East,* vol. 13 (Oxford: Clarendon Press, 1881).
806 *Samādhirājasūtra,* chap. 36, Toh 127 Kangyur, mdo sde, *da,* 128b6.
807 Ibid., 128b2. Wording in Degé is a little different.
808 *Susthitamatidevaputraparipṛcchā,* chap. 22, Toh 66 Kangyur, bkon rtsegs, *ca,* 48b2.
809 *Treatise on the Classification of the Three Vows,* Collected Works, *na,* 14a6.
810 *Ornament of Mahayana Sutras (Mahāyānasūtralaṃkāra),* 18:10, Toh 4020 Tengyur, sems tsam, *phi,* 25b2.
811 *Precious Garland (Ratnāvalī),* 5:92, Toh 4158 Tengyur, skyes rabs, *ge,* 125b4. These two citations were quoted in full above.
812 Atiśa, *Light on the Path (Bodhipathapradīpa),* v. 20, Toh 3947 Tengyur, dbu ma, *khi,* 239a4.
813 Collected Works, *nya,* 71b4.
814 Ibid., 82a6.
815 Asaṅga, *Bodhisattvabhūmi,* chap. 10, Toh 4037 Tengyur, sems tsam *wi,* 73b6.
816 *Bodhisattvasaṃvaraviṃśaka,* v. 1, Toh 4081 Tengyur, sems tsam, *hi,* 166b2.
817 Asaṅga, *Bodhisattvabhūmi,* chap. 10, Toh 4037 Tengyur, sems tsam, *wi,* 83b2.
818 *Rituals for Taking the Bodhisattva Vows and Meditation Deity (Bodhicittotpādasamādānavidhi),* Toh 3968 Tengyur, dbu ma, *gi,* 242b5.
819 *Broom of the Buddha's Precious Doctrine,* Collected Works, *nya,* 64b1. The "seven

cause-and-effect transmitted instructions" refers to the tradition of developing bodhicitta involving the six causes of recognizing living beings as your mothers, remembering their kindness, resolving to repay that kindness, developing affectionate love, developing compassion, and developing the special attitude, followed by the result of bodhicitta.

820 *Bodhipathapradīpa,* v. 20, Toh 3947 Tengyur, dbu ma, *khi,* 239a4.

821 If by his nature he does not kill, steal, and so on.

822 Collected Works, *ka,* 10a2.

823 *Bhadrakalpika,* fascicle 23, Toh 94 Kangyur, mdo sde *ka,* 293b2. Degé reading preferred.

824 Chap. 4, Toh 353 Kangyur, mdo sde, *ah,* 117b1. Translated from the Chinese.

825 *Triskandhakasūtra,* Toh 284 Kangyur, mdo sde, *ya,* 68a6.

826 *Karuṇāpuṇḍarīka,* chap. 3, Toh 112 Kangyur, mdo sde, *cha,* 149a3.

827 *Māyopamāsamādhisūtra,* Toh 130 Kangyur, mdo sde, *da,* 226a3.

828 *Dharmārthavibhaṅgasūtra,* Toh 247 Kangyur, mdo sde, *za,* 45a7.

829 *Stages of the Bodhisattva (Bodhisattvabhūmi),* chap. 10, Toh 4037 Tengyur, sems tsam, *wi,* 74b6.

830 Therefore, the term "vow" *(sdom pa)* is being used in its more literal sense of "restraint" and not as some formal commitment.

831 *Śikṣāsamuccaya,* Toh 3939 Tengyur, dbu ma, *khi,* 1a3.

832 Ibid., 2a1.

833 Asaṅga, *Mahāyānasaṃgraha,* fascicle 3, Toh 4048 Tengyur, sems tsam, *ri,* 32a5.

834 *Bodhisattvasaṃvaraviṃśakapañjikā,* Toh 4083 Tengyur, sems tsam, *hi,* 186a7.

835 *Bhaiṣajyagurusūtra,* Toh 504 Kangyur, rgyud, *da,* 280a3.

836 *Saṃvaraviṃśakavṛtti,* Toh 4082 Tengyur, sems tsam, *hi,* 170a6.

837 Bhāvaviveka, *Tarkajvāla,* chap. 4, Toh 3856 Tengyur, dbu ma, *dza,* 166a3.

838 Nāgārjuna, *Ratnāvalī.* Citation not traced.

839 Toh 256 Kangyur, mdo sde, *za,* 79b2.

840 *Twenty Verses on the Bodhisattva Vow (Bodhisattvasaṃvaraviṃśaka),* Toh 4081 Tengyur, sems tsam, *hi,* 166b3.

841 *Śikṣāsamuccaya,* chap. 3, Toh 3940 Tengyur, dbu ma, *khi,* 43a5.

842 Toh 260 Kangyur, mdo sde, *za,* 272b4.

843 "Defeats" *(pham pa)* here refers to the defeats of the fully ordained monk. "Cause" *(gnas)* refers to the mental afflictions such as desire that bring about defeats. See Tatz, p. 51. To be a complete severing of the vow, there must be four binding factors *(kun dkris chen po):* habitually repeating of the fault, having no sense of shame, taking joy in the fault, not regarding it as a fault.

844 Śāntideva, *Bodhicaryāvatāra,* 4:4, Toh 3871 Tengyur, dbu ma, *la,* 8a4.

845 Candragomin, *Bodhisattvasaṃvaraviṃśaka,* Toh 4081 Tengyur, sems tsam, *hi,* 166b5. Śāntarakṣita'a commentary to the *Twenty Verses* explains this phrase as meaning that if there is no suitable person present, you should confess in front of your own mind, and then later if possible, you should confess again to another person. Sakya Drakpa Gyaltsen's commentary explains it to mean that faults driven by afflictions should be confessed before another person and those not driven by affliction may be confessed internally (Tatz, p. 29).

846 *Treatise on the Classification of the Three Vows,* Collected Works, *na,* 2b2.

847 *Mañjuśrīmūlakalpa,* Toh 543 Kangyur, rgyud, *na,* 107a3.

848 Toh 480 Kangyur, rgyud, *nya,* 211b6.

849 Toh 424 Kangyur, rgyud, *nga,* 53b5. In the Degé Tengyur this verse is written in its better-known form used for the generation of the aspiring bodhi mind in ceremonies, empowerments, and the like.
850 *Gaṇḍavyūhasūtra,* fascicle 19, Toh 44 Kangyur, phal chen, *a,* 317b4.
851 Found in *Gaṇḍavyūhasūtra,* fascicle 20, Toh 44 Kangyur, phal chen, *a,* 323a5.
852 *Maitreyaprasthāna,* Toh 198 Kangyur, mdo sde, *tsa,* 287a3.
853 *Bodhicaryāvatāra,* 1:9, Toh 3871 Tengyur, dbu ma, *la,* 2a6.
854 *Bodhipathapradīpa,* vv. 15, 18. Toh 3947 Tengyur, dbu ma, *khi,* 239a1.
855 *Ugraparipṛcchā,* fascicle 1, Toh 63 Kangyur, bkon brtsegs, *nga,* 259a2.
856 Ibid., 261b4.
857 *Vinayaviniścayaupāliparipṛcchā,* fascicle 21, Toh 68 Kangyur, bkon brtsegs, *ca,* 23a7.
858 Ibid., 124a1.
859 *Vinayaviniścayaupāliparipṛcchā,* fascicle 2, Toh 68 Kangyur, bkon brtsegs, *ca,* 120a3. The sutra excerpt beginning with the address to Śāriputra and containing the *Sutra of the Three Heaps* is quoted in full in Śāntideva's *Compendium of Practice,* but in the Degé edition of the sutra, only the passages addressed to Upāli are found.
860 These are the four enlightened bodies or forms of a buddha.
861 *Treatise on the Classification of the Three Vows,* Collected Works, *na,* 18a2.
862 *Seka;* corrected by the editor of the new Tibetan redaction to *sarga,* which according to the *Great Tibetan-Chinese Dictionary* means "outline" or "chapter" but according to Monier-Williams also means stream or emission. This is preferred because the four oral transmissions use the metaphor of a river and its water.
863 *Hevajratantra,* chap. 3, Toh 417 Kangyur, rgyud, *nga,* 17a3.
864 Text untraced. Because early Tibetan translators decided to translate *abhiṣeka,* meaning to "wash" or "cleanse," with the Tibetan word *dbang,* meaning "power," then the etymological explanation of this verse does not quite follow. "Empowerment" is a direct translation of the Tibetan, but etymologically "initiation" might be better.
865 *Thob bya rang gnas kyi gnyug ma'i rdo rje bzhi.* These are the vajras of body, speech, mind, and exalted wisdom. Their gradual purification results in the emergence of the four bodies of a buddha.
866 *Rang bzhin du gnas pa'i rigs;* sometimes translated as "buddha nature."
867 *Mahāmudrātilakayoginītantra,* chap. 2, Toh 420 Kangyur, rgyud, *nga,* 66b4.
868 *Vajramālābhidhāna,* chap. 2, Toh 445 Kangyur, rgyud, *ca,* 212a2.
869 *Sarvabuddhasamāyogatantra,* chap. 37, Toh 366 Kangyur, rgyud, *ka,* 164b2.
870 *Laghusaṃvaratantra,* chap. 3, Toh 368, Kangyur, rgyud, *ka,* 216a2.
871 Untraced.
872 *Blossom Cluster of Siddhis: Teachings on Tantric Ethics,* Collected Works, *ka,* 69a5.
873 Vows *(sdom pa, saṃvara)* and pledges *(dam tshig, samaya).* Although Tsongkhapa in his *Blossom Cluster of Siddhis* cites a passage defining differences between the two, they are used interchangeably in the discussion here.
874 *Vajraśekhara Tantra,* Toh 480 Kangyur, rgyud, *nya,* 183a7.
875 This refers to the verse as cited by Tsongkhapa in his *Blossom Cluster of Siddhis.* The words *dag pa* meaning "pure" and *dga' ba* meaning "joyful" are close in spelling.

876 *Vajraśekhara Tantra,* Toh 480 Kangyur, rgyud, *nya,* 183b1.
877 Ibid., 183b2.
878 *Phyi nang gsang ba theg pa gsum.* In this *Vajraśekha* line as cited by Tsongkhapa, the *nang* (inner) becomes *dang* (a conjunctive particle) and so reads *phyi dang gsang ba theg pa gsum:* "The outer and secret vehicles." Tsongkhapa's comments on this line are based on this reading.
879 *Vajraśekhara Tantra,* Toh 480 Kangyur, rgyud, *nya,* 183b2.
880 Ibid., 183b3.
881 Ibid., 183b3. "Gross" *(sbom po, stüla)* is a term normally used for the eight secondary downfalls. It means "thick," "heavy," "bulky," and so on. "Fault" here is *kha na ma tho ba (avadya)* and is usually of two kinds: natural and proscribed.
882 All fourteen are listed by Tsongkhapa in his *Blossom Cluster of Siddhis.*
883 *Vajraśekhara Tantra,* Toh 480 Kangyur, rgyud, *nya,* 183b4.
884 Ibid., 183b5.
885 Ibid., 183b6.
886 Ibid., 183b7.
887 Ibid., 183b7.
888 Ibid., 183b7.
889 Ibid., 183a2.
890 Ibid., 183a6.
891 Ibid., 184a1.
892 Ibid., 184a1.
893 See previous note on the pledges of Amitābha.
894 In this section the verses from the *Vajraśekhara Tantra* run from 184a2–4.
895 *Vajraśekhara Tantra,* Toh 480 Kangyur, rgyud, *nya,* 184a5.
896 In the Mahayana, *nonabiding nirvana (mi gnas pa'i mya ngan las 'das pa, apratiṣṭanirvāṇa)* is the enlightenment of a buddha, who is free of both the turmoil of samsara and the quietism of an arhat's nirvana. It signifies that while Mahayana enlightened beings remain active in the world, they are not stained by it.
897 *Vajradhātumahāmaṇḍalavidhisarvavajrodaya,* Toh 2516 Tengyur, rgyud 'grel, *ku,* 44a3.
898 This abrupt style of commentary is the author quickly running through Tsongkhapa's *Blossom Cluster of Siddhis,* which is followed closely in this topic.
899 Abhayākaragupta, *Vajrāvalīmaṇḍalasādhana,* Toh 3140 Tengyur, rgyud 'grel, *phu,* 76b2.
900 Ibid., 85b7.
901 Aśvaghoṣa [Śūra], *Compilation of Vajrayana Root Downfalls (Vajrayānamūlāpattisaṃgraha),* Toh 2478 Tengyur, rgyud 'grel, *zi,* 179a7.
902 Śūra is Aśvaghoṣa. Here and throughout this topic the author closely follows his *Compilation of Vajrayana Root Downfalls,* which in turn is quoted in Tsongkhapa's commentary. The voice here is therefore primarily that of Aśvaghoṣa.
903 *Compilation of Vajrayana Root Downfalls,* Toh 2478 Tengyur, rgyud 'grel, *zi,* 179a7.
904 Dharmakīrti, *Pramāṇavārttika,* 2:142, Toh 4210 Tengyur, tshad ma, *ce,* 112b6.
905 Aśvaghoṣa, *Compilation of Vajrayana Root Downfalls,* Toh 2478 Tengyur, rgyud 'grel, *zi,* 179a7. In this version of these two lines, the word "anger" is not in the

instrumental case, and in the second line Sangyé Gyatso does not take it to mean that the anger that causes us to verbalize the faults of our vajra brothers and sisters. In the commentary in *Blossom Cluster,* Tsongkhapa reads the second line as a verbalizing of faults that is brought on by anger, and his text has the first line in the instrumental, which when translated would read, "Becoming angry at a vajra brother or sister/ and speaking of his or her faults is the third." Both interpretations of this vow are discussed by Jé Tsongkhapa. Degé reads "Becoming angry and speaking of the faults of vajra brothers and sisters."

906 Ibid., 179b1.

907 Ibid., 179b1.

908 *Avataṃsakasūtra,* chap. 9, Toh 44 Kangyur, phal chen, *a,* 309b1.

909 Aśvaghoṣa, *Compilation of Vajrayana Root Downfalls,* Toh 2478 Tengyur, rgyud 'grel, *zi,* 179b1.

910 Untraced.

911 Aśvaghoṣa, *Compilation of Vajrayana Root Downfalls,* Toh 2478 Tengyur, rgyud 'grel, *zi,* 179b1.

912 Ibid., 179b1.

913 The text here on the examples of despising the body appears to be corrupt. Therefore, as the author follows Tsongkhapa very closely in the whole of this topic, I have translated his sentence according to Tsongkhapa.

914 Aśvaghoṣa, *Compilation of Vajrayana Root Downfalls,* Toh 2478 Tengyur, rgyud 'grel, *zi,* 179b2.

915 Probably a reference to the fact that the Fifth Dalai Lama practiced extensively in the Nyingma tradition as well as in the Geluk, and there may have been some who expressed doubts over the authenticity and purity of such practices.

916 Aśvaghoṣa, *Compilation of Vajrayana Root Downfalls,* Toh 2478 Tengyur, rgyud 'grel, *zi,* 179b2.

917 *Bsgral:* to liberate, to kill legally, to banish. The sense here is to kill through the use of tantric powers, as Tsongkhapa cites passages here promoting the use of violent methods in such cases.

918 Bhavila, or Bhabilha, is another name for Aśvaghoṣa, though it does not appear in the list of his twenty-one names listed previously.

919 Aśvaghoṣa, *Compilation of Vajrayana Root Downfalls,* Toh 2478 Tengyur, rgyud 'grel, *zi,* 179b2.

920 Ibid., 179b2.

921 Ibid., 179b2.

922 Ibid., 179b3.

923 *Vajrapañjaratantra,* chap. 15, Toh 419 Kangyur, rgyud, *nga,* 64b3.

924 Aśvaghoṣa, *Compilation of Vajrayana Root Downfalls,* Toh 2478 Tengyur, rgyud 'grel, *zi,* 179b3.

925 Tsongkhapa in his *Blossom Cluster of Siddhis* (p. 52a6) states this quote was cited by Saraha in his *Commentary on the Buddhakapāla Tantra* (Toh 1652 Tengyur, rgyud 'grel *ra*).

926 Padmasambhava, *Samayapañca,* Toh 1224 Tengyur, rgyud 'grel, *nya,* 28b2.

927 *Garland of Light on the Three Vows (Trisaṃvaraprabhāmālā),* Toh 3727 Tengyur, rgyud 'grel, *tshu,* 56b6.

928 Aśvaghoṣa, *Compilation of Vajrayana Root Downfalls,* Toh 2478 Tengyur, rgyud 'grel *zi,* 179b3.
929 *Buddhakapāla Mandala Ritual,* Toh 1657 Tengyur, rgyud 'grel, *ra,* 243a7.
930 Aśvaghoṣa, *Compilation of Vajrayana Root Downfalls,* Toh 2478 Tengyur, rgyud 'grel *zi,* 179b4.
931 Toh 480 Kangyur, rgyud, *nya,* 211a7.
932 Aśvaghoṣa, *Compilation of Vajrayana Root Downfalls,* Toh 2478 Tengyur, rgyud 'grel, *zi,* 179b4.
933 *Song of Realization,* chap. 1, Collected Works, *kha,* 53b5.
934 *Kālacakra Tantra,* 3:86, Toh 362 Kangyur, *ka,* 66a7.
935 *Kālacakra Tantra,* 3:102, Toh 362 Kangyur, *ka,* 68a1.
936 Untraced.
937 Untraced. *Tshig pa* also means "burn," and other commentators have glossed the term *dam tshig* to mean "bound and burn."
938 Collected Tantras of the Nyingma, vol. *da,* chap. 10, 176b7.
939 Ibid., chap. 9, 175a6.
940 Ibid., chap. 10, 177b7.
941 Ibid., 178a1.
942 These etymologies are for purposes of practice rather than scholastic precision. Another approach would be to say that *slob dpon* means "master of learning," qualified by *slob* with its dual meaning of "to teach" and "to learn." Also the *ma* of *slob ma* is more typically construed as a nominative ending rather than meaning "mother."
943 Collected Tantras of the Nyingma, vol. *da,* chap. 10, 178a1.
944 Ibid., 178a3.
945 Untraced.
946 Collected Tantras of the Nyingma, vol. *da,* chap. 10, 176b7.
947 Ibid., 178b4.
948 Ibid., 178a5. "Three-circle purity" refers to the fact that for any act, the object, action, and agent all lack true existence.
949 Ibid., 178a7.
950 *Hundred Prostration Abandonment Reparations,* Toh 267, mdo sde, *ya.* One of the texts that fell from the sky during the reign of the early Tibetan king Lha Thothori Nyenshal as a sign that the Dharma would spread to Tibet. It was eventually translated into Tibetan by Thönmi Sambhota but has no Sanskrit title.
951 *Naraka* ("hell") here refers to the fruits of breaking pledges.
952 *Tantra of the Self-Appearing Mind,* Collected Tantras of the Nyingma, vol. *da,* chap. 10, 178b3.
953 Ibid., 177b3.
954 Ibid., 177b4.
955 *Gross Downfalls in the Vajrayana (Vajrayānasthūlāpatti),* Toh 2482 Tengyur, rgyud 'grel, *zi,* 180b1.
956 Ibid., 180b1.
957 *Song of Realization,* chap. 1, Collected Works, *kha,* 53b1.
958 Ibid., 54b4.
959 *Book of Kadam: Father Teachings* (in "Extensive Biography of Glorious Atiśa"), 92.5.
960 *Gnas 'gyur ba.*

961 *Rnam par rig byed ma yin pa.* The *pratimokṣa* vows are nonrevelatory because they are conceptualized forms known only by the mental consciousness that conceptualizes them.
962 Untraced.
963 *Analysis of the Vinaya Sutra: Elucidation of the Essence of the Ocean of Vinaya,* Collected Works, *zha,* 7a7.
964 Chim Jampaiyang, *Ornament to Commentary on Abhidharmakośa,* chap. 4, 195b4.
965 Collected Works, *nya,* 121a1.
966 Puṇḍarīka, *Stainless Light Great Commentary (Vimalaprabhā),* chap. 4, Toh 845 Kangyur, rgyud, *śrī,* 262a4.
967 *Rdzas tha dad.*
968 *Garland of Light on the Three Vows (Trisaṃvaraprabhāmālā),* Toh 3727 Tengyur, rgyud 'grel, *tshu,* 56b6.
969 Ibid., 56a4. Quotes together with the commentary found in Ngawang Losang Gyatso, *Golden Victorious Myrobalan Vinaya Ceremonies,* Collected Works, *pha,* 82b4.
970 I have added the two previous lines as found in the Degé Tengyur edition here to give reference to the next line beginning, "the first...."
971 Vibhūticandra, *Trisaṃvaraprabhāmālā,* Toh 3727 Tengyur, rgyud 'grel, *tshu,* 55b4.
972 *Guhyagarbhatantra,* chap. 19, Toh 832 Kangyur, rnying rgyud, *kha,* 129b6.
973 In Degé found in fascicle 2.
974 *Ugraparipṛcchā,* Toh 63 Kangyur, dkon brtsegs, *nga,* 275b5.
975 *Srin kālā.* Possibly *sṛkāla* ("jackal").
976 *Daśacakrakṣitigarbha,* chap. 3, Toh 239 Kangyur, mdo sde, *zha,* 138.
977 Untraced. In this discussion on what constitutes being a monk, the term used is *dge slong, bhikṣu.*
978 Found in *Biography of Ra Lotsāwa* by Ra Yeshé Sengé, p. 267.
979 Shangdro Yudrakpa Tsöndrü Drakpa (1123–93), founder of the Tsalpa Kagyü sect.
980 Jikdral Namtrül Jampa Chönyi (fifteenth century).
981 Better known as Tāranātha.
982 *Avataṃsakasūtra,* chap. 45, Toh 44 Kangyur, phal chen, *ga,* 317b7.
983 *Adhyāśayasañcodana,* Toh 69 Kangyur, dkon brtsegs, *ca,* 133b5.
984 *Aśokadattavyākaraṇa,* Toh 76 Kangyur, dkon brtsegs, *ca,* 236a6.
985 *Pañcapāramitānirdeśa,* Toh 181 Kangyur, mdo sde, *tsa,* 32b7.
986 *Avataṃsakasūtra,* Toh 44 Kangyur, phal chen, *a,* 23a3.
987 Or osprey, according to Monier-Williams.
988 *Avataṃsakasūtra,* Toh 44 Kangyur, phal chen, *a,* 23a3ff.
989 *Legs bshad.* The king's name, Subhāṣitagaveṣa, means "in search of wise counsel."
990 The name of the hunter means "cruel hunter."
991 *Bodhisattvāvadānakalpalatā,* story 53, Toh 4155 Tengyur, skyes rabs, *khe,* 30a2.
992 Ibid., 30a2.
993 Ibid., 31b2.
994 Only the first line of the verse is reproduced here. The rendering in the text seems a little corrupt, and so I have given the sense of this verse that appears in the Degé edition and in the commentary by Somendra.

995 Kṣemendra, *Bodhisattvāvadānakalpalatā,* story 107, Toh 4155 Tengyur, skyes rabs, *khe,* 290a6.

996 "Object" *(yul)* here means a recognized and formal object from whom one receives vows and teachings, such as a monk. The author's main point here, which he has been making over many pages, is that that the presence of a *pratimokṣa*-holding monk is not necessary for the imparting of teachings and vows. This has now been extended to include the point that an intention to teach is not necessary for a teaching to be imparted. In the first account, the hunter only gave his counsel because, according to the commentary, he wanted the jewel, and he had the king jump off a cliff because he feared that if the king remained alive he would take the jewel back. In the second story Śuddhodana heard the wise counsel being sung by the king's daughter as he walked past her room. In neither account was there an intention to give teachings. Mere reverence on the part of the listener was enough to receive them, a point emphasized below in the account of the queen's servant girl.

997 Found in fascicle 4 in Degé.

998 *Karaṇḍavyūha,* fascicle 4, Toh 116 Kangyur, mdo sde, *ja,* 235b1.

999 This is told in the *Prophecy of Aśokadatta (Aśokadattavyākaraṇa),* Kangyur Toh 76, dkon brtsegs, *ca.*

1000 Untraced.

1001 The three white-robed practitioners are Sachen Künga Nyingpo (1092–1158) and his sons Sönam Tsemo and Drakpa Gyaltsen.

1002 Ngawang Losang Gyatso, Collected Works, *ca,* 129b4.

1003 *Maitreyamahāsiṃhanāda,* Toh 67 Kangyur, dkon brtsegs, *ca,* 82a1.

1004 Ibid., 82a4.

1005 *Dānānuśaṃsānirdeśa,* Toh 183 Kangyur, mdo sde, *ca,* 96a3.

1006 *Daśasāhasrikāprajñāpāramitā,* chap. 19, Toh 11 Kangyur, sher phyin, *nga,* 207b4.

1007 *Adhyāśayasañcodana,* Toh 69 Kangyur, dkon brtsegs, *ca,* 150a4.

1008 Although there is some slight variation in the wording, this verse is a repetition of the verse above in the *Maitreyamahāsiṃhanāda,* Toh 67 Kangyur, dkon brtsegs, *ca,* 82a4.

1009 *Madhyantavibhaṅga,* 5:9, Toh 4021 Tengyur, sems tsam, *phi,* 5a4.

1010 *Chos spyod.* These ten causes are known as the *ten Dharma activities.* The term is often used these days to refer to liturgical books of prayers and praises.

1011 Sthiramati, *Madhyāntavibhaṅgaṭīkā,* chap. 5, Toh 4032 Tengyur, sems tsam, *bi,* 295a5.

1012 *Pūrṇaparipṛcchā,* chap. 5, Toh 61 Kangyur, dkon brtsegs, *nga,* 206a2.

1013 *Pitāputrasamāgamasūtra,* chap. 27, Toh 60 Kangyur, dkon brtsegs, *nga,* 167b6.

1014 *Mañjuśrībuddhakṣetraguṇavyūha,* Toh 59 Kangyur, dkon brtsegs, *ga,* 295b6.

1015 *Ugraparipṛcchā,* Toh 63 Kangyur, dkon brtsegs, *nga,* 287b6.

1016 Untraced.

1017 *Maitreyamahāsiṃhanāda,* Toh 67 Kangyur, dkon brtsegs, *ca,* 91a3.

1018 *Adhyāśayasañcodana,* Toh 69 Kangyur, dkon brtsegs, *ca,* 144a2.

1019 *Sumatidārikāparipṛcchā,* Toh 74 Kangyur, dkon brtsegs, *ca,* 221b6.

1020 *Aśokadattavyākaraṇa,* Toh 76 Kangyur, dkon brtsegs, *ca,* 240b4.

1021 *Vimaladattāparipṛcchā,* Toh 77 Kangyur, dkon brtsegs, *ca,* 256a1.

1022 *Kāśyapaparivarta,* Toh 87 Kangyur, dkon brtsegs, *cha,* 150b1.

1023 Found in the Gaining Immeasurable Qualities chapter; *Aṣṭasāhasrikāprajñāpāramitā,* chap. 3, Toh 12 Kangyur, sher phyin, *ka,* 35a3.
1024 *Moonlight: A Commentary on the Essence of Eight Branches,* Toh 4312 Tengyur, gso rig, *ko,* 16b1.
1025 *Madhyāntavibhaṅgaṭīkā,* Toh 4032 Tengyur, sems tsam, *bi,* 294a5.
1026 Both editions of the text have "twenty-first chapter" but the passage is clearly from the thirty-first chapter.
1027 *Four Tantras,* Explanatory Tantra, 31.95.16.
1028 Ibid., 31.95.17.
1029 Ibid., 31.96.2.
1030 Ibid., 31.96.8.
1031 Ibid., 31.96.9. These last two lines are omitted in both editions of the text, but because they are commented on later, I have inserted them as found in *Four Tantras.*
1032 The doctor should not be squeamish or repulsed by blood and pus but regard them as dogs and pigs would.
1033 *Phud.* A term usually referring to a portion of food and drink separated out as an offering at the beginnings of meals, festivities, etc.
1034 *Four Tantras,* Explanatory Tantra, 31.97.14.
1035 Ibid., 31.97.17.
1036 Thönmi Sambhota, *Vyākaraṇaliṅgāvataraṇa,* Toh 4348 Tengyur, sna tshogs, *co,* 160b2.
1037 Ibid., 161b2.
1038 Ngawang Losang Gyatso, *Letters Arranged in Verse to Various Persons in China, Tibet, and Mongolia Containing Many Oral Transmissions,* Collected Works, *dza,* 26a3.
1039 Chap. 9, Toh 353 Kangyur, mdo sde, *ah,* 189b2. Translated from the Chinese.
1040 Ibid., 189a7.
1041 In other words, merely asserting and firmly believing that which is true is not enough to cut deep-seated doubts.
1042 *Words Composed on the Three Jewels,* Collected Works, *kha,* 58a6.
1043 Ngawang Losang Gyatso, *Letters Arranged in Verse,* Collected Works, *dza,* 58a2.
1044 Untraced.
1045 Untraced.
1046 A garuḍa-faced protector often invoked in medical practices, such as those found in Yuthok's *Heartdrop.*
1047 Untraced.
1048 Moods *('gyur)* are internal and made external through expression *(nyams)* by way of the many verbal adornments *(tshig rgyan)* taught in the treatises on poetics *(snyan ngag, kāvya).*
1049 Ngawang Losang Gyatso, *Letters Arranged in Verse,* Collected Works, *dza,* 57b4.
1050 *Mngon brjod, abhidhāna.* This term is often used to mean a thesaurus.
1051 By the Indian lexicographer Amarasiṃha, *Amarakośa,* Toh 4299 Tengyur, sgra mdo, *se.*
1052 Śrīdhara, *Various Clarifications: A Work on Lexicography, Abhidhānaśāstraviśvalocana(ityaparābhidhānamuktāvalī). Mngon brjod kyi bstan bcos sna tshogs gsal ba,* Toh 4453 Tengyur, sna tshogs, *po.*
1053 Ngawang Losang Gyatso, *Letters Arranged in Verse to Various Persons in China, Tibet and Mongolia containing Many Oral Transmissions.* Collected Works, *dza,* 63b4.

1054 Ibid., 57b5. The last line is clearly a tease.

1055 Ibid., 57b6.

1056 *Zla snyigs,* a subdivision of the zodiac sign occupied by the moon. My thanks to Edward Henning for this information.

1057 Astrology is *skar rtsis,* which I have elsewhere translated as "astronomy," and in its function of calculating the calendar, phases of the moon, eclipses, and so on, "astronomy" would be a preferable translation. After all, the term does mean "calculations from the stars." However, in this context, its function is more divinatory, in the sense of predicting outcomes and auspicious times.

1058 "Planetary and stellar combinations" *(skar rtsis 'phrod sbyor)* refers to the correspondence of element combinations with the planets and constellations. Each correspondence portends a particular outcome.

1059 *Nag rtsis.* It is also known as elemental calculation *('byung rtsis).* The country of black clothes is China *(rgya nag),* often juxtaposed with India *(rgya dkar),* the land of white clothes.

1060 *Sa bdag.* Spirits, usually nāgas, that have domain over land and are especially linked to astrological influences.

1061 The life force *(bla)* travels about the body, and its position can be mapped out by recourse to astrology.

1062 *Four Tantras,* Explanatory Tantra, 31.98.2.

1063 The verse has *gsog cung,* which could mean "of simple means" as Clarke has translated it, because the verb *gsog pa* means "to accumulate," and *cung* means "few," but here the author understands it as *gsog po,* meaning "hollow," "without essence," and "false." He has also paired it with *gsob pa,* which has the same meaning.

1064 *Four Tantras,* Explanatory Tantra, 31.98.6.

1065 Ibid., 31.98.8.

1066 Ibid., 31.98.9.

1067 Ibid., 31.98.10.

1068 Ibid., 31.98.15.

1069 The ten vulnerable bodily phenomena, or objects of harm *(gnod bya),* are the seven bodily constituents—plasma, blood, flesh, fat, marrow, bone, and semen—and the three excretions or impurities—sweat, excrement, and urine.

1070 *Four Tantras,* Explanatory Tantra, 31.98.15.

1071 *Sman pa; sman* means medicine and *pa* as it is spelled here is usually a nominative particle indicating a male noun. Sometimes, however, it is spelled *dpa'* when it means hero (as in *byang chub sems dpa',* bodhisattva, in the sense of being a compassionate hero).

1072 According to Surkhar Lodrö Gyalpo in his *General Compendium of Knowledge Indispensable to Physicians* (478b6), as a verb *sman* can also mean "to help," and a physician is "one who helps" *(sman pa).* Of course *sman pa* could also just be read as "medicine man."

1073 *Four Tantras,* Explanatory Tantra, 31.98.17.

1074 Found in *Names of Mañjuśrī, Mañjuśrīnāmasaṃgīti,* Toh 360 Kangyur, rgyud, *ka,* 6a3.

1075 "Upright and true" *(drang srong, ṛṣi)* is the etymology of the term *rishi.* This is the etymology used by Clark (p. 228).

1076 Untraced.

1077 By Sumtön Yeshé Sung.

1078 Found in *Eighteen Auxiliary Texts,* 290.5. The second of the four, "the physician limited by scrolls," is missing from the text as has been added from the source text.

1079 *Four Tantras,* Explanatory Tantra, 31.99.3.

1080 Ibid., 26.85.4.

1081 *Four Tantras,* Final Tantra, 27.666.10.

1082 Sukhar Lodrö Gyalpo.

1083 Untraced.

1084 Pitṛceṭa, *Aṣṭāṅgahṛdayasaṃhita,* chap. 1, Toh 4310 Tengyur, gso rig, *he,* 45b3.

1085 Untraced.

1086 Pitṛceṭa, *Aṣṭāṅgahṛdayasaṃhita,* chap. 40, Toh 4310 Tengyur, gso rig, *he,* 334b4. Translated according to Degé reading.

1087 Puṇḍarīka, *Paramārthasevā,* Toh 1348 Tengyur, rgyud 'grel, *na,* 4b2.

1088 Aśvaghoṣa, *Gurupañcāśikā,* Toh 3721 Tengyur, rgyud 'grel, *tshu,* 10a5.

1089 *Vajramālābhidhānatantra,* chap. 2, Toh 445 Kangyur, rgyud, *ca,* 212a6.

1090 *Vajramālābhidhānatantra,* chap. 15, Toh 445 Kangyur, rgyud, *ca,* 273a3.

1091 *Subāhuparipṛcchā,* chap. 1, Toh 805 Kangyur, rgyud, *wa,* 119b4.

1092 *Vajraḍākatantra,* chap. 32, Toh 370 Kangyur, rgyud, *kha,* 70b1.

1093 *Sāmānyavidhiguhyatantra,* Toh 806 Kangyur, rgyud, *wa;* but verse untraced.

1094 Ibid.

1095 *Vajraḍākatantra,* chap. 21, Toh 370 Kangyur, rgyud, *kha,* 70b2.

1096 Found in *Secrets of All Tathāgatas (Sarvatathāgataguhya).* Toh 830 Kangyur, rnying rgyud, *ka,* 344a1.

1097 *Māyājālatantra,* chap. 1, Toh 466 Kangyur, rgyud, *ja,* 95a4. Wording of first line slightly different in Degé, which states, "Taking joy in the vows and virtue." The third line also has "deities" instead of "gurus."

1098 Untraced, but he is probably referring to the *Great Illusion Tantra (Mahāmāyātantra),* Toh 425 Kangyur, rgyud 'bum, *nga.*

1099 *Guhyagarbha,* chap. 9. Toh 832 Kangyur, rnying rgyud, *kha,* 120a6.

1100 *Vajraśekhara Tantra,* Toh 480 Kangyur, rgyud, *nya,* 163a2.

1101 Āryadeva, *Catuḥśatakaśāstra,* 12:1, Toh 3846 Tengyur, dbu ma, *tsha,* 13a4.

1102 Untraced.

1103 *Tshangs par spyod pa, brahmacaryā;* often refers to the chaste life of a religious student, or more specifically to celibacy.

1104 Pitṛceṭa, *Aṣṭāṅgahṛdayasaṃhita,* chap. 3, Toh 4310, gso rig, *he,* 118a2. Last line translated according to Degé.

1105 Untraced.

1106 Pitṛceṭa, *Essence of Eight Branches (Aṣṭāṅgahṛdayasaṃhita),* chap. 40, Toh 4310, gso rig, *he,* 334b4. The term for "poison" here *(halāhala)* in Sanskrit refers to the great poison spewed up by the churning of the ocean in the Vedic myth, and in Tibetan refers to the poisonous qualities of black aconite.

1107 Ibid.

1108 *Four Tantras,* Final Tantra, 27.665.17.

1109 *Four Tantras,* Explanatory Tantra, 31.99.8. "They are the levers that topple the fortress of life," translated with the addition of "fortress" from *Oral Transmission of Our Ancestors,* 481b3.

1110 *Four Tantras,* Final Tantra, 27.666.4.

1111 *Girth of an Elephant Mahayana Sutra (Hastikakṣyamahāyānasūtra),* Toh 207 Kangyur, mdo sde, *tsha,* 97b6.

1112 Asaṅga, *Bodhisattvabhūmi,* Toh 4037 Tengyur, sems tsam, *wi,* 57a1.

1113 *Avataṃsakasūtra,* chap. 17, Toh 44 Kangyur, phal chen, *a,* 286b7.

1114 Śāntideva, *Bodhicaryāvatāra,* 2:54, Toh 3871 Tengyur, dbu ma, *la,* 6a3.

1115 Found in *Abridged Perfection of Wisdom in Verse (Prajñāpāramitāsaṃcayagāthā),* Toh 13 Kangyur, shes phyin, *ka,* 13a7.

1116 *Samādhirājasūtra,* chap. 9, Toh 127 Kangyur, mdo sde, *da,* 27b4.

1117 *Samādhirājasūtra,* chap. 4, Toh 127 Kangyur, mdo sde, *da,* 14a5.

1118 Śāntideva, *Bodhicaryāvatāra,* 5:109, Toh 3871 Tengyur, dbu ma, *la,* 14b23.

1119 *Nan tan:* conscientious, earnest, careful.

1120 *Vyākhyāyukti,* Toh 4061 Tengyur, sems tsam, *shi,* 65b4.

1121 *Daśacakrakṣitigarbhasūtra,* chap. 7, Toh 239 Kangyur, mdo sde, *zha,* 223a5.

1122 Aśvaghoṣa, *Jātakamālā,* no. 31, Toh 4150 Tengyur, skyes rabs, *hu,* 125a1.

1123 Untraced.

1124 The Tibetan has *me long* (mirror) which seems strange. As the text is untraced, I have emended it to the more probable *le lo* (laziness). The whole verse is difficult to comprehend.

1125 Untraced.

1126 Untraced.

1127 Śāntideva, *Bodhicaryāvatāra,* 5:16, Toh 3871 Tengyur, dbu ma, *la,* 10b6.

1128 *Tathāgatācintyaguhyanirdeśa,* chap. 5, Toh 47 Kangyur, dkon brtsegs, *ka,* 119b1. Degé has slightly different wording.

1129 *Lalitavistarasūtra,* chap. 26, Toh 95 Kangyur, mdo sde, *kha,* 198a2.

1130 *Bodhisattvapiṭaka,* chap. 11, Toh 56 Kangyur, dkon brtsegs, *kha,* 160b5.

1131 *Udānavarga,* chap. 22, Toh 326 Kangyur, mdo sde, *sa,* 228b2.

1132 Ibid., 228b1.

1133 *Vinayavibhaṅga,* Toh 3 Kangyur, 'dul ba, *nya,* 119a7.

1134 Aśvaghoṣa, *Jātakamālā,* chap. 31, Toh 4150 Tengyur, skyes rabs, *hu,* 122a1.

1135 Ibid., 122a4.

1136 Maitreya, *Uttaratantra,* 5:9, Toh 4024 Tengyur, sems tsam, *phi,* 72a2.

1137 *Samādhirājasūtra,* chap. 9, Toh 127 Kangyur, mdo sde, *da,* 91b2.

1138 *Bhadrakalpika,* chap. 2, Toh 94 Kangyur, mdo sde, *ka,* 18a5.

1139 *Prajñāpāramitāsaṃcayagāthā,* Toh 13 Kangyur, sher phyin, *ka,* 2a2.

1140 *Lcags ri bai dūrya 'gro phan lta na ngo mtshar rig byed gling.*

1141 *Rtsi,* short for *rtsi tog/thog,* according to Surkhar Lodrö Gyalpo.

1142 *Four Tantras,* Final Tantra, 12.604.13.

1143 The time of the rishis is either the first or the third month of autumn. According to Prof. Losang Tenzin, the "face of the rishis" may refer to the appearance of the rishi constellation in the night sky.

1144 *Rāṣṭrapālaparipṛcchā,* Toh 62 Kangyur, dkon brtsegs, *nga,* 240a6.

1145 Ibid., 241a7.

1146 Ibid., 241a5. Degé wording somewhat different.

1147 Atiśa (revealer), 280.13.

1148 *Unborn, Uncontrived, Self-Arising Self-Appearing Precious Enlightened Activities Tantra,* vol. *khu,* 6b4; from *Unobstructed Enlightened Mind and Primordially Pure Self-Arising Self-Appearing Collection,* vol. *trāṃ.*

1149 Untraced.
1150 In other words, barely studying at all.
1151 *Candragarbhaparipṛcchā*, Toh 356 Kangyur, mdo sde, *ah*, 217a6.
1152 *Treasury of Wise Sayings*, chap. 3, Collected Works, *tha*, 5a4.
1153 *Shoots of Wisdom (Nītiśāstrajantupoṣanabindu)*, Toh 4329 Tengyur, lugs kyi bstan bcos, *ngo*, 109a7.
1154 *Eliminating Wrong Views*, Collected Works, *dza*, 31a2. Wording slightly different in Collected Works.
1155 *Ltar snang nad;* a disorder that has the appearance of an illness and from which the patient will recover without treatment; one of the four types of disorder.
1156 Sakya Paṇḍita, *Treasury of Wise Sayings*, chap 3, Collected Works, *tha*, 4b2.
1157 *Candragarbhaparipṛcchā*, Toh 356 Kangyur, mdo sde, *ah*, 217a2.
1158 Ibid., 217b1.
1159 *Kaliyugaparikathā*, Toh 4170 Tengyur, skyes rabs, *ge*, 192a6.
1160 Ibid., 192b1.
1161 Ibid., 193a1. The line sequence is different in Degé.
1162 *The'u brang/rang*. Type of spirit that flies through the air, or a kind of ghost (*Great Tibetan-Chinese Dictionary*, p. 1187).
1163 Orgyen Lingpa, *Five Chronicles*, Future Occurrences chapter, 517.21.
1164 *Sāgaramatiparipṛcchā*, chap. 2, Toh 152 Kangyur, mdo sde, *pa*, 18b2.
1165 *Shoots of Wisdom (Nītiśāstrajantupoṣanabindu)*, Tengyur 4329, Tengyur, lugs kyi bstan bcos, *ngo*, 105b3.
1166 The reliquary constructed for the Fifth Dalai Lama's remains.
1167 These are astrological calculations made for the purpose of determining auspicious times for medical procedures, compounding medicines, and so on.
1168 Sakya Paṇḍita, *Treasury of Wise Sayings*, chap. 3, Sakya Collection, vol. 5, 5a6.
1169 Desi Sangyé Gyatso was a great medical scholar but, as Prof. Losang Tenzin points out, he was not a qualified doctor.
1170 *Rang blos tsha grang ha lam mi 'gal lam snyam pa kha yar gtad*. I am still not sure if my understanding of the second half of this sentence is correct.
1171 Bamboo concretion, saffron, clove, nutmeg, small cardamom, and greater cardamom (Pasang and Clark).
1172 *Four Tantras*, Final Tantra, 27.666.10.
1173 *Subāhuparipṛcchā*, chap. 9, Toh 405 Kangyur, rgyud, *wa*, 135b2.
1174 *Ratnolkādhāraṇī*, Toh 145 Kangyur, mdo sde, *pa*, 69b4.
1175 *Vimalakīrtinirdeśa*, chap. 7, Toh 176 Kangyur mdo sde, *ma*, 217a2.
1176 *Pāramitāsamāsa*, chap. 4, Toh 3944 Tengyur, dbu ma, *khi*, 220a1.
1177 The whole dedication has annotations inserted in the text explaining poetical references. Here it states that this verse makes reference to the story of Kumāra pulling out the fangs of Gaṇapati.
1178 Annotation here states that the allegory is of the peahen who conceives at the sound of thunder.
1179 *Dga' ba rdzogs ldan pho brang*, which is usually written *dga' ldan pho brang* (Ganden Podang), referring to the rule over Tibet established by the Fifth Dalai Lama. Ganden usually refers to the celestial realm of Tuṣita and is an alternative name for the Geluk *(dge lugs)* tradition and of course the monastery of the same name. By inserting *rdzogs* here, the author also offers the possibility of reading the term

rdzogs ldan, which is a translation of the Sanskrit *kṛtayuga* (era of completion) or *caturyuga* (era of four), the first and best of the four eras. This is again referred to in the last line.

1180 Usually attributed to the later Yuthok Yönten Gönpo; first of the Eighteen Auxiliary Texts.

1181 Attributed to the later Yuthok.

1182 Also known as *History of Medicine: Sun that Blossoms the White Lotus.*

1183 To be identified with Jangdak Tashi Topgyal (1550–1603)

1184 This refers to his *Well-Compiled History of Medicine.*

1185 Author's name is not mentioned.

1186 According to Trinlé (p. 256) this work was composed by Namkha Delek, the uncle of Tsarong Chöjé Palden.

1187 Possibly his *Accounts from History.*

1188 Possibly by Shangtön Siji Bar. See bibliography.

1189 In other words, all the same (Prof. Losang Tenzin).

1190 The male water horse year of the twelfth sixty-year cycle is 1702, three years before he died. The *aṣaḍha* month is usually the sixth Tibetan month and corresponds to the months of July and August. The auspicious combination *('grub sbyor)* of the *śrāvana* constellation is one seven auspicious stellar combinations matched to the days of the week. Therefore, *śrāvana,* which is also the name of a month, is always linked to a Monday.

1191 Untraced. These regions (*khri skor,* literally "myriarchy," an area of around ten thousand households) were first drawn up by Drogön Chögyal Phakpa when he was appointed ruler of Tibet by Kublai Khan in the thirteenth century.

1192 According to Dungkar (p. 1533), this is to be identified with upper and lower Kyi *(skyid stod skyid smad).*

1193 An eleventh-century disciple of Marpa Lotsāwa.

1194 Although the root *ap* is usually translated as "water," rather than "ocean."

1195 Vyākaraṇa is the study of Sanskrit grammar. Explainer of All *(kun bshad)* is a title given to those competent in their studies of grammar.

1196 Vajrapāṇi, *Cakrasaṃvara Commentary,* Toh 1402, rgyud 'grel, *ba.* Commentary on the first fifty chapters of the *Shorter Cakrasaṃvara;* one of the *Three Bodhisattva Commentaries.*

1197 This is 1703. Therefore, he completed this work in a year. With this date as a fixed reference, the other dates mentioned can be calculated; e.g., Rudracakrin's coming in 2424.

1198 This is the thirteenth lunar day. The thirty days of the month share five names between them, each repeated six times. Victory *(rgyal ba)* is third in the list, and so its third occurrence is on the thirteenth.

1199 Anurādhā is the fifteenth lunar mansion.

1200 *Nyi ma me stag.* I am not sure what this refers to.

1201 I have sought to understand these astrological terms through research and questioning scholars, but it may be that some are translated literally without depth of understanding.

Materia Medica

THE CROSS-REFERENCES in this list indicate the entry or entries where the term is mentioned in the glossary that follows.

a ba. See carex sp
a la. See yellow orpiment
a ru ra. See chebulic myrobalan
a svadtha. See *aśvattha* figs
agaru. See aloe or eagle wood
akaru. See aloe or eagle wood
bā la ka, bā li ka. See *bālaka, balika, hrivera, jala, udaka*
ba lang lca ba. See bull angelica
ba ru ra. See baleric myrobalan
bal gul dza. See *avalguja*
bde ba. See *sukha*
bdud rtsi (a ru ra). See chebulic myrobalan
bdud rtsi 'o ma 'dzin pa. See ambrosia holder of milk
bhe ru ṇḍa va ṣiṭa. See *bheruṇḍaviṣṭha*
'bigs byed. See *vindhya* preparation
bong dkar. See seven female relatives
bong nga dkar po. See white aconite
bong nga nag po. See black aconite
'bra go. See date
brag shun. See mineral exudate
brag zhun. See *śaileya*
'bras bu can. See *priyaṅgu*
bu len. See *mākṣika*
bya rog. See black aloe
byang ba. See *jangwa*
bzang po drug. See six excellent medicinal plants
chu rtsa. See Himalayan rhubarb
chu shing. See plantain
cong zhi. See calcite
cu gang. See six excellent medicinal plants
da byid. See snow frog
da lis bcud len. See *dali* elixir
'dam bu mda'. See arrow-reed grass
dan rog. See castor oil plant
dar yak an. See *daryakan*
dbang po'i lag. See *markata/margada/markada*
dbang ril. See bezoars
dbyi mong. See clematis
dhā tri. See *dhātri*
dkar khra man. See banded agate
dkar po chig thub. See white powerful single medicine
dkar po mdung rtsi. See white powerful single medicine
dngul chu. See *mercury*
dngul tig. See silver spot
dpa' bo chen po. See white powerful single medicine
dpa' rgod. See zedoary
drod sman. See black pepper; pepper resin
dub dmar rdzad. See *mākṣika*
dva lis. See white rhododendron

pi pi ling. See long pepper / black medicine
pra tshil. See beeswax
pri ka. See *prika* flower
pu shel rtse. See *uśīra*
pū ti. See *putrakeśa/pūti*
pu tra ke sha. See *putrakeśa/pūti*
pu tse shel. See seven female relatives
ra dug. See goat poison
ral ba. See *relwa* ambrosia
rdo drag ga. See *śaileya*
rdul can ma. See black zedorary; *rajanī/rajasvas*
rgya mtsho'i lan tshwa. See salts
rgya shug. See Indian juniper
rgya skyeg. See *lac*
rgya spos. See *tagara/takara*
rgya tshva. See salts
rgyal blon. See king and minister medicine
rgyam tshwa. See salts
rgyan 'khor. See *gyenkhor*
ri bdag skyes. See musk
ri skyes. See *śaileya*
rmigs pa. See lizard
rnam rgyal (a ru ra). See chebulic myrobalan
rnam rgyal. See *vijaya* myrobalan
rong skyes nag po. See black valley plant
ru rta. See costus root
sa ga bhe ta. See *pakabheta* ambrosia
sa zhag. See natural ambrosia
sbal gyab. See hematite
sbal mdung ma. See *beldung ma*
sbra tshil. See beeswax
sbur len. See amber
se 'bru. See pomegranate
seng ldeng. See *khadira*
sga tig. See *gatik*
sgam bse. See *gamsé*
sgeu gsher. See wild ginger
sgog skya. See garlic
sha che (a ru ra). See chebulic myrobalan
sha dar ya kan. See flesh *daryakan* / flesh-king daryakan
sha la ki. See *silhaka/sihalaka*
sha med (a ru ra). See chebulic myrobalan
sha rgyal dar ya kan. See flesh *daryakan* / flesh-king daryakan
shing kun. See asafetida
shing sa rdzi ka. See corn smut
shog shing. See *lāṅgalī*
shu dag. See sweet flag
shug pa. See juniper
siddha mu le. See *siddhimūla*
siha la ka. See *silhaka/sihalaka*
singha mū tra. See *siṃhamūtra*
skye bdun. See seven-births compound
skyer pa. See Indian barberry
skyu ru ra. See emblic myrobalan
sle tres. See heart-leaved moonseed
sman dkar. See white radish medicine
smyo byed mda'. See *unmatta/unmādana*
smyung ba (a ru ra). See chebulic myrobalan
sne dmar. See *nemar*
sne rgod. See wild goosefoot
sngo'i bu mo sbun bdun. See seven female relatives
snyi ba. See *mṛdu*
sor mo la spyod. See *aṅgulacarya*
spang rtsi do bo. See seven female relatives
spang spos. See *māṃsa/māṃsī*
spos dkar. See sal-tree resin
spos shel. See amber
spra tshil. See beeswax
sra rtsi. See sal-tree resin
sta ri ma. See *tarima*
stag ma kha ral. See torn-mouthed rhododendron
stong zil. See seven female relatives
sug smel. See cardamom; six excellent medicinal plants
ta ma la. See *tamāla*
tar nu. See ambrosia holder of milk
thang khrom dkar po. See white powerful single medicine
thang khrom. See *datura, dhustura, unmatta*

Glossary

Sources

Butön	Butön Rinchen Drup, *Annotations on Vimalaprabhā*
Clark	Dr. Barry Clark, *The Quintessence Tantras of Tibetan Medicine*
Dash	Vaidya Bhagwan Dash, *Encyclopedia of Tibetan Medicine*
Dash 2	Vaidya Bhagwan Dash, *Tibetan Medicine with Special Reference to Yoga Śataka*
Dash 3	Vaidya Bhagwan Dash, *Materia Medica of Tibetan Medicine*
Doc	Unsourced Tibetan-English materia medica document
Drungtso	Dr. Tsering Thakchoe Drungtso, *Tibetan Medicine: The Healing Science of Tibet*
Dungkar	Dungkar Losang Trinlé. *Dungkar Tibetological Great Dictionary*
Dutt	Uday Chand Dutt, *Materia Medica of the Hindus*
GTD	*Great Tibetan-Chinese Dictionary*
Him	http://www.himalayahealthcare.com/herbfinder
Khare	C.P. Khare, Indian Medicinal Herbs
LC	Lokesh Chandra, *Tibetan-Sanskrit Dictionary*
LT	Prof. Losang Tenzin, Central Institute of Higher Tibetan Studies, Sarnath
Mon	Monier Monier-Williams, *A Sanskrit-English Dictionary*
Norbu	Kachupa Tsering Norbu, *Sman ming tshig mdzod blo gsar sgo 'byed lde mig*
Pasang	Dr. Pasang Yonten Arya, *Dictionary of Tibetan Materia Medica*
RR	Rechung Rinpoché, *Tibetan Medicine*
THDL	Tibetan and Himalayan Digital Library Preliminary Glossary of Tibetan Medical Terms: http://www.thdl.org/collections/medicine/med_glossary.html
TMI	*Rgyun du mkho gnad che ba'i nad ming dbyin bod snan sbyor,* a document put out by Tibetan Astro-Medical Institute, Dharamsala, India, listing the more important diseases in both English and Tibetan
TMP	Desi Sangyé Gyatso, *Tibetan Medical Paintings*
Trungpé	Gawai Dorjé, *'Khrungs dpe dri med shel gyi me long*

Tsarong T. J. Tsarong, *Handbook of Traditional Tibetan Drugs*
VP Synonym or translation according to Puṇḍarīka's *Vimalaprabhā* commentary on the passage in the *Condensed Kālacakra Tantra* where the listing of this medical substance occurs
Wallace Vesna Wallace, *The Inner Kālacakratantra*

abdominal dropsy *(dmu rdzings).* See *muchu*
ācārya *(slob dpon).* Title given to a learned scholar and spiritual teacher.
acidity *(skyur khu, amla drava)*
activity deity yoga *(las bsnyen)*
āgama. In Sanskrit grammar: grammatical augment or meaningless added syllable.
air spirits *(theu rang).* Kind of flying elemental *(bhūta)* or hungry ghost.
Akaniṣṭha *('og min).* Highest of the form realms.
alkali powders *(thal sman, kṣāra)*
allegorical tree of medicine *(sdong 'grems).* A way of explaining medical texts by dividing the text up into the root, trunk, branches, leaves, and fruit of a wish-fulfilling tree.
aloe or eagle wood *(agaru, akaru).* Aquilaria agallocha Roxb; *Lci med / 'ba' shig ka.* Of three kinds: white: Aquilaria sinensi Lour; black: Aquilaria agallocha Roxb; and red: Cinnamomum parthenoxylon Tack (Clark). Amyris Agallocha (Mon). Dysoxylum malabaricum (Khare).
amber *(sbur len / spos shel)*
ambrosia holder of milk *(bdud rtsi 'o ma 'dzin pa).* Synonym of Euphorbia nematocypa Hand-Mazz *(tar nu),* Fritillaria delavayi Franch and Gallium aparine L. *(zang rtsi dkar po)* (Pasang).
amnesia *(brjed byed)*
anatomical layout of the channels *(rtsa yul gyi thig)*
anatomical layout, body dimensions *(yul thig)*
angelica *(lca ba).* Angelica archangelica (Clark). Pignut or hog's fennel: Changium smyrniodes Wolff (TMP).
angelica coraka *(tsa ron / tsi rong / tso ra; coraka, dhanar, taskara).* Angelica glauca Edgw.
aṅgulacarya *(sor mo la spyod)*
anubandha. In Sanskrit grammar: indicatory letter or syllable attached to roots.
anudātta. In Sanskrit grammar: accentless, neutral, or low tone.
anuresis, dysuria *(gcin 'gags).* Inability to urinate.
anusvāra *(rje su nga ro).* In Sanskrit grammar: nasalization of previous contiguous vowel.
arrow-reed grass *('dam bu mda', śara, munja).* Saccharum Sara/Munja Roxb.
arthritis and gout *(dreg nad)*

ārya *('phags pa).* Strictly, one who has attained the path of seeing of either of the two vehicles.

asafetida *(shing kun, hiṅgu).* Ferula narthex.

aśvattha **figs.** Ficus religiosa (Dash).

atiyoga *(shin tu rnal 'byor).* The highest of nine vehicles of practice according to the Nyingma school; synonymous with Dzokchen *(rdzogs chen).* Unlike the lower vehicles, atiyoga takes the pristine nature of the primordial mind as the path.

ātmanepada. In Sanskrit grammar: form of the verb implying action belonging or reverting to oneself.

aural purgatives *(rna bshal)*

avalguja. Veronia Anthelmintica Willd (Dutt, Mon).

bālaka, balika, hrivera, jala, udaka. Coleus vettiveroides K. C. Jacob (Dash, Khare).

baleric myrobalan *(ba ru ra, bibhītakī).* Terminalia belerica.

balneology, medical bath *(lums)*

banded agate *(dkar khra man)*

bardo *(bar do).* The intermediate state of existence between death and rebirth.

beeswax *(pra tshil, sbra tshil, spra tshil; madhūcchiśṭa)*

beké *(beg/be ge).* A condition characterized as serious and infectious; another name for *sibi (sib bi)* (GTD). Possibly measles.

belch *(sgreg dri)*

beldung ma *(sbal mdung ma).* Head medicine.

bezoars *(dbang ril)*

bhāva *(dngos po).* In Sanskrit grammar: action *per se* as expressed by the verbal root. Also means "state" when defining the semantics of certain suffixes.

bheruṇḍaviṣṭha. Sweet-smelling droppings of a yellow crow-like bird (Butön).

bhṛṅga rāja, mārkava. Trailing eclipta plant, Eclipta alba Hassk (Dash 3).

birch tree *(grog ga, kṛtti).* Bark used for writing on.

black aconite *(bong nga nag po, halāhala).* Aconitum richardsonanium Lauener var, crispulum W. T. Lang (Pasang).

black aloe *(bya rog, agaru). See* aloe or eagle wood

black magic *(yad stems)*

black ***mingchen*** *(ming can nag po).* Pulicaria insignis Drumm (Pasang).

black pepper *(na le sham, drod sman, marica).* Piper nigrum.

black skin bile disorder *(sha ya nag po).* The stage of jaundice when the whole body is permeated with bile (LT).

black valley plant *(rong skyes nag po).* A plant found in shady valleys in China with leaves like tiger ears and white, red, and blue flowers.

black zedorary *(rdul can ma; rajanī niśā, rātri, haldi).* Curcuma caesia Roxb (Khare).

bloodletting instrument *(gtsag bu)*

bloodletting point in elbow joint *(ru thung)*
bloodletting, phlebotomy, venesection *(gtar ga / gtar kha)*
blue poppy *(tsher ngon; gul-e-nilam, kunda, gudi, kanderi, kalihāri).* Meconopsis horridula Hook f. et Thoms/aculeata Royle.
brain membrane *(klad rgyas)*
bull angelica *(ba lang lca ba).* Anthriscus nemerosa (M. Bieb); Spreng (Pasang); Angelica dahurica Peucedanum sp. (TMP).
bull sores *(glang shu).* Skin disease that sees the skin become covered with small, pale, soft, and itchy pustules. The swellings resemble the neck of a bull (GTD).
cakravartin *('khor lo sgyur ba'i rgyal po).* Universal emperors who rule over the four continents of a world realm and who only appear when human lifespan has increased to at least 80,000 years.
calcite *(cong zhi)*
camphor *(ga pur, kapūra).* Cinnamomun camphora: Nees and Eberm.
caṇḍālī *(gtum mo).* An inner heat produced at the navel through advanced tantric practices.
canon *(sde snod, piṭaka)*
cardamom *(sug smel; elā, truṭī, sūkṣmaila).* Elettaria Cardamomum.
carex sp *(a ba).* Lloydia serotina Reichb. An arctic lily.
castor oil plant *(dan rog).* Croton tiglium L.
catarrh, mucus *(smug po)*
cauterization *(sreg dpyad)*
cauterization tool *(me thur)*
channel cleansing *(rtsa sbyongs)*
channel openings *(rtsa mig).* The small openings in the intestine walls for the pathways of plasma.
channels
life channel *(srog rtsa),* spinal cord
white channels *(rtsa dkar),* nerves and tendons running off from spinal cord
red channels *(rtsa dmar),* pulsating veins and arteries
black channels *(rtsa nag),* non-pulsating veins and arteries
water channels *(chu rtsa),* same as white channels
wind channels *(rlung rtsa),* mostly same as white channels
charm circle *('khor lo).* Mystical diagrams drawn to produce extraordinary effects.
chebulic myrobalan *(a ru ra; abhaya haritaki, haritaka, paritaki, harita, munibhesaja, papant, visva).* Terminalia chebula Retz. Myrobalan. Of **seven types:** oval *(smyung ba),* fearless *('jigs med, abhaya),* life or golden *('tsho, jivantī),* ambrosia or fleshy *(bdud rtsi* or *sha che),* victorious *(rnam rgyal),* increase *('phel, vṛddhihari),* purity or non-fleshy *(gtsang ma* or *sha med).*
chief physician / titled physician *(lha rje)*

Chinese medical system *(krung yus)*
chiretta *(tig ta; bhūnimba, kirātta, trinimba).* Swertia chirata.
chokgyal/chokgyel *(lcog 'gyal / cog 'gyel).* Unconsciousness, collapse.
chong *(gcong).* Class of serious chronic degenerative diseases of which there are four main types.
chronic pain *(ther gzug na)*
***cittamaṇi* jewel.** A wish-fulfilling jewel.
clematis *(dbyi mong, cavya).* Clematis montana.
coca *(tso tsa).* Identified variously as apple, coconut, fan-palm, banana.
combined or dual disorder *(ldan pa)*
commitments *(dam tshig, samaya)*
compendium *('khrugs sdebs)*
compilation *(be bum)*
complete cure *(rjes gcod)*
complex or combination disorder *('dus pa)*
complications or secondary disorder *(bla gbyan).* An illness arriving on top of an existing disorder.
concoction, decoction *(thang)*
constitutional/legal document *(bca' yig)*
contraction of the stomach *(gsus chung)*
copper *(zangs / nyi ma)*
core/oral instructions *(man ngag, upadeśa)*
coriander *('u su, dhānyaka).* Coriandrum sativum.
corn smut *(shing sa rdzi ka, svarjika).* Ustilago nuda Rostr. (Clark, Pasang); sodium bicarbonate alkali preparation, *svarji kṣāra* (Dash 3).
costus root *(ru rta, kuṣṭha).* Saussurea lappa.
court physician / foremost physician *(bla sman)*
crystal *(spug, sphaṭika)*
cupping *(nad sdud pa rngab ru / rngam ru sti ba).* Technique for removing toxins through suction; performed in earlier times with a horn.
ḍākinī/ḍāka. Supernatural being, usually female, called upon to be of assistance in tantric practices.
***dali* elixir** *(da lis bcud len)*
darada, dardva. White cinnabar *(mtshal dkar)* (Butön).
daryakan *(dar yak an).* According to Pasang, a generic term of Greek origin for panacea-like medicines. There are twenty-five types. For more, see introduction, p. 3.
date *('bra go, kharju).* Polygonum convolvulus (Clark); Phoenix dactylefera (Pasang); Phoenix sylvestris (Dash 3).
datura, dhustura, unmatta *(thang phrom, thang khrom).* Datura alba, Rumpf, and Fatuosa L. (Dutt).
decoction *(khaṇḍa)*
defining characteristics *(mtshan nyid)*

demoness *('dre mo)*
deodar *(thang shing, devadaru)*. Cedrus deodara Loud.
descending cold *(grang ba thur babs)*
destructive power/forces *(mi mthun phyogs)*
dhāraṇī. Spells or mantras recited and concentrated upon to produce special effects.
dhātri. *See* emblic myrobalan
dhustura. See *datura, dhustura, unmatta*
diabetes *(gcin snyi, meha)*. Involuntary and frequent urination due to build up of phlegm (GTD).
disorder-changing *(kha bsgyur)*
dré *('dre)*. According to Bön, a personal protector or a malicious spirit who takes over a person's life. According to Buddhism, a person reborn as a spirit because of adverse circumstances at death.
dropsy. See *muchu*
drumbu *(drum bu)*. Rheumatoid arthritis (Drungtso); Rheumatism (Clark); Increase of *chuser* (serum, lymph) in the joints due to prolonged exposure to wet conditions, causing the connecting phlegm *(bad kan 'byor byed)* to weaken, resulting in the feeling and appearance of the joints being broken *(grum)* (GTD).
dual and complex disorders *(ldan 'dus pa)*
dysentery and diarrhea *(tshad 'khru)*
eight branches *(yan lag brgyad, āṣṭāṅga)*. Physical or internal disorders *(lus, kāya)*, children's disorders *(byis pa, bāla)*, women's disorders *(mo nad, mātṛ roga)*, demonic disorders *(gdon, bhūta vidyā)*, surgery for injuries from weapons or wounds *(mtshon/rma, śalyatantra)*, poisons *(dug, agada)*, remedies for aging *(rgas, jarā)*, and aphrodisiacs *(ro tsa ba, vājikaraṇa)*.
eight branches *(yan lag)*, **eleven sections** *(gnas)*, **fifteen topics** *(skabs)*, **four divisions** *(mdo)*: ways that *Four Tantras* is classified.
eight powers of medicines *(nus pa)*. Heavy *(lci)*, oily *(snum pa)*, cool *(bsil)*, blunt *(rtul ba)*, light *(yang po)*, coarse *(rtsub)*, hot *(tsha)*, and sharp *(rno ba)*.
eight śubha jewels. Eight auspicious jewels that appeared during the Vedic legend of churning of the great ocean and whose power can cure illnesses and so on.
eight worldly attitudes. Reacting with delight or despair at small occurrences of the good and bad in life: praise and criticism, gain and loss, renown and disgrace, and pleasure and pain.
elixirs *(bcud len, rasāyana)*
elixirs / essence medicine *(bcud len, rasāyana)*. The practice of extracting and isolating the powerful constituents of a substance for a particular use, such as longevity.
emblic myrobalan *(skyu ru ra; āmla/āmlakī/dhātri)*. Emblica officinalis.
emetic *(skyugs sman, sbrag/sgyags pa)*

emetics and purgatives *(rlon khrus)*
empty fever *(stong tshad)*
enema *(ni ru ha)*
epigastric region *(lhan sna'i 'og)*
epilepsy *(gza'i gdon nad, apasmāra)*
erysipelas *(me dbal)*
exceptional insight *(lhag mthong, vipaśanyā)*
extracted medicines *(rtsi sman).* E.g., musk.
familiar with medical practice *(las la gom).* Refers to a physician who has learned by observing his master's practice.
fault *(kha na ma tho ba / nyes byas, avadya)*
female stones *(mo rdo/rde'u).* Gall stones, kidney stones, urinary stones, and so on removed from the male or female body to treat similar disorders in the opposite gender.
fire and water reversal *(me chu mzlog).* Examining one patient in order to diagnose another.
first-stage edema. See *kyabap*
five ambrosias. In tantric rituals these are excrement, urine, blood, semen, and marrow. In medicine, according to Pasang, they are Sabina przewalskii Kom *(shug pa),* Rhododendron primulaeflorum Bur et franch / Rhododendron nivale Hook *(ba lu),* Artemisia sps. *(mkhan pa),* Ephedra sps. *(mtshe),* and Myricaria bracteata Rotle *('om bu).*
five cleansing therapies *(sbyong byed las lnga, pañcakarma).* Purgative *(bshal),* emetics *(skyugs),* nasal purgatives *(sna sman),* suppository *('jam rtsi),* and enema *(niruha).*
five external therapies *(dpyad lnga).* Bloodletting, venesection *(gtar ga);* cauterization, moxabustion *(me btsa');* fomentation, compress therapy, sudation *(dugs);* balneology, embrocation *(lums);* and ointments *(byugs).*
five parenchymatous or vital organs *(don lnga).* Heart *(snying),* liver *(mchin pa),* lungs *(glo ba),* spleen *(mcher),* and kidneys *(mkhal ma).*
five-garuḍa compound *(khyung lnga).* Compound of five ingredients; according to early traditions, these five were *arura,* costus root, sweet flag, black aconite, and musk.
flatulence, inflation *(sbo ldeng)*
flesh *daryakan* / flesh-king *daryakan* *(sha dar ya kan / sha rgyal dar ya kan).* One of the twenty-five types of *daryakan* ambrosia. Oxtropis reniformis PC Li. / Oxtropis microphylla (Pall) DC (Pasang), and identified as tiger flesh.
forceps *(skam pa)*
four ambrosia garlands. Untraced.
four types of disease. Fatal *(gzhan dbang bcos kyang 'chi);* spirit-caused *(kun brtags gdon nad);* not fatal if treated *(yongs grub ma bcos na 'chi);* and minor, cured without treatment *(ltar snang ma bcos).*
fumigation *(bdug)*

***gaklhok** (gag lhog).* Combination of *gagpa* and *lhokpa.* Diphtheria (Clark).

***gakpa/gakser** (gag pa / gag gzer).* Serious condition characterized by a swollen tongue and loss of voice (GTD); an infectious disease of the throat and uvula, with obstruction of the cavity as the main symptom (THDL); tonsillitis (Clark).

gallbladder *(mkhris snod)*

***gamsé** (sgam bse).* Cockroach with a foul smell.

gaṇacakra. Tantric festivity.

gandharva. Celestial musician or type of spirit that lives off smells

gaṇḍi. A thick wooden plank that when beaten produces a ringing sound; used to summon monks in a monastery.

gaṇḍola. Small Buddhist temple.

gargle therapy *(mkhur bkang ba)*

garlic *(sgog skya, laśuna).* Allium sativum.

gastroenteritis *(tshad 'khru).* Dysentery brought on by heat disorder (Drungtso).

***gatik** (sga tig).* Androsace mariae Kaniz var. Tibetica Hand Mazz. (Pasang).

general commentary on the words of the Buddha *(bka' 'grel)*

geshé *(dge bshes).* Lit. "spiritual friend." In old Tibet used as a general title for Buddhist teachers; but more recently in the Geluk tradition it is a degree awarded to monks who have passed a rigorous examination of their studies.

***girikarṇā** (= aparājitā).* Clitorea Ternatea (Mon, Dutt); = *kṣudra śvetā* (Dash). = Butterfly Pea, āsphota, kokilā, yonipuṣpa (Khare)

goat poison *(ra dug, zimpa).* Polyanthum aconite. Aconitum polyanthum (F. et G.); H-M. var. purborulum W. T. Wang (Pasang).

goiter *(lba)*

***gojé/goji** (go bye).* Semecarpus anacardium: Momordica cochinchinensis (Clark).

gold spot / golden gentian *(gser tig).* Swertia augustifolia. Swertia wolfgangiara, Swertia vacillans (Clark); Erysimum longisiliquum Hook F. (Pasang).

golden sand. A type of medicine.

***goshöl** (go shol).* No clear identification; may be a form of small pox.

***gośīrṣa** (tsan dan sa mchog).* Best type of sandalwood.

gout *(dreg nad, vāta rakta / vāta śoṇita)*

Great Perfection *(rdzog chen).* See *atiyoga*

greater cardamom. See *kakkola*

growth *('bras).* Solidification of impure blood by the winds to form tumors resembling the *vidara* fruit *('bras)* (GTD). "The *'bras* diseases arise due to a disturbance of the three humors in the stomach induced by unsuitable diet and behavior. The digestive processes are disturbed, and impure blood and *chuser* are produced. The impure blood and *chuser* enter the circulatory system and spread throughout the body. As the humors are imbalanced, the influence of imbalanced wind causes the impure blood to solidify, manifesting tumors in different parts of the body (THDL).

growth *(khong/'bras, vṛddhi/apacī).* Often tumor or cancerous growth.

guhyaka *(gsang ba pa).* Class of demigod, like *yakṣas.*

gulgak *(mgul 'gags).* Throat constriction causing loss of voice (GTD).

guṇa *(yon tan).* In Sanskrit grammar: gradation of vowel strength.

gyazer *(rgya mdzer).* Skin disease similar to warts (LT); skin disease that feels as if the skin has been pricked with nails (GTD); possibly originating in China *(rgya).*

gyenkhor *(rgyan 'khor).* Untraced.

gyugen *(rgyu rgan).* Chronic ailment of the small intestines, brought on by a fever in the intestines or poor digestion (GTD).

gyuser *(rgyu gzer atisāra).* Colic (Drungtso, Clark); serious condition characterized by pain in the intestines and diarrhea tinged with blood (GTD).

hala chokgyal *(ha la lcog 'gyal).* Demonic illness causing sudden death.

Hayagrīva *(rta mgrin).* Horse-headed tantric deity.

head compresses *(bzlum bcos)*

healer *('tsho byed)*

heart-leaved moonseed *(sle tres).* Tinospora cordifolia (Clark); Tinospora sinensis (Lour) Merr (Pasang).

hematite *(sbal gyab).* White and brown varieties.

hemorrhoids *(bzhang 'brum)*

Hevajra. A tantric meditation deity.

Himalayan rhubarb *(chu rtsa; amlaparni, pitamūli).* Rheum emodi (TMP).

Indian barberry *(skyer pa; dāru, vrahitapahla, valliphala, somāka).* Berberis aristata/asiatica (Clark).

Indian bdellium tree *(gu gul, guggulu).* Commiohora mukul (Clark); Frankincense Balsamodendron (TMP); Balsamodendron Mukul Hooker (Dutt).

Indian juniper *(rgya shug)*

individual capability *(rkyang sel).* What individual medical substances are capable of.

individually trained physician *(rjes sbyang rigs).* Physician not conferred by royal appointment.

indravāruṇi. Cucumis colocynthis, wild bitter gourd / wild cucumber (Mon, Dutt).

infectious fever *(rims nad)*

intestinal worm *(grol ma)*

iron pyrites *(mākṣika)*

jambū *('dzam bu).* Syzygium cumini (Dash); rose apple (Mon).

jangwa. Type of beetle, Mylabris phalerata (Clark).

jātisāra. Possibly Jasmine essence.

jinchung *(byin chung).* See *jinlok*

***jinlok** (byin log/ nywa log).* Condition in which the calf muscles are contorted against the shinbone; accompanied by vomiting and diarrhea (GTD, LT).

juniper *(shug pa).* Sabina recurva, Juniperus recurva, Empetrum niger (Clark); Juniperus formosana Hayata (Pasang).

***kairava* flower** *(kun da).* May refer to the white lotus flower that blossoms at night. See also *utpala.*

kakkola. Greater cardamom, Amomum sabulatum Roxb.

***kaliyuga** (brtsod ldan gyi dus).* Literally, "age of troubles." One of the four great eras described in ancient India. The length of these eras varies according to tradition.

***kangbam** (rkang 'bam).* Often translated as elephantiasis, but according to Professor Losang Tenzin, it is a disorder caused by high blood pressure affecting all joints, especially the knees, which become severely swollen.

***Kangyur** (bka' 'gyur).* The canon of Buddha's teachings translated into Tibetan.

karkoṭī/karkoṭaka. Bur cucumber. Mormordica mixta (Mon); non-fruit-bearing *khenpa (mkhan pa)* (Butön); = mugwort, Artemesia sieversiana (Clark).

kaseru. Nepalese sweet potato *(gro ma)* (Butön).

kaśeru/kaseruś. Root of Scirpus Kysoor (Mon).

***kaustubha* jewel.** Celebrated jewel worn by Krishna that arose during the Vedic churning of the ocean.

***khadira** (seng ldeng).* Acacia catechu Willd. = somavalka, gāyatri (Khare).

khaṇḍa. Decoction.

***kheldrum** (mkhal grum).* Arthritis-like disorder affecting the kidneys, knees, and other joints (LT).

king and minister medicine *(rgyal blon)*

knowledge holders *(rig 'dzin vidyādhara).* Refers to those tantric practitioners who have direct knowledge of exalted wisdom of great bliss, and who hold onto this wisdom with profound methods.

knowledge, insight realization *(rtogs pa)*

knowledge/practice of healing *(gso ba'i dpyad pa, cikitsita)*

kodrava. Grain mash.

***kośam** (ko sham pa).* Untraced.

kośātaka. Trichosanthes dioica (Mon); Luffa acutangula Roxb. (Dash); a cucumber-like ribbed gourd, = *katukoshataki* (Khare).

***kramuka** (go yu / gu yu).* Betel; Areca catechu L.

krośa. Ancient Indian measurement equivalent to five hundred armspans, or one eighth of a league *(yojana).*

kṛta. In Sanskrit grammar: primary affixes added to roots to form nouns or nominal stems *(nāmin).*

***kulika** (rigs ldan, kalkī).* Lord of the lineage.

***kumuda* flower** *(ku mu da).* See *utpala*

kuva. Said to be a type of gourd, possibly the squash.

***kyabap** (skya rbab).* Fluid disorder arising from a loss of body heat in which the skin becomes mottled and swollen. Types include *kyabap* of the lungs, liver, spleen, serum, and winds (GTD). First-stage edema or dropsy (Clark, Drungtso, and others).

***lac** (rgya skyeg, lākṣā).* Laccifer lacca Kerr (Clark).

***lado* preparation** *(la do)*

lāṅgalī. Coconut palm, cocos nucifera L. = *nārikela, tunga, skandhaphala,* (Khare). Methonia superba (Wallace); Atlercanthera sessilis (Dash); *shokshing (shog shing)* (Butön).

***langshu** (glang shu, maṇḍala).* LC; skin infections; psoriasis TMI; cutaneous eruption (Mon).

leprosy *(mdze)*

***leser** (klad gzer).* Infectious disease affecting the brain, often resulting in death (GTD); possibly meningitis.

lexicography *(mngon brjod, abhidhāna)*

***lhok/lhokpa** (lhog pa).* One of the eighteen serious conditions particularly affecting the muscles and leading to a feeling of numbness in them. General symptoms are shivering, swelling, headache, pain in the joints, bitter taste, lethargy, a depressed feeling, and incoherent speech and thought (THDL). A disease of the muscle tissue caused by an infection that is like bubbling water in appearance, hence the name, which means "bubble-like" (THDL).

lhokser. See *lhok/lhokpa*

ligament *(chu ba)*

lineage physician / physician by royal appointment *(gnang ba rigs).* Includes descendents.

lingro. Cataracts.

***lingro raling** (ling ro rwa ling).* Untraced.

***lingtok** (ling tog).* The growth of fatty deposits on the eye.

liver *(mchin pa)*

lizard *(rmigs pa).* Eremias argus.

local governor *(sde pa)*

lodestone *(khab len, jumbaka)*

***loma** (lo ma)*

long pepper / black medicine *(pi pi ling, pippalī).* Piper longum L.

loosening the back *(rked pa gcag).* Tigerskin placed on back.

lotus filament *(padma ke sar).* (Mon).

***lukmur** (lug mur).* Phlomis younghusbandii Mukerj. (Pasang); Phlomis kawaguchii Murata (Clark); wickweed (TMP).

lymph caused tumors and glandular swellings *(rmen bu, granthi)*

mākṣika. *"Stone containing flecks of gold" (gser zil gyi rdo)* (Butön); iron or copper pyrites *(bu len, dub dmar rdzad)* (Dash); pyrites (Wallace).

mālā. = *spṛkka, priyaka* (VP). Khare identifies *spṛkka* with Malabar catmint, Anisomeles malabarica L.
māṃsa/māṃsī. = *spang spos* (Butön); Nardostachys jatamansi (Dash 2); *Spang spos* = Nardostachys grandiflora (Pasang).
mandala *(khyil khor, maṇḍala)*
manu. Trigonella corniculata (Mon); According to Pasang this is a term meaning "beautiful" and is prefixed to a variety of medicines.
manufacture of medicine *(sbyor ba)*
markata/margada/markada *(dbang po'i lag).* Dactylorhiza hatagirea Soo (Pasang). = *takrā, pañcānguli.*
master/celestial physician *(lha rje)*
meaning of the term, description *(sgra don)*
medical practice *(lag len)*
medicinal incense *(phur ma).* Rather like potpourri.
medicine goddess *(sman gyi lha mo)*
memorization and recitation examination *(rgyugs)*
Menrampa *(sman ram pa).* Title awarded to learned medical scholars.
mental affliction *(nyon rmongs)*
mercury *(dngul chu)*
metrics *(sdeb sbyor, chandas)*
mica *(lhang tsher, nam mkha' las skyes, pa ṭa las skyes, abhraka)*
michü *(mid 'chus/'phyus).* Breathing disorder brought on by grief, depression, and other mental problems (GTD).
mikser *(mig ser).* Lit. "yellow eyes"; presumably a form of jaundice.
mineral exudate *(brag shun, śilājatu).* (Clark); bitumen (Pasang).
mingchen *(ming can).* Ambrosia. There are three types of this plant: black *mingchen,* Pulicaria insignis Drumm ex Dunn; little yellow *mingchen,* Chrysanthemum tatsinense Bur et Franch; and yellow *mingchen,* Cremanthodium humile Maxim (Pasang).
minor surgery, external therapies *(dpyad).* Defined in the Eighteen Auxiliary Texts as expelling and pacifying the inner disease through external means. Sometimes it means medical practice in general.
mother of pearl *(nya phyis)*
moxabustion/cauterization *(me btsa' / me rgyag)*
mṛdu *(snyi ba).* Vine with red grapes (Mon); bellflower (TMP); Codonopsis convolvulacea Kurz (Pasang).
muchu *(dmu chu/ dmu rdzings, udara).* A fluid-retention disorder or dropsy named after the demon that causes it; *mu* is one of the eight pernicious demons (GTD). Third-stage edema; a type of phlegm that afflicts all the vital and vessel organs of the body (THDL, Clark, and others).
mucus *(be snabs).* Especially in urine indicating labor.
mud-horn cupping *('dam ru). See* cupping

***munjā* reed.** Saccharum munja Roxb. = *vāna, rāmśara* (Khare).

murā. = *daidra* (VP); = Selinum Sp (Dash); = white sweet flag (Butön). Selinium monnieri L. (Khare).

musk *(gla rtsi, ri bdag skyes; kastūri)*

musk creeper *(khril shing gi gla rtsi, latā)*

myrobalan. Of three main types: chebulic, baleric, and emblic. See individual entries.

nāga *(lto phye, klu, nāga)*

nāgakesara. Mesea ferrea L. (Dash 2); Mesua Roxburghi (Mon); Stamen of the red flower of the Bombax ceiba tree (Pasang); Petals of Ironwood tree Mesua ferrea (Clark).

nāgarṣi *(klu'i drang srong).* Rishi whose practice involves nāgas.

nāmin. The nine vowels minus *a.*

nasal purgative *(sna sman)*

natural ambrosia *(sa zhag, pṛthivī pārvataka)*

neem tree *(nimba).* Azadirachta Indica (Dash/Mon); Sophora subprostrata (Pasang).

nemar *(sne dmar).* Red chenopodium, Red goosefoot, chenopodium aristatum (TMP).

Nepali illness *(bal nad).* Infectious fever said to have been spread by the Nepalese woman Halé Barma *(ha le 'bar ma),* a manifestation of Palden Lhamo (GTD).

nervous system *(dbang rtsa)*

nirguṇdi. Vitex negundo (Dash, Dutt, Him); = Five-Leafed Chaste Tree (Him, Khare).

nonmaterial *(bem min)*

novice monastic *(śramaṇera dge tshul)*

nutgrass *(gla sgang, musta).* Cyperus rotundus. Polygonum sphaerostachyum Meissn / geranium pylzowianum Maxim (Pasang).

nutmeg *(dzā ti; jātī/jātiphala)*

nyalok. See *jinlok*

nyenkhamé *(gnyan kha med).* One of the eighteen serious conditions; causes pain in the kidneys; urine and feces mixed with blood (GTD).

offering feast. Same as *gaṇacakra.*

oil massage *(bsku snye)*

ointments *(byug)*

oral instruction *(zhal shes)*

oral/whispered tradition *(snyan brgyud)*

orné *('or nad).* Second-stage edema, dropsy of the skin vesicles (Clark, Drungtso, Dash). A metabolic disorder in which the essential nutrients *(dangs ma)* and the bodily wastes (sweat, urine, etc.) are mixed up and go into the liver (THDL). Fluid disorder in which the plasma and waste are mixed because of nondigestion of food. This mixture enters the plasma routes polluting the blood, spreading to the muscles and the skin, and bringing about an increase and descent in serum (GTD).

owl-hand plant *('ug pa lag pa).* Yellow *mingchen.* See *mingchen.*

***pakabheta/kabheta* ambrosia.** *Honglen* (Pasang); *kṛṣna bhedā* (Norbu).

pancreas *(gsher ma)*

pāramitā *(phe rol tu phyin pa).* Literally, "gone beyond"; perfected state.

parasmaipāda. In Sanskrit grammar: "word for another." When the verb is conjugated by using the terminations pertaining to this *pada,* the action denoted by it is "theoretically" done "for the sake of another."

pārijāta. Celestial wish-fulfilling tree *(shing yongs 'du).*

***parūṣaka* berries.** Grewia Asiatica L. (Dash).

paṭola. Small cucumber, pointed gourd. Trichosanthes Dioeca (Mon/Khare). = *kulaka, rājiphala* (Khare).

pepper resin *(drod sman).* Black and long pepper; although the Vinaya describes *drod sman* as the resin of trees other than those listed in the text (Toh 1, *ka,* 279a3).

peripheric nerves *(phyi rtsa).* Nerves near the skin.

phala. Fruit (especially of trees).

piṇḍataka. = *piṇḍitaka* = *piṇḍitailaka* (?), Randia dumetorum Lam. (Dash 2).

planetary demonic illness *(gza' nad)*

plantain *(chu shing, kadala)*

plaster *('dam 'ching)*

pledge breaker *(dam sri).* Person who broke samaya and was reborn a spirit.

polok *(pho log).* Digestive heat goes into reverse and disturbs the organisms of the intestines; characterized by a distended stomach, severe pain, and heartburn (GTD).

pomegranate *(se 'bru).* Punica granatum.

prāṇāyāma *(srog rtsol).* Yogic practices involving breath and inner wind control.

pratimokṣa *(so sor thar pa).* The vows of "individual liberation," which includes those of monks and nuns. See the discussion in the vows section of the text.

preceptor *(mkhan po, upādhyāya)*

preliminary diagnosis *(sad mda' / nyam se)*

***prika* flower.** Possibly *spṛkka,* for which see *mālā* above.

priyaṅgu *(khre, 'bras bu can).* Dracocephalum tanguticum Maxim (Pasang); Perfumed cherry, Callicarpa macrophylla Vahl. (Dash 2 / Khare).

prognosis *(kha smar / kha dmar)*

pulse analysis *(reg pa rtsa)*

purgative *(bshal/bkru sman)*

putrakeśa/pūti. = Pongamia pinnata Merr. (Dash 2).

quiescence *(gzhi gnas, śamatha)*

rajanī/rajasvas *(rdul can ma).* Curcuma longa L. (Dash 2). *See also* turmeric

rākṣa *(srin po).* Class of demonic spirit or cannibal, often female.

reaction imbalance *(ldog rgyu).* An adverse reaction to treatment.
realgar, red orpiment *(ldong ros, śilā)* (Clark).
rectal fistula *(mtshan bar rdol ba)*
rectum *(gzhang dkar nag)*
rejuvenation *(ro tsa)*
rejuvenation and impotency *(ro tsa ba, vajikaraṇa)*
relwa **ambrosia** *(ral ba)*
restorative medicine for prevention of side effects and to reverse any adverse reaction to medicine *(kha 'dzin)*
revelatory explanation *(pra 'khrid)*
reversal suppressants *(log gnon).* Treatment given to suppress unwanted side effects of original medicine, or opposite type of treatment given when original treatment fails. *See also* reversal treatment
reversal treatment *(ja log / bya log).* Opposite treatment given when the original treatment fails. For example, giving cold-power medicine to treat a cold disorder when hot-power medicine fails.
rheumatic gout *(dreg grum)*
sādhana *(sgrub thabs).* Literally, "means of accomplishment"; a tantric daily practice ritual.
saffron *(gur kum/gum, kesara).* Crocus sativus.
śaileya *(ri skyes).* Bitumen *(brag zhun)* (Butön); Vallisneria spiralis L. (Dutt); = *rdo drag ga,* Parmelia perlata (Dash); = Parmela tinctorium Desp. (Pasang); = Parmelia saxatilis, a type of lichen (Clark).
sakong *(za rkong).* Contagious skin disease characterized by a shedding of bodily hair, itching, and the skin turning blue (GTD).
saku *(za khu).* Diabetes-related urinary disease, in which the plasma does not travel to bodily tissue but falls to the urinary bladder and is discharged with urine (GTD). Pathologically transformed urine; a harmful liquid that is produced owing to a disturbance in the digestive processes. Wrong diet and behavior leads to an increase in fat that cannot be transformed into bone tissue and descends directly to the urinary bladder. There, the mixture of urine and fat causes the formation of *saku.* There are twenty different types (THDL).
sal-tree resin *(sra rtsi / spos dkar, sāla sarjarasa/sarjaka).* Shorea robusta.
salts *(lan tshwa, lavaṇa).*
lake salt *(rgya tshva)* (Clark); Sal ammoniac (Pasang, TMP)
white salt *(lan tshwa, lavaṇa)* (Dash)
sea salt *(rgya mtsho'i lan tshwa, sāmudra lavaṇa)*
sanchal salt / halite *(kha ru tshwa, sauvarcala).* Halitum violaceum
rock salt *(rgyam tshwa)*
brown salt *(lan tshwa smug po)*
samādhi *(ting nge 'dzin).* A meditative and powerful concentration of mind.

samprasāraṇa. Mutual interchange of vowels: *i u ṛ* becoming *ya, va,* and *ra,* and vice versa.

sandalwood *(tsan dan)*

sané gaklok *(sa nad gag lhog).* Serious disease affecting cattle or humans (GTD); possibly anthrax.

śata *(me tog brgya pa).* Cabbage rose, hundred-leaved rose, provence rose, Rosa centifolia L. (Khare). Fennel, Foeniculum vulgare Mill (Dash). Anetheum sowa Kurz (Dash 2).

śaṭī. = *zur pa dkar po,* Hedychium spicatum Ham. ex Smith (Dash). = Circuma Zerumbet Roxb. (Dutt). Ginger Lily, Hedychium coronarium Koenig (Khare).

science of healing *(gso ba rig pa, cikitsā vidyā)*

science of life *(tshe yi rig byed, āyurveda)*

scripture *(gzhung lugs, lung)*

second-stage edema. See *orné*

semok *(bse mog).* A sexually transmitted disease (GTD); illness of the prostate (LT); Syphilis (TMI).

serious condition *(gnyan nad).* A condition caused by the coming together of harmful external organisms and innate internal blood organisms. There are eighteen kinds (GTD).

sertung *(gzer thung).* One of the eighteen serious conditions, characterized by bronchial inflammation.

serum *(chu ser)*

seven births *(skye ba bdun).* The flesh of one who has been a brahman for seven lives.

seven bodily constituents *(lus zungs bdun sapta dhātu)*

plasma *dangs ma (rasa).* Chyle, essence, protoplasmic substance of albumin and globulin

blood *(khrag rakta)*

flesh, muscle *(sha māṃsa)*

fat *(tshil medo)*

marrow *(rkang majjā)*

fluid, semen *(khu ba, śukra).* Could refer to hormones (LT)

bone *(rus, asthi)*

seven female relatives *(sngo'i bu mo sbun bdun)*

1. *yakyima (g.ya' kyi ma).* Pyrola incarnate / Pyrola rotundifolia / Chrysoplenium nepalense (Clark); Chrysoplenium carnosum Hook. f. et Thoms (Pasang). Also *g.ya'i bdud rtsi ma lha mo'i khrag.* Identified (GTD, p. 2616) as a synonym for *daryakan.* (Although there are twenty-five types of *daryakan,* this is not among them.)
2. *tongsil (stong zil).* Corydalis govaniana (Doc).
3. *gangā chung (gang gā chung).* Gentiana urnula H.sim; Gentiana depressa (Clark).

4. *honglen (hong len; kutki/kaṭuka/katurohiṇi).* Picrorhiza Kurroa (Doc); Lagotis yumnanensis Franch (Pasang); Picrorhiza *(= pu tse shel)* (Clark).
5. chiretta *(tig ta, bhūnimba).* Swertia chirata.
6. white aconite *(bong dkar).* Aconitum naviculare Atapf. (Clark); aconitum tanguticum (Pasang).
7. *pangtsi dowo (spang rtsi do bo).* Pterocephalus hookeri Hook.

seven-births compound *(skye bdun)*

seven-leaved tree *(lo ma bdun, saptaparṇa).* Devil's tree, Dita bark tree, Alstonia scholaris (Khare).

sharo *(sha ro).* Numbness or swelling that develops around wounds and pustules of other skin disorders.

shatrek *(sha mkhreg).* Same as *sharo.*

shazer *(sha mdzer).* White excrescence on the eyes (GTD).

siddha *(grub thob).* One accomplished in tantric practices, especially supernatural powers.

siddhi *(dngos grub).* The powers possessed by the siddha.

siddhimūla. Radish (LT); Cannabis Sativa (Pasang).

silhaka/sihalaka. Liquid amber orientalis, liquid storax, Miller (Dutt); olibanum tree (Monier); possibly *śallaki, sha la ki* = Boswellia serrata Frankincense (Him).

silver spot *(dngul tig).* Silver cerastium, Cerastium arvense (TMP).

siṃhamūtra. = *jayanti* tree (Butön).

single disorder *(rkyang pa)*

single-word examination *(mnan/gnan rgyugs).* Test on the memorization of each word of the text with no omissions or additions.

sinlang *(srin glang/glang 'thab).* "Bull-like worms"; severe stomach pains akin to being gored by a bull *(glang)* due to disturbance of the internal organisms *(srin)* (GTD); abdominal or stomach cramps (Drungtso, Clark).

śirīṣa. Siris tree, East Indian walnut, Albizzia lebbeck (Khare/Dash).

śita. White sugar.

six excellent medicinal plants *(bzang po drug)*

1. bamboo concretion *(cu gang).* (Clark); nodal silica of Bambusa textiles McClure/Calciosinter/Kaolin (Pasang).
2. saffron *(gur gum)*
3. clove *(li shi).* Syzygium aromaticum Merr. and L.M.Perry, *lavaṅga* (Dash); Eugenia aromatica Baill. (Pasang).
4. nutmeg *(dzā ti, jātiphala).* Myristica fragrans (Clark).
5. small cardamon *(sug smel).* Elettaria cardamomum. *Sūkṣmailā.* (Dash); *elā* (Dutt).
6. *kakola (ka ko la, kakkola).* Greater cardamom, Amomum subulatum Roxb (Clark, Dash). Piper cubeba L. (Dash).

six tastes *(ro drug).* Bitter *(kha ba);* astringent *(bska ba);* sour *(skyur ba);* hot, pungent, or acrid *(tsha ba);* sweet *(mngar ba);* and salty *(lan tswa ba).*

six vessel organs *(snod drug).* Large intestine *(long),* gallbladder *(mkhris snod),* small intestine *(rgyu ma),* urinary bladder *(lgang ba),* stomach *(pho ba),* endocrine system *(bsam se),* and small intestine *(rgyu ma).*

skin sores, coarse and cracked skin *(shu ba)*

smallpox and other poxes *('brum).* Serious and infectious condition, of which there are three white and three black kinds (GTD).

sneezing *(sprid)*

snow frog *(da byid).* (Clark).

Sogdian. Relating to Sogdiana, a kingdom of ancient Persia.

solidified animal bile *(gi wang / ghiu dbang / gi hang / gi wam / ghi wang; gorocanā)*

sore, abscess *(phol mig)*

spasms *(sha 'phrig)*

spinal cord *(srog rtsa dkar po, rgyungs rtsa, rgyung pa, klad gzhung, sgal klad)*

spleen *(mcher)*

spṛkka. See *mālā*

śrāvaka *(nyan thos).* Literally, "listeners"; followers of the Buddha belonging to the lesser vehicle.

stomach *(pho ba)*

stone layout *(rdel 'grems).* Examination on medicine using stones as markers

stroke *(steng grib)*

sukha *(bde ba).* Untraced but equated with *vṛddhi* (Mon); = Habernia intermedia D. Don (Khare).

sukhuk *(su khugs).*Untraced.

śukra. Generally juice of any kind; also semen.

sulphur *(mu zi; gandha, saugandhika)*

supplement *(kha skong)*

suppository / light enema *('jam rtsi / mas btang)*

suppressant *(kha gnon / mgo gnon).* When treating one humor, medicine given to prevent the other two humors from arising.

surgery *(thur ma)*

sūrya. Ulcerous growths, similar in shape and color to the sun *(sūrya),* forming in the lungs, stomach, kidneys, and liver (GTD); metastatic cancer (Clark).

svarita. In Sanskrit grammar: an intermediate tone or accent often indicated by the letter *ñ* attached to the form, e.g., *kṛñ.*

swastika *(g.yung drung)*

sweet flag *(shu dag, vacā).* Acorus calamus.

swelling *(skrang).* Noticeable swelling of the skin due to a particular disorder (GTD).

swelling and rumbling *(sbo 'khrog)*

swelling of the stomach *(spo ldeng)*

tagara/takara. = *rgya spos,* Indian Valerian, Valleriana wallichilli (Dash/Khare); = Tabernaemontana coronaria (Mon, Dutt); *rgya spos* = Melilotus suaveolens (Clark).

tamāla. Cinnamomum zeylanicum Blume (Dash 2); *khadira* tree, Xanthochymus pictorius MBh Hariv (Mon); Garcinia Xanthochymus Hook.f. (Dutt); *tamālpatra* = Cinnamomum Tamala (Khare).

tarima *(sta ri ma).* Expensive preparation; literally, "That which costs the price of a horse."

teaching, word, speech of the Buddha *(bka', buddhavacana)*

tendon *(rgyus pa)*

tetanus *('dzum kha rtseg / 'dzum ltag 'gye)*

three excretions/impurities *(dri ma gsum).* Sweat, excrement, and urine.

three humors/constituents *(nyes pa / 'du ba rnam pa gsum / skyon, dośa).* Wind *(rlung, vāyu),* bile *(mkhris pa, pitta),* and phlegm *(bad kan, kapha).*

tintirā. = *bandhūka* flower (VP). Tamarind tree, tamarindus indica L. (Dutt).

torn-mouthed rhododendron *(stag ma kha ral)*

töser *(stod gzer).* A bile illness affecting the upper part of the body brought on by excessive blood; similar to *sertung* (GTD). Described in the revealed treasure *Ambrosia Vase* as producing pain in the heart or armpits, headache, yellow eyes, and shortness of breath.

tötsang *(stod 'tshang).* Illness in which the winds gather in the upper part of the body (GTD).

trainee nun *(śikṣamāṇā dge slob ma)*

treatise *(bstan bcos)*

troublesome spirit *('gong po).* Person who fought against his lama and was reborn a spirit (Dungkar).

tuberculosis *(glo gcong zad byed)*

tumor *(skran).* Usually the term *skran* is translated as "tumor," but this may be misleading as not all types of *skran* refer to swellings. *Skran* can be defined as concretions, swellings, cysts, or blood clots. It is classified into two types, differentiated by the presence or absence of a coating (THDL). An external or internal concretion brought on by undigested waste or plasma. There are eighteen kinds (GTD).

turmeric *(yung ba; haridrā, haldi, rajanī).* Curcuma longa.

(turtle) diagrams *('khor lo).* Diagrams drawn on a template of an upside-down spread-eagled turtle, used for various divination purposes.

udumbara. Ficus racemosa L. (Dash); Ficus glomerata (Dutt).

unmatta/unmādana *(smyo byed mda').* See *datura, dhustura, unmatta.*

upadhā. In Sanskrit grammar: the penultimate vowel.

urinary bladder *(lgang ba)*

urinary stones *(rdel rde'u nad, aśmarī)*

urine retention *(gcin 'gags)*

uśīra *(pu shel rtse).* Dendrobium nobile Lind (Pasang); Vetiveria zizanioides Nash (Dash); Andropogon Muricatus (Mon); Vetiver or khus khus grass (Him).

utpala. Meconopsis, of four varieties: white, blue, yellow, and red (Clark, Pasang); blue lotus, Nelumbo nucifera (Clark); species of Nymphoea including white *kumuda,* Nymphoea lotus; blue *nilopala,* Nymphoea stellata; red *raktopala,* Nymphoea rubra (Dutt).

***Utta* roar.** Sanskrit term possibly from *uttam;* "highest tone."

vaidūrya. Beryl; precious stone associated with Medicine Buddha.

Vajrāsana. The locale where Buddha attained enlightenment, what is today the Indian town of Bodhgāya.

vidyādhara. *See* knowledge holders

***vijaya* myrobalan.** The best chebulic myrobalan.

***vindhya* preparation** *('bigs byed)*

visarga *(rnam bcad).* In Sanskrit grammar: aspiraton of the preceding vowel.

vulnerable points *(gnyan gnad)*

white aconite *(bong nga dkar po).* Aconitum tanguticum (Pasang).

white and red dysentery *(dkar shal dmar bshal)*

white leprosy / eucoderma *(sha bkra, kilāsa)*

white powerful single medicine *(dkar po chig thub).* Generally agreed to refer to a variety of medicinal plants. "Powerful single" refers to the fact that a plant of this type treats a variety of disorders. According to Pasang, examples of this type of medicinal plant are Iris goniocarpa Bakor *(koṭha),* Przewalskia tangutica Maxim *(thang khrom dkar po),* Panax ginseng C. A. Mey. *(dpa' bo chen po),* and White pyrolusite *(dkar po mdung rtsi).*

white radish medicine *(sman dkar, la phug)*

white rhododendron *(dva lis).* Rhododendron primulaeflorum Bur et Franch.

white sister *(go sring gi).* Unidentified plant.

wild ginger *(sgeu gsher).* (Clark); fresh ginger (Pasang).

wild goosefoot *(sne rgod).* Cheopodium album (Clark, TMP); Amaranthus viridis (Pasang).

wind, bile, and phlegm in a (un)balanced state *(rnam pa (ma) gyur pa)*

wolf-face wind *(rlung ce spyang).* Where the knees swell up and resemble the face of a wolf.

word/textual commentary *(tshig 'grel)*

word-by-word explanation *('bru snon/bsnan)*

yantra *('phrul 'khor / 'khrul 'khor).* Machination, magic wheel, etc. Here usually a magic diagram used for remedial purposes.

yavakṣara. Potash (Dutt, Clark); Saltpeter (Pasang); alkali from barley corn ashes (Butön); alkali preparation from Hordeum vulgare L. (Dash).

yellow flower *(me tog ser po).* Possibly marigold.

yellow orpiment *(āla, tāla).* (Mon, Wallace).

yenpa *(g.yan pa, kacchū).* Scab, itch, etc.

yugas. The four great eras described in ancient India. Their duration varies according to tradition, but thematically they describe a golden age replete with the four features of a perfect society—Dharma, wealth, pleasures, and happiness—that gradually declines and loses these features to become an era of strife and troubles. They are called, therefore, the era of completion *(rdzogs ldan, caturyuga),* the era of three *(gsum ldan, tretāyuga),* the era of two *(gnyis ldan, dvāparayuga),* and the era of troubles *(rtsod ldan, kaliyuga).*

yumo. Arrowhead expeller plant *(yu mo mde'u 'byin).* Paraquilegia microphylla Royle.

yumo. Disorder similar to dropsy, of which there are three distinct types.

zedoary *(dpa' rgod, śaṭi).* Curcuma zedoaria (Pasang).

Bibliography

A NOTE ON THIS BIBLIOGRAPHY: In *Mirror of Beryl,* Desi Sangyé Gyatso refers to an enormous number of texts. Some appear in the Tibetan canon—the *Kangyur* collection of scriptures and the *Tengyur* collection of classsical treatises—and for these, the appropriate bibliographic details have been provided, as it has for many of the Tibetan texts that are extant today. But for many of the texts he mentions, scant additional information is available elsewhere. For these texts, only the Tibetan transcription from Desi's text is provided. When a group of such titles connected to a particular author are listed only once in the book, these are here run together in single entries.

To provide the easiest access for readers, anonymous texts are listed in alphabetical order by title alongside works from the Kangyur, such as sutras and tantras. The texts that Desi mentions with known authors—whether Tibetan, Indian, or otherwise—are listed alphabetically by author name in the subsequent section. Please note that many works that are technically anonymous may be listed under the translator's name in the authored texts section. In addition, some works attributed to particular authors may also be listed under the translator's name if this was the way they were primarily identified in Desi's text.

Rather than reproduce all the text names again in the index, we have instead provided page references at the end of each entry here to indicate where the works are mentioned in the translation.

Works cited by the translator of the present volume are listed in a separate section at the end of the bibliography.

Works Cited or Mentioned by the Author

KANGYUR AND ANONYMOUS AUTHORSHIP

Abhidhana Later Tantra. Abhidhana-uttaratantra. Mngon par brjod pa'i rgyud bla ma zhes bya ba. Toh 369, rgyud 'bum *ka.* [85]

Abridged Perfection of Wisdom in Verse. Prajñāpāramitāsaṃcayagāthā. Shes rab kyi pha rol tu phyin pa sdud pa tshigs su bcad pa. Toh 13, shes phyin *ka.* [472, 479, 529n535, 551n1115]

Ākāśagarbha Sutra. Nam mkha'i snying po'i mdo. Toh 260, mdo sde *za.* [380–81]

Ambrosia Tree: The Root Tantra on Meat Elixir Preparation. Bcud lens ha sbyor rtsa ba'i rgyud bdud rtsi ljon shing. [168]

Amṛtakuṇḍalī Tantra. Kuṇḍalyamṛtahṛdayacaturtha. Bdud rtsi thab sbyor gyi snying po bzhi pa. Toh 755, rgyud 'bum *wa.*

Arising Letters: Victory in Battle Tantra. Yuddhajayanāmatantrarājasvarodaya. G.yul las rnam par rgyal ba zhes bya ba'i rgyud kyi rgyal po dbyangs 'char ba. Toh 4322, bzo rig pa *ngo.* [330, 453, 454, 504, 505]

Avataṃsaka Sutra. Buddha-avataṃsaka-nāmamahāvaipūlyasūtra. Sangs rgyas phal po che zhes bya ba shin tu rgyas pa chen po'i mdo. Toh 44, phal chen *ga.* [215, 224, 228, 404, 428, 429–32, 472]

Basic Vinaya. Vinayavastu. 'Dul ba gzhi. Toh 1, 'dul ba *ka.* [70, 79, 242, 336, 366]

Beryl Light Dhāraṇī Developing the Power of the Tathāgata Meditative Concentration. Tathāgatavaidūryaprabhānāmabalādhānasamādhi. De bzhin gshegs pa'i ting nge 'dzin gyi stobs bskyed pa vai dūr ya 'od. Toh 505. rgyud 'bum *da.* [78]

Black Īśvara Tantra. Dbang phyug nag po'i rgyud. [86, 103]

Black Yamāri Tantra. Yamārikṛṣṇakarmasarvacakrasiddhikara. Gshin rje'i gshed dgra nag po'i 'khor lo las thams cad grub par byed pa. Toh 473, rgyud 'bum *ja.* [408]

Blazing Fire Commentary. From the speech tantra of the Maheśvara tantras. [327]

Bodhisattva Basket of Scripture. Bodhisattvapiṭaka. Byang chub sems dpa'i sde snod. Toh 56, dkon brtsegs *kha/ga.* [353, 476]

Book of Kadam: Father Teachings and *Book of Kadam: Son Teachings. Bka' gdams glegs bam pha chos bu chos.* Kokonor: Mtsho sngon mi rigs dpe skrun khang, 1993. [157, 323–24, 329, 418–19]

Boxed Arrangement. Karaṇḍavyūha. Za ma tog bkod pa. Toh 116, mdo sde *ja.* [433]

Buddha Skull Tantra. Buddhakapālanāmayoginītantrarāja. Sangs rgyas thod pa zhes bya ba rnal 'byor ma'i rgyud kyi rgyal po. Toh 424, rgyud 'bum *nga.* [219]

Buddha Vairocana's Teachings on Bodhisattva Practice. Sangs rgyas rnam par snang mdzad kyis byang chub sems dpa'i sems kyi gnas bshad pa le'u bcu pa / Chos kyi rgya mo. Translated from the Chinese. Toh 256, mdo sde *za.* [365, 380]

Cakrasaṃvara/Saṃvarodaya Tantra. Śrīsaṃvarodayamahātantrarāja. Dpal sdom pa 'byung ba'i rgyud kyi rgyal po chen po / Bde mchog byung ba'i rgyud kyi rgyal po chen po. Toh 373, rgyud 'bum *kha.* [93–94, 219, 356, 434]

Candravyākaraṇa Sutra. See under Candragomin
Caraka Aṣṭavarga Great Tantra. Rgyud chen po tsa ra ka sde brgyad.
Caraka Sutra. Tsa ra ka'i mdo. Untraced. [216]
Chronicles of Ministers. Blon po'i bka' thang. See Orgyen Lingpa, *Five Chronicles.* [80, 149, 324, 486]
Chronicles of the Kings. Rgyal po'i bka' thang. See Orgyen Lingpa, *Five Chronicles.* [329–30]
Clarifying Lamp Inventory. Dkar chag sgron gsal. An index of the later Yuthok's works. [251]
Clearly Seeing Knowledge Tantra. Gcer mthong rig pa'i brgyud. [71, 501]
Collection of Aphorisms. Udānavarga. Ched du brjod pa'i tshoms. Toh 326, mdo sde *sa.* [476–77, 551n1131]
Compilation of the Enlightened Mind / Sutra Gathering All Intentions. Dgongs pa 'dus pa. Vol. 11, No. 160, *Collected Tantras of the Nyingmapa.* Thimpu: Jamyang Khyentse Rinpoche, 1973. [217]
Concise Meaning of the Dharmasaṃgīti. Sdud pa'i bsdus don.
Consecration Tantra. Rab gnas kyi rgyud. [358]
Consequence. Thal 'gyur. Untraced. [213]
Crystal Mirror Medicine Tantra. Mman gyi rgyud shel gyi me long. [87]
Cure for Rabies. Khyi dug gso thabs. Received by Atiśa from his guru Avadhūtipa in the land of Kampoché. [87]
Ḍāka Liberation. Dpa' bo 'ching grol. [207]
Ḍāka Ocean Tantra. Ḍākārṇavamahāyoginītantrarāja. Mkha' 'gro rgya mtsho rnal 'byor ma'i rgyud kyi rgyal po chen po zhes bya ba. Toh 372, rgyud 'bum *kha.* [93, 218, 336]
Dense Array Sutra. Ghanavyūhasūtra. Rgyan stug po bkod pa'i mdo. Toh 110, mdo sde *cha.*
Destruction of the Four Māras. Bdud bzhi rab bcom. [331]
Destruction of the Great Thousand Sutra. Mahāsahasrapramardana. Stong chen mo rab tu 'joms pa. Toh 558, rgyud 'bum *pha.* [84–85]
Detailed Vinaya. Vinayavibhaṅga. 'Dul ba rnam par 'byed pa. Toh 3, 'dul ba *ca–nya.* [242, 477]
Dharma Compendium. Dharmasaṃgitī. Chos yang dag par sdud pa. Toh 238, mdo sde *zha.* [228]
Differentiating Dharma and Meaning. Dharmārthavibhaṅga. Chos dang don rnam par 'byed pa. Toh 247, mdo sde *za.* [377]
Drangti Multicolored Works. Brang ti'i pod khra. [261]
Drangti Red Works. Brang ti' pod dmar. [261, 319]
Drop from the Heart of Mañjuśrī. 'Jam dpal snying gi zur thig. [102]
Eight Branches in 20,000 Fascicles. Yan lag brgyad pa bam po nyi khri ba.[70]
Eight Thousand Perfection of Wisdom Sutra. Aṣṭasāhasrikāprajñāpāramitā. Shes rab kyi pha rol tu phyin pa brgyad stong pa. Toh 12, shes phyin *ka.* [442–43]

Eighteen Ambrosia Drop Tantras. Bdud rtsi thigs pa'i rgyud bco brgyad. [87]

Encouraging the Exceptional Thought. Adhyāśayasañcodana. Lhag pa'i bsam pa bskul ba. Toh 69, dkon brtsegs *ca.* [87, 428, 438, 441]

Enlightened Qualities Ambrosia Tantras. Bdud rtsi yon tan gyi rgyud. From the *bka' brgyad* of the Mahāyoga series of the Collected Works of the Nyingma. [499]

Entering Gnosis. Ye shes la 'jug pa. [527n494]

Entering Laṅka Sutra. Laṅkāvatārasūtra. Lang kar gshegs pa'i theg pa chen po'i mdo. Toh 107, mdo sde *ca.* [123]

History. Bdud rtsi snying po'i khog 'bugs. [501]

Instruction Tantra on Eight Branches / Four Tantras: Bdud rtsi snying po yan lag brgyad pa gsang ba man ngag gi rgyud / Rgyud bzhi. A Treasure *(gter ma)* also asserted as being Transmission *(bka' ma),* or a treatise written by Indian and/or Tibetan masters. [2, 6–9, 138, 261, 262, 279, 286, 288, 289, 293, 311, 312, 318, 321, 325, 336, 351–52, 501, 507n4; ambrosia sought out, 57; auxiliary texts for understanding, 248–50; causes of doctor, 445–47, 488; characteristics of master of medicine, 445–49; companions, endeavor with regard to, 455; devotion to the master, 454–55; Drathang redaction of, 312, 321, 334–35, 337; eight branches of, 6; given to Yeshé Sung, 256, 257, 259; greatest medical work but generally spoiled, 334; and histories of medicine, 497–501; ignorant doctor, 469–71; medicinal plants collection, 481–82; medicines listed in, 3; patient, endeavoring for, 456; place where taught, 76–80, 81; and Ngawang Losang Gyatso, 325, 326; physician, nature, and types of, 457–63; reception of, 87; redaction of/commentary (Blue Beryl) on/paintings/supplement (Camphor to Cool the Burning Torment of Pain) by Desi Sangyé Gyatso, 14, 335, 337–44; redaction of by Surkar, 13, 14; revealed by Drapa Ngönshé, 191–92; science of healing, 47; *Somarāja* in, 4, 7, 247; taught by Buddha, 76, 209–28, 313, 519n543, 534n646; taught in Oḍḍiyāna, 80, 247; time in Buddha's life when taught, 81; in Transmission vs. Treasure traditions, 164; and Vairocana, 163–64, 201; various editions studied by Desi Sangyé Gyatso, 336–37; wisdom in world traditions, 456–57; as word of the Buddha, 247–48; and Yuthok Yönten, 206, 209, 247–50]

Essence of Secrets Tantra. Guhyagarbhatattvaviniścaya. Rgyud gsang ba'i snying po de kho na nyid rnam par nges pa. Toh 832, rnying rgyud *kha.* [425, 467]

Extensive Commentary on the Sutra of Liberation. Pratimokṣasūtraṭīkāvinayasamuccaya. So sor thar ba'i mdo rgya cher 'grel pa 'dul ba kun las btus pa. Toh 4106, 'dul ba *pu.* [244]

Four Branches. Yan lag bzhi ba. [336]

Four Tantras. See *Essence of Ambrosia Secret Instruction Tantra on Eight Branches*

Gaṇḍavyūhasūtra. Sdong po bkod pa. Chapter 45 of the *Avataṃsakasūtra.* [353, 384]

Garland of Core Instructions. Man ngag 'phreng ba. A Root Tantra commentary from the Sur tradition. [501]

Garland of Narrative. Sgrung 'phreng. [501]

General Rituals Secret Tantra. Sarvamaṇḍalasāmānyavidhiguhyatantra. Dkyil 'khor thams cad kyi spyi'i cho ga gsang ba'i rgyud. Toh 806, gyud 'bum *wa.* [466]

Girth of an Elephant Mahayana Sutra. Hastikakṣya. Glang po'i rtsal. Toh 207, mdo sde *tsha.* [471, 551n1111]

Great Cloud Sutra. Mahāmeghasūtra. Sprin chen po'i mdo. Toh 232/235, mdo sde *wa.* [124, 224]

Great Exposition on Medicinal Plant Preparation. Sngo sbyor chen mo. [171–72]

Great Illusion Tantra. Mahāmāyātantrarāja. Sgyu 'phrul chen po zhes bya ba'i rgyud kyi rgyal po. Toh 425, rgyud 'bum *nga.* [467]

Great Nirvana Sutra. Mahāparinirvāṇasūtra. Yongs su mya ngan las 'das pa. Toh 119, mdo sde *tha.* Translation from Chinese. [88–91, 377]

Great Peacock Tantra. Mahāmayūrīvidyārājñī. Rig sngags kyi rgyal mo rma bya chen mo. Toh 559, rgyud *pha.* [103]

Great Presentation of Atiyoga. A ti bkod pa chen po. Untraced. [212]

Great Treasury of Detailed Explanation. Mahāvibhāṣa. Bye brag bshad mdzod chen mo. [77–78, 242]

Great Treatise on Medicine. Sman dpyad chen mo. Brought by princess Weng Cheng; translated into Tibetan by Hvashang Mahādeva and Dharmakośa. [148]

Guardian of the Three Lineages Collection. Rigs gsum dgon po'i skor. [86]

Heart Sutra. Bhagavatīprajñāpāramitāhṛdaya. Shes rab kyi pha rol tu phyin pa'i snying po. Toh 21, shes phyin ka. [228]

Hevajra Root Tantra. Hevajratantrarājanāma. Kye rdo rje zhes bya ba rgyud kyi rgyalpo / Brtags gnyis pa. / Kye'i rdo rje mkha' 'gro ma dra ba'i sdom pa'i rgyud kyi rgyal po. Toh 417/418, rgyud 'bum *nga.* [390]

Hundred Prostration Abandonment Reparations. Dpang skong phyag brgya pa. Toh 267, mdo sde *ya.* [416, 545n950]

Hundred Thousand Versed Science of Healing Collection. Gso dpyad 'bum pa sde. [69, 71, 86]

Illuminating Lamp of Thirty Instructions. Sgron gsal gdams pa sum cu. [336]

Illusion-Like Samādhi Sutra. Māyopamāsamādhisūtra. Sgyu ma lta bu'i ting nge 'dzin gyi mdo. Toh 130, mdo sde *da.* [85, 377]

Illusory Net Tantra. Māyājālamahātantrarāja. Rgyud kyi rgyal po chen po sgyu 'phrul dra ba. Toh 466, rgyud 'bum *ja.* [83, 358, 467]

Instructions on the Four Categories of Chong Diseases. Cong sde gzhi'i man ngag. Handed down from Virūpa and written down by Tharpa Lotsāwa. [260]

Jewel Lamp Dhāraṇī. Ratnolkānāmadhāraṇī. Dkon mchog ta la la'i gzungs. Toh 145, mdo sde *pa.* [215, 488–89]

Mañjuśrī Root Tantra. Mañjuśrīmūlakalpa. 'Jam dpal gyi rtsa ba'i rgyud. Toh 543, rgyud 'bum *na.* [58, 123, 128, 323, 358, 383, 534–35n663]

Marvelous Eon. Ngo mtshar bskal pa ma. [331]

Māyā Tantra. Sgyu 'phrul. Untraced. [415]

Medicine Buddha Sutra. Bhagavatobhaiṣajyaguruvaidūryaprabhāsyapūrvapraṇid hānaviśeṣavistārasūtra. Bcom ldan 'das sman gyi bla bai dūr+ya'i 'od kyi sngon gyi smon lam gyi khyad par rgyas pa. Toh 504, rgyud 'bum *da.* [379]

Medicine Sutras in Eight Hundred Verses. Sman mdo brgyad brgya ba zhes bya ba theg pa chen po'i mdo. [80, 82–83]

Meeting of Father and Son Sutra. Pītaputrasamāgamasūtra. Yab dang sras mjal ba. Toh 60, dkon brtsegs *ga.* [439–40]

Mine of Jewels Sutra. Ratnākarasūtra. Dkon mchog 'byung gnas. Toh 124, mdo sde *tha.* [83]

Miscellany of Beneficial Advice and Practices. Phan byed man ngag lag len thor bu. [327]

Moon Sutra. Candrasūtra. Toh 42, sher phyin sna tshogs *ka.* [64]

Names of Mañjuśrī. Mañjuśrījñānasattvasyaparamārthanāmasaṃgīti. 'Jam dpal ye shes sems dpa'i don dam pa'i mtshan yang dag par brjod pa. Toh 360, rgyud 'bum *ka.* [218, 459]

Notes Explaining the Text of the Questions of Subāhu. Dpung bzangs kyis zhus pa'i rgyud kyi tshig gi don bshad pa'i brjed byang. Toh 2672, rgyud *thu.* [217, 527n491]

Ocean of Wealth. Dpal 'byor rgya mtsho. [216]

One Hundred Thousand Perfection of Wisdom Sutra. Śatasāhasrikāprajñā-pāramitā. Shes rab kyi pha rol tu phyin pa stong phrag brgya pa. Toh 8, shes phyin *ka.* [125, 206]

Opening the Eyes: A Lamp Dispelling Darkness. Mig 'byed mun sel sgron ma. From the tradition of Mitrayogi. [260]

Ornament of Vajra Essence Tantra. Vajrahṛdayālaṃkāratantra. Dpal rdo rje sny-ing po rgyan gyi rgyud. Toh 451, rgyud 'bum *cha.* [355–56, 358]

Overview. Stong thun. [501]

Pramāṇa Sutra. Tsad ma'i mdo. Untraced. [216]

Pratimokṣa Sutra. Pratimokṣasūtra. So sor thar ba'i mdo. Toh 2, 'dul ba *ca.* [365]

Prophecy of Aśokadatta. Aśokadattavyākaraṇa. Mya ngan med kyis byin pa lung bstan pa. Toh 76, dkon brtsegs *ca.* [428–29, 433, 441]

Prophecy of Bhadra Māyākāra. Bhadramāyākāravyākaraṇa. Sgyu ma mkhan bzang po lung bstan pa. Toh 65, dkon brtsegs *ca.* [363]

Protecting the Country. Srid bsrungs. [100]

Qualities of the Buddha Realm of Mañjuśrī. Mañjuśrībuddhakṣetraguṇavyūha. 'Jam dpal gyi sangs rgyas kyi zhing gi yon tan bkod pa. Toh 59, dkon brtsegs *ga.* [440]

Questions of Mañjuśrī. Mañjuśrīparipṛcchā. 'Jam dpal gyis dris pa. Toh 172, mdo sde *ma.* [85]

Red Ink Son and Mother Texts. Smar byang ma bu. [261]

Red Yamāri Tantra. Raktayamāritantrarāja. Gshin rje'i gshed dmar po zhes bya ba'i rgyud kyi rgyal pa. Toh 474/75, rgyud 'bum *ja.* [408]

Rising Letters Tantra. See *Arising Letters: Victory in Battle Tantra.*

Samādhi of Śūraṅgama Sutra. Śūraṅgamasamādhisūtra. Dpa' bar 'gro ba'i ting nge 'dzin. Toh 132, mdo sde *da.* [83, 224]

Saṃghāṭasūtradharmaparyāya. Zung gi mdo'i chos kyi rnam grangs. Toh 102, mdo sde *nga.* [85]

Sarasvatī Grammar Sutra. Sarasvatīvyākaraṇasūtra. Brda sprod pa dbyangs can gyi mdo. Toh 4297, sgra mdo *se.* [61, 528n507, 539n786]

Scripture on Tastes. Ro brjod pa'i gzhung. [100]

Secret Body, Speech, and Mind Tantra of Ambrosia Preparation of Medicinal Plants. Ngo sbyor bdud rtsi 'chi med gsang ba sku gsung thugs kyi rgyud. A dialogue between Mañjuśrī and four rishis. [167]

Secret Quintessence. Gsang ba'i yang tig. A commentary on *Brown Compilation* by Hvashang Mahākyinda. [168]

Secrets of All Tathāgatas. Sarvatathāgataguhyamahāguhyakośakṣayanidhadīpamahāpratapasādhanatantrajñānāścaryadyuticakra. De bzhin gshegs pa thams cad kyi gsang ba gsang ba'i mdzod chen po mi zad pa gter gyi sgron ma brtul shugs chen po bsgrub pa'i rgyud ye shes rngam pa glog gi 'khor lo. Toh 830, rnying rgyud *ka.* [467, 500n1097]

Seven Ambrosia Fasicles. Bdud rtsi bam po bdun. [336]

Seven Dharmas Requested by Avalokiteśvara. Avalokiteśvaraparipṛcchāsaptadha rmaka. Spyan ras gzigs dbang phyug gis zhus pa chos bdun pa. Toh 150, mdo sde *pa.* [438]

Seventy Chapters. Le'u bdun cu ba. Compiled from Caraka's *Illuminated Jeweled Throne Treasury Āyurveda Tantra.* [168]

Short Vinaya. Vinayakṣudrakavastu. 'Dul ba phran tshegs. Toh 6, 'dul ba *tha.* [79, 116, 242, 336]

Silver Measuring Dish of Instructions. Man ngag dngul bre. By unnamed son of Drangti Paljor Döndrup. [263, 264, 311]

Sixteen Drops of the Kadampa. Bka' gdams thig le bcu drug. [248]

Somarāja. Zla ba'i rgyal po / Sman dpyad so ma rā dza. Attributed to Nāgārjuna or Mañjuśrī but translated from the Chinese by Hvashang Mahāyāna and Vairocana. See also *Somaraja: Sman dpyad zla ba'i rgyal po.* Beijing: Mi rigs dpe skrun khang, 1985. [4, 7, 101, 149–152, 206, 247, 279, 336, 343]

Special Treatments for the Head. Mgo'i lhag chos. [172]

Supreme Ambrosia Scriptures. Bdud rtsi mchog gi gzhung lugs. Collected Works of the Nyingma, Tingkyé edition, Mahayoga Series, vol. 26, *la.* [336]

Supreme Ambrosia Tantras. Che mchog bdud rtsi rgyud. Untraced. [80]

Supreme Pledges Tantra. Dam tshig mchog gi rgyud. Untraced. [412]

Sutra Collection of Dharma. Chos kyi phung po'i mdo. Abhidharma tradition credits the compilation of this collection to Śāriputra. [222]

Sutra Dispelling the Remorse of Ajātaśatru. Ajātaśatrukaukṛtyavinodana. Ma skyes dgra'i 'gyod pa bsal ba. Toh 216, mdo sde *tsha.* [228]

Sutra of Firmly Remembering the Sacred Dharma. Saddharmasmṛtyupasthāna. Dam pa'i chos dran pa nyer gzhag. Toh 287, mdo sde *ra.* [64]

Sutra of Going Forth. Abhiniṣkramaṇasūtra. Mngon par 'byung ba'i mdo. Toh 301, mdo sde *sa.* [79, 349]

Sutra of Golden Light: King of the Supremely Victorious Sutras. Gser 'od dam pa mchog tu rnam par rgyal bar mdo sde'i rgyal po. Translated from the Chinese. Toh 555, rgyud 'bum *pa.* [71, 76, 81, 336, 514n149]

Sutra of Golden Light: Mighty King of Sutras. Suvarṇaprabhāsottamasūtrendrarāja. Gser 'od dam pa mdo sde dbang po'i rgyal po. (Two versions with the same title.) Toh 556 and 557, rgyud 'bum *pa* and *pha.* [76, 81, 336, 350, 514n149]

Sutra of Great Play. Lalitavistarasūtra. Rgya cher rol pa. Toh 95, mdo sde *kha.* [79, 476]

Sutra of Inconceivable Secrets. Tathāgatācintyaguhyanirdeśa. De bzhin gshegs pa'i gsang ba bsam gyis mi khyab pa bstan pa. Toh 47, dkon brtsegs *ka.* [476]

Sutra of Limitless Life and Gnosis. Aparimitāyurjñāna. Tshe dang ye shes dpag tu med pa. Toh 675, rgyud 'bum *ba.* [209]

Sutra of Pure Morality. Śīlasaṃyuktasūtra. Tshul khrims yang dag par ldan pa'i mdo. Toh 303, mdo sde *sa.* [365]

Sutra of Repaying the Kindness of the Skillful Buddha. Thab mkhas chen po sangs rgyas drin lan bsab pa'i mdo. Toh 353, mdo sde *ah.* Translated from the Chinese. [41–42, 46, 223, 377, 450]

Sutra of Secret Prophecies. See *King of the Teachings on the Sutras*

Sutra of the Definitive Explanation of the Buddha's Thought. Saṃdhinirmocanasūtra. Mdo sde dgongs pa nges 'grel. Toh 106, mdo sde *ca.* [228]

Sutra of the Good Eon. Bhadrakalpika. Bskal ba bzang po. Toh 94, mdo sde *ka.* [377, 479]

Sutra of the Gradual Arising of Enlightenment. Rim gyis byang chub yang dag par 'byung ba'i mdo. Untraced. [440]

Sutra of the Great Mantra Protection. Mahāmantrānudhārisūtra. Gsang sngags chen po rjes su 'dzin pa'i mdo. Toh 563, rgyud 'bum *pha.* [64]

Sutra of the Ten Levels. Daśabhūmikāsūtra. Sa bcu pa'i mdo. Twenty-sixth chapter of *Avataṃsaka Sutra.* [228]

Sutra of the Three Heaps. Triskandhakasūtra. Phung po gsum pa. Toh 284, mdo sde *ya.I* [377, 387, 542n859]

Sutra on What Is Precious to a Monk. Bhikṣupriyasūtra. Dge slong la rab tu gces pa'i mdo. Toh 302, mdo sde *sa.* [365, 377]

Sutra Requested by Candragarbha. Candragarbhaparipṛcchā. Zla ba'i snying pos zhus pa'i mdo. Toh 356, mdo sde *aḥ*. [484, 485]

Sutra Requested by the Girl Sumati. Sumatidārikāparipṛcchā. Bu mo blo gros bzang mos zhus pa. Toh 74 dkon brtsegs *ca*. [441]

Sutra Requested by the Householder Ugra. Gṛhapati-ugraparipṛcchā. Khyim bdag drag shul can gyis zhus pa. Toh 63, kon brtsegs *nga*. [385, 425–26, 440]

Sutra Requested by Kāśyapa / Kāśyapa Chapter. Kāśyapaparipṛcchāsūtra / Kāśyapaparivarta. 'Od srung gi le'u. Toh 87, dkon brtsegs *cha*. [442]

Sutra Requested by Pūrṇa. Pūrṇaparipṛcchā. Gang pos zhus pa. Toh 61, dkon brtsegs *nga*. [439]

Sutra Requested by Rāṣṭrapāla. Rāṣṭrapālaparipṛcchā. Yul 'khor skyong gis zhus pa. Toh 62, dkon brtsegs *nga*. [482]

Sutra Requested by Rishi Vyāsa. Ṛṣivyāsaparipṛcchā. Drang srong rgyas pas zhus pa'i mdo. Toh 93, dkon brtsegs *cha*. [80]

Sutra Requested by Rāṣṭrapāla. Sāgaramatiparipṛcchā. Blo gros rgya mtshos zhus pa. Toh 152, mdo sde *pha*. [482, 486]

Sutra Requested by Susthitamati Devaputra. Susthitamatidevaputraparipṛcchā. Lha'i bu blo gros rab gnas kyis zhus pa. Toh 80, dkon brtsegs *ca*. [372]

Sutra Requested by Upāli on Determining the Vinaya. Vinayaviniścaya-upāliparipṛcchā. 'Dul ba rnam par gtan la dbab pa nye bar 'khor gyis zhus pa. Toh 68, dkon brtsegs *ca*. [385–87]

Sutra Requested by Vimaladatta. Vimaladattāparipṛcchā. Dri ma med kyis byin pas zhus pa. Toh 77, dkon brtsegs *ca*. [441–42]

Sutra Teaching the Benefits of Giving. Dānānuśaṃsānirdeśa. Sbyin pa'i phan yon bstan pa. Toh 183, mdo sde *tsa*. [437–38]

Tantra of Eight Branches. Yan lag brgyad pa'i rgyud. [87]

Tantra of the Fierce and Wrathful. Ekavīrākhyāśrīcaṇḍamahāroṣaṇatantrarāja. Gtum po khro bo chen po'i rgyud kyi rgyal po dpa' bo gcig pa. Toh 431, rgyud 'bum *nga*. [85]

Tantra of the Self-Appearing Mind. Rig pa rang shar gyi rgyud. Collected Tantras of the Nyingma, vol. 10, no. 153. Thimpu: Jamyang Khyentsé Rinpoché 1973. Mtsham brgag edition, vol. 11, *da*, p. 323. [210, 413, 414, 415–16, 417]

Tantra Requested by Subāhu. Subāhuparipṛcchātantra. Dpung bzang gis zhus pa. Toh 805, rgyud 'bum *wa*. [220, 466, 488]

Tatvasaṃgraha Root Tantra. De nyid 'dus pa'i rtsa rgyud. [216]

Tārākurulullekalpa. Ku ru kulle rtogs pa. Toh. 437, rgyud *ca*. [125]

Teaching the Five Perfections Sutra. Pañcapāramitānirdeśa. Pha rol tu phyin pa lnga bstan pa. Toh 181, mdo sde *tsa*. [429]

Ten Cakra Kṣitigarbha Sutra. Daśacakrakṣitigarbhasūtra. Sa'i snying po'i 'khor lo bcu pa. Toh 239, mdo sde *zha*. [426–27, 474]

Ten Thousand Perfection of Wisdom Sutra. Daśasāhasrikāprajñāpāramitā. Shes rab kyi pha rol tu phyin pa khri pa. Toh 11, shes phyin *ga/nga*. [438]

Three Ācārya Medical Collections. A tsa rya'i gso dpyad skor gsum. [261]

Treasury of Jewels: A General Explanation of the Science of Medicine. Gso rig spyi'i rnam bshad rin chen bang mdzod. By a disciple of the Dakpo physician Karma Künphen. [499]

Treasury of Secrets. Guhyakośa. Gsang ba'i mdzod. Quoted by Saraha in his *Commentary on the Difficult Points of the Buddha Skull Tantra.* [409]

Unborn, Uncontrived Self-Arising Self-Appearing Precious Enlightened Activities Tantra. Skye med ma bcos rang byung rang shar ba rin po che phrin las kyi rgyud; found in *Unobstructed Enlightened Mind and Primordially Pure Self-Arising Self-Appearing Collection, Zang thal dang ka dag rang byung rang shar gyi chos skor,* vol. *traṃ.* [483]

Understanding the Language of All Creatures. 'Byung po thams cad kyi skad shes pa. [110]

Universal Emperor Compilation. 'Khor lo rgyal po be bum. A Shangshung text. [336]

Vairocana Enlightenment Sutra. Mahāvairocanābhisaṃbodhivikurvitādhiṣṭānavaipulyasūtrendrarājanāmadharmaparyāya. Rnam par snang mdzad chen po mngon par rdzogs par byang chub pa rnam par sprul pa byin gyis rlob pa shin tu rgyas pa mdo sde'i dbang po'i rgyal po. Toh 494, gyud 'bum *tha.* [80, 218]

Vajra Essence Ornament Tantra. Vajrahṛdayālaṃkaratantra. Rdo rje snying po'i rgyan gyi rgyud. Toh 451, rgyud 'bum *cha.* [209, 220, 408]

Vajra Garland Tantra. Vajramālābhidhānamahāyogatantrasarvatantrahṛdayarahasyavibhaṅganāma. Rnal 'byor chen po'i rgyud dpal rdo rje phreng ba mngon par brjod pa rgyud thams cad kyi snying po gsang ba rnam par phye ba. Toh 445, rgyud 'bum *ca.* [209, 356, 358, 392, 465]

Vajra Gnosis Compendium Tantra. Vajrajñānasamuccaya. Ye shes rdo rje kun las btus pa. Toh 447, rgyud 'bum *ca.* [216–17, 220]

Vajraḍāka Tantra. Vajraḍākanāmamahātantrarāja. Rgyud kyi rgyal po chen po dpal rdo rje mkha' 'gro zhes bya ba. Toh 370, rgyud 'bum *kha.* [91–93, 336, 466–67]

Vajrapañjara Tantra. Ḍākinīvajrapañjaranāmamahātantrarājākalpa. Mkha 'gro ma rdo rje gur zhes bya ba'i rgyud kyi rgyal po chen po'i brtag pa. Toh 419, rgyud 'bum *nga.* [355, 356, 383, 408]

Vajraśekhara Tantra. Vajraśekharamahāguhyayogatantra. Gsang ba rnal 'byor chen po' rgyud rdo rje rtse mo. Toh 480, rgyud 'bum *nya.* [61–62, 383, 393, 395, 396–400, 408, 411, 467]

Vajravārahī Tantra. Ḍākinīsarvacittādvayācintyajñānavajravarāhyabhibhavatantrarāja. Mkha' 'gro ma thams cad kyi thugs gnyis su med pa bsam gyis mi khyab pa'i ye shes rdo rje phag mo mngon par 'byung ba'i rgyud kyi rgyal po. Toh 378, rgyud 'bum *ga.* [217]

Vidyottama-mahātantra. Rig pa mchog gi rgyud chen po. Toh 746, rgyud 'bum *dza.*

Vimalagutra Medical Collection in 72,000 Chapters. Bi ma la bu tra le'u bdun khri nyis stong. [70]

Vimalakīrti Sutra. Vimalakīrtinirdeśa. Dri ma med par grags pas bstan pa. Toh 176, mdo sde *ma.* [489]

Wheel of the Great Chariot of Limbs. Yan lag shing chen 'khor lo. [171]

White Lotus of Compassion. Karuṇāpuṇḍarīka. Snying rje pad ma dkar po. Toh 112, mdo sde *cha.* [377]

Wondrous Eon. Rmad byung bskal pa ma. [331]

Yoga Equal to All Buddhas Later Tantra. Sarvabuddhasamāyogaḍākinījāla-saṃvaranāma-uttaratantra. Sangs rgyas thams cad dang mnyam par sbyor ba mkha' 'gro ma sgyu ma bde ba'i mchog ces bya ba'i rgyud phyi ma. Toh 366, rgyud 'bum *ka.* [85, 392]

Authored texts

The author marked with an asterisk (*) below has many aliases, including Pitṛceṭa, Mātṛceṭa, Śūra, and Aśvaghoṣa, among others. As the author of *Essence* (or *Treatise*) *of Eight Branches,* he is identified in Sanskrit literature as Vāgbhaṭa.

Abhyākaragupta. *Lesser Stalks of Oral Instruction. Man ngag chung ba.* [391]

———. *Ornament to the Thought of the Buddha. Munimatālaṃkara. Thub pa'i dgongs pa'i rgyan.* Toh 3903, dbu ma *a.* [376]

———. *Stalks of Oral Instruction. Śrīsaṃpuṭatantrarājaṭīkāmnāyamañjarī. Dpal yang dag par sbyor ba'i rgyud kyi rgyal po'i rgya cher 'grel pa man ngag gi snye ma zhes bya ba.* Toh 1198, rgyud *cha.*

———. *Vajra Garland of Mandala Rituals. Vajrāvalīnāmamaṇḍalasādhana. Dkyil 'khor gyi cho ga rdo rje phreng ba.* Toh 3140, rgyud *phu.* [357–58, 401, 402]

Achö. *Treatment of Wounds of the Head. Mgo sogs rma yi bcos pa.* [267]

Amarasiṃha. *Treasury of Immortality. Amarakoṣa. 'Chi ba med pa'i mdzod.* Toh 4299, sgra mdo *se.* [453]

Ānandagarbha. *Commentary on the Illusory Net Tantra. Māyājālamahātantra-rājaṭīkā-ākhyā. Rgyud kyi rgyal po chen po sgyul 'phrul dra ba'i rgya cher bshad pa.* Toh 2513, rgyud *i.* [355]

———. *Sarvavajrodaya Vajradhātu Mandala Ritual. Vajradhātumahāmaṇḍala-vidhisarvavajrodaya. Rdo rje dbyings kyi dkyil 'khor chen po'i cho ga rdo rje thams cad byung ba.* Toh 2516, rgyud 'grel *ku.* [401]

Anara/Ānanda (Nepalese or Central Indian). *Three Translocations. Gnas bsgyur gsum pa.* [144, 169]

Anupamarakṣita. *Commentary to Names of Mañjuśrī. Mañjuśrīnāmasaṃgītya-*

mṛtabindupradīpālokavṛtti. 'Jam dpal gyi mtshan yang dag par brjod pa'i 'grel pa bdud rtsi'i thig pa sgron ma gsal ba. Toh 1396, rgyud *pha.*

Āryadeva. *Essentials of the Mandala Rite of the Four Seat Tantra. Śrīcatuḥpīṭhatantrarājamaṇḍalavidhisārasamuccaya. Rgyud kyi rgyal po dpal gdan bzhi pa zhes bya ba'i dkyil 'khor gyi cho ga snying po mdor bsags pa.* Toh 1613, rgyud *ya.* [357]

———. *Four Hundred Verses. Catuḥśatakaśāstrakārika. Bstan bcos bzhi brgya pa zhes bya ba'i tshig le'ur byas pa.* Toh 3846, dbu ma *tsha.* [468]

Asaṇga. *Ascertainment from Stages of the Yogacaryā. Yogacaryābhūmiviniścayasaṃgraha. Rnal 'byor spyod pa'i sa rnam par gtan la dbab pa bsdu ba.* Toh 4038, sems tsam *zhi.* [42, 225, 240–41, 245]

———. *Commentary to the Sutra Unraveling the Intent of the Buddha. Saṃdhinirmocanabhāṣya. Dgongs pa nges par 'grel pa'i rnam par bshad pa.* Toh 3981, mdo 'grel *ngi.* [243]

———. *Compendium of the Mahayana. Mahāyānasaṃgraha. Theg pa chen po bsdus pa.* Toh 4048, sems tsam *ri.* [243, 379]

———. *Compendium on Abhidharma. Abhidharmasamuccaya. Chos mngon pa kun las btus pa.* Toh 4049, sems tsam *ri.* [243]

———. *Stages of the Bodhisattva from Stages of the Yogacaryā. Yogacaryābhūmaubodhisattvabhūmi. Byang chub sems dpa'i sa'i gzhi'i rnal 'byor gyi gnas.* Toh 4037, sems tsam *wi.* [42–45, 46, 374, 375, 379, 381, 471]

———. *Stages of Yogacaryā. Yogacaryābhūmi. Rnal 'byor spyod pa'i sa.* Toh 4035, sems tsam *tshi.* [46]

Aśvaghoṣa.* *Compilation of Vajrayana Root Downfalls. Vajrayānamūlāpattisaṃgraha. Rdo rje theg pa rtsa ba'i ltung ba bsdus pa.* Toh 2478, rgyud *zi.* [138, 403–4, 405–7, 409, 410, 411]

———. *Engaging in Eight Branches. Yan lag brgyad pa la 'jug pa.* [138, 143]

———. *Extensive Exposition of Eight Branches. Yan lag brgyad pa chen po.* [138, 143]

———. *Fifty Verses on the Guru. Gurupañcāśikā. Bla ma lnga bcu pa.* Toh 3721, rgyud *tshu.* [389, 465]

———. *Garland of Past Lives. Jātakamālā. Skyes pa'i rabs kyi rgyud.* Toh 4150, skyes rabs *hu.* [138, 475, 477]

———. *Praise of the Praiseworthy. Varṇārhavarṇebhagavatobuddhasyastotreaśakyastavanāma. Sangs rgyas bcom ldan 'das la bstod pa bsngags par 'os pa bsngags pa las bstod par mi nus yar bstod pa zhes bya ba.* Toh 1138, bstod tshogs *ka.* [138]

Aśvinīputra (from the Fortunate Eon Deva Tradition). *Siddhasāra Saṃhita. Gces grub pa.* [102]

Atiśa, revealer. *King's Chronicle Extracted from a Pillar. Rgyal po bka' chems ka khol ma.* History attributed to King Songtsen Gampo. [483]

———. *Light on the Path. Bodhipathapradīpa. Byang chub lam gyi sgron ma.* Toh 3947, dbu ma *khi.* [376, 385]

Atiśa Dīpaṃkara and Naktso Lotsāwa, translators. *Daryakan Ambrosia Meat Preparations (Sha sbyor bdud rtsi dar ya kan); Net of Treatments for the Head (Mgo dpyad dra ba sdom pa).* [171]

Avalokiteśvara. *Treating Infectious Bile and Poisons. Mkhris rims dug thabs gso ba.* Taught to Tārā. [168]

Avalokiteśvara (from the Bodhisattva Tradition). *Clear Mirror (Gsal byed me long); Clearly Understanding on Seeing (Mthong ba don gsal); Drop of Ambrosia (Bdud rtsi thigs pa); Essential Surgery (Dpyad gces gzungs); Greater and Lesser Stream of Ambrosia (Bdud rtsi chu rgyun che chung); Greater and Lesser Commentary on Fundamental Topics (Gal mdo'i 'grel ba che chung); Red and Black Treatise on the Abdomen (Byang khog 'grel ba dmar nag); Supreme Adornment (Rgyan dam pa); Supreme Victory Standard: Treatise on Head Ailments (Mgo bcos rgyal mtshan dam pa).* [101–2]

Balmen Karnak. *Treatments for Stones. Rde ma'i bcos.* [267]

Balmen Nyima Pal. *Wish-Fulfilling Jewel of Essentials. Gces bsdus yid bzhin norbu.* [263]

Bari Lotsāwa. *Miscellaneous Knowledge Collection (Rig pa'i thor bu 'bum); Small Collection on Knowledge (Rig pa 'bum chung).* [260, 268]

Barmenpa (Parmenpa). *Bag of Instructions for Entering. 'Jug khug ma.* [260]

Bhalipa (Vyādipāda). *Treatise on Mercury Preparation. Rasasiddhiśāstranāma. Dngul chu grub pa'i bstan bcos.* Toh 4313, bzo rig pa *ngo.* [304–5, 336]

Bharadhaja, translator. *Bushak Divided into Wind, Bile, and Phlegm: Extensive and Short Exposition (Rlung mkhris bad kan gsum du phye ba'i 'bu shag ma bu); Fresh Ghee Preparation (Sbyor bar mar gsar).* [148]

Bharo of Amputated Hand / Puruṣa Agnideva. *Blue Compilation of Children's Disorders. Chung dpyad be bum sngon po.* [260]

———. *Fistful Collection. 'Bum khu tshur.* Beijing: Mi rigs dpe skrun khang, 2006. [260]

———. *Outer, Inner, and Secret Stone-Removal Collection. Rde [dhe] skor phyi nang gsang gsum.* [260]

———. *Whispered Tradition Black Compilation. Snyan brgyud be bum nag po.* Beijing: Mi rigs dpe skrun khang, 2006. [260]

Bhavabhadra. *Commentary to the Vajraḍāka Tantra. Vajraḍākanāmamahātantrarājāvivṛtti. Rgyud kyi rgyal po chen po dpal rdo rje mkha' 'gro zhes bya ba'i rnam par bshad pa.* Toh 1415, rgyud *tsha.* [355]

Bhāvaviveka. *Blaze of Reasoning. Madhyamakahṛdayavṛttitarkajvālā. Dbu ma'i snying po'i 'grel pa rtog ge 'bar ba.* Toh 3856, dbu ma *dza.* [62, 380]

Biji. *See* Tsenpashila[ha]

Biji Leklo / Chejé Gyalwa. *Essentials of Knowledge. Rig byed don bsdus.* [266]

Bodhibhadra. *Commentary to Twenty Verses on the Bodhisattva Vows. Bodhi-*

sattvasaṃvaravimśakapañjikā. Byang chub sems dpa'i sdom pa nyi shu pa'i dka' 'grel. Toh 4083, sems tsam *hi.* [379]

Bodong Choklé Namgyal. *Compendium of Reality. De nyid 'dus pa / dpal de kho na nyid 'dus pa'i chos spyod rab tu gsal ba.* Collected Works, *traṁ.* Delhi: Tibet House, d.u. [215]

Bönlep. *Compilation of Various Teachings. Man ngag sna tshogs bsdus.* [267]

Bönpo Draktsal. *Ambrosia Vase of Healing (Bdud rtsi bum pa); Four Great Perfection Gurus (Rdzogs chen gu ru bzhi ba).* [175]

Brahmā (from the Fortunate Eon Deva Tradition). *Guhyagarbha Saṃhita (Gsang ba snying po don bsdus); Guṇaśāstra (Gu ṇa sha skra'i rgyud).* [102]

Brahmaputra Hāsavajra. *Essence of Āyurveda. Āyurvedasarvasvasārasaṃgraha. Tshe'i rig byed mtha' dag gi snying po bsdus pa.* Toh 4438, sna tshogs *no.* [327]

Buddhaguhya. *Brief Commentary on Tantra Requested by Subāhu. Subāhuparipṛcchānāmatantrapiṇḍārtha. Dpung bzang gis zhus pa rgyud kyi bsdus pa'i don.* Toh 2671, rgyud *thu.*

Buddhaśrījñāna. *Commentary on the Collected Verses. Sañcayagāthāpañjikā. Sdud pa tshigs su bcad pa'i dka' 'grel.* Toh 3798, shes phyin *nya.* [244]

Butön Rinpoché. *Analysis of the Vinaya Sutra Elucidation of the Essence of the Ocean of Vinaya: 'Dul ba mdo'i rnam par 'byed pa rgya 'dul ba'i mtsho'i snying po rab tu gsal bar byed pa.* Lhasa Shöl Collected Works *zha.* [421–22]

———. *General Presentation on the Tantras: Shedding Light on the Secrets of All Classes of Tantra. Rgyud sde spyi'i rnam bzhag rgyud sde thams cad kyi gsang ba gsal bar byed pa.* Lhasa Shöl Collected Works, *ba.* Delhi: Lokesh Chandra, 1971. [214]

———. *Eliminating Wrong Views. Lta ba ngan sel.* Lhasa Shöl Collected Works *dza.* [484]

———. *History of the Dharma: Clarity on the Doctrine of the Sugata, a Treasury of Precious Teachings. Bde bar gshegs pa'i gsal byed chos kyi 'byung gnas gsung rab rin po che'i mdzod.* Kokonor: Mtsho sngon mi rigs dpe skrung khang, 2004. [77–78]

Candragomin. *Candravyākaraṇasūtra. Lung ston tsandra pa'i mdo.* Toh 4269, sgra mdo *re.* [216]

———. *Drama: Beloved by the World. Lokānandanāṭaka. 'Jig rten kun du dga' ba'i zlos gar.* Toh 4153, skyes rabs *u.* [244]

———. *Twenty Verses on the Bodhisattva Vow. Bodhisattvasaṃvaraviṃśaka. Byang chub sems dpa'i sdom pa nyi shu pa.* Toh 4081, sems tsam *hi.* [358, 375, 380, 382]

Candrakīrti. *Bright Lamp. Pradīpodyotananāmaṭīkā. Sgron ma gsal bar byed pa zhes bya ba'i rgya cher bshad.* Toh 1785, rgyud 'grel *ha.* [63, 84]

———. *Commentary on Four Hundred Verses. Bodhisattvayogācāracatuḥśatakaṭīkā. Byang chub sems dpa'i rnal 'byor spyod pa bzhi brgya pa'i rgya cher 'grel pa.* Toh 3865, dbu ma *ya.* [358–59]

Candranandana. *Lexicon of Medical Terms from the Commentary on the Essence of Eight Branches. Vaidyāṣṭāṅgahṛdayavṛttaubheṣajanāmaparyāyanāma. Sman dpyad yan lag brgyad pa'i snying po'i 'grel pa las sman gyi min gis rnam grangs zhes bya ba/sgra sbyor nges pa.* Toh 4309, gso rig pa *he.* [8, 143, 144, 173, 311]

———. *Moonlight: A Commentary on the Essence of Eight Branches. Padārtha-candrikāprabhāsanāma-aṣṭāṅgahṛdayavivṛtti. Yan lag brgyad pa'i snying po'i rnam par 'grel pa tshig don gyi zla zer zhes bya ba.* Toh 4312, gso rig pa *ko.* [5, 61, 143, 144, 170, 205, 246, 279, 311, 336, 340, 344, 443]

Caraka. *Eight Caraka Collections (Caraka Aṣṭavarga; tsa ra ka sde brgyad)* attributed to the eight human rishis: *Ambrosia Accomplishment Collection (Bdud rtsi sgrub pa'i sde); Āyurveda Tantra: An Illuminated Treasury of Jewels (Tshe'i rig byed kyi rgyud rin po che khri mdzod 'od ldan); Box of Life Collection (Srog gi sgrom bu'i sde); Carved Collection (Rkos gdab pa'i sde); Fundamentals Collection (Gzhi sgrub pa'i sde); Great Ambrosia Collection (Bdud rtsi chen po'i sde); Preparation of Medicine Collection (Gso dpyad sman sbyor gyi sde); Weapons of Fearlessness Collection (Mi 'jigs mtshon cha'i sde).* [2, 6, 86, 87, 102–3, 144, 148, 168, 350–51, 352, 459, 462, 468]

Chakdor Gönpo. *Precious Garland Quintessence of Medicine. Man gyi gces bsdus rin chen 'phreng ba.* [321]

Chakmen Rinchen Gyaltsen and Shakya Yeshé. *Pearl Garland Compilation of Instructions* or *Fistful Collection. Phyogs bsgrigs mu tig 'phreng ba / 'Bum khu tshur.* [260]

Changmen Sangyé Gönpo. *Thirty-Two Instructions of the Fistful Collection. 'Bum khu tshur gdams oa sum cu ba.* [260]

Chejé Gyalwa. *Charms. Rten 'brel.* [266] *See also* Biji Leklo

Chejé Śākya Pal. *Moonlight Flower Commentary to the First Chapter. Le'u dang po'i ṭikka zla zer me tog.* [264]

Chejé Shangtön Shikpo. *Compendium of Knowledge Blazing from the Top of a Victory Banner (Shes bya spyi'i khog 'bugs rgyal mtshan rtser 'bar); Drop of Ambrosia Direct Instruction on Practice in the Manner of an Old Woman Pointing Her Finger (Lag len mar khrid rgan mo mdzub tshugs kyi tshul du 'chad pa bdud rtsi thigs pa); Illuminating Beacon (Gsal byed sgron ma); Meteor Destruction of the Hindrance of Difficulties and Doubts (Dka'tshom gegs sel gnam lcags 'khor lo); Outline: A Key to Open the Content (Sa bcad don 'khrigs 'byed pa'i lde mig); The Pearl Garland: A Detailed and Extensive Word Commentary (Tshig don zhib rgyas su 'grel bam mu tig gi 'phreng ba).* [129, 170, 267, 501]

Cheyu Sher. *Brown Casket Branch Treasure. Yan lag gter sgrom smug po.* [189]

Chikmen Gawo. *Extensive Work on Medical Plant Preparation (Sngo sbyor che); Words of a Simpleton (Man ngag blun tshig).* [267, 269]

Chim Jampaiyang. *Ornament to Commentary on Abhidharmakośa. Chos mngon mdzod kyi 'grel ba'i rgyan.* Delhi: Loseling Library, 1988. [422]

Chipa Palgön Dorjé. *Commentary to the Explanatory Medical Tantra: Light Rays of Validity Radiating Afar. Bshad rgyud kyi 'grel pa 'thad ldan 'od zer rab tu 'phro ba.* [260]

Chomden Rikpai Raldri. *Commentary to Compendium of Knowledge (Chos mngon pa kun las btus pa'i rgyan gyi me tog); Flower Ornament Medical Text (Gso dpyad rgyan gyi me tog).* [225, 264, 268]

Chösé. *Jewel Heap of Miscellany. Kha 'thor rin chen spung.* [266]

Dampa. *Eighty Charms. Rten 'brel brgyad cu.* [267]

Dampa Marpo. *See* Trülku Dampa Marpo

Dānadāsa. *The Remedies of Dānadāsa. Āryadeśaphahabhiṣagdānadāsabheṣajasaṃskāra. 'Phags yul pha ha'i sman pa da na da sa'i sman bcos.* Toh 4439, sna tshogs *no.* [327]

Daṇḍin. *Mirror of Poetics. Kāvyādarśa. Nyan ngag me long ma.* Toh 4301, sgra mdo *se.* [244, 245, 314, 361, 536n687]

———. *Wheel of Samantrabhadra. Samantabhadracakra. Kun bzang 'khor lo.* A subsection of the *Mirror of Poetics.* [330]

Darma Drak. *Collection on Urine and Pulse. Rtsa chu'i skor.* [267]

Darma Gönpo. *Essential Instructions (Zin tig); Quintessential Instructions (Yang tig).* [170–71]

Darmo Menrampa. *Biography of Yuthok the Elder and the Younger. G.yu thog gsar rnying gi rnam thar.* Kokonor: Mtsho sngon mi rigs dpe skrun khang, 2005. Also Beijing: Mi rigs dpe skrun khang, 1982. Translated in Rechung Rinpoche, *Tibetan Medicine* (Delhi: Sri Satguru Publications, 2001). [535n681]

———. *Brilliant Jewel Treasury: The Sealed Manuscript Biography of the Elder Noble Yuthok Yönten Gönpo. Rje btsun g.yu thog yon tan mgon po rnying ma'i rnam par thar pa bka' rgya ma gzi brjid rin po che'i gter mdzod.* From *Biography of Yuthok the Elder and the Younger.* [2, 202]

———. *Biography of the Younger Yuthok Yönten Gönpo: Personification of the Wisdom and Compasssion of the Buddhas of the Three Times and Their Bodhisattva Princes Who Has Traveled to the Further Shore of Scholarship and Practice; Master of a Hundred Buddha Families. Dus gsum gyi rgyal ba sras dang bcas kyi mkhyen brtse'i spyi gzugs mkhas pa dang grub pa'i pha rol tu son pa rigs brgya'i khab bdag g.yu thog gsar ma yon tan mgon po'i rnam par thar ba.* From *Biography of Yuthok the Elder and the Younger.* [206, 208, 254–55]

Darmo Menrampa Losang Chödrak, Mermo Lodrö Chöpel, and Larawa Losang Dönden. *Golden Ornament of Excellent Explanation. Legs bshad gser rgyan.* [328]

Darmo Menrampa Losang Chödrak and Namling Panchen. *Loosening the Vajra Knots. Rdo rje mdud 'grol.* [328]

Darseng Gönpo. *Treatments. Bcos kha.* [265]

Dawa Shönu. *Essence of Eight Branches. Brgyad pa'i don bsdus.* [267]

Depa Rongtso. *Garland of Ambrosia Drops: Abridgement of Profound Instructions (Man ngag zab bsdus bdud rtsi thigs 'phreng); Mandala of Wisdom (Rig pa'i 'khor lo).* [321]

Desi Sangyé Gyatso. *Cleaning the Dirt from Vaidūrya to Reveal Its True Face. Bai dūrya g.ya' sel don gyi bzhin ras ston byed.* Collected Works of Desi Sangyé Gyatso, vol. 4. [129]

———. *Answers to the Questions: The Arrow of Arjuna that Illuminates the True Flight. Dri lan nam gsal byed drang thig srid sgrub kyi mda'.* [345]

———. *Camphor to Cool the Burning Torment of Pain: A Sword to Cut the Noose of Untimely Death; Supplementary Material to the Core Instruction or Enlightened Qualities Tantra. Man ngag yon tan rgyud kyi lhan thabs zug rngu'i tsha gdung sel ba'i kar pū ra dus min 'chi zhags bcod pa'i ral gri.* Leh: T. S. Tashigangpa, 1978. Vol. 7 of Potala Collected Works. [344]

———. *Ornament to the Mind of Medicine Buddha: Blue Beryl Lamp Illuminating Four Tantras. Sman bla'i dgongs rgyan rgud bzhi'i gsal byed bai dūrya sngon po'i ma lli ka.* Leh: T. S. Tashigangpa, 1974. [14, 21, 337–44, 345]

———. *White Beryl. Phug lugs rtsis kyi legs bshad mkhas pa'i mgul rgyan bai dūrya dkar po'i do shal dpyod ldan snying nor.* Zi ling: Krung po bod kyi shes rig dpe skrun khang, 1996. [14, 64]

Deva Sarvajña. *Blazing Like Fire (Me ltar 'bar ba); Matted Hair (Skra shad 'dzings pa); Mountain Stack (Ri bo brtsegs pa); Vajra Voice (Rdo rje kha smra).* [103]

Devacandra. *Ambrosia Drop Oral Transmission. Snyan rgyud bdud rtsi'i thigs pa.* [175]

Dharmakīrti. *Ascertaining Valid Cognition. Pramāṇaviniścaya. Tshad ma rnam par nges pa.* Toh 4211, tshad ma *ce.* [242]

———. *Treatise of Valid Cognition. Pramāṇavārttikakārikā. Tshad ma rnam 'grel gyi tshig le'ur byas pa.* Toh 4210, tshad ma *ce.* [57–58, 403]

Dharmamitra. *Clear Words Commentary to Ornament of Realization. Abhisamayālaṃkārakārikā-prajñāpāramitopadeśaśāstraṭīkā-prasphuṭapadā. Shes rab kyi pha rol tu phyin pa'i man ngag gi bstan bcos mngon par rtogs pa'i rgyan gyi tshig le'ur byas pa'i 'grel bshad tshig rab tu gsal ba.* Toh 3796, shes phyin *nya.* [223]

Dharmapāla. *Collection on Knowledge. Rig pa 'bum.* [264]

Dharmarāja, Hvashang Mahākyinda, and Tsenpashilaha (the three manifested sons), translators and compilers of Indian, Chinese, and Taksik texts. The collection on internal diseases, a.k.a. the twenty-seven short commentaries: *Ambrosia Drop of Cauterization (Me btsa' bdud rtsi'i thigs pa); Bushak Copper Vase Medical Lexicon (Sman ming 'bu shag zangs kyi bum pa); Commentary on the Healing of the Three Roots of Disease (Nad gzhi gsum gso thabs kyi 'grel ba); Compilation of Medicine Places (Sman gnas mdor bsdus); Conch Pus Cleanser (Rnag bshal dung gi phyags shing); Eye of the Conch Illustrations ('Dra yig dung gi mig); Fire and Water Needles of Massage (Byug pa me chu'i *gzer); From the Ocean of Dropsy to Dry Land (Dmu chu rgya mtsho 'dren skems); Golden Chisel Beacon on the Powers of Medicinal Substances (Sman nus sgron ma gser gzong); Golden Door Bolt of Prognosis and Abridged Iron Axe of Prognosis (Kha dmar rgyas pa gser gyi gtan pa phyis bsdus pa lcags kyi sta re); Golden Mirror Analysis of Urine (Chu brtags pa gser gyi me long); Golden Sun Vase of Suppositories ('Jam rtsi nyi ma'i gser bum); Iron Cup of Strong Enemas (Ni ru ha lcags kyi par bu); Iron Door Bolt of the Chinese Oral Tradition of Pulse Examination (Sgo gtan lcags kyi gzer rtsa dpyad rgya'i smra mchu); Iron Garland of Tastes (Ro skor lcags kyi phreng ba); Iron Lotus of Bloodletting (Gtar kha lcags kyi padma); Medical Baths: A Drop of the Sun and Moon (Lums nyi zla'i thigs pa); Calculation of the Orbits of the Sun and Moon: An Essential Root of Medicine (Gso ba'i rig pa'i rtsa ba rtsis nyi zla'i 'khor lo); Pearl Garland of Pacification Remedies (Zhi byed mu tig phreng ba); Precious Crystal Rosary Elixir (Bcud len rin chen shel 'phreng); Precious Hook of Emetics (Skyugs rin chen lcags kyu); Secret Transmission of Precious Ambrosia (Rin po che bdud rtsi gsang ba'i lung); Silver Mirror Charm Circle of Instruction (Gdams pa'i 'phrul 'khor dngul gyi me long); Silver Vase of Purgatives (Bshal dngul gyi bum pa); Turquoise Network Compendium ('Khrugs sdebs g.yu'i dra ba); Turquoise Network: Entering the Forest of Medical Plants (Sngo sman nags su 'jug pa g.yu'i dra ba); Weapon Wheel of Minor Surgery (Thur dpyad mtshon cha 'khor lo).* [154–55]

———. *Heap of Jewels (Rin chen spung pa)* collection. [100–101, 155, 206, 336, 363, 372, 385, 425–26, 437, 440, 442, 501]

———. *King of Khotan Treatment for the Neck (Li'i rgyal po'i ske'i bcos).* Discovered by the Mongolian Menpa Jangchup. [155, 189]

Dharmaśīla (Nepalese doctor of the nine royal physicians), compiler and translator. *Drampati ('Gram pa ti); Illustrations of Precious Medicine (Rin po che'i sman gyi 'khrung dpe); Minor Surgery and Treatment of Lhokpa (Thur dpyad dang lhog pa'i gso thabs); Yogaśataka (Sbyor ba brgya ba), see also under* Nāgārjuna. [167]

Dharmaśreṣthin. *Praise of Vinaya. Vinayastotra. 'Dul ba la bstod pa.* Toh 4136, 'dul ba *su.* [365–66]

Dölpa Ringmo. *Essential Transmission of the Thirty Instructions (Gdams pa zum cu pa'i zhal shes); Main Points Word Commentary ('Bru 'grel stong thun); Important Rivets for Fever (Tshad la gal 'gag gzer chen); Thirteen Paths of Fever (Tshad 'phrang bcu gsum).* [172]

Dondrup Gönpo. *Treatment of Infectious Diseases. Rims bcos.* [265]

Dongnak Chemen Dargyé. *Great Commentary to the Root Medical Tantra. Rtsa rgyud la 'grel chen.* [260]

Dorbum Chökyi Drakpa. Essential mind-treasure collection compiled by Chögyal Tashi Topgyal; includes: *Deity Meditation: A Wish-Fulfilling Tree Ornament (Lha sgom kha brgyan dpag bsam ljon shing); Pāñcalika-Necklace Mind*

Recitation ('Dzab/jap dgongs mgul rgyan panyja li ka); Peacock-Feather Fire-Offering Ornament (Sbyin sreg kha brgyan rma bya'i mdongs). [185]

———. *Great Vase of Ambrosia. Bdud rtsi bum chen.* Revealed by Hayagrīva. The three tantras of the root collection of this are *Ambrosia Vase of Immortality Root Tantra [Three Collections] ('Chi med bdud rtsi'i bum pa rtsa rgyud [Don skor gsum]); Essence of the Mind of Mañjuśrī (Jam dbyangs kyi thugs bcud)* counted as one with *Illuminating Mandala of the Sun (Snang gsal nyi ma'i dkyil 'khor);* and *Vajra Armor [of Thunderbolt Iron] Explanatory Tantra (Bshad rgyud [gnam lcags] rdo rje'i khrab ring).* [177–85, 325–26, 336]

———. Supplementary teachings: *Ambrosia Vase Secret Magic: Mantra Fulfilling to Behold (Bdud rtsi bum pa'i 'phrul gsang sngags byang mthong chog ma); Arrowhead Essence (Mde thung gnad kyi khu ba); Bright Lamp of Oral Instruction Teachings (Zhal shes gsal sgron); Charm-Circle Force ('Khor lo gyad); Garuḍa (Khyung); Stream of the Pure Initiations: The Vase-Elixir Initiation Rituals (Rnam dag dbang gi chu rgyun bum bcud ma'i dbang chog); Three Garuḍa Self-Sustaining Wheel Collection on the Practices of the Root Forces (Chig rkya thub pa'i 'khor lo khyung gsum ma'i phyag len skor); Twenty Essences of Charm Circle Mudra ('Khor lo phyag rgya'i yang ti nyi shu).* [185]

Dorjé Bum. *Fever Collection. Tshad pa'i skor.* [267]

Dorjé Lingpa (revealer). *Great Mask: A Biography of the Translator Vairocana. Lo tsā chen po vai ro tsa na'i rnam thar 'dra 'bag chen mo.* [159, 160–61]

Drakpa Dorjé. *Six Beneficial Clarifications. Phan gsal drug.* [267]

Drangti Dorjé Palsang. *Illuminating Commentary to the Explanatory Tantra (Bshad rgyud 'grel ba don gsal); Shorter Golden Measuring Dish [of Instructions] (Gser bre chung ba).* [263]

Drangti Dréu. *Medical History. Khog 'bugs.* [266]

Drangti Gyalnyé. *Secret Treasury of Ambrosia. Bdud rtsi gsang mdzod.* [266]

Drangti Jampal Sangpo. *Five-Section Commentary / Small Volume on Practice (Sde tshan lnga grel / Lag len pod chung); Treatment of Bird-Like Demons (Bya 'dre'i bcos pa).* [261–62]

Drangti Palden Tsojé. *See* Palden Tsojé, Drangti

Drapa Ngönshé. *Essence of the Tantra. Rgyud kyi bdus don.* [192, 267]

Drö Tsoknyi Gyatso. *See* Tsoknyi Gyatso of Phenyül Drosawa

Dru Sengé, a.k.a. Drangsong Thutop Dorjé. *Ambrosia Treasury of Medical Practice. Sman dpyad bdud rtsi'i gter.* [315]

Drukpa Pema Karpo. *Chapter on Treatment of Poisoning. Dug bcos le tshan.* [322]

———. *Chos 'byung bstan pa'i padma rgyas pa'i nyin byed,* Collected Works, *kha.* Darjeeling: Publishing House for the Restoration of Kagyü Works, 1973.

———. *Treasure for the Benefit of Others: A Presentation of the Four Tantras. Rgyud bzhi'i rnam bzhag bshad pa gzhan la phan pa'i gter.* [321–22, 499]

Drungtso Wangdenpa. *Hook of Wisdom: Messenger in Search of Excellent Explanation. Legs bshad 'tshol ba'i pho nya rig pa'i lcags kyu.* [321]

Dütsi Gyurmé. *Practices of the Science of Medicine: Fulfilling All Needs and Wishes. Gso dpyad kyi lag len dgos 'dod kun 'byung.* [289, 336]

Dzajo Sung. *Clear Overview. Spyi khog gsal ba.* [264]

Gadé. *Teachings in the Field of Knowledge. Man ngag rig pa'i sde.* [267]

Galenos. *Blue Head Collection (Mgo sngon bsdus pa); Dissection of Cockerels, Peacocks, and Parrots (De pho rma bva ne co gsum).* [148]

Galenos, Hsüan Yüan Huang, and Bharadhaja. *Heap of Jewels (Rin chen spung pa); Weapons of Fearlessness ('Jigs pa'i mtshon cha).* [2, 148, 169]

Gangpa Palgön Lhündrup. *Garland of Excellent Explanation: An Overview of the Science of Medicine (Gso rig gi spyi don legs bshad 'phreng ba); Method to Avoid Errors in Identifying the Four Times (Dus bzhi'i ngos 'dzin la 'khrul ba spong thabs).* [321]

Geshé Marpo. *Fire Circle. Me yi 'khor lo.* [267]

Geshé Roktön. *Clarifying the Meaning of the Text. Tshig don gsal byed.* [264]

Gongmen Könchok Delek. *Beacon Illuminating All Places: Commentary on the Difficult Points of the Final Tantra (Phyi rgyud la bka' 'grel gnas thams cad gsal ba'i sgron me); Biographies of the Lineage (Brgyud pa'i rnam thar); Black Volume of Instructions (Man ngag pod nag); Brief Illustrative Descriptions of Medical Plants (Sngo'i 'khrung dpe don bsdus); Compilation of Tastes and Powers (Ro nus kyi sdeb sbyor); Direct Teachings on Disentangling the Main Points of Pulse and Urine Analysis (Rtsa chu'i gnad 'grol zhal gyi gdams pa dmar 'byin); Khadira Tree Multicolored Compilation on the Great Tantra (Rgyud chen khra mo be bum seng ldeng ma); Medical Lexicon (Sman ming brda sprod); Multicolored Volume of Instructions (Man ngag pod khra); Red Volume of Instructions (Man ngag po ti dmar po); Yellow Scroll that Disentangles the Precipice Path of the Difficult Points of the Tantra (Rgyud kyi dka' 'phrang 'grol ba'i shog ser).* [319–20]

Gongmen Könchok Phendar. *Caturyoga Requests to the Rishi Lineage (Drang srong brgyud pa'i gsol 'debs rdzogs ldan ma); Clear Mirror: Commentary on the Root Tantra (Rtsa rgyud kyi 'grel ba me long mthong gsal); Collection on Medicine Goddess Practices (Sman gyi lha mo'i sgrub skor); Compilation of the Essentials (Dgos pa kun bsdus); Consecration Ritual for Calling Down Blessings for Medicine (Sman gyi byin 'bebs rab gnas kyi cho ga); Hundred Works of Experience (Nyams yig brgya rtsa); Jeweled Garland Fulfilling All Needs within the Science of Medicine (Gso rig dgos 'dod 'byung ba nor bu'i 'phreng ba); Summarizing the Thoughts (Dgongs don 'dus pa); Table of Contents for the Extensive, Intermediate, and Abridged Preparation of Great Black Medicine (Sman nag chen mo'i sbyor ba rgyas 'bring bsdus gsum gyi dkar chag); Treatise on Preparing Mercury (Dngul chu grub pa'i bstan bcos).* [320]

Gönpo Dorjé. *Thirty Chapters on Examination by Charms. Brten 'brel gyi brtag pa sum cu ba.* [265]

Gönpo Drakpa. *Collection on Practice. Lag len skor.* [266]

Gönpo Rinchen. *Son Teachings in Ninety-Four Chapters. Bu gdams le'u dgu bcu bzhi.* [266]

Gönseng. *Brief Work on the Abdomen. Byang khog yig chung.* [266]

Gopadatta. *Teachings of Respect for the Teacher of Dharma and for Listening to Dharma. Dharmavacanasaddharmaśrāvakasatyakṛtyakathā. Chos smra ba dang dam pa'i chos nyan par gus par bya ba'i gtam.* Toh 4172, spring yig, *nge.* [353–54]

Great Fifth (Dalai Lama). *See* Ngawang Losang Gyatso

Guhyavajra (Kashmiri doctor from the nine royal physicians), compiler and translator. *Beacon Dispelling the Darkness of the Difficulties of Medical Practice (Dpyad 'phrang sel bar byed pa mun pa'i sgron me); Essential Prognostic Manuscript on Instruction (Man ngag gnad kyi pra yig); Nine Works on Medicine (Dpyad mdo dgu).* [166]

Guṇaprabha. Commentary on the Five Aggregates. *Pañcaskandhavivaraṇa. Phung po lnga'i rnam par 'grel ba.* Toh 4067, sems tsam *si.* [239–40]

———. *Vinaya Sutra. Vinayasūtra. 'Dul ba'i mdo.* Toh 4117, 'dul ba *wu* [241, 242, 244]

Guru Chökyi Wangchuk. *Ambrosia-Vase Heartdrop Treatise in Twenty Chapters: A Storehouse of Jewels and Compilation of the Thoughts of the Twenty-One Rishis. Drang srong nyer gcig gi dgongs 'dus gzhung snying tig rin po che'i khri mdzod bdud rtsi'i bum pa.* [187]

———. *Sealed Vase Producing Ambrosia Medicine. Bdud rtsi sman sgrub bum pa'i rgya can.* [187]

———, revealed by. *Consummation of Secrets. Gsang ba yongs su rdzogs pa.* [332]

Guru Jotsé. *Liquid Butter Collection. Mar khu'i skor.* [189]

Gyaben Dorjé Ö. *Elixir of Sadāprarudita. Rtag tu ngu'i bcud len.* [189]

Gyalbum. *Treatments for the Head. Mgo bo'i bcos.* [267]

Gyaltsen Jungné. *Stream of Ambrosia Compilation on Fevers. Stong thun bdud rtsi chu rgyun.* [264]

Gyalwa Dorjé. *Seven Branches. Yan lag bdun pa.* [169]

Halaśānti (Taksik doctor of the nine royal physicians), compiler and translator. *Eight Outsider Root and Commentary Collections on Treatments for the Head (Mgo bcos mu stegs kyi skor brgyad pa rtsa 'grel); Greater and Lesser Tree of Instructions on Channel Treatment (Rtsa bcos man ngag ljon shing che chung); Precious Wheel of Life Treatment for Humor Combination Disorders ('Dus pa bcos thabs rin chen srog gi 'khor lo); Saving the Life of the King of Garlok: Treatment for Poisoning (Dug gso ba gar log rgyal po shi gsos); Sogdian Tantra (Sog po sha stag can gyi rgyud).* [166]

Haribhadra. *Bhagavān Jewel Qualities / Commentary to the Collected Verses on*

Precious Qualities of the Bhagavān. Bhagavadratnaguṇasañcayagāthānāma-pañjikā. Bcom ldan 'das yon tan rin po che sdud pa'i tshigs su bcad pa'i dka' 'grel. Toh 3792, shes phyin *ja.* [244, 472]

Hsüan Yüan Huang. *Extensive and Short Expositions of Various Chinese Treatments. Rgya dpyad thor bu che chung.* [148]

Hvashang Mahākyinda. *Brown Compilation. Be bum smug po.*

Hvashang Penatseta. *Beacon-Like Commentary on Difficult Points of the Root Text (Rtsa ba dka' 'grel sgron me); Brilliant Jewel (Rin po che 'bar ba); Dispelling Immediate Hindrances (Gnas skabs gegs sel); Forty-Two Magic Keys ('Phrul lde zhe gnyis); Fundamental Treasury of the Five Collections (Rtsa ba rin po che'i mdzod skor); Heart-Peak Amulet (Snying rtse ga'u); Heart-Shaped Amulet (Snying 'dra ga'u); Hidden Treasury (Gab pa'i bang mdzod); Key Instructions (Lde mig dmar 'khrid); Large and Small Magic Keys of Instruction (Man ngag 'phrul lde che chung); Lifesaving Armor against Strong Poisons (Btsan dug srog skyabs go cha); Quintessential Instructions (Yang tig dmar 'khrid).* [156–57]

———. The collection on internal illnesses: *Clear Mirror for Fevers (Tshad pa gsal byed me long); Cloudless Sunrays for Meat Poisoning (Sha dug nyi zer sprin bral); Precious Cleanser for Dysentery (Bshal rin po che'i phyags shing); Precious Meat Compound for Cold Diseases (Grang ba rin po che sha sbyor); Precious Vase of Poison Treatments (Dug bcos rin po che'i bum pa).* [156]

———, translator. *Key to Precious Titles (Kha byang rin po che).*

Indra (from the Fortunate Eon Deva Tradition). *Condensed Siddhasāra (Gces pa bsdus pa); Structure of the Abdomen: A Radiant Transmission (Byang khog khrem kyi lung 'od gsal).* [102]

Indrabodhi. *Gnosis Accomplishment Sādhana. Jñānasiddhināmasādhana. Ye shes grub pa zhes bya ba'i sgrub pa'i thabs.* Toh 2219, rgyud 'grel *wi.* [354]

Jagaddarpaṇa. *Kriyāsamuccaya. Rdo rje slob dpon gyi bya ba kun la btus pa.* Toh 3305, rgyud 'grel *bu.* [358]

Jampa Tsönseng. *Mercury Preparation. Dngul chu'i sbyor.* [267]

Jampal Sangpo. *See* Drangti Jampal Sangpo

Jamyang. *Compilation of Miscellaneous Treatments. Thor dpyad sna tshogs.* [265]

Janadhara. *Magic Draining of Dropsy Instructions. Dmu chu'i 'phrul tshags man ngag.* [264]

Jangchup Pal. *Treatment for Urinary Stones. Rde bcos.* [265]

Jangchup Sherap. *Refutation of Arguments. Rtsod bzlog.* [265]

Jangmo Khyüpa and Melingpa. *Head Compresses without Surgery. Mgo bo dras med zlum bcos.* [268]

Jangmo Khyüpa Yeshé Sangmo. *Clarifying Explanation: Essence of the Sun. Don gsal nyi ma'i snying po.* [264]

Jangpa Namgyal Draksang. *Beacon Illuminating the Meaning of the Tantra: Explanation of the Root Tantra. Rtsa rgyud kyi 'grel pa rgyud don gsal byed sgron ma.* [277]

———. *Beacon Illuminating the Meaning of the Tantra. Rtsa bshad gsal ba'i sgron me.* [277]

———. *Body Mandala Completion Stage of the Path. Lus dkyil rdzogs rim lam.* [277]

———. *Clarification of Phenomena. Shes bya rab gsal.* [277]

———. *Divisions of the Nine Fatal Illnesses. Srog gcod nad dgu'i dbye ba.* [277]

———. *Easy to Understand Astronomical Treatise. Rtsis kyi bstan bcos byis pa bde blag tu 'jug pa.* [276–77]

———. *Essence of All Eight Branches: A Precious Wish-Fulfilling Jewel. Yan lag brgyad thams cad kyi snying po bsdus pa yid bzhin nor bu rin po che.* Beijing: Mi rigs dpe skrun khang, 2004. [277]

———. *Explanation of the First Summary of the Kālacakra Tantra. Mdor bsdus dan po'i rnam bshad.* [277]

———. *Fulfilling All Needs and Wishes: Textual Commentary on the Final Tantra. Phyi ma rgyud kyi dka' 'grel dgos 'dod 'byung ba.* [277]

———. *Heartfelt Magical Manuscript for Doctors. 'Tsho byed rnams la snying nas brtse ba'i 'phrul gyi yig chung.* [277]

———. *Identifying the 360 Healing Methods. Gso thabs sum brgya drug cu'i ngos 'dzin.* [277]

———. *Measurements of the Form of the Tathāgata. De bzhin gshegs pa'i sku gzugs kyi cha tshad.* [277]

———. *Ornament to the Kalāpa Sutra. Ka lā pa'i mdo rgyan.* [277]

———. *Precious Casket Medical Text. Sman gzhung rin chen sgrom bu.* [277]

———. *Response to the Physician Sengé Tsé. Seng ge rtse 'tsho byed kyi dris lan.* [277]

———. *Short Commentary Illuminating the Meaning of the Explanatory Tantra. Bshad rgyud kyi 'grel pa ṭik chung don gsal.* [277]

———. *Short Text Dispelling the Darkness on the Difficult Path of Four Tantras. Rtsom pa chung ba rgyud bzhi'i dka' 'phrang mun sel.* [277]

———. *Stream of Ambrosia: Extensive Commentary on the Explanatory Tantra. Bshad rgyud kyi 'grel chen bdud rtsi'i chu rgyun.* Chengdu: Si khron mi rigs dpe skrun khang, 2001. [277, 328]

———. *Stream of Great Bliss Initiation Procedure. Dbang chog bde chen chu rgyun.* [277]

———. *Word Commentary on the Text of the Entrustment Section. Yongs gtad kyi 'grel pa tshig don rnam par gsal ba.* [277]

Jarpo Panchen (Dorjé Palam). *Golden Sheaves: A Well-Composed History of Medicine (Khog 'bugs legs bshad gser gyi snye ma); Table of Contents for "Relic of Millions" (Bye ba rang bsrel gyi dkar chag).* [311, 313, 498]

Jetāri. *Rituals for Taking the Bodhisattva Vows and Meditation Deity. Bodhicittotpādasamādānavidhi. Byang chub kyi sems bskyed pa dang yi dam blang ba'i cho ga.* Toh 3968, dbu ma *gi*. [375]

Jetsün Drakpa Gyaltsen. *Medical Treasury of the King (Gso dpyad rgyal po'i dkor mdzod); Treasury of the King (Rgyal po'i dkor mdzod).* [264, 268]

Jinamitra (Oḍḍiyāna). *One Thousand and Ninety-Nine Treatments. Gso ba stong dgu bcu rtsa gcig.* [144, 169]

Jñānaśrī. *Eliminating the Two Extremes in Vajrayana. Vajrayānāntadvayāpoha. Rdo rje theg pa'i mtha' gnyis sel ba.* Toh 3714, rgyud 'grel *tsu.* [217, 227]

Josung. *Divisions of the Tantra Auxiliary Work (Rgyud kyi dbye ba cha lag); Five Bodies Biography (Lo rgyus ku lnga).* [267]

Kalyāṇamitra. *Extensive Commentary on Basic Vinaya. Vinayavastuṭīkā. 'Dul ba gzhi rgya cher 'grel pa.* Toh 4113, 'dul ba *tsu.* [62]

Kamalaśīla. *Fifty Verses for the Monk. Śramaṇapañcāśatkārikāpadābhismaraṇa. Dge byong gi kā ri kā lnga bcu pa'i tshig gi brjed byang du byas pa.* Toh 4128, 'dul ba *su.* [244]

———. *Stages of Meditation. Bhāvanākrama. Sgom pa'i rim pa.* Toh 4567, jo bo'i chos chung. [243]

Karma Künphen. *Golden Rosary of Ambrosia: Quintessence of All the Profound Points of the Instruction Collections (Zab gnad mtha' dag bsdus pa'i snying po bdud rtsi gser 'phreng); Treatment of Kangbam ('Bam bcos).* [315]

Karmapa Rangjung Dorjé. *Bezoars (Dbang ril); Brief Essence of Eight Branches (Brgyad pa'i snying po bsdus pa); Ocean of Medicine Names (Sman ming rgya mtsho); Vajra Diamond Expelling and Protecting against Poisons (Dug 'dred bsrung bar rdo rje pha lam).* [260, 298]

Kawa Śākya Wangchuk. *Commentary on the Final Tantra: An Illuminating Lamp on Its Difficult Points (Phyi rgyud 'grel ba dka' gnad gsal sgron); Explicit and Essential Compilation of Practices (Lag len smar 'khrid du sdebs pa snying po bsdus pa); Flower Garland: Clarification of the Five Families (Rigs lnga gsal byed me tog 'phreng ba); Mirror of White Silver: A Well-Composed History of Medicine (Khog 'bugs legs bshad dngul dkar me long).* [310, 328, 498]

Kāyastha. *Commentary to the Saṃpuṭa Tantra. Suvīsadasaṃpuṭaṭīkā. Rab tu gsal ba'i kha sbyor gyi rgya cher 'grel pa.* Toh 1190, rgyud 'grel *nga.* [63]

Khedrup (Jé) Gelek Palsangpo. *Broom of the Buddha's Precious Doctrine: A Brief Presentation on the Three Sets of Vows. Sdom gsum gyi rnam bzhag mdor bsdus te gtan la dbab pa'i rab tu byed pa thub bstan rin po che'i byi dor.* Potala Collection, vol. *nya.* [373–74, 422]

———. *General Aspects of the Classes of Tantra. Rgyud sde spyi'i rnam par bzhag pa rgyas par bshad pa.* Collected Works, *nya.* [214–15]

———. *Illuminating Reality: An Extensive Explanation of the Stainless Light, the Great Commentary on the Glorious Kālacakra. Dpal dus kyi 'khor lo'i 'grel chen dri med 'od kyi rgya cher bshad pa de kho na nyid snang bar byed pa.* Collected Works, *kha/ga.* New Delhi: Mongolian Lama Guru Deva, 1980. [147, 210, 214]

Khorlo Gyalpo / Sherap Ö. *Golden Treasury History of the Buddha. Sangs rgyas khog 'bugs gser gyi bang mdzod.* [171]

Khyölma Rutsi (one of the nine royal physicians), compiler and translator. *Bloodletting Therapy (Gtar kha'i dpyad); Clarifying the Hidden (Gab bsal byed); Chapter on Signs of Life and Death ('Tsho 'chi rtags kyi le'u); Pulse Signs (Rtsa'i la nye); Weapons of the Eight Kinds of Fearlessness (Mi 'jigs pa brgyad kyi mtshon cha).* [167]

Khyung Tri. *Essence of the Enlightened Mind. Thugs kyi snying po.* [267]

Khyungwo. *Commentary on Eight Branches. Brgyad pa'i 'grel ba.* [266]

Könchok Gyaltsen. *Chapters and Commentary to Eight Branches. Brgyad pa'i le dang 'grel ba.* [265]

Kongpo Degyal. *Brilliant Jewel Treasury Biography. Rnam thar gzi brjid rin po che'i gter.* [260]

Kṛṣṇacarya. *Cakrasaṃvara Mandala Ritual / Sādhana. Śrīcakrasaṃvarasādhana. Bcom ldan 'das dpal bde mchog 'khor lo'i dkyil 'khor gyi cho ga.* Toh 1446, rgyud 'grel *wa.*

Kṣemendra. *Wish-Fulfilling Tree of the Bodhisattva's Lives. Bodhisattvāvadāna-kalpalatā. Byang chub sems dpa'i rtogs pa brjod rin po che dpag bsam gyi 'khri shing. Skyes rabs.* Toh 4155, skyes rab *khe.* [56, 432–33]

Künga Nyingpo. *Types of Elixir. Bcud len rigs.* [265]

Künga Wangchuk. *Magic Mirror Compilation on Pulse and Urine. Rtsa chu yi stong thun 'phrul gyi me long.* [264]

Kusa Menpa. *Pile of Jewels. Rin chen spung pa.* [189]

Kyempa Tsewang. *Appearance of the Essence (Snying po snang ba); Clarification of Practice (Lag len gsal byed); Granting Wishes: Well-Explained Overview of Medicine (Gso dpyad spyi don legs bshad 'dod 'jo); Granting Wishes of Happiness (Bde ba'i 'dod 'jo); Medical Practices: Hundreds of Life-Granting Empowerments (Sman dpyad lag len tshe dbang brgya rtsa); Sun Word Commentary (Tshig don nyi ma).* [310, 499]

Lata Tsewang. *See* Kyempa Tsewang

Latö Marpo. *Liquid-Butter Ambrosia Treasure Collection. Gter ma bdud rtsi mar khu'i skor.* [189]

Lekden Gönpo. *Treatments for Poisoning. Dug bcos skor.* [265]

Lekpa Gyaltsen. *Thirty-Five Methods of Bursting from Gagön. Ga gon gyi brdol thabs su co rtsa lnga.* [169]

Lhabar, revealed by. *Commentary on Meanings of Treasure Writing. Gter yig don 'brel.* [267]

Lhajé Mipham Sangpo. *History of Medicine: Endowed with the Five Ambrosia Perfections. Khog 'bugs 'chi med phun tshogs lnga ldan.* [499]

Lhasé. *Ambrosia Essence. Bdud rtsi bcud bsdus.* [266]

Lhatsün Drong Tsewa. *Drangtsé Compilation. 'Brong rste be bum.* Contains the *Black Exposition on Medicine (Sman nag chen mo).* [260]

Lhatsün Tashi Palsang. *Jewel of Excellent Explanation: A Commentary on the Explanatory Tantra (Bshad rgyud kyi 'grel ba legs bshad nor bu); Shorter Blazing from Atop a Victory Banner (Rgyal mtshan rtser 'bar chung ba); Treasury of Jewels Fulfilling All Needs: A Commentary on the Final Tantra / All-Knowing When Studied (Phyi rgyud kyi 'grel ba 'dod 'byung ba rin po che bang mdzod / bklags pa kun shes); White Smile of the Sun: A History of Medicine (Khog 'bugs 'dzum dkar bzhad pa'i nyi ma); Wish-Granting Tree: Verses on the Ascertainment of Four Tantras [as Word of the Buddha] (Rgyud bzhi'i [bka' sgrub] rnam nges dpag bsam ljon shing).* [286, 498, 501]

Lhünding Namgyal Dorjé. *Great Adornment of the Stone Pillar. Rdo ring rgyan mchog.* [328]

Lhuné. *Ocean Garland Treatments for the Head. Mgo dpyad rgya mtsho'i 'phreng ba.* [266]

Lodrö. *History of Medicine. Khog dbubs.* [267]

Lodrö Gyalpo. *See* Surkhar Lodrö Gyalpo

Lodrö Tenpa of Kyishö / Rinchen Ding Bodhisattva Losang Gyatso. *Clear Mirror: A Word Commentary to the Final Tantra (Phyi rgyud la bka' 'grel gsal ba'i me long); Ornament to the Thoughts of the Rishis: A History of Medicine (Sman gyi chos 'byung drang srong dgongs rgyan).* [315, 499]

Lodrö Tsungmé. *Annotations on Eight Branches. Brgyad pa'i mchan.* [268]

Longchen Rapjampa. *Treasury of the Supreme Vehicle. Theg mchog mdzod.* Collected Works, *ga*. Shes rab rgyal mtshan and mkhyen brtse bla brang: 1983. [210–11]

Lotsāwa Drakpa Sengé. *Compilation of Essentials. Nyer kho phyogs bsdus be bum.* [260]

Mahādeva Maheśvara. *Black and White Frog Tantra (Sbal pa dkar nag gi rgyud); Heroic Rescuer Tantra (Dpa' bo 'ching 'grol gyi rgyud); Fast-Moving Tantra (Khyug pa'i rgyud); Profound and Secret Black and White Tantras (Zab gsang dkar nag gi rgyud); Red and Blue Life-Channel Tantra (Srog rtsa sngo dmar gyi rgyud); Wheel of Fire Tantra (Me lce 'khor lo'i rgyud).* [103]

Maitreya. *Differentiating the Middle Way and the Extremes. Madhyantavibhaṅgakārikā. Dbus dang mtha' rnam par 'byed pa'i tshig le'ur byas pa.* Toh 4021, sems tsam *phi*. [243, 264, 439]

———. *Examination of Phenomena and the Nature of Phenomena. Dharmadharmatāvibhaṅga. Chos dang chos nyid rnam par 'byed pa.* Toh 4022, sems tsam *phi*. [243]

———. *Ornament of Mahayana Sutras. Mahāyānasūtralaṃkārakārikā. Theg pa chen po'i mdo sde'i rgyan gyi tshig le'ur byas pa.* Toh 4020, sems tsam *phi*. [42, 226, 241, 243, 359–60, 360–61]

———. *Ornament of Realization. Abhisamayālaṃkāranāmaprajñāpāramitopadeśāśāstrakārikā. Shes rab kyi pha rol tu phyin pa'i man ngag gi bstan bcos *mngon par rtogs pa'i rgyan zhes bya ba'i tshig le'ur byas pa.* Toh 3786, shes phyin *ka.* [85, 243, 244, 359]

———. *Uttaratantra/Mahāyānottaratantraśāstra/Ratnagotravibhāga. Theg pa chen po rgyud bla ma 'i bstan bcos.* Toh 4024, sems tsam *phi.* [41, 229, 477–78]

Manaho. *Meaningful to Behold: Opening the Eyes. Amoghadarśinetravibhaṅga. Mig 'byed mthong ba don ldan.* Toh 4443, sna tshogs *no.* [327]

Mañjuśrī (attributed). *Alms Bowl of Ambrosia: Treatment of Head Ailments (Mgo bcos bdud rtsi'i lhung bzed); Charms for the Abdomen (Rten 'brel byang khog); Clear and Concise Manuscript on Diagnosis (Kha smar gsal ba'i yig chung); Five Jewel Treasuries (Rin chen bang mdzod lnga ba); Jeweled Box (Rin chen sgrom bu); Life Treatment: Opening the Mouths of the Mute (Srog bcos lkug pa kha 'byed); Medical Plants Collection (Sngo 'bum); Ocean of Ambrosia: A Treatment of Head Ailments (Mgo bcos bdud rtsi rgya mtsho); Quintessence: The Magic Fourfold Collection (Yang thig 'phrul gyi bzhi skor); Special Treatment of Head Ailments (Dkyus bzlog mgo bcos); Supreme Magic: A Treatment of Womb Disorders (Mngal nad gso ba 'phrul gyi rgyal po); Three Sections of the Greater and Lesser Mineral Tantra (Rdo rgyud che chung rnam gsum).* [101]

Mañjuśrīkīrti. *Commentary to the King of Meditative Concentrations Sutra. Sarvadharmasvabhāvasamatāvipañcitasamādhirājanāmamahāyānasūtra-ṭīkākīrtimālā. Chos thams cad kyi rang bzhin mnyam pa nyid rnam par spros pa'i ting nge 'dzin kyi rgyal po zhes bya ba theg pa chen po'i mdo'i 'grel pa grags pa'i phreng ba.* Toh 4010, mdo 'grel *nyi.* [243, 372]

Mara Gomchen. *Revealing Mirror Commentary. Tikka gsal byed me long.* [263]

Marlo. *Peacock* and *Parrot* collections. *Rma bya ne tso'i skor.* [266]

Maticitra. *Tales of the Kaliyuga. Kaliyugaparikathā. Rtsod pa'i 'dus kyi gtam.* Toh 4513, jo bo'i chos chung / Toh 4170, skyes rabs *ge.* [485–86]

Maudgalyāyana. *Cause Terminology. Kāraṇaprajñapti. Rgyu gdags pa.* Toh 4087, mngon pa [336]

———. *Karma Terminology. Karmaprajñapti. Las gdags pa.* Toh 4088, mngon pa. [336]

Mentön Shönu Rinchen. *Great Overview. Stong thun chen mo.* [501]

Minyak Dawa Drakpa. *Great Compilation. Stong thun rgyas bshad.* [268]

Minyak Dorjé Bum. *Profound Commentary. Zab 'grel.* [264]

Minyak Mikyö Dorjé. *Accounts from History (Chos 'byung lo rgyus); Fifteen Difficult Paths of Illness ('Phrang bco lnga); Golden Garland Word Commentary (Bru 'grel par bkab gser phreng); Main Point Overviews (Stong thun); Nine Treatments (Dpyad dgu); Pearl Necklace (Mu tig 'phreng ba); Supplement to Scriptural Explanation (Gzhung bshad thabs kyi yan lag).* [172–73, 501]

Minyak Rongjé Gaga. *Mountain Stack Commentary. Ri bo brtsegs pa'i 'grel ba.* [265]

Minyima Thongwa Dönden. *Ascertainment of Four Tantras / Established as Enlightened Speech (Gyud bzhi'i rnam nges / bka' sgrub); Exalted General*

Medicine (Khyad 'phags spyi sman); Extraordinary General Medicine (Ngo mtshar spyi sman); Four Presentations (Bkod pa rnam bzhi); Four Streams (Rgyun rnam bzhi); Illumination of the Truth: A Commentary on the Fourth Chapter of the Explanatory Tantra (Bshad rgyud le'u bzhi pa'i 'grel ba gnas lugs rab gsal); King of Medical Practice (Gso dpyad rgyal po); Large and Small Wish-Granting Cow Commentary on the Difficult Points of Mālaya (Mā la ya'i dka' 'grel 'dod 'jo che hung); Precious Garland Quintessence (Gces bsdus rin chen 'phreng ba); Realization Requests (Mngon par rtogs pa'i gsol 'debs); Treatments of Infectious Diseases: Giving Life to Mankind (Rims bcos mi la srog sbyin); Vajra Verse Oral Transmission Commentary on the Pulse Section (Rtsa mdo'i 'grel ba snyan brgyud rdo rje'i tshig rkang). [285]

Mipham Gelek. *Anatomy of the Torso (Byang khog yul thig); Explanation of the Tastes and Powers of Medicines (Sman gyi ro nus).* [328]

Mitra Miwang Chandra and Hvashang Devabodhi, translators. *Eight Verses (Tshig rkang brgyad); Precious Beacon: A Magic Treasury of Medicine (Gso byed 'phrul gyi mdzod rin po che'i sgron ma)* reputed to be the speech of Mañjuśrī; *Root Tantra (Rtsa ba'i rgyud)* attributed to Vajrapāṇi; *Siddhi of Rishi Śūrya (Drang srong nyi ma'i dngos grub); Twenty-Two Chapters on Treatments (Bcos thabs nyer gnyis).* [155–56]

Mönlam Gyaltsen. *Collection on Stone Removal. Sde ma'i skor.* [267]

Nāgārjuna. *Compendium of Sutra. Sūtrasamuccaya. Mdo kun las btus pa.* Toh 3934, dbu ma *ki.* [243]

———. Compendium of Tantra (Rgyud kun la btus pa). Untraced. [126]

———. *Establishing the Conventional. Tha snyad grub pa.* Untraced. [243]

———. *Finely Woven Scripture. Vaidalyasūtra. Zhib mo rnam par 'thag pa.* Toh 3826, dbu ma *tsa.* [243]

———. *Friendly Letter. Suhṛllekha. Bshes pa'i spring yig.* Toh 4182, spring yig *nge.* [244]

———. *Fundamental Stanzas on the Middle Way. Mūlamadhyamakakārikā. Dbu ma rtsa ba'i tshig le'ur byas pa shes rab ces bya ba.* Toh 3824, dbu ma *tsa.* [242, 253]

———. *Gross Downfalls in the Vajrayana. Vajrayānasthūlāpatti. Rdo rje theg pa'i sbom po'i ltung ba.* Toh 2482, rgyud 'grel, *zi.* [418–19]

———. *Hundred Medical Preparations. Yogaśataka. Sbyor ba brgya pa.* Toh 4306, gso rig *he.* [126–27, 173, 279, 336]

———. *No Fear from Anywhere: Commentary on Fundamental Stanzas on the Middle Way. Mūlamadhyamakavṛttyakutobhaya. Dbu ma rtsa ba'i 'grel pa ga las 'jigs med.* Toh 3829, dbu ma *tsa.* [243]

———. *Precious Garland of Advice for the King. Ratnāvalī/Rājaparikathāratnamālā. Rgyal po la gtam bya bar in po che'i phreng ba.* Toh 4158, spring yig *ge.* [243, 358, 380]

———. *Refutation of Arguments. Vigrahavyāvartanīkārikā. Rtsod pa bzlog pa'i tshig le'ur byas pa.* Toh 3828, dbu ma *tsa.* [242]

———. *Ritual of Ava Medicine Ācāryanāgārjunabhāṣitāvabheṣajakalpa. Slob dpon klu sgrub kyis bshad pa sman a ba'i cho ga.* Toh 4308, gso rig pa *he.* [127]

———. *Seventy Verses on Emptiness. Śūnyatāsaptatikārikā. Stong pa nyid bdun cu pa'i tshig le'ur byas pa.* Toh 3827, dbu ma *tsa.* [242–43]

———. *Shoots of Wisdom: Treatise on Ethics. Nītiśāstrajantupoṣanabindu. Lugs kyi bstan bcos shes rab sdong po.* Toh 4329, thun mong ba lugs kyi bstan bcos *ngo.* [354, 484, 486]

———. *Sixty Verses of Reasoning. Yuktiṣaṣṭikākārikā. Rigs pa drug cu pa'i tshig le'ur byas pa.* Toh 3825, dbu ma *tsa.* [243]

———. *Sutra of Life. Jīvasūtra. Sman 'tsho ba'i mdo.* Toh 4307, gso rig *he.* [127, 336]

Nāgārjuna (attributed). *Curing Illnesses of the Five Aggregates (Phung po lnga'i nad gso ba); Descriptions of the Organs (Don snod ti ka); Drop of Ambrosia (Bdud rtsi thigs pa); Four Limbs Treatise (Yan lag rnam bzhi); Jewel Garland Preparation of Mercury (Dngul chu'i sbyor bar rin chen 'phreng ba); Magic Black Key Treatise on the Abdomen (Byang khog gi ti ka 'phrul lde nag po); Precious Essential Points Commentary on the Anatomy of the Head (Mgo thig rin chen gnad 'grel); Precious Medicine (Sman rin po che'i rim pa); Secret Ambrosia: Preparation of Medicinal Plants (Sngo sbyor bdud rtsi gsang ba); Secret Commentary on the Precious Stones Treatise (Mdo rin po che'i gsang ba'i 'grel chen); Secret Essence Beacon of Ambrosia Gem Medicine (Bdud rtsi'i sman rin po che gsang tig sgron ma); Short Gold Treatise (Phran bu ser gyi ti ka); Treatise on the Four Humors ('Du ba rnam bzhi'i ti ka); Treatise on the Four Limbs (Yan lag rnam bzhi'i ti ka); Treatise on the Head (Mgo'i ti ka); Treatment for the Four Kinds of Lhok and Infectious Fevers (Lhog pa spun gzhi gnyan bnyan bcas kyi bcos); Vase of Ambrosia (Bdud rtsi bum pa).* [127, 149, 155, 199–200, 279, 296, 318, 332]

Namgyal Draksang. *See* Jangpa Namgyal Draksang

Namkha Delek. *Abridged Outline of the Pulse Section from Four Tantras (Rtsa mdo'i sa dpyad); Ambrosia Garland (Bdud rtsi 'phreng ba); Diamonds (Rdo rje pha lam); Divisions and Abridgements of the Ailments, Remedies, and Healing Methods of the Final Tantra (Phyi rgyud kyi nad dang gnyen po gso thabs gsum gyi dbye bsdu); Identification of the Four Classes of Chronic Degenerative Disorders (Gcong sde bzhi'i ngos 'dzin mdzub tshugs ma); Light of Excellent Explanation: An Overview of Four Tantras (Rgyud bzhi'i spyi don legs bshad snang ba).* [320]

Nāropa. *Commentary on a Short Teaching on Initiation. Paramārthasaṃgrahanāmasekoddeśaṭīkā. Dbang mdor bstan gyi 'grel bshad don dam pa bsdus pa zhes bya ba.* Toh 1351, rgyud 'grel *na.* [218]

Ngawang Losang Gyatso (The Great Fifth Dalai Lama). *Golden Victorious*

Myrobalan Vinaya Ceremonies. Bstan pa'i rtsa ba rab byung dang khyim pa la phan gdags pa'i las kyi cho ga mtha' dpyod dang bcas pa 'khrul spong rnam rgyal gser mdog. Potala Collection, *pha.* Gangtok: Bod kyi rig gzhung nyams zhib khang (Tibetan Cultural Research Center), 1991. [367, 423, 540n794]

———. *Letters Arranged in Verse to Various Persons in China, Tibet, and Mongolia Containing Many Oral Transmissions. Rgya bod hor sog gi mchog dman bar ma rnams la 'phrin yig snyan ngag tu bkod pa rab snyan rgyud mang,* Collected Works, *dza.* Mtsho sngon mi rigs dpe skrun khang, 1993. Thimphu: Künsang Topgay, 1975. [450, 451, 453]

———. *Monastic Regulations. Bca' yig.* [80–82]

———. *Silken Robe Biography. Za hor gyi bande ngag dbang blo bzang rgya mtsho'i 'di snang 'khrul pa'i rol rtsed rtogs brjod kyi tshul du bkod pa du kū la'i gos bzang.* Potala Collection, *ca, cha, ja.* [435]

———. *Stream of the Ganges: An Account of Teachings Received. Gsan yig ganga chu'i rgyun.* Potala Collection, *ka, kha, ga, nga.* [80, 177, 187, 217, 317, 318]

———. *Wish-Fulfilling Tree: List of Practices from the Yuthok Heartdrop. G.yu thog syning thig gi las byang dpag bsam ljon shing.* Collected Works, *nga.* [10, 21, 253]

Nup Sangyé Yeshé, translator. *Ambrosia Drop Treatments of the Head in Seven Chapters. Mgo dpyad bdud rtsi thigs pa.* By Ketu Prajñā. [167]

———, translator. *Ambrosia Mirror in Eight Chapters. Mgo dpyad bdud rtsi me long le'u brgyad pa.* By Vedura. [167]

———, translator. *Candraguhya Weapon Wheel Activity Tantra in Ten Chapters. Zla gsang 'khor lo mtshon cha las kyi rgyud.* [167]

———, translator. *Fire Wheel Treatments for Poison. Dug dpyad me lce 'khor lo.* By Śuka, a manifestation of Mañjuśrī. [167]

———, translator. *Five Beacon Collection. Sgron ma lnga skor.* Attributed to Nāgārjuna. [167]

———, translator. *Fungi Treatment for Poisons. Dug dpyad sha mo las dkyus.* By Rishi/Ācārya Sūryasiṃha (translation also attributed to Vairocana). [162, 167]

———, translator. *Precious Belt of Liberation. Rin po che ske rags 'ching 'grol.* [167]

———, translator. *Precious Compilation on Medicine and Treatment in Seven Fasicles. Sman dpyad rin po che 'dus pa bam po bdun.* Attributed to Nāgārjuna. [167]

———. *Precious Examination: Light Reflection. Brtag pa rin po che 'od kyi gzugs brnyan.* [167]

———. *Precious Protection: The Light of Instruction. Bsrung ba rin po che 'od kyi gdams pa.* [167]

———. *Traveling Lamp of Good Remedies. Gso ba dkar po lam gyi sgron ma.* [167]

Nuptön. *Treatment for Bird Demons. Bya 'dre'i bcod thabs.* [189]
Nyah. *Six Traditions on Reversal Treatment (Ja log don khrigs sde drug); True Illumination Commentary to the Heart Tantra (Snying rgyud 'grel ba yang dag gsal).* [265]
Nyang Ralpachen. *Tantra on Shining Ambrosia in Sixty Chapters (Bdud rtsi 'od ldan gyi rgyud le'u drug cu); Three Warrior Deities (Dpa' bo lha gsum).* [187]
Nyemo Chökyi Wangchuk. *Lamp Illuminating the Four Points. Don bzhi gsal sgron.* [267, 501]
Nyemo Künga Döndrup. *Histories. Lo rgyus 'byung tshul.* [501]
Nyima Pal. *Cauterization. Me btsa'.* [267]
Orgyen Lingpa. *Five Chronicles. Bka' thang lnga.* New Delhi: International Academy of Indian Culture, 1982. Beijing: Mi rigs dpe skrun khang, 1986. Delhi: Tibetan Cultural and Religious Publication Centre, 2007. [3, 80, 486]
———. *Lotus Chronicles / Crystal Rock Chronicles: The Past Lives and Extensive Biography of the Orgyen Padma Sambhava. Gu ru pad ma 'byung gnas kyi skyes rabs rnam par thar pa rgyas par bkod pa pad ma bka'i thang yig / Thang yig shel brag ma.* Chengdu: Si khron mi rigs dpe khang, 1993. [5, 161–62, 163, 175, 176, 189–90, 210, 215, 291]
Orgyenpa. *Black Medicine Text. Sman nag.* [268]
Özer Gönpo. *Elixirs. Bcud len.* [265]
Padmasambhava. *Ambrosia Essence. Bdud rtsi snying po.* [144]
———. *Ambrosia Vase Treatments. Gso ba bdud rtsi bum pa.* [144]
———. *Five Pledges. Samayapañca. Dam tshig lnga pa.* Toh 1224, rgyud *nya.* [409]
———. *Lotus Precious Garland: A Short Work on Medicinal Treatments. Chung dpyad pad ma bces phreng.* [144, 189]
———. *Sun and Moon Union. Brtag pa nyi zla kha sbyor* [144].
———. *Vajra Armor Prevention. Rdo rje khrab ring.* [144]
Pal Khachö Wangpo. *Short Work on Sources. Khungs kyi yig chung.* [501]
Palchen. *Three Fundamental Collections. Rtsa ba don skor gsum.* [266]
Palchen Öpo. *Sun Circle Commentary on the Shorter Eight Branches. Brgyad chung nyi ma'i 'khor lo.* [264, 268]
Palden Gyaltsen, Drangti. *Compound of the Six White Ingredients (Dkar po drug sbyor); Golden Measuring Dish of Instructions (Man ngag gser bre).* [263, 264, 311, 328]
Palden Tsojé, Drangti. *Commentary on Decoctions and Powders (Thang phye'i 'grel ba); Commentary on Difficult Points on the Malaya (Ma la ya'i dka' 'grel); Compilation of Essentials (Gces bsdus); Exposition of Eight Branches (Brgyad pa'i khog 'bugs); Illumination of Knowledge: A History of Medicine (Khog 'bugs shes bya rab gsal); Illumination of the Meanings of the Tantra (Rgyud don rab gsal),* a commentary to the Root Tantra; *Illumination of the Three Ways (Tshul gsum snang ba),* a commentary to the Final Tantra; *Illustrations*

of Medicinal Preparations from the Final Tantra (Phyi ma'i rgyud sman sbyor dpe'u ris); Lamp Illuminating the Structure of the Torso (Byang khog gi thig 'grems gsal sgron); Rays of the Sun (Nyi ma'i 'od zer), a commentary to the *Pulse Section; Rishi Chronicles (Drang srong gi rtogs brjod); Sādhana of the Pulse Goddess (Rtsa'i lha mo'i sgrub thabs); Thirty-Chapter Wooden-Board Commentary to the Compilations and Sections of the Tantra (Mdo gnas le'u sum cu'i sa ma 'grel); Wish-Fulfilling Jewel Clarifying the Text (Tshig don gsal byed yid bzhin nor bu),* a commentary to the *Urine Treatise.* [87, 262–63, 497, 498]

Palgön Dorjé. *See* Chipa Palgön Dorjé

Palgön Sherap. *Treatments for Women's Diseases: Fulfilling to Behold. Mo nad bcos skor bltas chog.* [265]

Palpoché. *See* Palchen Öpo

Palshé. *Essence of Eight Branches. Brgyad pa'i bsdus don.* [5, 265]

Panchen Jaliwa (from Droding). *Precious Pill Collection (Rin chen ril bu skor); Three Collections on Mercury (Dngul chu gzhung skor gsum).* [260]

Pawo Tsuklak Trengwa. *Illuminating Beacon on Mineral Exudates (Rdo zhun gsal sgron); Quintessential Notes on Medical Practice (Sman dpyad zin bris snying po bsdus pa).* [315]

Pema Karpo. *See* Drukpa Pema Karpo

Pené. *Stainless Brilliance. Dri med gzi brjid.* [267]

Phadampa Sangyé. *Charm Collections (Rten 'grel skor); Lantern of Pacification (Zhi byed sgron ma); White, Black, and Multicolored Magic Treatments (Khyug dpyad dkar nag khra gsum).* [190, 260]

Phaktön Śākya Gönpo. *Sunlight Clarity of Meaning. Don gsal nyi ma'i o'd ldan.* [260, 501]

Pitṛceṭa.* *Medical Commentary to Essence of Eight Branches. Aṣṭāṅgahṛdaya-nāmavaiduryakabhāṣya. Yan lag brgyad pa'i snying po zhes bya ba'i sman dpyad kyi bshad pa.* Toh 4311, gso rig *he.* [138]

———. *Treatise of Eight Branches / Essence of Eight Branches. Aṣṭāṅgahṛdaya-saṃhitanāma. Yan lag brgyad pa'i snying po bsdus pa zhes bya ba.* Toh 4310, gso rig *he.* [5, 47, 51, 60, 138, 206, 261, 262, 279, 336, 352; description of chapters of, 138–42; Desi Sangyé Gyatso's study of, 333; histories on the theme of, 501; physicians, 462, 463; qualities of disciple, 468–69; science of healing/doctors, 351; search for ambrosia, 57, translation of, 169, 170]

Pönsé Khyungö. *Intermediate Ambrosia Vase. Bdud rtsi bum pa 'bring po.* [189]

Prajāpati (from the Fortunate Eon Deva Tradition). *Magic Mirror. 'Phrul gyi me long.* [102]

Prajñāvarman. *Commentary on Praise of the Exalted. Viśeṣastavanāmaṭīkā. Khyad par du 'phags pa bstod pa'i 'grel pa.* Toh 1110, bstod tshogs *ka.* [51–52]

———. *Commentary on Praises from the Gods. Devātiśayastotraṭīkā. Lha las phul du byung bar bstod pa'i rgya cher 'grel pa.* Toh 1113, bstod tshogs *ka.* [52–53]

———. *Commentary to the Collection of Aphorisms. Udānavargavivaraṇa. Ched du brjod pa'i tshoms kyi rnam par 'grel pa.* Toh 4100, mngon pa *tu.* [244]

Puṇḍarīka. *Great Commentary / Stainless Light. Vimalaprabhānamamūlatantrānusāriṇīdvādaśasāhasrikālaghukālacakratantrarajaṭīkā. Bsdus pa'i rgyud kyi rgyal po dus kyi 'khor lo'i 'grel bshad rtsa ba'i rgyud kyi rjes su 'jug pa stong phrag bcu gnyis pa dri ma med pa'i 'od ces bya ba.* Toh 845, rgyud *śrī* (Dro Lotsāwa translation, found in Kangyur). Also Toh 1347, rgyud 'grel *da* (Shong Lotsāwa translation in Tengyur). [228]

———. *In Devotion to the Ultimate Truth Paramārthasevā. Don dam pa'i bsnyen pa.* Toh 1348, rgyud 'grel *na.* [463]

———. *Stainless Light Commentary on the Mañjuśrī Saṃgīti. Mañjuśīnāmasaṃgīṭikāvimalaprabhā. 'Jam dpal gyi mtshan yang dag par brjod pa'i 'grel pa dri ma med pa'i 'od.* Toh 1398, rgyud 'grel *pha.* [213]

Pūrṇacandra. *Sutra of Roots. Dhātusūtra. Dbyings kyi mdo.* Toh 4424, sna tshogs *no.* [61]

Ra Yeshé Sengé. *Biography of Ra Lotsāwa. Rva lo tsā ba'i rnam thar.* Kokonor: Mtsho sngon mi rigs dpe skrun khang, 1989. [427]

Ragunātha. *Advice from the Royal Āyurvedic Practitioner Ragunātha from Mathurā. Āryadeśamagadhamathurākṣatriyabhiṣak Rakunāthāmnaya. 'Phags yul dbus 'gyur ma thu ra'i rgyal rigs kyi sman pa ra ku nā tha'i gdams pa.* Toh 4442 sna tshongs, *no.* [327, 535n678]

Rakshak Tertön. *Padma Transmission Holder Compendium. Pad ma lung 'chang bsdus pa.* [267]

Ralpatra. *Black Moonlight (Zla zer nag po); Black Tome (Dum pa nag po); Black Fasicle (Bam po nag po).* [103]

Rangjung Dorjé. *See* Karmapa Rangjung Dorjé

Ratna Lingpa. *Creation of Medicine: The Complete Secrets (Sman sgrub gsang ba yongs rdzogs); Extensive General Transmissions (Spyi lung chen mo).* [189, 324]

Ratna Mingchen. *Well-Compiled History of Medicine. Gso ba rig pa'i khog 'bugs legs bsdus.* [499]

Ratnākara. *Jewel Source Treatise of Metrics. Chandoratnākara. Sdeb sbyor rin chen 'byung gnas.* Toh 4303, sgra mdo *se.* [453]

Ravigupta. *Essential Medical Siddha. Vaidyasiddhasāra. Dpyad gces pa grub pa.* Toh 4434, sna tshogs *no.* [336]

Rikzin Gödem. *Brilliant Lamp (Snang gsal sgron me); Essential Instruction for the Treatment of Infectious Fevers (Gnad kyi man ngag gnyan tshad bcos thabs); Small Vase of Ambrosia (Bdud rtsi bum chung).* [177]

Rinchen Ding Bodhisattva Losang Gyatso. *See* Lodrö Tenpa of Kyishö

Rinchen Gyalpo. *Collections. Skor tshoms.* [266]

Rinchen Lingpa. *Ambrosia Mercury Elixir (Bdud rtsi ngul chu'i bcud len); Eye Medicine (Mig sman).* [189]

Rishi Khadyota, translator. *Beacon Illuminating the Meaning (Don gsal sgron ma); Beacon of the Heart ('Thugs kyi sgron ma); Bright Beacon Quintessential Treatment for Planetary Disorder (Gza' bcos snying tig gsal sgron); Clear Insight (Mngon par rtogs pa); Clear Mirror (Me long rab gsal); Extensive Question and Answer in Thirty-Four Chapters (Zhu lan che ba le'u sum cu so bzhi); Illuminating Beacon (Gsal byed sgron ma); Magic Mirror ('Phrul gyi me long); Signs of Leprosy Manuscript (Mdze rtags mig yig)* attributed to Vetālaḍākinī. [167]

Rishi Tsewang Rikzin. *Swift Path Traveled by the Fortunate. Bskal bzang bgrod pa'i myur lam.* [321]

Rishi Śrīmālā. *Magic Key. 'Phrul gyi lde mig.* Commentary to the second part of the *Eight Caraka Collections* in forty fascicles. [103]

———. *Replicating Sun and Moon. Nyi zla par bkab.* Commentary to the first part of the *Eight Caraka Collections* in eighty fascicles [103]

Rokchung. *Draining and Drying Dropsy Procedure. Dmu chu 'tshags skems 'grems.* [267]

Ruddha Ānanda. *Well-Explained Ocean-Like Overview: A Dance to Delight the Rishis. Spyi don legs bshad rgya mtsho drang srong kun tu dga' ba'i zlos gar.* [500]

Sakya Paṇḍita Künga Gyaltsen. *Essence of Eight Branches. [Yan lag] brgyad pa'i don bsdus.* [264, 268]

———. *Treasury of Wise Sayings. Legs par bshad pa rin po che'i gter.* Collected Works, *tha.* Collected Works of the Sakya, vol. 5. Tokyo: Tōyō Bunko, 1968–69. [289, 484, 485, 487]

———. *Treatise on the Classification of the Three Vows. Sdom pa gsum gyi rab tu dbye ba'i bstan bcos.* Collected Works, *na.* Collected Works of the Sakya, vol. 5. Tokyo: Tōyō Bunko, 1968–69. [389]

———. *Various Compositions: A Bouquet of Flowers. Sdeb sbyor sna tshogs me tog gi chun po.* Collected Works, *tha.* Collected Works of the Sakya, vol. 5. Tokyo: Tōyō Bunko, 1968–69. [45]

Śākyaprabha. *Vinaya Light / Commentary on Verses on the Novice Monk of the Mūlasarvāstivādin Traditon. Āryamūlasarvāstivādiśrāmaṇerakārikāvṛttiprabhāvati. 'Phags pa gzhi thams cad yod par smra ba'i dge tshul gyi tshig le'ur byas pa'i 'grel pa 'od ldan.* Toh 4125, 'dul ba *shu.* [359]

Śālihotra. *Horse Āyurveda Compiled by the Sage Śālihotra. Śālihotrīyāśvāyurvedasaṃhitā. Rta'i tshe'i rig byed drang srong śālihotras bsdus pa.* Toh 4345, lugs kyi bstan bcos *ngo.* [54–55]

Samten Sherap. *Magic Circle of Water Surgical Removal. Dpyad dbyung chu'i 'phrul 'khor.* [265]

Sangyé Lingpa. *Eye Medicine (Mig sman); Oral Testament in the Outer Tradition of the King (Phyi rgyal po lugs kyi gtam rgyud bka' chems).* [189]

Śāntideva. *Compendium of Practice. Śikṣāsamuccaya. Bslab pa kun las btus pa.* Toh 3940, dbu ma *khi.* [241, 244, 378–79]

———. *Engaging in the Practices of the Bodhisattva. Bodhicaryāvatāra. Byang chub sems pa'i spyod pa la 'jug pa.* Toh 3871, dbu ma *la.* [241, 242, 352, 382, 384–85, 472, 474, 475–76]

———. *Verses on Compendium of Practice. Śikṣāsamuccayakārikā. Bslab pa kun las btus pa'i tshig le'ur byas pa.* Toh 3939, dbu ma *khi.* [380–81]

Śāntigarbha, translator and compiler. *Begging Bowl of Ambrosia (Bdud rtsi lhung bzed),* attributed to Buddha; *Essence of Vase of Ambrosia (Bdud rtsi bum snying),* attributed to Buddha; *Five Collections (Spung pa sde lnga),* attributed to Avalokiteśvara; *Five Treatises (Mdo lnga),* attributed to Nāgārjuna; *Four Collections of Verses (Shlo ka sde bzhi),* attributed to Buddha; *One Hundred Thousand Medicinal Plants in 120 Chapters (Sngo 'bum le'u brgya dang nyi shu),* attributed to Tārā; *Tantra of the Brown Casket (Bal/bse sgrom smug po'i rgyud),* attributed to Buddha. [166]

———, translator. *Pacification of Infectious Bile and Poisoning (Mkhris rims dugs thabs zhi byed),* attributed to Tārā; *Precious Beacon of Materia Medica (Sngo'i 'khrungs dpe rin chen); Precious Beacon Treasury (Rin po che sgron ma'i mdzod),* attributed to Mañjuśrī. [167]

Śāntipa. *Supreme Essence Commentary to the Eight Thousand Perfection of Wisdom Sutra. Aṣṭasāhasrikāprajñāpāramitāpañjikāsārottamā. Shes rab kyi pha rol tu phyin pa brgyad stong pa'i dka' 'grel snying po mchog.* Toh 3803, shes phyin *tha.* [228]

Śāntarakṣita. *Commentary on Twenty Verses on the Bodhisattva Vows. Saṃvaraviṃśakavṛtti. Sdom pa nyi shu pa'i 'grel pa.* Toh 4082, sems tsam *hi.* [379–80, 541n845]

———. *Ornament of the Middle Way. Madhyamakālaṃkārakārikā. Dbu ma rgyan gyi tshig le'ur byas pa.* Toh 3884, dbu ma *sa.* [242]

Saraha. *Buddhakapāla Mandala Ritual. Buddhakapālamaṇḍalavidhikramapradyotana. Sangs rgyas thod pa zhes bya ba'i dkyil 'khor gyi cho ga'i rim pa gsal ba.* Toh 1657, rgyud *ra.* [410]

———. *Commentary on the Buddhakapāla Tantra.* Toh 1652, rgyud 'grel *ra.* [544n925]

———. *Commentary on the Difficult Points of the Buddha Skull Tantra. Buddhakapālatantrapañjikājñānavatī. Sangs rgyas thod pa'i rgyud kyi dka' 'grel ye shes ldan pa.* Toh 1652, rgyud 'grel *ra.*

Sarvavarmā. *Kalāpa Sutra. Kalāpasūtra. Ka lā pa'i mdo.* Toh 4282, sgra mdo *le.* [216]

Sarvahitāmṛta Datta. *Caraka Supplement to the Ocean-Like Brahmā Āyurveda. Brahmavedasāraṅgadharacarakanāma. Tshangs pa'i rig byed rgya mtsho'i yan lag 'dzin pa gyo ba can.* Toh 4440, sna tshogs *no.* Attributed in the text to Raghunātha. [327]

Sasang Mati Paṇchen. *Well-Composed and Illuminating Commentary on the Kalāpasūtra Grammar Work. Sgra'i bstan bcos ka lā pa'i mdo'i rnam bshad legs sbyar rab gsal snang ba.* Collected Works of the Sakya, vol. 8. Tokyo: Tōyō Bunko, 1968–69. [45]

Sengdo Öchen (one of nine royal physicians), compiler and translator. *Guṇaśata in Five Hundred Fasicles (Gu ṇa shat a bam po lnga brgya ba); Eye of the Conch Illustrations ('Dra yig dung gi mig); Greater and Lesser Annotations on the Three Black Tantras (Nag po rgyud gsum gyi mdo byang che chung); Mirror of Equine Medicine in Three Collections (Rta'i dpyad me long skor gsum); Three Black Tantras (Nag po rgyud gsum); Turquoise Network: Entering the Forest of Medical Plants (Nags su 'jug pa g.yu yi dra ba).* [166–67]

Shāka Lo. *Structure of the Torso. Khog thig khrems.* [264]

Shakrampa Nyima Pal. *Sunlight Commentary. 'Grel bshad nyi ma'i 'od zer.* [264]

Shamarpa Chökyi Wangchuk. *Death-Defying Ambrosia: Treatise on Medical Science. Gso rig gi bstan bcos 'chi ba med pa'i bdud rtsi.* [322]

Shangtön Shikpo. *See* Chejé Shangtön Shikpo

Shangtön Siji Bar. *Mother and Son Stainless Radiance (Dri med gzi brjid ma bu); Outer and Inner Collections (Phyi skor nang skor); Rosary of Illustration and Meaning (Dpe don grangs kyi phreng ba); Stainless Radiance (Dri med gzi brjid); Sun Rays (Nyi ma'i 'od zer); Thirty Instructions (Gdams pa zum cu pa); Three Heart-Like Continuous Writings (Khong snying dang 'dra ba'i dkyus bkod rnam gsum); Six Illuminating Lamps (Sgron gsal drug).* [172, 267, 501]

Sherap Lodrö. *Essential Instructions (Man ngag don bsdus); Treatments for Naga Illness (Klu bcos).* [266]

Sherap Öser. *Secret Commentary to the Heart Tantra. Snying rgyud kyi don 'grel.* [265]

Shikpo. *Fourfold Exposition Collection. Don khrigs bzhi skor.* [266]

Shikpo Lingpa. *Treasure Transmissions. Gter lung.* [325]

Shönu Samten. *Treatment and Prevention of Epidemics from Guru Padma's Journey to Wild Boar Mountain. Gu ru pad ma phag rgod la chibs pa'i rims srungs bcos thabs kyi rgyun.* [177]

Shönu Wangchuk. *Essence of Somarāja. Sau ma rā ja'i bsdus don.* [265]

Siji Bar. *See* Shangtön Siji Bar

Śīlabhadra. *Presentation of the Levels to Enlightenment. Buddhabhūmivyākhyāna. Sangs rgyas kyi sa'i rnam par bshad pa.* Toh 3997, mdo 'grel *chi.* [243]

Sokdokpa Lodrö Gyaltsen. *Essence of the Definitive: Four Tantras as Enlightened Speech. Rgyud bzhi'i bka' sgrub nges don snying po.* [322]

Sönam Yeshé Gyaltsen. *History of Medicine: Sun that Nourishes the White Lotus / Sunlight that Opens the Lotus Grove of the Science of Medicine. Khog 'bugs pad dkar rgyas pa'i nyin byed / Gso rig pad tshal 'byed pa'i nyi 'od.* [286]

Śraddhakara Varman. *Understanding Highest Yoga Tantras. Yogānuttaratantārthāvatārasaṃgraha. Rnal 'byor bla na med pa'i rgyud kyi don la 'jug pa bsdus pa.* Toh 3713, rgyud, *tsu.* [210, 214]

Śrīdhara. *Various Clarifications: A Work on Lexicography. Abhidhānaśāstra-viśvalocana (ityaparābhidhānamuktāvalī). Mngon brjod kyi bstan cos sna tshogs gsal ba.* Toh 4453, sna tshogs *po.* [63, 453]

Śrīvajra and Chökyi Wangchuk, translators. *Rainbow Light Flash Tantra (Gzha' 'od 'khyug pa'i rgyud); Viramuni Tantra on Treatment for Poisons. (Dug bcos dpa' bo thub pa),* attributed to Nāgārjuna. [167]

Sthiramati. *Commentary to Differentiating the Middle Way and the Extremes. Madhyāntavibhaṅgaṭīkā. Dbus dang mtha' rnam par 'byed pa'i 'grel bshad.* Toh 4032, sems tsam *bi.* [265, 444]

———. *Explanation of the Kāśyapa Chapter from the Heap of Jewels Sutra. Mahāratnakūṭadharmaparyāyasatasāhasrikakāśyapaparivartaṭīkā. Dkon mchog brtsegs pa chen po chos kyi rnam grangs le'u stong phrag brgya pa las 'od srungs kyi le'u rgya cher 'grel pa.* Toh 4009, mdo 'grel *ji.* [243]

Sthiramati (Kashmir). *Stainless Radiance. Dri med gzi brjid.* [144, 169]

Subhūticandra. *The Wish-Fulfilling Cow: A Commentary to the Treasury of Immortality. Amarakoṣaṭīkākamadhenu. 'Chi ba med pa'i mdzod kyi rgya cher 'grel pa 'dod 'jo'i ba mo.* Toh 4300, sgra mdo *se.* [56]

Sumatikīrti (Nepal). *Three Preparations Compilation. Bsdus sbyor gsum.* [169]

Sumtön Yeshé Sung. *Effortless Accomplishment of the Five Bodies* or *Sealed Biography of Yuthok. Sku lnga lhun drub ma / Gyu thog pa'i rnam thar bka' rgya ma.* [256–59]

———. *Illuminating Beacon Small (Black) Collection: Commentary on the Explanatory Tantra. Bshad rgyud kyi 'grel ba 'bum chung (nag) gsal sgron.* [259, 459–60]

———. *Secret Biography. Gsang ba rnam thar.* [259]

———. *Sunlight of Compassion Clearing the Darkness of Suffering: History of the Heartdrop: Hook of Virtue. Sdug bsngal mun sel thugs rje nyi 'od snying tig lo rgyus dge ba'i lgags kyu.* Leh, Ladakh: D. L. Tashigang, Smanrtsis shesrig spendzod, vol. 106. [247, 256, 295]

———. *Treatment of Kangbam: Notes from the Whispered Tradition. Rkang 'bam gso ba snyan rgyud zin bris.* [259, 315]

Śūra.* *Pāramitā Synthesis. Pāramitāsamāsa. Pha rol tu phyin pa bsdus pa.* Toh 3944, dbu ma *khi.* [489]

Surkhar Lodrö Gyalpo. *Boiling Water. Chu skol rnam bshad.* [314]

———. *Clear Crystal Vase. Snang gsal shel bum pa.* [336]

———. *The Cuta Vine: Questions Put to Gongmen Könchok Phendar. Gong sman dkon cog phan dar la dri ba tsu ta'i 'khri shing.* [314]

———. *Dispelling the Torment of Sorrow: Entreating the Compassion of the Two Rishis. Drang srong rnam gnyis la thugs rje bskul ba mya ngan gdung sel.* [313]

———. *Eliminating Mistakes: Comments after the Printing of Four Tantras. Rgyud bzhi par bkod mjug rtsom gyi skyon sel.* [314]

———. *Eliminating the Impurities of Camphor, Saffron, Eaglewood, Sandalwood, and the Like. Ga bur gur kum a gar tsan dan sogs kyi skyon sel.* [314]

———. *Flower in the Cupped Palms of the Faithful. Dad ldan snyim pa'i me tog.* [313]

———. *Ford for Those of Bright Minds: Questions to the Panam Physician Künga Lekpa. Pa snam 'tsho byed kun legs par dri ba blos gsal 'jug ngogs.* [314]

———. *General Compendium of Knowledge Indispensable to Physicians (Sman pa rnams kyis mi shes su mi rung ba'i spyi'i khog dbubs). General Knowledge History: A Presentation on the External, Internal, and Other, Indispensable for Physicians Wishing to Engage in the Practices of the Bodhisattvas, the Wide Open Door to the Unending Ceremonial Offering, a Dance Delighting the Rishis. Gang dag byang chub sems dpa'i spyad par spyod par 'dod pa'i sman pa rnams kyis mi shes su mi rung ba'i phyi nang gzhan gsum gyi rnam bzhag shes bya'i spyi'i khog 'bugs drang srong kun du dga' ba'i zlos gar gtan pa med pa'i mchod sbyin gyi sgo 'phar yangs po.* [314, 499–500, 534n646]

———. *Golden Ornament Autocommentary. Rang 'grel gser gyi phra tshoms.* [312]

———. *Irrefutable and Extensive Written Account of the Life and Liberation of Rishi Nyamnyi Dorjé. Drang srong mnyam nyid rdo rje'i rnam thar 'gog pa med pa yi ge'i gtam chen mo.* Kun ming: Yun nan mi rigs dpe skrun khang, 2003. [309, 312]

———. *Lamp Dispelling Darkness: Presentation of Four Tantras as Being the Word of the Buddha and Treatise. Rgyud bzhi bka' dang bstan bcos rnam par dbye ba mun sel sgron me.* [534n646]

———. *Moondrops: An Ocean of Light. Zla thig nyin byed 'od mtsho.* [314]

———. *My Own Response: The Testament of an Old Man, a Flash of Lightning on a Dark Night. Rang lan rgan po kha chems mtshan mo mun nag gi glog 'od lta bu.* [311, 312, 315]

———. *Oral Transmission of Our Ancestors. Mes po'i zhal lung.* Leh: T. S. Tashigang, 1980–85. [77, 312, 314, 315, 326, 328]

———. *An Outline to Captivate the Minds of the Wise: The Contents of Relic of Millions—Great Dispeller of Hindrances. Bye ba ring bsrel bzhugs tshul gegs sel chen mo'i nang ltar dkar chag mkhas pa'i yid 'phrog.* [313, 315]

———. *Questions and Answers on Manu. Ma nu'i dris lan.* [314]

———. *Questions and Answers: A Well-Composed Emetic. Dris lan legs bshad skyugs pa.* [314]

———. *Questions Beautifying a Stone Pillar: A Flash of Lightning on a Dark Night: The Testament of an Old Man. Rdo ring mdzes byed kyi dris lan rgan po kha chems mtshan mo mun nag gi glog 'od lta bu.* [311, 315]

———. *Refined Drop of Summer Sun: Answers to Questions from a Phenyül Doctor on the Rising of the Wind Element. 'Phan yul gyi sman pa rlung khams langs pa'i dris lan dbyar nyi'i zhun thig.* [314]

———. *Requests Based on Biography: A New Enjoyment Ocean of Faith. Rnam thar gsol 'debs dad pa'i rol mtsho gsar pa.* [313]

———. *Table of the Powers, Tastes, and Post-Digestive Tastes of Medicines. Sman gyi ro nus zhus rjes kyi re'u mig.* [314]

———. *Thunder: The Rousing Drum of Summer. Dbyar skyes rnga sangs.* [314]

———. *White Singly Powerful Medicine or the Vajra of Indra: Reply to the Jang Position on Establishing the Tantra as the Word of the Buddha. Byang pa'i bka' sgrub kyi lan dkar po chig thub bam dbang po'i lag nyal.* [313]

Surkhar Nyamnyi Dorjé. *Advice Beneficial for Others and Myself. Rang bzhan la phan pa'i bslab bya.* [308]

———. *Ambrosia Pool. Bdud rtsi rdzing bu.* [308]

———. *Ambrosia Treasury. Bdud rtsi gter mdzod.* [308]

———. *Commentary on the Kālacakra Tantra. Dpal dus kyi 'khor lo'i 'grel chen.* [308]

———. *Fundamentals of Medicines. Sman gyi byings.* [308]

———. *Golden Spoon of Excellent Explanation. Legs bshad ser thur.* [308]

———. *Guidance on Mahāmudrā and on Places for Cutting-Off Practice. Phyag chen dang gcod yul gyi 'khrid yig.* [308]

———. *Iron Garland Collection on Tastes. Ro skor lcags kyi 'phreng ba.* [308]

———. *A Letter to Far-Flung Physicians. Phyogs kyi sman pa rnams la springs yig.* [308]

———. *Mirror of White Mercury: Questions on the Difficult Points of the Tantra / Overview. Rgyud kyi dka' gnad rnams la dri tsig dngul dkar me long / Spyi don.* [308, 313]

———. *Precious Illustrations / Identification and Clarification of Medicines. Rin chen 'khrungs dpe / Sman ngo gsal byed.* [308]

———. *Relic of Millions. Bye ba ring bsrel.* New Delhi: Tibet House, 1985 and Leh: S. W. Tashigangpa, 1974. [13, 295–309, 311, 313, 325, 498]

———. *Sunrays: A Well-Composed Work. Legs bshad nyi zer.* [308]

———. *Vajra Songs of Experience and Collection of Praises. Nyams kyi rdo rje'i glu dang bstod tshogs skor.* [308]

———. *Well-Composed Work Called Sunrays. Legs bshad nyi zer.* [308]

———. *A Work of Fine Crystal: Extensive Commentary on the Four Glorious Tantras. Dpal ldan rgyud bzhi'i 'grel chen pod shal khra mo.* [308, 313]

Sūryasiṃha. *Fungi Therapy for Poisons. Dug bcos sha mo las dkyus.* Translated by Vairocana, hidden by Muné Tsenpo, and revealed by Nanam Thupa Gyalpo. [189]

Takgom Ngönshé Chen. *Compilation of Essential Miscellaneous Treatments. Thor dpyad snying gi don bsdud.* [267]

Takla Gah. *Laying Out the Keys to Eight Branches. Brgyad pa'i lde mig don khrigs.* [266]

Taktsang Lotsāwa Sherap Rinchen. *Essence of Medical Practices. Sman gyi lag len gces bdus pa.* [264]

———. *Exposition on the History of Medicine. Gso dpyad byung tshul gyi lo rgyus khog 'bugs.* [264]

———. *Knowledge of All Sciences. Rig gnas kun shes. Quintessence of the Ten Sciences of Tibet. Gangs ljongs rig bcu'i snying bcud chen mo.* Vol. 1. Beijing: Mi rigs dpe skrun khang, 2006. [215–16, 217, 501]

———. *Ocean Overview of Kālacakra. Dus 'khor spyi don bstan pa'i rgya mtsho.* New Delhi: Trayang and Jamyang Samten, 1973. [216]

Tārā (from the Bodhisattva Tradition). *Illustrative Work on Medicinal Plants in 120 Chapters (Sngo shing gi 'khrung dpe le'u brgya dang nyi shu); Preparing Medicinal Plants (Sngo sbyor); Six Methods for Dealing with Pain (Zug rngu rtsal thabs drug).* [102]

Tashi Dar. *Short Essential Work on Fevers. Tshad pa'i tig chung.* [267]

Tashi Dorjé. *Precious Garland. Rin chen 'phreng wa.* [267]

Tertön Gyashang Trom. *Compilation of Essential Profound Treasures. Zab gter bcud kyi don bsdus.* [267]

Thangmen Drangsong Döndrup. *Tarima Death-Defying Ambrosia. Bdud rtsi 'chi gsos rta ri ma.* [189]

Thar Lotsāwa Nyima Gyaltsen. *Instructions on Calcite. Cong zhi'i gdams pa.* [173]

Thazhi Rinchen. *Matted-Hair Core Instructions. Skra shad 'dzings pa'i don bsdus.* [265]

Thazhi Śīlasaṃgha. *Stream of Ambrosia Medical History. Khog 'bugs 'dud rtsi'i chu rgyun.* [264, 501]

Thönmi Sambhota. *Thirty Verses. Vyākaraṇamūlatriṃśaka. Lung du ston pa'i rtsa ba sum cu pa.* Toh 4348, sna tshogs *co.* [330, 361, 449]

———. *Use of Affixes. Vyākaraṇaliṅgāvataraṇa. Lung du ston pa rtags kyi 'jug pa.* Toh 4349, sna tshogs *co.* [330]

Thukjé Triö. *See* Chejé Shangtön Shikpo

Thumi Sambhota. *See* Thönmi Sambhota

Tisang. *Essentials of Eight Branches. Brgyad pa'i don bsdus.* [266]

Tongmen Tsojé Shönu. *Compilation of Essentials of the Eight Branches (Brgyad pa'i snying po bsdus pa); Treatise on Mercury Preparation (Dngul chu grub pa'i bstan bcos).* [264]

Tongsum Gangwa. *Four Refined Ingredients Compound from the Tradition of the Surrounding Countries (Mtha' bzhi'i lugs zhu ba bzhi ldan); Traveling Lamp of Good Medicine (Gso ba dkar po lam gyi sgron me).* [168]

Tongsum Gangwa, Hvashang Bala, and Hangti Pata (Chinese doctors from the nine royal physicians), compilers and translators. *Garland of Medicinal Compounds (Sbyor ba'i phreng ba); Magic Mirror Exposition on Anatomy (Byang khog don 'grel/'grems 'phrul gyi me long); Treatment of the Limbs: Five Jewel*

Treasuries Arising from Gestures of the Hand (Yan lag phyag gi brda las byung wa); Untainted Jewel of Remedial Treatment (Ja log nor bu dri ma med pa); Fire and Water Reversal (Me chu go bzlog); Wheel of Fire Treatment for Poisons (Dug dpyad me lce 'khor lo); Specific Treatments for Miscellaneous Ailments (Thor bu'i nad kyi sgos bcos); Urine Analysis (Chu dpyad); Magical Treatments (Mkhyud dpyad); Beacon of Cauterization Practice (Me btsa'i lag len sgron me). All attributed to Mañjuśrī. [166]

Tötön Könchok Kyap. *Jeweled Net Outline (of Eight Branches). Gzhung gi sa bcad bsdus don rin po che'i dra ba.* [173]

Trikhu. *Six Chapters on Fever. Tshad pa'i skabs drug.* [266]

Trülku Dampa Marpo, revealer. *Great Ambrosia Elixir Collection: Root of All Siddhis (Dngos grub kun gyi rtsa ba bdud rtsi chen po'i bcud len gyi skor).* This includes: *Ambrosia Practice of Precious Garland Preparations (Bdud rtsi lag len rin chen 'phreng sbyor); Tantra on Ambrosia-Producing Teachings (Lung bdud rtsi 'byung pa'i rgyud); Ambrosia Teachings (Bdud rtsi lung 'bogs); Blessings of Ambrosia (Bdud rtsi byin rlabs); Clearing the Difficult Paths of Medicine (Sman gyi 'phrang bsal); Excrement Ambrosia Accomplishment (Bdud rtsi dri chen sgrub thabs); Instructions on Ambrosia in the Form of Butter (Bdud rtsi mar du drangs pa'i zhal gdams);* and *Instructions on the Use of Elixirs (Bcud len lag tu blangs pa'i zhal gdams).* This last text includes: *Mañjuśrī Secret Moon ('Jam dpal zla gsang* from *Dpal zla gsang nag po'i rgyud)* and *Vairocana Method of Producing Elixir from Liquid Butter (Rnam par snang mdzad mar khu bcud 'byung ba'i thabs).* [186]

Tsarong Aü. *Quick Path for the Fortunate: A Religious History. Chos 'byung skal bzang bgrod pa'i myur lam.* [500]

Tsarong Chöjé Palden Gyaltsen. *Overview of Medicine / Lamp Dispelling the Darkness: A New Tradition of Teaching. Gso rig spyi don / Bshad pa'i srol 'byed mun sel sgron me.* [320]

Tsenpashila[ha]. *Biji's Yellow Collection / Radiant Documents of the King (Bi ji'i po ti kha ser / Rgyal po'i bla yig 'od 'bar),* includes seventy-eight instructional works as well as *Black Compilation Collection with Units of Measurements (Be bum nag po'i skor 'jal tshad dang bcas pa)* and *Three Collections on Clear Descriptions of Head, Abdomen, and Limbs from Caraka's Rishi Essence Tantra (Tsa ra kas mdzad pa drang srong snying rgyud mgo byang khog yan lag gi pra 'khrid skor gsum).* [156, 336]

———. *Collection on Health: Higher Texts on Medical Practice (Bla dpyad kyi gzhung 'tsho ba'i mdo).* Refers to the entire corpus of translations and compositions that Tsenpashila offered to the Tibetan king. [153]

———. *Crystal Mirror Tantra. Rgyud shel gyi me long,* with ancillary texts and commentaries: *Heart-Like Network (Snying gi dra ba); Red Ink Illuminating Beacon on the Upper Abdomen (Byang khog stod kyi dmar byang gsal ba'i sgron me); Red Ink Magic Key to the Lower Abdomen (Smad kyi dmar byang 'phrul kyi lde mig); Teachings on Treatment of the Limbs (Yan lag gi bcos them byang).* [152–53, 154]

———. The four secret and exclusive son texts: *Essential Beacon for the Elimination of Hindrances (Bgegs sel gnad kyi sgron ma); Four Conclusions from Examinations of Pus (Rnag brtag thag chod bzhi ba); Gentle Ambrosia Emetic for Pus (Rnag skyug 'jam 'dren); Precious Base Emaciation Medicine (Skem sman rin chen gzhi bzhag).* [153]

———. *Heartdrop Collection (Snying tig bsdus pa),* which consists of: *The Beacon (Sgron ma); Lesser Network (Dra chung); Lesser Treatise on Pacification (Zhi chung); Small Commentary (Ṭik chung).* [153, 293]

———, translator. *Abdomen of Humans and Rishis (Drang srong mi'i khog pa); Bones of the Rishis (Drang srong gi keng rus); Chapter on Restoring Joints (Tshigs kyi sdoms kyi le'u); Chasing Fever (Tshad pa 'bros 'ded); Clear Drop Treatise on the Threefold Classification of Wounds (Rma skor gsum ston pa thig le gsal ba'i mdo); Combining the Nine Anatomical Threads (Ro bkra thi gu dgu sbyor); Essential and Quintessential Versions of Brown Compilation (Be bum smug po tig yang tig gnyis); Feminine Gem (Mo dbyig); Four Chapters on Essentials for Physicians (Sman pa la rab tu gces le'u bzhi); Great* and *Lesser Concise Annotations (Mdo byang che chung)* composed by Hvashang Kyinda; *Lesser Red Ink Text (Yi ge dmar chung); Magic Almsbowl of Daryakan Ambrosia (Bdud rtsi dar ya kan lhung bzed),* composed by Trulpai Khyeu; *Magic Mirror of Anatomy (Ro bkra 'phrul gyi me long); Measurements of Living and Dead Bodies (Gson thig ro thig gi rnam gzhag); Mirror of Ambrosia (Bdud rtsi me long); Precious Garland (Rin po che'i phreng ba); Precious Gem (Rin chen dbyig / Rin po che'i dbyig); Resolving Disputes Concerning the Head (Mgo ba'i rtsod bzlog),* composed by Vajrapāṇi; *Restoring Joints (Tshigs kyi sdoms); Structure of the Abdomen (Byang khog khrems kyi mdo),* reputedly by Ātreya; *Suspended Rope of Five Essentials (Don snying rnam pa lnga'i dpyang thag); Thirteen Chapters (Le'u bcu gsum); Thirty-Five Faults (Nyes dmigs sum cu rtsa lnga); Three Secret Commentaries (Gsang ṭik gsum); Treasure Mine: Ten Chapters of Beneficial Medicine (Rin po che'i mdzod phan pa sman gyi le'u bcu ba).* [153, 154, 169]

Tsojé Drupa. *Arrowhead Treatment for Eyes and Urinary Stones (Mig dang rde'u'i sgos bcos mde thung sbyar); Treatment of Growths ('Bras bcos).* [264, 265]

Tsojé Könchok Kyap. *Compilation on Hot and Cold Disorders. Tsha grang gi stong thun.* [267]

Tsojé Namkha Gyaltsen. *Essence of Eight Branches. Brgyad pa'i don bsdus.* [265]

Tsoknyi Gyatso of Phenyül Drosawa. *Stream of Beryl: A History of Four Tantras. Rgyud bzhi'i khog 'bubs bai dūrya'i chu rgyun.* [313, 497]

Tsomé Khenchen. *See* Kawa Śākya Wangchuk

Tsöndrü Nyingpo. *Sukhuk. Su khugs.* [169]

Tsöndrü Sengé. *Essence of Madhyāntavibhaṅga. Dbus mtha'i don bsdus.* [265]

Tsongkhapa (Losang Drakpa). *Blossom Cluster of Siddhis: Teachings on Tantric Ethics. Gsang sngags kyi tshul khrims rnam bshad dngos grub kyi snye ma.* Shöl Parkhang Collection, vol. *ka.* Translated as *Tantric Ethics* by Gareth Sparham (Boston: Wisdom Publications, 2005). [393, 395, 543–44n905, 544n925]

———. *Essence of the Ocean of Vinaya. 'Dul ba rgya mtsho'i snying po bsdus pa.* Shöl Parkhang Collection, vol. *ka.* [368]

———. *Fulfilling All Hopes of the Disciples: A Commentary on Fifty Verses on the Guru. Bla ma lnga bcu pa'i rnam bshad slob ma'i re ba kun skong shes bya ba.* Shöl Parkhang Collection, vol. *ka.* [355, 538n752]

———. *Golden Rosary of Eloquence. Legs bshad gser gyi phreng ba / Shes rab kyi pha rol tu phyin pa'i man ngag gi bstan cos mngon par rtogs pa'i rgyan 'grel pa dang bcas pa'i rgya cher bshad pa.* Shöl Parkhang Collection, vols. *tsa, tsha.* [243]

———. *Highway to Enlightenment: An Exposition of Bodhisattva Ethics. Byang chub sems dpa' tshul khrims kyi rnam bshad byang chub gzhung lam.* Shöl Parkhang Collection, *ka.* [376, 380]

———. *Ocean of Reasoning. Dbu ma rtsa ba'i tshig le'ur byas pa shes rab ces bya ba'i rnam bshad rigs pa'i rgya mtsho.* Shöl Parkhang Collection, vol. *ba.* [243]

———. *Song of Realization. Rtogs brjod mdun legs ma.* Shöl Parkhang Collection, *kha.* [411, 418]

———. *Stages of Mantra / Great Exposition of Secret Mantra. Rgyal ba khyab bdag rdo rje 'chang chen po'i lam gyi rim pa gsang ba kun gyi gnad rnam par phye ba.* Shöl Parkhang Collection, *ga.* Delhi: Sokpo Lama (Mongolian Lama), 1978. [214, 539n765]

———. *Words Composed on the Three Jewels. Rin po che gsum gyi gtam gyi sbyor ba.* Shöl Parkhang Collection, *kha.* [450–51]

Ukpa Chösang. *Crystal Jewel Commentary. Dbyig shel don 'grel.* [266]

Ulang. *History of Medicine. Khog dbubs.* [266]

Urbaya/Urvaya. *Six Narratives. Chos 'byung drug.* [169]

Vairocana. *Darkness-Dispelling Lamp of Explanation (Tikka mun sel sgron ma); Medical Dictionary in Five Parts (Ming don brda sprod rnam lnga).* [163]

———, translator. *Instructions on Medicinal Plants (Hundred Thousand Medicinal Plants of Mañjuśrī). Sngo'i man ngag ('Jam dbyangs sngo 'bum).* [162]

Vairocana and Pandit Ratnavajra, translators. *Jewel Heap Planet Tantra. Gza' rgyud rin chen spungs pa.* Composed as a dialogue between Vajrapāṇi and Nāgārjuna. [167]

Vajramati. *Extraordinary and Profound Ḍākinī Treasures. Mkha' 'gro zab gter ngo mtshar can.* [176]

Vajrapāṇi. *Cakrasaṃvara Commentary / Vajrapāṇi Commentary. Lakṣābhidhānāduddhṛtalaghutantrapiṇḍārthavivaraṇanāma. Mngon par brjod pa 'bum pa las phyung pa nyung ba'i rgyud kyi bsdus pa'i don rnam par bshad pa / Phyag rdor stod 'grel.* Toh 1402, rgyud 'grel *ba.* [504]

Vajrapāṇi (from the Bodhisattva Tradition). *Black Jaṭila (Lcang lo nag po); Charms for Pain (Zug rngu rten 'brel brtag pa); Curing All Miscellaneous Disorders (Kha thor kun 'joms); Magic Mirror of Anatomy (Ro bkra 'phrul gyi me long),* received by earlier Yuthok; *Precious Wheel of the Eight Planets (Gza' brgyad 'khor lo rin chen); Settling Arguments over Head Ailments (Mgo'i rtsod bzlog); Upturned Lotus (Pad ma sbubs pa).* [102]

Vasubandhu. *Commentary to Sutra Requested by Akṣayamati. Akṣayamatinirdeśaṭīkā. Blo gros mi zad pas bstan pa rgya cher 'grel pa.* Toh 3994, mdo 'grel *ci.* [243]

———. *Science of Explanation. Vyākhyāyukti. Rnam par bshad pa'i rigs pa.* Toh 4061, sems tsam *shi.* [226, 239, 360, 361, 474]

———. *Thirty Verses. Triṃśikākārikā. Sum cu pa'i tshig le'ur byas pa.* Toh 4055, sems tsam *shi.* [242]

———. *Treasury of Abhidharma. Abhidharmakośa. Chos mngon pa'i mdzod kyi tshig le'ur byas pa.* Toh 4089, mngon pa *ku.* [77, 221–22, 226, 241, 242, 336, 421]

Vasudhāra Medicine Goddess (from the Fortunate Eon Deva Tradition). *Precious Garland. Rin po che'i 'phreng ba.* [102]

Vibhūticandra. *Garland of Light on the Three Vows. Trisaṃvaraprabhāmālā. Sdom gsum 'od kyi phreng ba.* Toh 3727, rgyud *tshu.* [409, 423–25, 544n927]

Vinītadeva. *Three Hundred Verses Commentary. Triśatakārikavyākhyāna. Tshig le'ur byas pa sum brgya pa'i rnam par bshad pa.* Toh 4126, 'dul ba *shu.* [242]

Viśākhadeva. *Vinaya Flower Garland. Vinayakārikā. 'Dul ba tshig le'ur byas pa me tog phreng rgyud.* Toh 4123, 'dul ba *shu.* [105, 242]

Wangchuk. *Commentary on the Causes of Purification. Dag rgyu'i tik ka.* [266]

Yaśomitra. *Bodhisattva Abhidharma Commentary. Abhidharmakośaṭīkā. Chos mngon pa'i mdzod kyi 'grel bshad.* Toh 4092, mngon pa *gu/ngu.* [222–23]

Yeshé Khadro. *Instructions on Curing Illness. Nad sel gdams pa.* Translated by Jalipa and Tropu Lotsāwa. [175]

Yeshé Lodrö. *Treatments for Poisoning. Dug bcos.* [267]

Yeshé Wangchuk. *Ambrosia Drops Collection on Gaklhok Treatments. Gag lhog gi bcos skor bdud rtsi'i thigs pa.* [264]

Yiwong Lekpa. *Eight Ambrosia Chapters. Bdud rtsi le brgyad.* [267]

Yungdrung Tönpa Shenrap. *Mottled Naga Collection. Klu 'bum khra bo.* Published in Delhi, 1977, by Khedrup Gyatso. [64]

Yuthok Gönpo. *Annotations and Accounts from the Golden Jewel Tantra. Ratna gser rgyud las mchan dang lo rgyus.* [266]

Yuthok Gönpo Dorjé. *Auxiliary Texts for the Tantra. Rgyud kyi cha lag.* [266]

Yuthok Gönpo Drupa. *Commentary Clarifying the Meaning. 'Grel ba don gsal.* [266]

Yuthok Gönpo Sherap. *Ambrosia Essence Instructions. Man ngag bdud rtsi bcud.* [266]

Yuthok Gyaltsa. *Great Compilation (Stong thun chen mo); Scripture Count: Essence of the Sun (Lung grangs nyi ma'i snying po).* [263]

Yuthok Kharak Lhajé. *Jewel Garland Biography of Yönten Gönpo. Yon tan mgon po'i rnam thar nor bur in chen 'phreng ba.* [260]

Yuthok Tashi Gön. *Brief Work on the Number of Chapters (Le grangs bsdus don); Increase and Diminution ('Phel zad); Stages of the Niruha Enema Therapy (Ni ru ha'i las rim); Taste Preparations (Ro sbyor); Twenty Characteristics (Mtshan nyid ni shu).* [263]

Yuthok Yönten Gönpo (Earlier), received from Agniśa. *Collection on the Science of Healing (Gso dpyad 'bum pa); Crystal Mirror Tantra (Rgyud shel gyi me long); Essential Charm Circle (Gnad kyi 'phrul 'khor); Essential Key to Surgery (Thur dpyad gnad kyi lde mig); One Hundred and Eighteen Clear Instructions on Chasing Disease (Dmar 'ded brgya dang bco brgyad); One Thousand and One Commentaries on the Tantra (Rgyud 'grel stong dang rtsa gcig); Pointing Out Secret Divisions of the Torso (Byang khog gsang dbye mdzub btsug); Secret Measurements (Gsang thig).* [201, 202]

———, received from Candrabhīra. *Whispered Transmission of the Rishis. Drang srong snyan rgyud.* [202]

———, received from Mañjuśrī. *Exposition on the Abdomen (Byang khog don khrems); Garland of Medical Compounds (Sbyor ba'i 'phreng ba).* [205]

———, received from Medicine Buddha. *Ambrosia Medicine Practice* [205] *(Dud rtsi sman sgrub); Garland of Ambrosia Medicine (Bdud rtsi sman phreng); Medical Teachings on Practices of the Five Sword Collections (Sman khrid ral skor lnga'i phyag len).* [201, 205]

———, received by. *Bright Beacon Table of Contents (Dkar chag gsal sgron); Hundred Manuals ('Khrid yig brgya rtsa); Magic Mirror of Anatomy (Ro bkra 'phrul gyi me long); Pearl Garland Supplement to the Four Glorious Tantras (Dpal ldan rgyud bzhi'i kha skong mu tig phreng ba).* [201, 202]

Yuthok Yönten Gönpo (Later), received from Kanakavarman. *Ambrosia Inscriptions Threshold Manuscript on Presentation of the Body (Lus kyi rnam bzhag bdud rtsi them yig); Arising of Tārā (Sgrol ma 'byung); Brief Indian Work (Rgya yig smra chung); Chapter on Anatomy (Ro brka le'u); Craft of Precious Stones and Metals Such as Gold (Gser sogs rin po che'i bzo); Ḍāka Liberation (Dpa' bo 'ching 'gron); Examination of the Pulse (Reg pa rtsa dpyad); Fragment Transmission (Lung bsil bu); Guṇaśāstra (Gu ṇa sha skra'i rgyud); Hide Casket (Bse sgrom); Individual Elements ('Byung ba so so); Leaves of the Birch Tree (Gro kha'i 'debs ma); Liberation of Beings (Srog chags sgrol ba); Mañjuśrī Mother and Father ('Jam dpal yab yum); Nourishing Flesh and Blood (Sha khrag 'tsho ba); Teaching of the Essence (Snying po bstan pa); Three Hundred Fascicles (Bam po sum brgya); Union of Sun and Moon (Nyi zla kha sbyor).* [207]

———, received from the goddess Amṛtā. *Ambrosia Preparation for Healing*

Wounds (Rma rtsi 'chi med bcad sbyor); Beacon Medical Texts (Gso dpyad sgron ma skor gsum); Three Collections of Question and Answer (Zhu lan skor gsum). [207]

———, received by. *Ambrosia Vase (Bdud rtsi bum pa); Commentary on Protecting Life (Srog skyob ti ka); Essence of Ambrosia Eight Branches (Bdud rtsi snying po yan lag brgyad pa); Illustrations of Medical Plants ('Khrungs dpe che chung); Kumuda Flower (Ku mu da); Secret Preparations of Minerals (Rdo sbyor gab pa); Sutra of Help (Phan pa'i mdo); Sutra on Pulse (Reg pa rtsa mdo).* [202, 206, 207]

———. *Brief Document on the Work of the Doctor. Sman pa'i bya mdor bsdus pa.* [251]

———. *Clear Depiction of Channels of the Abdomen. Byang khog gi rtsa pra.* [250]

———. *Compositions for My Sons. Bu don ma.* [250, 336]

———. *Copper Annotations. Zangs mchan.* [209, 336]

———. The Eighteen Auxiliary Texts (ascribed to Yuthok and other early physicians). *Cha lag bco brgyad.* Gansu: People's Publications, 1999. The eighteen are: *Ambrosia Essence Short Tantra (Rgyud chung bdud rtsi snying po); Beautiful Rainbow Overview (Stong thun mdzes pa'i 'ja' ris); Darkness-Dispelling Lamp of Explanation (Ṭikka mun sel sgron me); Eighteen Secrets (Gab pa bco brgyad); Eleven Sectional Overviews (Skor tshoms stong thun bcu gcig); Four Wondrous Superior Features (Mkhas khyad ngo mtshar sprugs); Great Garuḍa History of Medicine (Khog 'bugs khyung chen lding ba); Great Treatise on the Pulse (Rtsa mdo chen po); Illuminating Beacon: Black Commentary Collection ('Grel pa 'bum nag gsal sgron); Lexicon in Five Parts (Min don brda sprod rnam lnga); Outline: Wrathful Pose of the Tigress (Sa bcad stag mo'i rngam thabs); Pearl Garland Medical Practice (Gso dpyad mu tig 'phreng ba); Precious Heap of Miscellany (Kha thor rin chen spung pa); Precious Jewel Heap of Medical Practice (Lag len rin chen gter spung); Refutation of Arguments: Hindrance-Destroying Wheel (Rtsod bzlog gegs sel 'khor lo); Short Works on Incisive Medical Practices (Lag len mar 'khrid yig chung); Three Indispensables (Med thabs med pa gsum); Three Profound Instructions (Zab pa rnam gsum); White Collection of Beneficial Mantras (Phan bya sngags 'bum dkar po).* [208, 249–50, 326, 335, 336, 459–60, 497, 498]

———. *Eliminating Bodily Disturbance Caused by the Elements. 'Byung ba lus 'khrugs kyi gegs sel.* [250]

———. *Essential Instructions. Zin tik.*

———. *Explicit Annotations. Smar mchan.* [336]

———. *Fistful Collection on the Gathered Essence of Instruction. Man ngag gi snying po drill ba khur tshur.* [250]

———. *Five-Ingredient Pain Medicine. Gzer sman gnyen po lnga sbyor.* [250–51]

———. *Fourteen Works on Women's Diseases. Mo nad ncos thabs yig sna bcu bzhi pa* [250].

———. *Golden Annotations. Gser mchan.* [209, 311–12, 336]

———. *Great Collection on Medicinal Plants. Sngo 'bum chen mo.* [250]

———. *Heap of Miscellany Jewels. Kha 'thor rin chen spungs pa.*

———, received from Śrīmālā. *Heart Blood of the Ḍākinī (Mkha 'gro'i snying khrag); Sixty-Five Classes of Moonbeam Essential Tantras on the Eight Branches (Yan lag brgyad pa bsil zer gyi gnad rgyud rigs drug cu rtsa lnga); Tantra of the Black Lock of Hair (Lcang lo nag po'i rgyud).* [208]

———. *Heartdrop Collection. G.yu thog snying thik skor.* [251–53, 311, 317, 318, 325, 335, 548n1046]

———. *Heat Lancing of Boils and So Forth. Thor bu me len.* [250]

———. *Illustrations of Bandages, Ties, and Splints. Deb chings rgyogs sogs kyi dpeu' ris.* [250]

———. *Mirror of Clear Image. Pra gsal ba' me long* [250].

———. *Naturally Illuminating Knowledge of Pulse Examination. Rtsa dpyad rig pa rang gsal.* [208]

———. *Pacifying Poisoning. Dug nad zhi ba.* [250]

———. *Quintessence. Yang snying bsdus pa.* [351]

———. *Quintessential Instructions. Yang tik.* [157]

———. *Six Key Collections. Lde mig skor drug.* [208]

———. *Small Volume on Practice. Lag len po ti chung.* [208, 250]

———. *Stream of Instructions on Treatment of Brown Phlegm Disorders. Smug po gso ba chu rgyun gyi gdams pa.* [250]

———. *Teachings on Medicinal Plants: Lamp Dispelling Error (Ngo'i man ngag 'khrul sel sgron me).* [250]

———. The Thirteen Auxiliary Texts (popularly ascribed to the later Yuthok Yönten Gonpo): *Collection of Beneficial Mantras (Phan byed sngags 'bum); Complete Heart-Teachings Collection (Gang ba snying gtam gyi skor); Hidden Document on Names (Gab yig ming brda sprod); Inventory without Fault (Dkar chag 'phyugs med); Investigation of Bezoar (Dbang po ril bu'i brtags thabs); Page on Compress Treatment for Head Injury (Mgo chag zlum bcos shog gcig); Rishi Treatment for Planetary Illness (Drang srong gza'i bcod thabs); Son Manuscript Supplement on the Body (Kha skong lus kyi bu yig); Sunlight of Wisdom Outline (Sa bcad shes rab nyin byed); Three Treatments for Lhok (Gnyan lhog bcos thabs rigs gsum); Way of Compiling the 404 Diseases (Bzhi brgya rtsa bzhi'i bsdus tshul); Word Commentary of the Three Humors (Nyes pa gsum gyi 'bru 'grel); Word Commentary on Causes of Excess and Deficiency (Zad 'phel byed pa'i 'bru 'grel).* [249–50]

———. *Three Scroll Collections. Shog dril skor gsum.* [208, 250]

———. *Urine Charm Circle. Chu'i 'khor lo.* [250]

Works Consulted by the Translator

Beckwith, Christopher I. "Tibetan Treacle: A Note on Theriac in Tibet." *Bulletin.* Bloomington, IN: The Tibet Society, 1980.

———. "The Introduction of Greek Medicine into Tibet in the Seventh and Eighth Centuries." *Journal of American Oriental Society* 99.2 (1979): 297–313.

Butön Rinchen Drup. *Annotations to the Inner Chapter of the Vimalaprabhā. Dri med 'od kyi mchan la nang gi le'u'i mchan 'grel.* Shöl Parkhang Collection, vol. *kha.*

Cabezón, José Ignacio, and Roger R. Jackson, eds. *Tibetan Literature: Studies in Genre.* Ithaca, NY: Snow Lion Publications, 1996.

Chandra, Lokesh. *Tibetan-Sanskrit Dictionary.* 7 volumes. New Delhi: Aditya Prakashan, 1992.

Chimpa, Lama, and Alaka Chattopadhyaya. *Tāranātha's History of Buddhism in India.* Delhi: Motilal Banarsidass, 1970.

Clark, Barry. *The Quintessence Tantras of Tibetan Medicine.* Ithaca, NY: Snow Lion Publications, 1995.

Cleary, Thomas, trans. *The Flower Ornament Scripture: A Translation of the Avatamsaka Sutra.* 3 vols. Boulder, CO: Shambhala, 1984–87.

Cotterell, Arthur. *China: A Concise Cultural History.* London: John Murray Publishers, 1988.

Dash, Vaidya Bhagwan. *Encyclopedia of Tibetan Medicine.* Delhi: Sri Satguru Publications, 1994.

———. *Materia Medica of Tibetan Medicine, with Illustrations.* New Delhi: Sri Satguru Publications, 1994.

———. *Tibetan Medicine Theory and Practice.* Delhi: Sri Satguru Publications, 1997.

———. *Tibetan Medicine with Special Reference to Yoga Śataka.* Dharamsala, India: Library of Tibetan Works and Archives, 1976.

Desi Sangyé Gyatso. *Tibetan Medical Paintings: Illustrations to the Blue Beryl Treatise of Sangye Gyamtso.* Eds. Yuri Parfionovitch, Gyurme Dorje, and Fernand Meyer. London: Serindia Publications, 1992. Published simultaneously at New York: H. N. Abrams, 1992.

———. *Yellow Beryl History of the Geluk School. Dga' ldan chos 'byung beryl ser po.* Beijing: Drungo Tibetan Educational Publication, 1987.

Dictionary of Medicine: Adornment to the Thoughts of Yuthok. Gso ba rig pa'i tshig mdzod g.yu thog dgong rgyan. Beijing: Mi rigs dpe skrun khang, 1982.

Drungtso, Tsering Thakchoe. *Tibetan Medicine: The Healing Science of Tibet.* Dharamsala, India: Drungtso Publications, 2004.

Dudjom Rinpoché, Gyurme Dorje, and Matthew Kapstein. *The Nyingma School of Tibetan Buddhism.* Boston: Wisdom Publications, 1991.

Dungkar Losang Trinlé. *Dungkar Tibetological Great Dictionary*. Beijing: Bod kyi shes rig dpe skrun khang, 2002.

Dutt, Uday Chand. *Materia Medica of the Hindus*. Varanasi: Chowkhamba Saraswati Bhawan, 1980 (Rev. ed. of 1877 publication).

Fairbank, John K., and Edwin O. Reischauer. *China: Tradition and Transformation*. Boston: Houghton Mifflin, 1989.

Gawa Dorjé. *'Khrungs dpe dri med shel gyi me long*. Beijing: Mi rigs dpe skrun khang, 1995.

Gö Lotsāwa Shönu Pal. *The Blue Annals. Deb ther sngon po*. New Delhi: International Academy of Indian Culture, 1974.

Great Tibetan-Chinese Dictionary. Bod rgya tshig mdzod chen mo, 3 vols. Beijing: Mi rigs dpe skrun khang, 1985.

Horner, I. B., trans. *Sacred Books of the Buddhists*, part 4. London: Luzac and Co., 1971.

Jamgön Kongtrül Lodrö Thayé. *Precious Treasury. Rin chen gter mdzod chen mo*. Tshurpu redaction. Paro, Bhutan: Ngödrup and Sherap Drimé, 1980.

Kachuwa Chölothar. *Bod kyi gso dpyad rig pa thog ma'i 'byung khung la rob tsam dpyad pa gzur gnas dgyes pa'i gtam*. Dharamsala, India: Tibetan Medical Institute, 2000.

Khare, C. P. *Indian Medicinal Herbs*. New York: Springer Science & Business Media, 2007.

Khedrup Norsang Gyatso. *Ornament of Stainless Light: An Exposition of the Kālacakra Tantra*. Translated by Gavin Kilty. Boston: Wisdom Publications, 2004.

Monier-Williams, Monier. *A Sanskrit-English Dictionary*. Delhi: Motilal Banarsidass, 1990 (1899).

Martin, Dan. "Greek and Islamic Medicines' Historical Contact with Tibet." Pre-publication version of paper. Jerusalem: 2007.

Norbu, Tsering. *Sman ming tshig mdzod blo gsar sgo 'byed lde mig* [*Medicine Lexicon Treasury: Key to Open the Doors of those with Fresh Minds*]. Dharamsala, India: Tibetan Medical Institute, 1998.

Pasang Yonten Arya. *Dictionary of Tibetan Materia Medica*. New Delhi: Motilal Banarsidass, 1998.

Pawo Tsukla Trengwa. *Feast for the Wise: An Historical Record (Chos 'byung mkhas pa'i dga' ston)*. Sarnath, India: Vajra Vidya Institute, 2003.

Rechung Rinpoché. *Tibetan Medicine*. Delhi: Sri Satguru Publications, 2001.

Shrestha, Romio, and Ian Baker. *The Tibetan Art of Healing*. San Francisco: Chronicle Books, 1997.

Sparham, Gareth, trans. *The Fulfillment of All Hopes* by Je Tsongkhapa. Boston: Wisdom Publications, 1999.

———, trans. *Tantric Ethics* by Je Tsongkhapa. Boston: Wisdom Publications, 2005.

Stearns, Cyrus. *King of the Empty Plain: The Tibetan Iron-Bridge Builder Tangtong Gyalpo.* Ithaca, NY: Snow Lion Publications, 2006.

Tatz, Mark. *Candragomin's "Twenty Verses on the Bodhisattva Vow" and Its Commentary by Sakya Dragpa Gyaltsen.* Dharamsala, India: Library of Tibetan Works and Archives, 1983.

Tibetan Medicine in Contemporary Tibet, Volume 2: Health and Health Care. London: Tibet Information Network, 2004.

Trinlé, Jampa. *Gangs ljongs gso rig bstan pa'i nyin byed rim byon gyi rnam thar phyogs bsgrigs zhes bya ba* [*Compiled Biographies of the Succession of Suns from the Medical Tradition of the Land of Snow*]. Dharamsala, India: Tibetan Medical Institute, 1991.

Troru Tsenam. *Short and Concise Commentary to Sarasvatī Grammar Sutra. Brda sprod pa dbyans can gi mdo'i 'grel pa nyung ngu rnam gsal.* Beijing: Krung go mi rigs dpe skrun khang, 1998.

———. *Khro ru tshe rnam gyi gsung rtsom thor bu phyogs bsgrigs* [*Compendium of the Shorter Miscellaneous Works of Troru Tsenam*]. Lhasa: Bod ljongs mi dmangs dpe skrun khang, 2003.

Tsarong, Tsewang Jigme. *Handbook of Traditional Tibetan Drugs: Their Nomenclature, Composition, Use, and Dosage.* Kalimpong, India: Tibetan Medical Publications, 1986.

Uttaratantra of Maitreya. E. H. Johnson's Sanskrit text, edited by H. S. Prasad. Delhi: Sri Satguru Publications, 1991.

Wallace, Vesna. *The Inner Kalacakratantra: A Buddhist Tantric View of the Individual.* New York: Oxford University Press, 2001.

Winder, Marianne. "Vaidurya." *Bulletin of Tibetology* (November 1990).

Index

N

O

R

About the Contributors

GAVIN KILTY spent thirteen years in Dharamsala, India (1971–84) studying Buddhism and learning the Tibetan language. Eight of those years were spent at the Institute of Buddhist Dialectics studying the Geluk monastic curriculum through classes and formal debate. After moving back to the United Kingdom in 1984, he worked into the 90s as an English language teacher, and since the mid 90s, he has worked as a Tibetan translator. He teaches with the Lotsawa Rinchen Zangpo Translator Programme in Dharamsala and also teaches beginner and intermediate Tibetan language courses at Jamyang Buddhist Center, London. He is married with three children and lives in Devon, UK.

Gavin's published translations include *The Key to Madhyamika* (Library of Tibetan Works and Archives, 1974), *Tibetan Traditions of Childbirth and Childcare* (Library of Tibetan Works and Archives, 1984), *The Splendor of an Autumn Moon: The Devotional Verse of Tsongkhapa* (Wisdom Publications, 2001), and *Ornament of Stainless Light* (Wisdom Publications, 2004).

GESHE THUPTEN JINPA was trained as a monk at the Shartse College of Ganden Monastic University, South India, where he received the Geshe Lharam degree. Jinpa also holds a B.A. honors in philosophy and a Ph.D. in religious studies, both from Cambridge University, England.

Jinpa has been the principal English-language translator for His Holiness the Dalai Lama for nearly two decades and has translated and edited numerous books by the Dalai Lama. His own works include *Songs of Spiritual Experience* (coauthored) and *Self, Reality and Reason in Tibetan Philosophy*. He is currently the president of the Institute of Tibetan Classics and lives in Montreal with his wife and two daughters.

The Institute of Tibetan Classics

The Institute of Tibetan Classics is a nonprofit, charitable educational organization based in Montreal, Canada. It is dedicated to two primary objectives: (1) to preserve and promote the study and deep appreciation of Tibet's rich intellectual, spiritual, and artistic heritage, especially among the Tibetan-speaking communities worldwide; and (2) to make the classical Tibetan knowledge and literature a truly global heritage, its spiritual and intellectual resources open to all.

To learn more about the Institute of Tibetan Classics and its various projects, please visit www.tibetanclassics.org or write to this address:

Institute of Tibetan Classics
304 Aberdare Road
Montreal (Quebec) H3P 3K3
Canada

The Library of Tibetan Classics

"THIS NEW SERIES edited by Thupten Jinpa and published by Wisdom Publications is a landmark in the study of Tibetan culture in general and Tibetan Buddhism in particular. Each volume contains a lucid introduction and outstanding translations that, while aimed at the general public, will benefit those in the field of Tibetan Studies immensely as well."

—Leonard van der Kuijp, Harvard University

"This is an invaluable set of translations by highly competent scholar-practitioners. The series spans the breadth of the history of Tibetan religion, providing entry to a vast culture of spiritual cultivation."

—Jeffrey Hopkins, University of Virginia

"Erudite in all respects, this series is at the same time accessible and engagingly translated. As such, it belongs in all college and university libraries as well as in good public libraries. *The Library of Tibetan Classics* is on its way to becoming a truly extraordinary spiritual and literary accomplishment."

—Janice D. Willis, Wesleyan University

Following is a list of the thirty-two proposed volumes in *The Library of Tibetan Classics*. Some volumes are translations of single texts, while others are compilations of multiple texts, and each volume will be roughly the same length. Except for those volumes already published, the renderings of titles below are tentative and liable to change. The Institute of Tibetan Classics has contracted numerous established translators in its efforts, and work is progressing on all the volumes concurrently.

1. *Mind Training: The Great Collection,* compiled by Shönu Gyalchok and Könchok Gyaltsen (fifteenth century). NOW AVAILABLE
2. *The Book of Kadam: The Core Texts,* attributed to Atiśa and Dromtönpa (eleventh century). NOW AVAILABLE
3. *The Great Chariot: A Treatise on the Great Perfection,* Longchen Rapjampa (1308–63)
4. *Taking the Result As the Path: Core Teachings of the Sakya Lamdré Tradition,* Jamyang Khyentsé Wangchuk (1524–68) et al. NOW AVAILABLE
5. *Mahāmudrā and Related Instructions: Core Teachings of the Kagyü School*
6. *Stages of the Path and the Ear-Whispered Instructions: Core Teachings of the Geluk School*
7. *Ocean of Definitive Meaning: A Teaching for the Mountain Hermit,* Dölpopa Sherap Gyaltsen (1292–1361)
8. *Miscellaneous Tibetan Buddhist Lineages: The Core Teachings,* Jamgön Kongtrül (1813–90)
9. *Sutra, Tantra, and the Mind Cycle: Core Teachings of the Bön School*
10. *The Stages of the Doctrine: Selected Key Texts*
11. *The Bodhisattva's Altruistic Ideal: Selected Key Texts*
12. *The Ethics of the Three Codes*
13. *Sādhanas: Vajrayana Buddhist Meditation Manuals*
14. *Ornament of Stainless Light: An Exposition of the Kālacakra Tantra,* Khedrup Norsang Gyatso (1423–1513). NOW AVAILABLE
15. *Lamp Thoroughly Illuminating the Five Stages of Completion,* Tsongkhapa (1357–1419)
16. *Studies in the Perfection of Wisdom*
17. *Treatises on Buddha Nature*
18. *Differentiations of the Profound View: Interpretations of Emptiness in Tibet*
19. *Elucidation of the Intent: A Thorough Exposition of "Entering the Middle Way,"* Tsongkhapa (1357–1419)
20. *Tibetan Buddhist Epistemology I: The Sakya School*

21. *Tibetan Buddhist Epistemology II: The Geluk School*
22. *Tibetan Buddhist Psychology and Phenomenology: Selected Texts*
23. *Ornament of Higher Knowledge: A Exposition of Vasubandhu's "Treasury of Higher Knowledge,"* Chim Jampalyang (thirteenth century)
24. *A Beautiful Adornment of Mount Meru: Presentation of Classical Indian Philosophies,* Changkya Rölpai Dorjé (1717–86)
25. *The Crystal Mirror of Philosophical Systems: A Tibetan Study of Asian Religious Thought,* Thuken Losang Chökyi Nyima (1737–1802). NOW AVAILABLE
26. *Gateway for Being Learned and Realized: Selected Texts*
27. *The Well-Uttered Insights: Advice on Everyday Wisdom, Civility, and Basic Human Values*
28. *A Mirror of Beryl: A Historical Introduction to Tibetan Medicine,* Desi Sangyé Gyatso (1653–1705). NOW AVAILABLE
29. *Selected Texts on Tibetan Astronomy and Astrology*
30. *Art and Literature: An Anthology*
31. *Tales from the Tibetan Operas*
32. *Selected Historical Works*

To receive a brochure describing all the volumes or to stay informed about *The Library of Tibetan Classics,* please write:

Wisdom Publications
Attn: Library of Tibetan Classics
199 Elm Street
Somerville, MA 02144 USA
or send a request by email to info@wisdompubs.org.

The complete catalog containing descriptions of each volume can also be found online at www.wisdompubs.org, where you can sign up for an email newsletter dedicated to *Library of Tibetan Classics* news.

Become a Benefactor of the Library of Tibetan Classics

The Library of Tibetan Classics' scope, importance, and commitment to quality make it a tremendous financial undertaking. Please consider becoming a benefactor. Contributors of US$2,000 or more will receive a copy of each volume as it becomes available and will have their names listed in all subsequent volumes. Simply send a check made out to Wisdom Publications or credit card information to the address below.

Library of Tibetan Classics Fund
Wisdom Publications
199 Elm Street
Somerville MA 02144
USA

Please note that contributions of lesser amounts are also welcome and are invaluable to the development of the series. Wisdom is a 501(c)3 nonprofit corporation, and all contributions are tax-deductible to the extent allowed by law.

To keep up to date on the status of the *Library of Tibetan Classics,* visit the series page on the Wisdom website, wisdompubs.org. Sign up for the email news list for the *Library of Tibetan Classics* while you are there.

About Wisdom Publications

Wisdom Publications is dedicated to making available authentic Buddhist works for the benefit of all. We publish translations of the sutras and tantras, commentaries and teachings of past and contemporary Buddhist masters, and original works by the world's leading Buddhist scholars. We publish our titles with the appreciation of Buddhism as a living philosophy and with the special commitment to preserve and transmit important works from all the major Buddhist traditions.

Wisdom Publications
199 Elm Street
Somerville, Massachusetts 02144 USA
Telephone: 617-776-7416
Fax: 617-776-7841
Email: info@wisdompubs.org
www.wisdompubs.org

Wisdom is a nonprofit, charitable 501(c)(3) organization affiliated with the Foundation for the Preservation of the Mahayana Tradition (FPMT).

Mind Training

The Great Collection

Translated and edited by Thupten Jinpa

720 pages, cloth, ISBN 0-86171-440-7, $49.95

"The practice of mind training *(lojong)* is based on the essential Mahayana teachings of impermanence, compassion, and the exchange of self and other that the eleventh-century master Atisha brought to Tibet from India. The *lojong* teachings are a source of inspiration and guidance shared by masters of all Tibetan traditions. This makes Thupten Jinpa's translation of *Mind Training: The Great Collection* a natural choice for publication as part of the *Library of Tibetan Classics* series. For the first time, this early collection of the instructions of the great Kadampa masters has been translated in its entirety. The clarity and raw power of these thousand-year-old teachings are astonishingly fresh, whether studied as a complete anthology or opened at random for inspiring verses on the heart of Buddhist practice."

—*Buddhadharma: The Practitioner's Quarterly*

"Thupten Jinpa has done us all a great service by editing and translating this marvelous volume. In an era when Buddhist meditation is largely equated with simply calming the mind and developing mindfulness, this compendium of methods for training the mind gives a glimpse of the tremendous richness and depth of the Buddhist tradition for enhancing mental health and balance and realizing the full potential of consciousness in terms of wisdom and compassion. With the current rise of positive psychology, in which researchers are seeking a fresh vision of genuine happiness and well-being, this volume can break new ground in bridging the ancient wisdom of Buddhism with cutting-edge psychology. Such collaborative inquiry between spirituality and science is especially timely in today's troubled and divisive world."

—B. Alan Wallace, author of *The Attention Revolution*

Taking the Result as the Path

Core Teachings of the Sakya Lamdré Tradition
Translated and edited by Cyrus Stearns
His Holiness Sakya Trizin, Foreword
784 pages, cloth, ISBN 0-86171-443-1, $59.95

"The Sakya school of Tibetan Buddhism has been the most conservative in maintaining the secrecy of its lineage's special practices. *Taking the Result as the Path* represents a major breakthrough by bringing these teachings to light with the full blessings of the Sakya masters. In nearly seven hundred pages of translation, the indefatigable Cyrus Stearns presents an anthology of essential texts on Lamdré. This collection will be an invaluable resource for practitioners of the Lamdré system."

—*Buddhadharma: The Practitioner's Quarterly*

"No one is better suited than Cyrus Stearns to offer the first major translation of Lamdré teachings to the world. He has studied intimately with the most revered leaders of the Sakya tradition for decades. Beyond this, Stearns possesses a quality that sets him apart from most translators today—he is a poet. Few have transmuted the verse or the prose, the earthy imagery or the celestial style of Tibetan Buddhist teachings, with comparable eloquence and inspiration; few are endowed with the capacity to inspire students of Tibetan Buddhism through force of the sheer beauty of the translated word. The Sakya tradition will henceforth be known to English audiences in all its splendor thanks to this new translation."

—Kurtis R. Schaeffer, University of Virginia

"In this volume, Stearns makes available for the first time a selection of key texts from the highly prized esoteric transmission of the great Tsarpa masters, translated with enormous effort and care. Students of the Lamdré will rejoice to see these often enigmatic Tibetan yoga manuals transformed into such lucid English."

—David P. Jackson, University of Hamburg

Ornament of Stainless Light

An Exposition of the Kālacakra Tantra
Khedrup Norsang Gyatso
736 pages, cloth, ISBN 0-86171-452-0, $49.95

"A radiant gem drawn from the vast ocean of Tibetan literature on the Kālacakra tantra. It provides a clear, comprehensive summary of the basic structure and essential features of this important system of mysticism. Also, Khedrup Norsang Gyatso's interpretations of controversial issues in the Kālacakra contribute to our understanding of the evolution of Tibetan theories of mysticism. Gavin Kilty's faithful translation makes this work easily accessible—it is a fitting inaugural volume for the *Library of Tibetan Classics*."

—John Newman, MacArthur Professor of
Asian Religions, New College of Florida

"When the Dalai Lama performed the Kālacakra initiation for a crowd of 20,000 at Madison Square Garden in 1991, a page was turned in the history of tantra. It was perhaps because of the popularity of this event and the success of others like it that when he was asked to select a text for the inaugural volume of the important new *Library of Tibetan Classics* series, the Dalai Lama chose a commentary on the Kālacakra tantra. The inaugural volume, *Ornament of Stainless Light,* is an important resource for anyone who has attended or will attend one of the many public performances of the Kālacakra initiation around the world."

—*Buddhadharma: The Practitioner's Quarterly*

The Book of Kadam

The Core Texts
Atiśa Dīpaṃkara (982–1054) and Dromtönpa (1005–64)
Translated by Thupten Jinpa
752 pages, cloth, ISBN 0-86171-441-5, $59.95

The Kadam school, which emerged from the teachings of the Indian master Atiśa and his principal student, Dromtönpa, is revered for its unique practical application of the bodhisattva's altruistic ideal in day-to-day life. One of the most well-known sets of spiritual teachings stemming from Atiśa and Dromtönpa is a special collection of oral transmissions enshrined in the two-volume *Book of Kadam (Bka' gdams glegs bam).* The texts in this volume include the core texts of *The Book of Kadam,* notably the twenty-three-chapter dialogue between Atiśa and Dromtönpa that is woven around Atiśa's *Bodhisattva's Jewel Garland.* Sometimes referred to as the "Kadam emanation scripture," *The Book of Kadam* is undisputedly one of the greatest works of Tibetan Buddhism. This volume contains (1) Atiśa's *Bodhisattva's Jewel Garland,* (2) the twenty-three chapters of the *Jewel Garland of Dialogues,* (3) Dromtönpa's *Self-Exhortation,* (4) *Elucidation of the Heart-Drop Practice* by Khenchen Nyima Gyaltsen (1223–1305), (5) four selected chapters from Dromtönpa's birth stories, (6) two brief verse summaries of the *Book of Kadam,* one by the second Dalai Lama (1476–1542) and the other by Yongzin Yeshé Gyaltsen (1713–93), and (7) *Sayings of the Kadam Masters,* compiled by Chegom Sherap Dorjé (ca. twelfth century). Although the Kadam school no longer exists as an autonomous lineage within Tibetan Buddhism, its teachings have become fully incorporated into the teachings of all four major schools of Tibetan Buddhism, especially the Geluk school.

The Crystal Mirror of Philosophical Systems

A Tibetan Study of Asian Religious Thought

Thuken Losang Chökyi Nyima

Translated by Geshé Lhundub Sopa et al.

Edited by Roger Jackson

696 pages, cloth, ISBN 0-86171-464-4, $59.95

The Crystal Mirror of Philosophical Systems by Thuken Losang Chökyi Nyima (1737–1802), is arguably the widest-ranging account of religious philosophies ever written in pre-modern Tibet. Like most Tibetan texts on philosophical systems, this work covers the major schools of India, both Buddhist and non-Buddhist, but then goes on to discuss in detail the entire range of Tibetan traditions as well, with separate chapters on the Nyingma, Kadam, Kagyü, Shijé, Sakya, Jonang, Geluk, and Bön schools. Not resting there, Thuken goes on to describe the major traditions of China—Confucian, Daoist, and the multiple varieties of Buddhist—as well as those of Mongolia, Khotan, and even Shambhala. *The Crystal Mirror of Philosophical Systems* is unusual, too, in its concern not just to describe and analyze doctrines, but to trace the historical development of the various traditions. *The Crystal Mirror of Philosophical Systems* offers evidence that the serious and sympathetic study of the history of religions has not been a monopoly of Western scholarship.

"An impressive translation of a fascinating and vitally important book. This will be of great interest to students of Tibetan Buddhism. Its broad scope and keen observation makes it an invaluable resource. And for scholars interested in the history of comparative religion, it shows how sophisticated, eighteenth-century Tibetan Buddhists could come to terms with diverse world religious traditions."

—Guy Newland, Central Michigan University,
author of *Introduction to Emptiness*

"Thuken's *Crystal Mirror of Philosophical Systems* is a unique work, seeking to document the full range of philosophical traditions known in Tibet, including Indian, Chinese, and, above all, indigenous Tibetan traditions. This translation is precise and a pleasure to read."

—Matthew T. Kapstein, Ecole Pratique des Hautes Etudes
and the University of Chicago,
editor of *Buddhism Between Tibet and China*

A Note About Dust Jackets

In response to readers' requests, Wisdom has elected to change the dust jackets on the *Library of Tibetan Classics* series from the vellum covers initially produced to conventional paper jackets. If you have purchased either of the first two releases in the series, *Ornament of Stainless Light* or *Mind Training*, and would like to receive a replacement jacket free of charge, please email us at info@wisdompubs.org with your mailing address. You can also send your request to Wisdom Publications, 199 Elm Street, Somerville MA 02144.